Healthcare Ethics and
Human Values

Healthcare Ethics and Human Values

An Introductory Text with Readings and Case Studies

EDITED BY

K. W. M. (Bill) Fulford,
Donna L. Dickenson,
and Thomas H. Murray

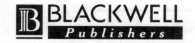

Copyright © Blackwell Publishers Ltd 2002

First published 2002

2 4 6 8 10 9 7 5 3 1

Blackwell Publishers Inc.
350 Main Street
Malden, Massachusetts 02148
USA

Blackwell Publishers Ltd
108 Cowley Road
Oxford OX4 1JF
UK

Library of Congress Cataloging-in-Publication Data has been applied for.

ISBN 0-631-20223-4 (hardback); 0-631-20224-2 (paperback)

British Library Cataloguing in Publication Data

A CIP catalogue record for this book is available from the British Library.

Typeset in 9.5 on 11.5pt Ehrhardt
by Kolam Information Services Pvt. Ltd, Pondicherry, India
Printed in Great Britain by MPG Books, Bodmin, Cornwall

This book is printed on acid-free paper.

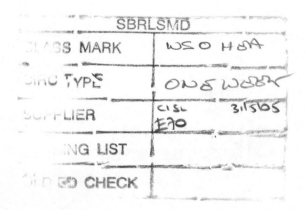

Contents

Acknowledgments

The publishers gratefully acknowledge the following for permission to reproduce copyright material. Every effort has been made to trace copyright holders, but in some cases has proved impossible. The publishers would be happy to hear from any copyright holder that has not been acknowledged.

1   Extract excerpted and reprinted from the chapter entitled "Toward a Feminist Ethics," included in *No Longer Patient: Feminist Ethics and Health Care*, by Susan Sherwin, published in 1992 by Temple University Press, Philadelphia. © 1992 by Temple University. All rights reserved. Reprinted with permission of Temple University Press.

2   Extract "A Deliberative Approach to Bioethics," in M. Parker and D. Dickenson, *The Cambridge Medical Ethics Workbook* (Cambridge: Cambridge University Press, 2000), pp. 304–10.

3   Extract "The Individual in Clinical Practice," by Dr. S. Kay Toombs, from *Allman-Medicin*, Argang 17, supplement 18 (1996). Used with permission of AllmanMedicin, Sweden.

7   Extract from *Journal of Medical Ethics* 21 (1995): 19–24; extract "Can There Be an Ethics of Care?" by Peter Allmark. Reprinted by permission of BMJ Publishing Group, London.

8   Extract from "From the Ethicist's Point of View: The Literary Nature of Ethical Inquiry," by Tod Chambers, in *Hastings Center Report* (January–February 1996). Reprinted with permission of the Hastings Center.

9   Extract from "Two Theories of Modernity," by Charles Taylor, in *Hastings Center Report* (March–April 1995). Reprinted by permission of the author.

10   Extract from *Journal of Medical Ethics* 19 (1993): 43–6; extract "What Counts as Success in Genetic Counselling?" by Ruth F. Chadwick. Reprinted by permission of BMJ Publishing Group, London.

11   Extract from "The Genetic Underclass" from the *Observer*, September 10, 1996. © The Observer. Used with permission.

13   Extract from "Public Health Then and Now: Eugenics and Public Health in American History," by Martin S. Pernick. In *American Journal of Public Health* 87/11 (November 1997): 1767–72, published by American Public Health Association. Reprinted with permission of APHA.

15 and 77 Extracts   "Do We Really Want to Know The Odds?" by David Runciman, in the *Guardian* (October 3, 1996) and "A Living Death," by Peter Lennon, in the *Guardian* (November 19, 1996). © The Guardian. Used with permission.

16, 23, 34, 42, 57, 68, 80   Various poems from *When I Became An Amazon*, by Jenny Lewis, illustrated by Tinker Mather (IRON Press, 1996). © Jenny Lewis 1996. Reprinted with permission of the author.

18   Extract "Healing and Incurable Illness," by Dr. S. Kay Toombs, in *Humane Medicine* 11/3 (August 1995). © S. Kay Toombs. Reprinted with permission of the author.

19   Extract from " 'My Story is Broken: Can You Help Me Fix It?' Medical Ethics and the Joint Construction of Narrative," by Howard Brody in *Literature and Medicine* 13/1 (1994): 79–92. © The Johns Hopkins University Press. Used with permission.

20   Extract "Spiritual Experience and Psychopathology," by Mike Jackson and K. W. M. Fulford, in *Philosophy, Psychiatry and Psychology* 4/1 (1997): 41–65. © The Johns Hopkins University Press. Used with permission.

21   Extract from "The Occurrence of High Levels of Acute Behavioral Distress in Children and Adolescents Undergoing Routine Venipunctures," by G. Bennett Humphrey, Chris M. J. Boon, G. F. E. Chiquit van Linden van den Heuvell, and Harry B. M. van de Wiel, in *Pediatrics* 90/1 (July 1992): 87–91, published by American Academy of Pediatrics. Reprinted with permission of American Academy of Pediatrics.

24   Extract from "Confidentiality in Child Psychiatry," by Emilio Mordini. Used with permission of the author.

26   Extract "Education and Debate: 'Not Clinically Indicated': Patients' Interests or Resource Allocation?" by Tony Hope, David Sprigings, and Roger Crisp, from *BMJ* 306 (6 February 1993). Reprinted with permission of BMJ Publishing Group, London.

27   Extract from "Body Language," by Priscilla Alderson, from *Nursing Times* 36 (September 4–10, 1996). Reprinted with permission of Nursing Times.

28 and 30   Extracts from *A Not Entirely Benign Procedure*, by Perri Klass, published by Penguin Putnam Inc. © 1987 by Perri Klass. Used by permission of Putnam Berkley, a division of Penguin Putnam Inc and Elaine Markson Literary Agency Inc.

29   Extract from "Ethnicity and Attitudes Toward Patient Autonomy," by Leslie J. Blackhall, Sheila T. Murphy, Gelya Frank, Vicki Michel, and Stanley Azen, in *JAMA* 274/10 (September 13, 1995). Reprinted by permission of the American Medical Association.

32   Extract from *The Stork and the Syringe: A Political History of Reproductive Medicine*, by Naomi Pfeffer, published by Polity. Reprinted with permission of Polity.

33   Extract from "Fertility Zone," by Patricia Eakins, first published in *Minnesota Review* (Fall 1987), reprinted in Jon Mukand (ed.), *Vital Lines* (St Martin's Press, 1990). Reprinted with permission of the author.

35   Extract from *The Hundred Secret Senses*, by Amy Tan. Reprinted with permission of Abner Stein, on behalf of the author.

36   "The Abortion," by Anne Sexton, from *The Selected Poems of Anne Sexton*, published by Virago. Reprinted by permission of the Peters Fraser and Dunlop Group Limited.

38   Extract from *Life-Size*, by Jenefer Shute, published by Houghton Mifflin. Copyright © 1992 by Jenefer Shute.

40   Extract from "Debating Point. Capable People: Empowering the Patient in the Assessment of Capacity," by Dermot Feenan, in *Health Care Analysis* 5/3 (1997): 227–36, published by Kluwer Academic Publishers. Reprinted with permission of Kluwer Academic Publishers.

41   Extract from *What the Body Told*, by Rafael Campo. © 1996 Rafael Campo (Duke University Press). Reprinted by permission of Georges Borchardt, Inc, for the author.

44   Extract from "Grief is Carved in Stone," by Sandra Gilbert, first published in *Times Higher Educational Supplement* (August 1996). Reprinted by permission of the author.

46   Extract from "The Ethics of Social Research With Children: An Overview," by Virginia Morrow and Martin Richards, in *Children and Society* 10 (1996): 90–105. Reprinted with permission of the author.

49   Extracts from *Nursing as a Therapeutic Activity*, by Steve Ersser, published by Ashgate Publishing, Aldershot. Reprinted by permission of the author and the publisher.

50   Extract from "Organ Salvage Policies," from *JAMA* 272/10 (September 14, 1994). Reprinted by permission of the American Medical Association.

53   Extract from *Journal of Medical Ethics* 23 (1997): 207–12, article "An Analysis of CPR Decision-making by Elderly Patients," by Gwen M. Sayers, Irene Schofield, and Michael Aziz. Reprinted with permission of BMJ Publishing Group, London.

54   Extract "Can the Elderly Tolerate Endoscopy Without Sedation?" by Sam A. Solomon, Vijay K. Kajla, and Arup K. Banerjee, in *Journal of the Royal College of Physicians of London* 28/5 (September/October 1994). Used with permission.

55   Extracts from *Fighting Spirit: The Stories of Women in the Bristol Breast Cancer Survey*, edited by Heather Goodare, published by Scarlet Press. Reprinted with permission of the publisher.

56   Extract from *Speaking Our Minds*, edited by Jim Read and Jill Reynolds, published by Macmillan. Reprinted with permission of Macmillan Press Limited.

58   "Flee on your Donkey," by Anne Sexton, from *The Selected Poems of Anne Sexton*, published by Virago. Reprinted by permission of the Peters Fraser and Dunlop Group Limited.

59   Extract from *A Leg to Stand On*, by Oliver Sacks. © 1984, by permission of The Wylie Agency (UK) Limited.

62   "When You Are Old," by W. B. Yeats, from *The Collected Poems of W. B. Yeats*, revised second edition, edited by Richard J. Finneran, published by Scribner. © 1983, 1989 by Anne Yeats. Reprinted with the permission of Scribner, a division of Simon and Schuster Inc, and A. P. Watt Limited, London.

63   Extract from *Setting Limits: Medical Goals in an Aging Society*, edited by Daniel Callahan, published by Simon and Schuster 1987. Reprinted with permission of Daniel Callahan.

64   Extract "Going Blind," from *The Best of Rilke*, translated by Walter Arndt. © 1989 by Walter Arndt, reprinted by permission of University Press of New England.

66   Extract from *The Memory Bird*, edited by Caroline Malone, Linda Farthing, and Lorrain Marce, published by Virago Press. Reprinted with permission of Little Brown.

67   Extract from "The Story of the Body" by Robert Hass, published in "Human Wishes" by Ecco Press.

69   Extract from *International Journal of Dermatology* 36 (1997): 2–9, article "Healthy Skin for All," by Terence J. Ryan and Vineet Kaur. Reprinted with permission of Blackwell Science Limited.

70   Extract from *The Politics of Aids*, by Virginia van der Vliet, published by Bowerdean Publishing Company Limited. Used with permission.

71   "Avon Mental Health Measure," reprinted by permission of Changing Minds Project, Bristol.

72 and 86   Extract from *Alzheimer's Disease: The Long Bereavement* (Faber and Faber, 1990), by Elizabeth Forsythe. Reprinted with permission of the author.

73   Extract "Caretakers' Views on Responsibilities for the Care of the Demented Elderly," by Mary Howell, in *Journal of the American Geriatrics Society* 32 (Sept 1984): 657–60. Reprinted with permission of Lippincott Williams and Wilkins.

74   Extract "Who Defines Futility," by Stuart J. Youngner, in *JAMA* 260/4 (October 14, 1998). Reprinted with permission of the American Medical Association.

75   Extract from *Nobody Nowhere*, by Donna Williams. © Donna Williams 1992, published by Doubleday, a division of Transworld Publishers. All rights reserved.

76   Extract from *The Body in Medical Thought and Practice*, edited by Drew Leder, pp. 127–37. © 1992 Kluwer Academic Publishers, article "The Body in Multiple Sclerosis: A Patient's Perspective," by S. Kay Toombs. Reprinted with permission of Kluwer Academic Publishers.

79   "Aids," by May Sarton, from *The Silence Now*, published by W. W. Norton Company. *New and Uncollected Earlier Poems by May Sarton*. Copyright © 1988 by May Sarton. Reprinted with permission of W. W. Norton Company, Inc, and A. M. Heath and Company Limited, on behalf of the Estate of the late May Sarton.

81 and 88   Extracts from *The Death of Ivan Ilyich*, by Leo Tolstoy, translated by Lynn Solotaroff. Copyright © 1981 by Bantam, a division of Bantam Doubleday Dell Publishing Group Inc. Used by permission of Bantam Books, a division of Random House Inc.

83   "Falls," by Edward Lowbury, from *Selected and New Poems 1935–1989*, published by Hippopotamus Press. Used with permission of the publisher.

84   Extract from "Decisions Near the End of Life," Council on Ethical and Judicial Affairs. Reprinted with permission of the American Medical Association.

85   Extract from *The Long Sleep: Young People and Suicide*, by Kate Hill, published by Virago Press. Reprinted with permission of Little Brown.

87   Extract "A Death of One's Own," by Martin Hollis, from *Philosophy and Medical Welfare*, J. M. Bell and Susan Mendus, Royal Institute of Philosophy Supplement 198. Reprinted with permission of Cambridge University Press.

89   Extract from *Journal of Palliative Medicine* 1/2 (1998). Essay "The Coevolution of Bioethics and the Medical Humanities with Palliative Medicine, 1967–1997," by David Barnard. Reprinted with permission of Mary Ann Liebert Inc.

90   Extract "Why I Don't Have a Living Will," by Joanne Lynn, in *Law, Medicine and Health Care* 19/1–2 (1991): 101–4. © 1991, Reprinted with the permission of the American Society of Law, Medicine and Ethics. All Rights Reserved.

91   Extract from *Mama Day*, by Gloria Naylor, published by Houghton Mifflin Company. Copyright. © 1988 by Gloria Naylor. Reprinted with permission of Houghton Mifflin Company and Sterling Lloyd Literistic Inc. Copyright. NULL. All rights reserved.

93   "Talking to the Family," from *The Smell of Matches*, by John Stone. Copyright © 1972 by John Stone. Reprinted by permission of Louisiana State University Press.

94   "To the Foot from its Child," by Pablo Neruda 1904–73, translated from the Spanish by Alistair Reid, from *European Poetry in Scotland*, edited by Peter France and Duncan Glen, published by Edinburgh University Press.

Introduction
Many Voices: Human Values in Healthcare Ethics

In an age of "ethics with everything," it may come as something of a surprise that there should be a need for a new reader on healthcare ethics and human values. In fact, this book is intended as a counterpoint (some might see it as a challenge!) to the growing legalism in many areas of bioethics. This quasi-legal ethics, as we will call it, is based on and gives expression to particular values (such as autonomy of patient choice). As such, quasi-legal ethics has been, and remains, an important part of bioethics' response to the ethical challenges of techno-logical advance in medicine. We will give a number of examples of the importance of quasi-legal ethics later in this Introduction. What is needed now, though, we will argue, is to draw together and to strengthen those aspects of bioethics which, in contrast to quasi-legal ethics, make central not particular values, but *diversity* of values.

It is the diversity of human values operative throughout healthcare that this book aims to illustrate. Hence the majority of contributions – canonical, newly commissioned, and first-hand narratives – are organized not according to "issues," but according to the main stages of the clinical encounter: they run from Staying Well (Part II), through Falling Ill (Part III), First Contact (Part IV), and Deciding What the Problem Is (Part V), to Negotiating a Treat-ment Plan (Part VI); and from there to Con-tinuing Contact, either Getting Well (Part VII), or Chronic Illness, Disability, Deformity, Re-mission, and Relapse (Part VIII), and, in our final Section, to Dying (Part IX).

In contrast to quasi-legal ethics, we will use the term "healthcare ethics" to cover the di-verse strands of scholarship and practice in bio-ethics, which, increasingly, start from and seek to make central the rich diversity of human values.[1] Healthcare ethics, understood in this way, and quasi-legal ethics are not sharply dis-tinct. They represent poles of bioethical think-ing, which, in theory and in practice, are woven together in varying proportions. There are, though, a number of important differences be-tween them, which, if both are to make their proper contributions to a balanced bioethics, it is important to keep clearly in mind.

In this Introduction, therefore, we set the contributions to this book in context by high-lighting some of the key differences between quasi-legal ethics and healthcare ethics, so defined. These differences are summarized in table I.1. As this indicates, and as we will describe in this chapter, quasi-legal ethics and healthcare ethics differ in their aims and in their scope of application, in their underlying conceptual models of medicine, in the use they make of ethical reasoning, and in their practical applications. The features of healthcare ethics are further illustrated by the readings from contemporary authors in Part I (Multidisciplinary Approaches). But it is in the remainder of the book, in the stages of the clinical encounter set out in Parts II–IX, in the many voices of patients, carers, and professionals, that the human values at the heart of healthcare ethics are brought fully into focus.

Aims

Bioethics developed originally, mainly in 1960s' America, as a response to the rapid growth of biomedicine. There were, no doubt, other factors at work. This was, after all, a period of rapid social change in all areas of life. But in medicine the particular challenge at this time was the emergence of new and more powerful technologies. With these technologies the "can do" of medicine expanded beyond all expectation. But with an enlarged "can do" went new and more urgent questions about what medicine *ought* to do. It was as a response to these questions that bioethics was born.

From regulation to partnership

Given the origins of bioethics, as a response to the growth of biomedical technology, it was natural that its initial aims should have been, in effect if not in intent, regulatory. Biotechnology, in itself morally neutral, was seen as being in need of control if it was to be directed to good purposes rather than bad. Again, wider social changes were important here: the rejection of received authority, widespread political cynicism, and loss of faith in the executive. In medicine the effect of these changes was a loss of confidence in its powers of self-regulation as an independent profession. Bioethics, corres-

Table I.1   Summary of differences between quasi-legal ethics and healthcare ethics

	Quasi-legal ethics	Healthcare ethics
Aims	Regulation	Partnership
	Advocacy of particular values	Respect for diversity of values
Scope of application	Treatment	Whole clinical encounter (including diagnosis)
	Secondary care	Primary (as well as secondary) care
Conceptual model of medicine	Medical-scientific model (fact-based)	Healthcare model (fact + value-based)
Ethical reasoning	Substantive ethical theory	Analytic ethical theory
	Value content	Empirical content
Practical applications	Ethical rules	Ethical process
	Law as external regulator	Law as framework for self-regulation
	Communication skills executive	Communication skills substantive

This table summarizes the differences between quasi-legal ethics, as it developed in response to the challenges of biomedicine, and healthcare ethics, as defined in this volume. Most of these differences are differences of emphasis. But the difference in value commitments, respectively to particular values (quasi-legal ethics) and to diversity of values (healthcare ethics), is a difference of kind (see text). It is the diversity of values operative at all stages of the clinical encounter that the readings in this volume seek to illustrate.

pondingly, developed its role on the model of moral guardian, protecting a vulnerable public from the predations of a technology which, otherwise, would run out of control. Biomedicine, with its new armoury of powerful technologies, required regulation. Bioethics would regulate it.

Regulation has been, and continues to be, an important aim of bioethics. The large and still growing library of codes and declarations, local, national, and international, has raised ethical awareness. In some cases, too, particularly in very adverse regimes, they have been effective in preventing abuses of medical power (Fulford and Bloch, 2000).

There is a growing feeling, though, that at least in some areas, regulation may have gone too far. In research ethics, for example, the requirements for consent adopted by some authorities are so elaborate as to be, in practice, unworkable. Researchers, therefore, are beginning to ignore them: not out of a desire to sidestep good practice, but because over-regulation, in this area, is perceived as a *barrier* to good practice (Osborn, 1999). Similar concerns, as we describe in more detail later in this Introduction (in the section on Practical Applications), have been surfacing in relation to confidentiality in mental health. Bioethical regulations aimed at promoting confidentiality have become so out of touch with the realities of practice, notably for multidisciplinary teams working in the community, that practitioners (social workers as well as doctors) have started to ignore them (Watson, 1999).[2] Good practice, again, is seen as being inhibited rather than promoted by over-zealous bioethical regulation.

Healthcare ethics differs from quasi-legal ethics in aiming for partnership rather than regulation. The difference is one of degree rather than kind. Regulation remains important. But the rules of engagement, which our codes and declarations embody, should be aimed as much at facilitating good practice as at preventing bad.

What does this mean? First, regulations, in so far as they have a role, should be framed to reflect the contingencies of real-life clinical care. Good practice is not promoted by unrealistic standards. To the contrary, if the standards

set are unrealistic, there is a real danger that well-motivated rule-breaking will let in just those abuses of medical power that bioethics has, properly, sought to prevent. Good practice, it should be said, can of course be frustrated by many factors external to the context of immediate clinical care, factors such as inadequate training and lack of resources (Agich, 1993). Such factors may thus be a proper target of ethical action by practitioners. Our codes should endorse such action, therefore, but they should not *require* it unless it is within the reasonable power of those concerned.

For those committed to a regulatory aim of bioethics, healthcare ethics, in requiring codes of ethics to be practically realistic, may appear to be taking the heat off practitioners. As Julian Savulescu (2001), a contributor to this volume (see chapter 14), has pointed out, ethics committees are at increasing risk of taking a paternalistic stand that is deeply inimical to the autonomy of patient choice. And individual cases of intrusive regulation are indeed far from uncommon (Dickenson and Fulford, 2000: ch. 6). The lesson they point to is not that we should abandon regulation. It is, rather, that what *counts* as good practice is far less settled than many in bioethics have recognized. In such cases, that is to say, what is good practice from one person's point of view may not be good practice from another person's point of view; and not because one is right and the other wrong, but because their values as such are, simply, different. Such cases, then, point to the importance of diversity of human values in healthcare.

From particular values to diversity of values

Closely related to the moral guardian model of bioethics, protecting patients from biomedicine, is that of the bioethicist as advocate, promoting patient choice. Like the moral guardian model, advocacy of patient choice was important in the early days of bioethics. At that time, faced with the growing power of biotechnology, a strong counterbalance to the established authority of medicine was needed. Hence medical paternalism, motivated by principles of beneficence, was counterbalanced by a principle of patient autonomy. To the accepted wisdom of "doctor knows

best" was opposed the strong principle of "patient knows best."

Patient autonomy is a strong principle essentially because of the primacy it gives to patients'
values. Against a background of widening technological options, it makes the patient, rather
than the doctor, the ultimate arbiter of what is
"for the best" in a given clinical (or research)
situation. In the "doctor knows best" model
what is "for the best" is the doctor's call. In
the "patient knows best" model it is the
patient's call. The doctor has a responsibility
to inform, even to advise, but not to choose on
the patient's behalf. In much bioethical thinking, however, respect for autonomy of patient
choice has become a value in its own right.
There are important exceptions, individual
and collective. The very name of the Society
for Health and Human Values, for example, of
which one of us (TM) has been President, suggests that even in the early days of the field
there were alternative conceptions of bioethics.
But many in bioethics, nonetheless, have come
to see themselves as campaigners for autonomy.

Campaigning has an important place in
ethics, of course. In chapter 1 Susan Sherwin
distinguishes feminist ethics from medical
ethics just in its campaigning stand against
what she calls "the structures of oppression."
There would indeed be little practical harm in
campaigning for patient autonomy if patient
autonomy were, as "western" bioethics has
tended to assume, a universal value. But it is
not. To the contrary, attitudes to autonomy
vary widely from culture to culture (Blackhall
et al., this volume, ch. 29). As the Egyptian
psychiatrist and ethicist Ahmed Okasha has
pointed out, autonomy is actually at odds with
the values of many "non-western" cultures
(Okasha, 2000). The imposition, therefore, of
supposedly universal codes of ethics based on
autonomy in such cultures, although well inten-
tioned, is blind to the values of those concerned.

These observations on autonomy illustrate
the wider point that campaigning for particular
values in ethics, especially if combined with a
legalistic "rules and regulation" approach to
implementation, risks being counter-productive
ethically. This will be necessarily so where the
values that are advocated clash with the values

of those to whom the rules and regulations
apply. The cases noted above mainly involved
clashes of values primarily between western and
non-western cultures. But it is important to
recognize that such clashes are endemic to
many areas of healthcare, arising as they do in
any situation in which human values differ.

In some areas of acute "high-tech" medicine,
it is true, values may be largely shared – a heart
attack, for example, is, in and of itself, a bad
condition for anyone (albeit that it may have
good or bad consequences). In the early days
of bioethics, then, when, as we described in the
previous section, the focus of concern was very
much on high-tech medicine, shared values
could be assumed. There were clear abuses of
biomedical technology to be tackled, i.e. uses of
such technology that were abusive by (almost)
everyone's values, as in Nazi concentration
camps, for example (Chodoff, 1999), and the
notorious Tuskagee incident (in which patients
with syphilis were left untreated without their
knowledge). But such cases are the exception
rather than the rule. In healthcare practice as a
whole the rule is diversity, not uniformity, of
values. Disability itself, as Sally French and
John Swain's study in chapter 78 shows, may
be a matter of positive rather than negative
value. Where there is diversity of values, then,
the bioethicist as advocate, in throwing down
the traditional idol of "doctor knows best," is at
risk of setting up a new idol of "ethicist knows
best."

Diversity of values is the core message of this
book. Diversity of values, though, as the range
of our readings illustrates, means diversity not
just among patients and carers but also among
professionals. In this respect healthcare ethics
generalizes the original bioethical principle of
respect for patients' values. It starts from a
recognition of the diversity of human values
operative in healthcare not only among patients
but among patients and professionals alike.

Where one goes in practice with this general-
ization of the principle of autonomy is a further
question. Basing healthcare ethics on a recognition of diversity of values (the values of professionals as well as patients) opens up crucial issues
of methodology (of how ethical reasoning should
be employed) and of practical application. We

return to these issues below. First, though, we will consider the implications of the shift in aims from a quasi-legal to a healthcare model for the scope of application of bioethics.

Scope of Application

The origins of bioethics, as a response to the challenges of biomedical science, are evident not only in its aims but also in its scope of application, viz., the areas of healthcare, and the kinds of clinical problem, with which it is concerned. It is in its scope of application, indeed, that bioethics' origins in biotechnology are most transparently evident. For bioethics has been concerned, primarily, with ethical problems in high-tech areas of secondary care, and with these problems as they arise mainly in relation to the applications of biomedical science in treatment. Healthcare ethics, by contrast, is concerned as much with primary as with secondary care; and with ethical issues as they arise not only in treatment but at all stages of the clinical encounter, including diagnosis. Both aspects of the wider scope of healthcare ethics are reflected in this volume.

From secondary to primary care

As noted above, dramatic advances in biotechnological science in the second half of the twentieth century created a raft of new ethical problems in healthcare. These problems have a high "gee-whiz" factor: heart transplants, brain implants, human cloning, cancer cures, fetal selection, genetic medicine, are all, rightly, headline-grabbing developments which challenge our deepest ethical intuitions about ourselves and the world in which we live. Small wonder, then, that the issues they raise have been and to a large extent remain at the top of bioethics' agenda.

Yet the high gee-whiz factor of these developments is out of all proportion to their significance, ethically speaking, in day-to-day healthcare practice. There is no sharp divide here, of course. Our readings, indeed, include problems in secondary as well as primary care. But we have sought to redress the balance. Thus

we have included no discussion of genetic selection of embryos, important as the ethical issues raised by this prospect may be. Instead, we cover the day-to-day experience of the implications of fetal screening (Julian Savulescu's "Letter from a doctor as a dad") and of the stigmatization of the new genetic underclass (ch. 11). Add to such issues, then, wider endemic problems such as poverty of resources (see Hope et al., this volume, ch. 26), and it becomes clear that, although they are less high profile, the ethical issues of primary care are far more significant practically than those of secondary care.

From treatment to all stages of the clinical encounter, including diagnosis

Neither the origins of bioethics as a response to the challenges of biomedicine nor its self-set aims of regulation and advocacy sufficiently explain its particular focus on treatment. "Treatment," in this context, should be broadly construed as covering any aspect of how a problem is dealt with: thus, besides direct interventions with drugs, surgery, and so forth, we use the term to cover prevention, screening, resource issues, and participation in research. All these come high on the bioethical agenda. But they have occupied bioethics largely to the exclusion of issues arising from how the problem itself is understood in the first place, namely, issues arising in the clinical encounter from diagnosis, aetiology (attribution of causes), and prognosis (prediction of outcome).

The focus in much of bioethics on treatment, we suggest, reflects the fact that, as is often the way with strong campaigners, it has unwittingly taken on the colours of its enemy. The enemy, then, metaphorically, is biomedicine: and the colours of the enemy are the elements of what has become widely known as the medical model. The medical model is biomedicine's underlying conceptual framework. It has been represented in various ways (see Macklin, 1973, and Fulford, 1998, for reviews). But it is essentially a medical *scientific* model. According to this model, medical *theory*, as the American philosopher Christopher Boorse put it, "is continuous with theory in biology and the other natural sciences" (1975: 55). Correspondingly, then, it is only when science is applied in medical *practice* that values (and hence ethical issues) come into the frame. Again, views differ as to exactly where the boundary between value-free theory and value-laden practice should be drawn (Fulford, 2001). But the broad consensus within the medical model is that the disease concepts on which medical diagnosis is based are value-free scientific concepts.

The medical model is plausible in high-tech secondary medicine. Here, it seems, diagnosis – coming to an understanding of the problem – is based simply on gathering facts: we take "a history," carry out a "physical examination," and organize laboratory tests. Even here, it should be said, the *process* of diagnosis may raise ethical issues. These, as Humphrey et al.'s work on venepuncture in children (ch. 21), and Solomon et al.'s study of endoscopy in the elderly (ch. 54) both show, may not be self-evident: procedures which appear trivial from the point of view of the professional may be highly problematic from that of the patient. All the same, the major ethical issues, on this model, arise not from diagnosis but from treatment. How the problem is understood, and hence the options available for doing something about it, are (according to the medical model) a matter for medical science. It is only when it comes to choosing between these options that the values of those concerned become relevant. Or, to put the point in terms of autonomy, the medical model allows patients to have a say in how their problems are treated, but it gives them no say at all in how their problems are understood in the first place.[3]

The medical model is considerably less plausible in primary care, however. In primary care, what is a problem for one person – an ache or pain, being a certain weight, having a given level of energy, or a particular sleep pattern – may not be a problem for another person. The facts are the same; it is how the facts are evaluated (good, bad, or indifferent) that varies. In psychiatry, as the case history of Simon (ch. 20) illustrates, the relevant value judgments (although not widely recognized for what they are) are actually explicit in the diagnostic criteria to be found in medical-scientific classifications such as the American DSM-IV (the

Diagnostic and Statistical Manual; American Psychiatric Association, 1994; see also Jackson and Fulford, 1997; and Fulford, 1994a). Medical diagnosis, we should add, is a matter not just of negative evaluation but of a particular *kind* of negative evaluation: disease has to be distinguished from other bad or unwelcome states (such as ugliness, foolishness, wickedness, etc.[4]). But in primary care, it seems, diagnosis is at least in part a matter of negative values.

If values are important in diagnosis, then, at the heart of the medical scientific model, values are likely to be important at all stages of the clinical encounter. With values, moreover, in a sense the very antithesis of scientific facts, will go a whole series of further "unscientific" but humanistically important elements of medicine – meaning, significance, understanding, empathy, responsibility, intuition, subjectivity, and an individual perspective. All this implies a theoretical model for healthcare ethics which is very different from the traditional medical model.

Conceptual Models of Medicine: From a Fact-based (Medical) Model to a Fact + Value-based (Healthcare) Model

There are a number of possible ways of interpreting the more value-laden nature of primary care, depending on how one understands the nature of medicine itself. Thus, according to the medical model, primary care is more value-laden because it is less scientific. Psychiatry, in particular, has been thought to be value-laden for this reason. Boorse, whose influential work we noted a moment ago, takes this line. He argues that psychiatry's continuing tendency (its disavowals notwithstanding) to make "social value judgments a test of normality" (1977: 380) stems from the absence of a "deep (biological) theory of psychological part function" (ibid: 382) which "takes physiology as a *model*" (ibid: 376; emphasis in original). Even some of psychiatry's friends have implicitly adopted a denigratory view of medical psychiatry (Phillips, 2000). Among anti-psychiatrists,

Thomas Szasz (1960) takes the more value-laden nature of psychiatric diagnosis to show that mental disorders are not really medical diseases at all but moral problems. In the popular imagination, similarly, the scientific cutting edge is perceived as being in secondary rather than primary care, epitomized by the technological wizardries of gene-sequencing, brain scanners, and the like.

A number of bioethicists, too, reflecting their implicit adoption of the medical model, have taken a similar line. Tom Beauchamp and James Childress, for example, to whose "principles" we return below, are unusual among bioethicists in offering a detailed analysis of how the concept of mental disorder underpins the ethics of involuntary psychiatric treatment. They connect the justification for such treatment, of a fully conscious adult patient of normal intelligence, to impaired capacity for autonomous choice; they analyze autonomy in terms of rationality; and they show that judgments of rationality are, in part, *value* judgments. But instead of concluding that value judgments are therefore integral to psychiatric diagnosis, they conclude that balancing autonomy with beneficence is a "moral *not a medical* problem" (Beauchamp and Childress, 1994: 84; emphasis added).

On this view, then, the values operative in diagnosis in primary but not (apparently) in secondary care are provisional on future developments in medical science. When medical science has developed sufficiently, therefore, there will be no need for healthcare ethics. There will be no need, indeed, for a book of this kind!

A different, indeed contrary, interpretation of the more value-laden nature of primary care is suggested by work in what is sometimes rather grandly called philosophical value theory, i.e., that part of ethical theory which is concerned with the logical properties – the meanings and implications – of value terms. Although not currently high profile in bioethics, nor indeed in ethics generally, philosophical value theory was the focus of a considerable research effort among analytic philosophers, notably in Oxford, in the middle decades of the twentieth century. Work from that period is highly relevant to our understanding of the relationship between fact and value (or, more precisely, descriptive and evaluative meaning) in the language of medicine.

We do not have space, here, to describe this work in detail. One of us has attempted this elsewhere (Fulford, 1989; and, in outline, Fulford and Bloch, 2000). The key point, though, for our present purposes is an observation, made most directly by a former Professor of Moral Philosophy in Oxford, R. M. Hare (see, e.g., Hare, 1952; and 1963), that value terms may come to look like factual terms where the value judgments they express are widely settled or agreed upon. Thus, "good" in "good eating apple," although expressing the value judgment "this apple is good to eat," carries the factual meaning "clean-skinned, sweet, grub-free, etc." This is because, straightforwardly, for most people in most contexts a clean-skinned, sweet, grub-free apple is a good eating apple. Hence this factual meaning has become stuck by association to the use of the value term "good" in respect of eating apples. Whereas, by contrast, "good" used of pictures, in respect of which people's values are highly diverse, has no consistent factual associations, and it thus remains overtly evaluative in meaning.

Hare's work on the way value judgments can come to look like descriptive or factual statements can be mapped directly onto the difference in evaluative connotations between primary and secondary care. According to the medical model, as we have seen, primary care is more value-laden because, essentially, it is scientifically primitive compared with secondary care. Hare's work suggests, to the contrary, that primary care is more value-laden, not because it is scientifically primitive compared with secondary care, but because it is *ethically more complex*.

It will be worth unpacking this suggestion a little, since it is the key both to the way in which ethical reasoning is employed in healthcare ethics and to its practical applications (to both of which we return in a moment). Thus, Hare's work suggests that secondary care is less value-laden not because it is more scientific, but because (as with "good" used of apples) the values operative in this area of healthcare are widely settled or agreed upon. We have already seen that this is broadly true at least of major pathology – a heart attack, as noted above, is in itself a *bad* condition for most people in most contexts. Hence, in respect of such conditions, because the relevant values are the same from person to person, there will rarely, if ever, be disagreements about them. Hence, such values can be ignored for practical purposes. Hence secondary care is, to this extent, uncomplicated ethically (to the extent that the relevant human values are shared). Conversely, then, Hare's work suggests that primary care is *more* value-laden, not because it is *less* scientific, but because (as with "good" used of pictures) the relevant human values are *highly diverse*. Hence in primary care the values (as well as the facts) *cannot* be ignored for practical purposes. Hence primary care is, to this extent, more *complex* ethically than secondary care.

The readings included in this book speak volumes to the diversity of human values operative in healthcare. Indeed, if there is a single message that we hope the book will convey, it is that these values are far more diverse than any of us, from our individual or professional perspectives, normally recognize. Raising our awareness of this given diversity of values, as we will indicate in the next two sections of this Introduction, is the first step to developing a practically effective healthcare ethics.

Two final points, though, need to be made before ending this section. The first is that primary care, in being more overtly value-laden, offers a window on secondary care. This, too, is clear from the chapters in this book. For while it is true that there are some areas of secondary care (like heart attacks) where the relevant values are shared, the contributions to this volume show that diversity of values is not restricted to primary care. There is a spectrum, certainly; and along this spectrum, secondary care, in tackling major pathology with high-tech scientific tools, is more towards the "shared values" end. But shared values are the exception rather than the rule. Hence, diversity of values, although more obvious in primary care, is important in all areas of medicine. Healthcare ethics is thus an ethics for all areas of healthcare.

The second point is that scientific advance will increase, not (as the medical model suggests) decrease, the importance of diversity of human values in healthcare. This is because one effect of scientific advance is to expand the remit of high-tech medicine into areas in which human values are highly diverse (Fulford, 2000a). In genetic medicine, for example, as Ruth Chadwick's work shows (ch. 10), the options opened up by the identification of genetic markers for an ever wider range of characteristics are ones in respect of which different groups, and indeed different individuals, will have very different values.

Scientific advance, then, will not make books of this kind redundant. Scientific advance itself will see to it that diversity of human values will become more, not less, important in all areas of healthcare in the years to come. But quasi-legal ethics, we argued earlier, was a response to the challenges of scientific advances in medicine. How, then, will healthcare ethics (as defined in this book) respond to these challenges? How will it differ from quasi-legal ethics in ethical reasoning? How will it differ from quasi-legal ethics in practical applications?

Ethical Reasoning

Quasi-legal ethics employs ethical reasoning substantively, that is, to draw ethical conclusions. This is consistent with both its aims and scope. If your aim is to regulate, you must have decided what people ought to do. If your aim is to advocate, you must have decided what it is you want to advocate. Regulation and advocacy, then, both depend on (or at any rate assume) shared values. And in secondary care, as we have seen, in particular as it involves high-tech treatments for major pathology, values are indeed (relatively) shared.

Healthcare ethics, by contrast, in starting from diversity of values, differs radically from quasi-legal ethics in the use it makes of ethical reasoning, in being, at one and the same time, both more abstract and more concrete. It is more abstract in its use of ethical theory; it is more concrete in the extent to which it relies on the results of empirical studies.

Ethical theory: from substantive to analytic

The difference between bioethics and health-care ethics in ethical reasoning is well illustrated by their two very different ways of using principles (we consider other forms of ethical reasoning below). A classic account of the use of principles in ethical reasoning in medicine is a book we mentioned earlier, Beauchamp and Childress's *Principles of Biomedical Ethics* (1994). This employs four ethical principles important in healthcare – autonomy, benefi-cence, non-maleficence, and justice. As we noted earlier, in their exclusion of values from diagnosis Beauchamp and Childress identify, implicitly, with the medical model. Their use of principles, though, perhaps somewhat sur-prisingly, is closer to (abstract) healthcare ethics than to (substantive) quasi-legal ethics.

Thus, one way to understand the use of prin-ciples in ethics is as a problem-solving algorithm: you feed in the problem, adjust the principles, and out comes the answer. This algorithmic ap-proach is similar to legal reasoning, at least where this is based on rules (explicit legal principles or statutes) as distinct from case law. As a method of ethical reasoning, however, the algorithmic approach has been rightly criticized for being too mechanical. It is said to be too insensitive to the nuanced subtleties of the particular situ-ations in which real-life ethical problems arise. Principles need not be used insensitively, of course; but there is certainly this danger. And the approach is anyway subject to a deeper meth-odological criticism, that "adjusting the prin-ciples," as we put it, the crucial weighing of principle against principle, has to be done intui-tively. In other words, the key step in the algo-rithm is not algorithmically defined. In its own terms, therefore, the approach (understood in this way) fails.

Beauchamp and Childress (1994) has been criticized on both these algorithmic counts (Cul-ver and Gert, 1982). "Principlism," indeed, has become a dirty word among many in bioethics! Yet what Beauchamp and Childress actually *say* about the use of principles in ethical reasoning in medicine is quite different. They emphasize (e.g. in their chapter 1) that principles reasoning, far from being used mechanically, as an algorithm,

must be carefully contextualized. This indeed follows directly from the very nature of prin-ciples, as Beauchamp and Childress define them. Their principles are prima facie: that is, they are principles that are *likely* to be relevant in some degree to any given ethical problem in practice; and their role, therefore, is to provide a *framework* for ethical reasoning rather than, in themselves, to generate ethical conclusions. Understood as a framework, therefore, the use of principles in ethical reasoning cannot be sep-arated from a careful consideration of the con-crete details of a given case; and the required intuitive weighing of principle against principle cannot be separated from the particular circum-stances of that case.

In healthcare ethics, then, we should under-stand principles reasoning not as generating ethical conclusions directly, but rather as pro-viding a four-dimensional "ethical space" in which the relevant particulars of a given situ-ation can be mapped out. This is the sense in which principles reasoning in healthcare ethics is abstract rather than substantive. It provides a way of analyzing ethical problems, a framework for ethical reasoning, rather than a mechanism for producing ethical answers as such.

Mark you, understood in this way, principles reasoning is far from being empty practically. In the first place, just in mapping out the space of values it may reveal aspects of the situation that are not immediately self-evident; and some eth-ical "problems" consist in simple failures fully to appreciate all aspects of the situation in question (the focus, say, has been on autonomy at the expense of issues of justice). Mapping out the "ethical space," then, may in itself help to re-solve the problem. At the very least, it will help to clarify the problem. This in turn may point the way to a solution: perhaps more information is needed, for example; or a deeper analysis of an underlying concept (as in Beauchamp and Child-ress's analysis of rationality noted above). And then, yes, if there is no solution, an intuitive weighing of values may in the end be necessary. Necessary because, in practice, matters cannot be left in the air. In practice, something has to be done (even if the "something" is just to leave well alone – see Fulford, 1994b). The problem, that is to say, if not solvable, still has to be resolved. Call the principles *values*, furthermore, and there is nothing in itself suspect about weighing them intuitively. How else, after all, can we *resolve* value issues? The alternative, certainly, is to impose a solution from a given value perspective. But this takes us back to the "rules and regulation" approach of quasi-legal ethics, which, as we have seen, although acceptable in situations in which values are shared, is inappropriate where values are not shared, where, as in primary (and increasingly in secondary) care, the relevant values are highly diverse.

Principles reasoning, then, as advocated by Beauchamp and Childress, is not an algorithm for producing ethical answers. It is one way of exploring the values which, although not always self-evident, are operative in a given situation. It helps us to map out the space of values. This may sometimes show the way to a solution (directly or indirectly); but it does not in itself produce solutions. To the contrary, it leaves resolution, in the contingencies of real clinical decision-making, firmly in the hands of those concerned. For the intuitive weighing of values to which principles reasoning points is, in the end, a matter for individual (value) judgment. This is why, as we noted a moment ago, principles reasoning in healthcare ethics is abstract rather than substantive. Principles reasoning contributes to clinical decision-making by giving us a thinking skill, a way of exploring and responding to ethical problems in practice, rather than by producing answers.

The importance of this distinction – between abstract and substantive, between improving thinking skills and handing down answers – in situations of value diversity is even clearer for one of the main rivals to principles reasoning, casuistry. Casuistry differs from principles reasoning in being bottom up (starting from particular cases) rather than top down (starting from general principles). It was introduced into bioethics by Albert Jonsen and Stephen Toulmin, in their ground-breaking book *The Abuse of Casuistry* (1988), as a way of producing answers. Jonsen was a philosopher and theologian and a member of the National Commission for the Protection of Human Subjects of Biomedical and Behavioral Research (in the USA). Toulmin, a philosopher, was on the Commis-

sion's professional staff. Both were struck by the fact that members of the Commission often agreed about *what* ought to be done in particular cases even though they disagreed widely about *why* it should be done. Hence, they argued, drawing on a deep vein of ethical theory, we should leave aside high level principles (concerned with reasons why) and focus on the contingencies of particular cases.

Casuistry is a powerful thinking skill for clinical decision-making. Understood substantively, though, as a way of producing answers to ethical problems, casuistry (like principles reasoning) depends on those concerned having shared values. It thus works well if the parties concerned are representative of those whose fate is under consideration. This is why the members of the National Commission, in Jonsen and Toulmin's original observation, agreed on what ought to be done. They differed in their political, religious, and ideological identifications; but their underlying values when it came to the ethical issues raised by biomedical advances were, nonetheless, the same.

The corollary, however, is that where those concerned are not representative, where their underlying values are not shared, casuistry can only produce answers if the values of the majority, or perhaps of a dominant minority, prevail. As the American philosopher, Loretta Kopelman, has pointed out, this may have adverse, even abusive, effects if the values operative in a given situation are left implicit rather than being made explicit in the casuistic process (Kopelman, 1994). Casuistry is not unique in this respect, of course. Hidden values (political in this case) lay behind the abusive uses of psychiatric diagnostic categories in the former USSR (Fulford et al., 1993). But the very strength of casuistry – its appeal to ethical intuitions rather than to explicit principles – puts it at perhaps particular risk of misuse in situations of value diversity (like primary care) if its basis in shared values is forgotten.

We do not wish to be misunderstood here. Casuistry is a powerful method of ethical reasoning. It is indeed particularly powerful in the context of clinical care. Being case-based, it is closely geared to clinical thinking; it is adaptable to the background and experiences of different clinical specialties, and indeed individuals; and it draws directly on the intuitive or craft knowledge by which professional expertise is (in part) characterized (Fulford and Bloch, 2000). In healthcare ethics, though, in situations of value diversity, its role may be as much to identify and characterize differences of values as to produce answers. Like principles reasoning, then, casuistry helps us to map out the "space of values" in a given case; as a form of ethical reasoning, this may contribute to clinical problem-solving in many ways (as above); principles and casuistry, indeed, in this respect may be highly complementary, notably in that most value-diverse area of primary care, psychiatry (Fulford and Hope, 1993); but neither form of ethical reasoning, as such, can produce ethical answers direct except where the values of those concerned are already shared.

Other more abstract forms of ethical reasoning can also be understood in this way, i.e., as contributing, in situations of value diversity, to the thinking skills of clinical problem-solving rather than producing answers to ethical problems as such: utilitarianism (consequences-driven) and deontology (rights-driven), for example; and virtue ethics (important especially in healthcare education – see Murray, 1994). Even more abstract, linguistic analysis, though relatively neglected in current philosophy, offers a powerful tool for unearthing hidden values in psychiatric diagnosis (Fulford, forthcoming), for example, and in our assumptions about clinical care (Peter Allmark, this volume, ch. 7).

Empirical studies: from informative to substantive

Abstract ethics has been criticized for eschewing substantive conclusions. Philosophical value theory, in particular, has been stigmatized as being trivial for this reason (Williams, 1985). Yet *all* theory is empty practically until it is combined with content. Theory is never productive in itself. That is why it is *theory*. The theory/content distinction (and its variants: form/content, analytic/synthetic, concept/data, etc.) is not without its philosophical critics (following Quine, 1948). But by analogy with mathematics in the natural sciences, ethical

theory, in providing thinking skills for clinical decision-making in healthcare ethics, must be combined with content if it is to have practical effect. Peter Allmark's critique of the "ethics of care" (ch. 7) makes this point directly. Care, as a framing concept, is ethically neutral: it is, as he points out, what we care *about* and *how* we care that make caring ethical or unethical.

There is much by way of content that may be relevant in a given case. The particular kind of content, though, relevant to ethical aspects of clinical problem-solving is human values. A key aim of this volume, as we have several times emphasized, is to illustrate the diversity of human values operative at all stages of the clinical encounter. Of the three kinds of reading included, the first-hand narratives are the most obviously relevant in this respect. Such narratives, as Howard Brody (ch. 19) was among the first to point out, in speaking directly to experience rarely fall short of achieving considerable dramatic impact. Elizabeth Forsythe's account of her husband's dementia, for example, presented here in two stages, his chronic illness (ch. 72) and subsequent death (ch. 86), is evocative in ways that no amount of secondary literature could achieve. But the work of novelists, too, may be deeply insightful, as in Tolstoy's account of the death of Ivan Illich (ch. 88). Poetry has a particular power of expressing ambiguous and implicit meanings (Kreitman, 1999). We have included a number of poems in this collection; Jenny Lewis's series of poems describing her experience of breast cancer provides a strong linking theme, introducing Parts II–IX of the book, and tracking the stages of the clinical encounter.

An important general point illustrated by these literary sources is the extent to which we fail to recognize just how different other people's values may be from our own. We noted a moment ago the dangers of unrecognized or hidden values. Hidden (or unacknowledged) values are particularly significant, though, in healthcare practice, in their effects on the relationships both between different professional groups and between professionals and their clients. Peter Campbell (ch. 56), for example, sets out, simply and directly, the oft-repeated but still not sufficiently heard view of the users of psychiatric services, that their values are all too often eclipsed by those of service providers.

First-hand accounts, therefore, can help to raise awareness of the actual – rather than imagined – values operative in the clinical encounter. Systematic methods may also be important here. Indeed, such methods, in providing general information, importantly complement the particular perspectives of first-hand narratives. There is no shortage of such methods. We illustrate in this volume, inter alia, surveys (e.g. Snowdon et al.'s study of the effects on parents of their babies being "randomized" in a research trial in chapter 45), direct clinical observations (Terence Ryan and Vineel Kaur's work with people with disfiguring skin diseases in chapter 69), ethnographic methods (Steve Ersser's study of differences between nurses and patients in their respective understandings of caring in chapter 49), and direct experimental designs (Veronica Thomas's work on patient-controlled analgesia in chapter 43).

Just why people should be obtuse about each other's values is a further question. As far as professionals are concerned, being value-pur-blind can be an effect of a dominant professional model: the medical model, as noted above, prioritizes facts; hence, doctors have tended to focus on impersonal facts about their patients' problems rather than seeking to understand what is important about them from their individual perspectives. Our obtuseness, though, is also a product of our values not being fully transparent even to ourselves. Besides explicit methods, then, deeper analytic forms of inquiry may be helpful: phenomenological philosophy (Kay Toombs's phenomenology of her own experience of multiple sclerosis in chapter 3); John McMillan and Grant Gillett's postmodern and discursive ethics (ch. 37); hermeneutic methods (three varieties of which are described by Guy Widdershoven in chapter 4 and illustrated in his account with Wies Weijts of diagnostic styles in clinical relationships in chapter 25); Tod Chambers's use of the techniques of literary analysis (ch. 8); and psychoanalytic insights (Joan Raphael-Leffs's work on the hidden emotions driving the experiences of both donor and recipient in assisted reproduction – see chapter 31).

An exciting recent development is the emergence of research paradigms combining philosophical-analytic and empirical methods. The rationale for this is the recognition that many of the problems with which we are concerned, in both clinical work and research, particularly in primary healthcare, are in part conceptual in nature.[5] Thus the Canadian social scientist (who subsequently trained as a doctor), David Robertson, in a ground-breaking combined methods study, explored the ethical concepts implicit in the day-to-day work of an old-age psychiatry unit in Oxford (Robertson, 1996). In psychiatry, generally, analytic philosophy is a powerful ally of empirical methods derived from the social sciences in the study of implicit models of disorder (Colombo, 1997; Fulford, forthcoming). Continental philosophy, too, is a potentially rich resource for combined methods studies. The British psychiatrist, Pat Bracken (1995), for example, has employed both Foucault's philosophy in developing a novel user-guided approach to community mental healthcare and Heidegger's phenomenology as the basis of more effective methods for the management of trauma in non-western countries (Bracken, forthcoming).

There is no shortage of content, then, for a healthcare ethics in which ethical theory is employed not in itself to draw substantive conclusions, but as a key thinking skill in clinical problem-solving. Take away, though, the rules and regulations of traditional bioethics, and how does all this work out in practice?

Practical Applications

In this section, we outline some of the practical implications of healthcare ethics, respectively, for ethics itself, for law, and for communication skills. As with our earlier points, these three aspects of healthcare ethics should be understood as a series of shifts of emphasis within bioethics, aimed not at dispensing with quasi-legal ethics, but at providing a more balanced approach.

The three shifts of emphasis are: (i) from rules to process in ethical thinking in healthcare; (ii) from external regulation to self-regulation as the basis of law; and (iii) from what might be called an executive to a substantive role for communication skills in ethical problem-solving.

Ethics: from rules to process

As we noted at the beginning of this Introduction, it was natural that in the early stages of its development, bioethics should have adopted a regulatory stance, defining and progressively refining the rules of engagement between healthcare professionals and their clients and patients. It is important to recognize, however, that the demand for rules and regulations has come from professionals no less than from patients. This, too, is natural enough. It is professionals, no less than patients, who are faced, daily, with ethically bewildering clinical dilemmas. It is professionals, therefore, no less than their patients, who feel the need for rules, externally validated and binding on them and their patients alike, to guide their choices. It is professionals, no less than their patients, who in cases of doubt or difficulty want to be able to turn the problem over to a regulatory body with powers of disposal, relieving them of responsibility for interpreting the rules.

All this is natural enough. But is it appropriate? At a recent conference in England, for example, on confidentiality and mental health, the call – from patients and healthcare professionals alike – was for more detailed guidance (Stern, 2001). Yet the problems they faced, as reflected in a book based in part on the conference (Cordess, 2001), were in large part themselves a direct result of the growing volume of ethical codes and legal regulation bearing on issues of confidentiality in healthcare. Contributor after contributor to Cordess's book, from psychiatry, social work, the law and so forth, called for further rules and regulations. But the problems they described arose from the rules themselves. The rules were now so all-embracing, they demanded such extreme standards, that they had become in some cases not only impractical but inimical to good practice. In multidisciplinary teamwork, for example, the relevant codes precluded sharing of information between agencies: but good practice in community care depends on just such sharing (Szmukler and Holloway, 2001). The result, in many cases,

was that practitioners had started to vote with their feet, honoring the codes more in the breach than in the observance (Pritchard, 2001).

This paradox, however, of ethical rules and regulations themselves becoming part of the problem is readily resolved once the diversity of values operative in healthcare is recognized. As one of us has argued elsewhere (Fulford, 2001), rules and regulations work well where values are shared. To the extent that values are shared, rules and regulations may indeed be a powerful mechanism for promoting ethical practice: they are a protection, notably, for healthcare practitioners working in abusive political regimes. Where values are *not* shared, however, rules and regulations, if they are intended to be substantive in effect, will necessarily be incompatible with the values of many of those to whom they apply.

We want to be clear about this. Rules and regulations have an important place. The point is that there is a great deal in ethics that cannot be done with rules and regulations alone. And ratcheting up the rules and regulations bearing on healthcare, although important in the early days of bioethics, shows signs, as we described in the first section of this Introduction (on Aims), of having reached the point of diminishing returns. It may be time to ratchet back, therefore. It may be time to stop producing ever more detailed substantive rules, expressing particular values. It may be time to balance up the rules and regulation approach with a model of ethics that aims to secure processes of clinical decision-making that respect, and as far as possible respond to, the diversity of human values operative in the particular circumstances of individual choices.

What a shift from rules to process will mean in practice is a large question to which, we believe, insufficient attention has been paid (Fulford, 2001). It will certainly involve an enlarged role for communication skills, to which we return in a moment. It will also require a shift in the relationship between ethics and law.

Law: from external regulation to self-regulation

Hand-in-hand with the rise of quasi-legal bioethics has gone a shift in medical law from self-regulation to external regulation of healthcare professionals. In the UK, this process has been fueled by a series of failures of self-regulation, particularly among doctors. The result of this has been that the principal self-regulatory body of the medical profession in England and Wales, the General Medical Council, is itself under threat.

A degree of external regulation is, of course, essential for any group in society. In healthcare, then, it is salutary, for example, that we have moved from a "doctor knows best" basis for clinical decision-making in the direction of "patient knows best." This has been reflected in medical law, in the UK, in a watering-down of what is known as the Bolam principle. The Bolam principle is the ultimate in professional self-regulation. It makes doctors themselves the measure of good standards of medical practice. More precisely, it defines good standards of medical practice as the standards to which any group of appropriately qualified practitioners subscribe. The Bolam principle, then, if not in theory inimical to patient autonomy (to which, after all, many practitioners subscribe), is perceived as being inimical to patient autonomy in practice (because the reference standard for good practice is professional-, not patient-, based). In the courts in the UK, in consequence, there has been a growing tendency to be guided not by what practitioners regard as right in a given situation (i.e. the Bolam principle), but by what the patient concerned wants (or would have wanted if appropriately informed).

But now the question arises, how far should this go? Will it be salutary if one extreme principle ("doctor knows best") ends up being replaced with another extreme principle ("patient knows best")? Would a consumer model of healthcare practice – interventions on demand (so long as you can pay for them) – be ethical? Clearly a balance is needed. But how, and on what basis, is the balance to be struck?

This is another large question to which we will not attempt a comprehensive answer. Self-regulation, though, albeit with an important twist on traditional models, has, we believe, a part to play. Again, the key is value diversity. But to see this we need to look in more detail at the Bolam principle and its relationship to professional expertise. Thus, the Bolam principle in effect accommodates value diversity so far as the values of professionals are concerned. The principle allows for, indeed it directly incorporates, differences of professional opinion. The Bolam principle requires not uniformity, nor even a consensus view, but only that a *group* of relevant professionals support the action in question. Professional opinion, then, may vary. This is partly a matter of differences of view on matters of fact. And professional expertise, it is worth noting, is under attack on its factual side: "evidence-based" practice, and management-led approaches to developing clinical practice guidelines, are increasingly subordinating individual clinical judgment to consensus opinion. But professional judgment is also a matter of values. Opinion on the facts (on what, say, the effects of a given treatment will be) may be the same; but there may still be wide differences of professional opinion on questions of value (on whether the treatment in question will be, in a given case, to *good* effect).

The parallel with evidence-based practice might now suggest that external regulation is, after all, the way to better standards of care. The assumption behind evidence-based practice is that science – in the form of computer-based meta-analyses of selected high-quality scientific research – is capable of providing more accurate opinion than the vagaries of individual clinical opinion. It is certainly true that such meta-analyses may supply important findings. But this general information, pooled across hundreds of studies, has always to be applied, in the context of clinical decision-making, to particular cases. Work from a variety of disciplines suggests that moving from the general to the particular requires expertise which is, in part, incapable of being reduced to a set of explicit rules (Fulford, 2001). Rather like riding a bicycle, or recognizing a face, applying general knowledge to particular cases depends on skills to which "craft" or implicit knowledge is as important as the explicit knowledge which evidence-based practice supplies.

If this is true of the "fact" side of professional expertise, then, if even this cannot be fully captured by a set of explicit regulations, how much more so will it be true of the value side? Here, though, comes the important twist to the self-regulation Bolam principle. For while the facts bearing on a given case may be a matter at least primarily for the professional (knowledge of causes, of available treatments, etc.), the relevant values are a matter as much for the patient as the professional. What is required, then, for a model of bioethics which starts from diversity of values, is not a return to "Bolam" per se. It is, rather, what one of us has called elsewhere "Bolam-plus" (Fulford, 2001). "Bolam-plus" is a framework of law that reflects not just diversity of professional opinion (Bolam), but diversity also of patients' values (Bolam-plus). Self-regulation, then, in healthcare ethics, aims to incorporate the values bearing on the decisions made together by individual professionals and patients within the contingencies of particular concrete clinical situations.

Communication skills: from an executive to a substantive role

Just how "Bolam plus" would work out in practice is yet another question to which we do not have a full answer. We should not be surprised to find open questions repeatedly cropping up like this in healthcare ethics. Open questions, rather than closed answers, are a feature of any subject at the cutting edge. One thing, though, is clear. Bolam-plus pushes the onus of decision back to those, patients and professionals, with the decisions to make. In contrast to the "calls for guidance" from both patients and professionals, noted at the start of this section, Bolam-plus is what a former professor of law in Oxford, H. L. A. Hart, called a "choosing system" (Hart, 1968). The function of law, Hart argued, is to provide a framework within which individual choices may be made as widely as possible and with a minimum of restrictions. "Bolam-plus" would thus be (part of) a choosing system for healthcare law. It would limit the role of law to providing a framework within which processes aimed at respecting diversity of values can operate to maximum effect. That such processes will depend crucially on good communication skills is self-evident. If diversity of values is to be respected, we must

at the very least understand the perspectives of those concerned. As the Oxford psychiatrist and Professor of Medical Ethics, Tony Hope, has pointed out, "perspectives," and our ability to understand and respect the often widely different perspectives of those concerned in clinical decision-making in healthcare, is a key component of the practice skills on which effective and ethically sound clinical decision-making critically depend (Hope et al., 1996).

Just how communication skills are taken to operate, however, depends on the model of bioethics adopted. In a quasi-legal model of bioethics, communication skills are, essentially, executive. They are required to give effect to ethical rules and regulations: to convey information, for example, as the basis of valid consent; to understand a given patient's wishes (out of respect for autonomy); or, in some cases, to "sell" a decision driven by a relevant ethical code, to someone who may disagree with it. On this quasi-legal model, then, the substantive ethical issues are determined by the rules. Communication skills are required only to execute the rules, to put them into effect.

In healthcare ethics, by contrast, ethical choices are determined, primarily, by the values of those concerned. Communication is central, therefore, where values are not shared. In such situations, rather than appealing to external rules and regulations, clinical decision-making depends on such communication skills as understanding each other's values, engaging in negotiation to agreed solutions, conflict resolution, and the like. In such situations, then, communication skills are the very essence of good clinical decision-making. It is in this sense that in healthcare ethics communication skills have a substantive rather than merely an executive role.

Conclusion: The Abuses of Absolutism

Mention diversity of values among traditionally minded doctors and the cry goes up "Relativism!" "Chaos!" Mention diversity of values among legally minded bioethicists and the cry goes up "Relativism!" "Chaos!" So is healthcare ethics, as we have defined it in this Introduction, a basis for a more balanced contribution of ethics to medicine? Or is it a recipe for relativism and chaos?

Quasi-legal bioethics, combined with the medical model, holds out the prospect of an orderly approach to healthcare practice. In this model, as we noted earlier, ethics and science have well-defined roles. Science is responsible for the knowledge infrastructure of medicine: it defines diseases, discovers causes and cures, develops new technologies, and so forth. Ethics regulates the applications of scientific knowledge in practice; its role is to ensure that science and technology are employed in medicine in ways that promote the best interests of patients. Best interests, moreover, whatever the practical difficulties of deciding what is "best" in particular cases, is defined in principle by certain substantive values, such as autonomy. These values, incorporated into ethical codes, and supported by law, provide an agreed set of standards against which the performance of practitioners can (in principle) be objectively measured.

Healthcare ethics, as we have described, offers a radically different model: it aims for partnership rather than regulation; it is concerned with primary as well as secondary care; it is concerned with each stage of the clinical encounter (including diagnosis) rather than just, or primarily, with treatment; it draws more deeply on both abstract ethical theory and empirical findings; and in its applications to practice it emphasizes ethical process rather than ethical rules, self-regulation rather than regulation by external bodies, and a substantive rather than merely executive role for communication skills.

We summarized this list of differences in table I.1 at the beginning of this Introduction. As we noted there, extensive as the list is, it is nonetheless a list mainly of differences of emphasis rather than of kind: many of the features of healthcare ethics are reflected to a greater or lesser degree in developments in bioethics itself; and healthcare ethics, in the way we have defined it here, could thus be understood as little more than a consolidation and drawing to a head of an evolution already under way in bioethics.

The sticking point, though, for those concerned by relativism, is the diversity of values from which healthcare ethics starts and on which its differences from quasi-legal ethics are built up. Surely, the quasi-legal bioethicist will say, this invites partnership to degenerate into collusion. Surely, the medical-model doctor will say, it makes diagnosis (to which on a healthcare model, values are relevant) a matter of perspective (like taste in food or preferences in pictures). It is all very well, then, both will say, to talk of drawing deeply on abstract theory and empirical findings; but if a substantive system of ethical norms is replaced with diversity of values, ethical process will be left rudderless. For self-regulation, then, read self-interest; and for communication skills, read rhetoric. Healthcare ethics, therefore, if it is based on diversity of values, risks ethical meltdown.

Healthcare ethics, as we have several times emphasized, certainly does put the locus of ethical decision-making back where it belongs: with those at the clinical coalface, with patients and informal carers and with professionals. Healthcare ethics relocates the locus of ethical control from the rules and regulations of an external ethic to the values of those directly concerned in healthcare practice. This, many may feel, is no bad thing. Bioethics has in some areas already gone too far towards, as we put it earlier, a culture of "ethicist knows best." All the same, the values of those concerned, as this book seeks to illustrate, may be highly diverse. Hence healthcare ethics does indeed, and uncompromisingly, place diversity of values at the centre of the ethical action.

There is no ducking this conclusion. Diversity of human values is central. And in this our model of healthcare ethics, although indeed a natural extension of established trends in ethical thinking in medicine, does involve a qualitative shift from the absolutism of quasi-legal ethics to relativism. There is little risk of ethical chaos here, though, still less of ethical meltdown. There are two reasons for this. First, and straightforwardly, human values, if diverse, are certainly not chaotic. Human values, after all, permeate every aspect of our lives – law, aesthetics, sport, and, not least, as Charles Taylor's article so ably reminds us (ch. 9), science itself. Yet none of these is chaotic. The second reason why there is no risk of ethical meltdown is because healthcare ethics, in showing the importance of values even in areas of medicine (like diagnosis) traditionally assumed to be "purely scientific," in no way undermines the importance of science. In so far as facts and values, description and evaluation, are separable, healthcare ethics conceives them as twin logical elements, woven together as warp and weft in the conceptual framework of healthcare as a whole.

Healthcare ethics, then, as one of us has put it elsewhere (Fulford and Bloch, 2000), adds values to, rather than subtracting facts from, medicine. All the same, it remains true that healthcare ethics, in being grounded in value diversity, precludes any a priori commitment to substantive values. In this sense it is, indeed, a relativistic rather than absolutist ethic. Yet this, in healthcare, is a strength not a weakness. For the hard lesson of history is that in medicine it is from absolutism, scientific as well as ethical, rather than from relativism that abusive practices have most often been born (Dickenson and Fulford, 2000: ch. 12). In the language of this book, the lesson of history is that abuses most often arise not from evil will, but from the spurious certainties of dogmatic conviction.

John Locke, the seventeenth-century political philosopher and philosopher of science, called such blind convictions "enthusiasms." In the twentieth century it was from the scientific enthusiasms generated by technological innovation that we had most to fear. Quasi-legal ethics, as we noted at the start of this introduction, was a proper response to these enthusiasms. In the twenty-first century, though, it is from the ethical enthusiasms driving quasi-legal thinking in bioethics that we have most to fear. This is because, as we described in the middle section of this introduction (Conceptual Models), technological advance itself is increasingly driving medicine as a whole into areas of human experience and behavior in which diversity of values is the norm.

NOTES

1   We are, of course, not the first to use the term "healthcare ethics." We adopt it here as reflecting the importance of diversity of values in all areas of healthcare.

2   Also see Szmukler and Holloway (2001) on community psychiatry; and for a corresponding concern about disclosure, Bollas (2001) on psychoanalysis.

3   We owe this clear way of marking the distinction to Dr V. Y. Alison-Bolger (personal communication).

4   See generally, Fulford (1989), especially chs 6 and 7. Subsequent chapters of this book explore the ethical and conceptual significance of the particular kind of negative value expressed by the medical concepts in psychiatry. See also, for a more clinical account, Dickenson and Fulford (2000).

5   In principle, of course, all research, not least in the natural sciences, is in part conceptual in nature (Lakatos, 1974). The point is that in psychiatry, and in other areas of primary care, the problems we face are in practice as well as in principle in part conceptual in nature. They involve not just problems of fact but of how the facts should be interpreted or understood. Psychiatry has been widely stigmatized in this regard as being conceptually muddled. But this is to mistake conceptual difficulty for conceptual deficiency. Psychiatry is, indeed, conceptually difficult, perhaps more so than any other area in healthcare. But far from being a mark of deficiency, conceptual difficulty is the mark of a discipline (like theoretical physics) at the very cutting edge of understanding (see Fulford (2000b) for a more extended treatment of this point).

REFERENCES

Agich, G. J. (1993) *Autonomy and Long-Term Care* (Oxford: Oxford University Press).

American Psychiatric Association (1994) *Diagnostic and statistical manual of mental disorders*, 4th edn (Washington, DC: American Psychiatric Association).

Beauchamp, T. L., and Childress, J. F. (1994) *Principles of Biomedical Ethics*, 4th edn (Oxford: Oxford University Press).

Bollas, C. (2001) The misapplication of "reasonable mindedness": Is psychoanalysis possible with the present reporting laws in the United States and the United Kingdom? In C. Cordess (ed.), *Confidentiality and Mental Health* (London: Jessica Kingsley Publishers), ch. 7.

Boorse, C. (1975) On the distinction between disease and illness. *Philosophy and Public Affairs* 5: 49–68.

Boorse, C. (1977) Health as a theoretical concept. *Philosophy of Science* 44: 542–73.

Bracken, P. J. (1995) Beyond liberation: Michel Foucault and the notion of a critical psychiatry. *Philosophy, Psychiatry, and Psychology* 2: 1–14.

Bracken, P. J. (forthcoming) *Meaning and Trauma in the Post-modern Age: Heidegger and a New Direction for Psychiatry* (London: Whurr Publishers).

Chodoff, P. (1999) Misuse and abuse of psychiatry: An overview. In S. Bloch, P. Chodoff, and S. A. Green, *Psychiatric Ethics*, 3rd edn (Oxford: Oxford University Press), ch. 4.

Colombo, A. (1997) *Understanding Mentally Disordered Offenders: a Multi-Agency Perspective* (Aldershot, UK: Ashgate).

Cordess, C. (ed.) (2001) *Confidentiality and Mental Health* (London: Jessica Kingsley Publishers).

Culver, C. M. and Gert, B. (1982) *Philosophy in Medicine: Conceptual and Ethical Issues in Medicine and Psychiatry* (New York: Oxford University Press).

Dickenson, D. and Fulford, K. W. M. (2000) Treatment: Trick or treat. In Dickenson and Fulford, *In Two Minds: A Casebook of Psychiatric Ethics* (Oxford: Oxford University Press), ch. 6.

Fulford, K. W. M. (1989, reprinted 1995; 2nd edn forthcoming) *Moral Theory and Medical Practice* (Cambridge: Cambridge University Press).

Fulford, K. W. M. (1994a) Closet logics: Hidden conceptual elements in the DSM and ICD classifications of mental disorders. In J. Z. Sadler, O. P. Wiggins, and M. A. Schwartz (eds.), *Philosophical Perspectives on Psychiatric Diagnostic Classification* (Baltimore: Johns Hopkins University Press).

Fulford, K. W. M. (1994b) Diverse ethics. In K. W. M. Fulford, G. Gillett, and J. Soskice (eds.), *Medicine And Moral Reasoning* (Cambridge: Cambridge University Press).

Fulford, K. W. M. (1998) Mental illness. In R. Chadwick (ed.), *Encyclopaedia of Applied Ethics* (San Diego: Academic Press).

Fulford, K. W. M. (2000a) Philosophy meets psychiatry in the twentieth century: Four looks back and a brief look forward. In P. Loutiala and S. Stenman (eds.), *Philosophy Meets Medicine* (Helsinki: Helsinki University Press), pp. 116–34.

Fulford, K. W. M. (2000b) Teleology without tears: Naturalism, neo-naturalism and evaluationism in the analysis of function statements in biology (and a bet on the twenty-first century). *Philosophy, Psychiatry, and Psychology* 7/1: 77–94.

Fulford, K. W. M. (2001) The paradoxes of confidentiality. A philosophical introduction. In C. Cordess (ed.), *Confidentiality and Medical Practice* (London: Jessica Kingsley Publishers), pp. 7–23.

Fulford, K. W. M. (forthcoming) Philosophy into practice: The case for ordinary language philosophy. In L. Nordenfelt (ed.), *Health, Science and Ordinary Language* (Amsterdam: Rodopi), ch. 2.

Fulford, K. W. M. and Bloch, S. (2000) Psychiatric ethics: Codes, concepts and clinical practice skills. In M. G. Gelder, J. López-Ibor, and N. Andreasen (eds.), *New Oxford Textbook of Psychiatry* (Oxford: Oxford University Press), pp. 27–32.

Fulford, K. W. M. and Hope, R. A. (1993) Psychiatric ethics: A bioethical ugly duckling? In R. Gillon and A. Lloyd (ed.), *Principles of Health Care Ethics* (Chichester, England: John Wiley and Sons), ch. 58.

Fulford, K. W. M., Smirnoff, A. Y. U., and Snow, E. (1993) Concepts of disease and the abuse of psychiatry in the USSR. *British Journal of Psychiatry* 162: 801–10.

Hare, R. M. (1952) *The Language of Morals* (Oxford: Oxford University Press).

Hare, R. M. (1963) Descriptivism. *Proceedings of the British Academy* 49: 115–34. Reprinted in R. M. Hare (1972) *Essays on the Moral Concepts* (London: Macmillan Press Ltd).

Hart, H. L. A. (1968) *Punishment and Responsibility: Essays in the philosophy of law* (Oxford: Oxford University Press).

Hope, T., Fulford, K. W. M., and Yates, A. (1996) *The Oxford Practice Skills Course: Ethics, Law and Communication Skills in Health Care Education* (Oxford: Oxford University Press).

Jackson, M. and Fulford, K. W. M. (1997) Spiritual experience and psychopathology. *Philosophy, Psychiatry, and Psychology* 4/1: 41–66.

Jonsen, A. R. and Toulmin, S. (1988) *The Abuse of Casuistry: A History of Moral Reasoning* (Berkeley, CA: University of California Press).

Kopelman, L. M. (1994) Case method and casuistry: The problem of bias. *Theoretical Medicine* 15/1: 21–38.

Kreitman, N. (1999) *The Roots of Metaphor: A Multidisciplinary Study in Aesthetics* (Aldershot, UK: Ashgate Publishing Limited).

Lakatos, I. (1974 [1969]) Falsification and the methodology of scientific research programmes. In I. Lakatos and A. Musgrave (eds.), *Criticism and the Growth of Knowledge* (Cambridge: Cambridge University Press), pp. 91–196.

Macklin, R. (1973) The medical model in psychoanalysis and psychotherapy. *Comprehensive Psychiatry* 14: 49–69.

Murray, T. H. (1994) Medical ethics, moral philosophy and moral tradition. In K. W. M. Fulford, G. Gillett, and J. M. Soskice (eds.), *Medicine and*

Moral Reasoning (Cambridge: Cambridge University Press), ch. 8.

Okasha, A. (2000) Ethics of psychiatric practice: Consent, compulsion and confidentiality. *Current Opinion in Psychiatry* 13: 693–8.

Osborn, D. (1999) Research and ethics: Leaving exclusion behind. *Current Opinion in Psychiatry* 12/5: 601–4.

Phillips, J. (2000) Conceptual models for psychiatry. *Current Opinion in Psychiatry* 13: 683–8.

Pritchard, J. (2001) The myth of confidentiality – A social work view. In C. Cordess (ed.), *Confidentiality and Mental Health* (London: Jessica Kingsley Publishers), ch. 8.

Robertson, D. (1996) Ethical theory, ethnography and differences between doctors and nurses in approaches to patient care. *Journal of Medical Ethics* 22: 292–9.

Quine, W. (1948) On what there is. *Review of Metaphysics* 2. Reprinted in W. Quine, *From a Logical Point of View* (Cambridge, MA: Harvard University Press, 1953).

Savulescu, J. (2001) Taking the plunge. *New Scientist* (3 March): 50–1.

Stern, J. (2001) Themes of confidentiality in clinical practice. In C. Cordess (ed.), *Confidentiality and Mental Health* (London: Jessica Kingsley Publishers), ch. 13.

Szasz, T. S. (1960) The myth of mental illness. *American Psychologist* 15: 113–18.

Szmukler, G. and Holloway, F. (2001) Confidentiality in community psychiatry. In C. Cordess (ed.), *Confidentiality and Mental Health* (London: Jessica Kingsley Publishers), ch. 3.

Watson, F. (1999) Overstepping our boundaries. Practice focus. *Professional Social Work*, September: 14–15.

Williams, B. (1985) *Ethics and the Limits of Philosophy* (London: Fontana).

Part I

Healthcare Ethics: Multidisciplinary Approaches

Introduction

The main aim of the first part of this book is to illustrate, through the work of a selection of key authors, the wide range of philosophical traditions relevant to healthcare ethics.

The distinctive feature of healthcare ethics, as we defined it in the volume Introduction, is that it makes central the diversity of human values operative in all areas of healthcare policy and practice. The dominant model within bioethics, at least in its interaction with practice, has been quasi-legal. Within quasi-legal ethics, as we described, philosophical reasoning is used primarily to give effect to particular values, such as autonomy of patient choice. The chapters in this first part of the book illustrate the extent of the reaction within bioethics against the quasi-legal model. Each shows in different ways, and to different degrees, the wide variety of philosophical approaches available for giving effect to the many voices at the heart of healthcare ethics.

As illustrations of these philosophical approaches, each chapter largely speaks for itself. Susan Sherwin (ch. 1) and Morwenna Griffiths (ch. 5) draw on feminist traditions to argue for a shift from individualism to a more relationship- or community-based ethic. Michael Parker (ch. 2) and Guy Widdershoven (ch. 4), while recognizing the dangers of individualism, note the equal and opposite threat (to the diversity of human values) from communitarianism: they offer, respectively, discursive and hermeneutic approaches to squaring the circle here. S. Kay Toombs (ch. 3) is a phenomenologist: she shows, through her account of her experiences as a multiple sclerosis sufferer, the extraordinary power of phenomenology to illuminate the experience of illness. Gwen Adshead (ch. 6), although consciously echoing the title of Carol Gilligan's foundational book on feminist ethics, *In a Different Voice* (1993), demonstrates with three cases from forensic psychiatry the limitations of relationship ethics.

The remaining chapters in this section illustrate the contributions to healthcare ethics of three more traditional philosophical approaches: linguistic analysis – Peter Allmark's sharp dissection of the concept of "care ethics" (ch. 7); literary discourse analysis – Tod Chambers's worked examples of the use of the narrative features of case histories to reveal the perspective, or point of view, of the narrator (ch. 8); and comparative scholarship in the history of ideas – Charles Taylor's authoritative demolition of the acultural (perspective-free) view of modernity (ch. 9).

Taken together, these chapters illustrate and indeed develop a number of the key themes of healthcare ethics outlined in our main Introduction. Besides the central point about diversity of values (noted explicitly by both Parker and Widdershoven, for example), these themes include the importance of partnership (Widdershoven's notion of Gadamerian dialogue as the basis of the doctor–patient relationship); the ethical significance of diagnosis (Adshead's identification of the difficulties presented for relationship ethics by psychiatric conditions, such as personality disorders, the very nature of which consists in relationship difficulties); the need for a full-field or fact+value conceptual model of medicine (Taylor's account of the "symbiotic relationship" between science and culture, culture being understood as "a constellation of understandings of person, nature, society, and the good"; and the substantive role of communication skills (in Parker's "discursive negotiation of meaning", and in Toombs's account of the unique individual present in "symptoms, diagnosis, and therapy").

A further key theme, which at first glance might seem to be inconsistent with the main thrust of this book, is the importance of quasi-legal ethics. In urging the need for healthcare ethics, we may at times have appeared to make quasi-legal ethics the villain of the piece. But quasi-legal ethics, as we emphasized at the start of our main Introduction, has a number of important roles.

One such role is to empower disadvantaged groups. Thus Sherwin, who is concerned to break the power of healthcare institutions "deeply implicated in the maintenance of structures of oppression" and thus to foster the agency of patients and non-professionals, argues that these ends will be achieved not by abandoning but by supplementing the principles approach. Griffiths, similarly, reconstructs the notion of autonomy, rather than rejecting it altogether. Like many feminist writers, she questions the lived experience of autonomy for women; yet she also finds it an essential component of women's liberation. Adshead, too, writing of what is arguably the most oppressed group of patients – those with mental disorders – argues that principles, although not in themselves sufficient, are nonetheless a necessary protection against abuses of the therapeutic relationship.

Our selection of philosophical approaches relevant to healthcare ethics is, of course, far from complete. This is a rapidly growing area with a number of significant recent publications (see, for example, Steven Sabat's (2001) application of discourse analysis to problems of meaning in old-age psychiatry). But we hope that our selection illustrates the range and power of the methods available for making healthcare ethics, with its focus on the diversity of human values, an equal partner with the dominant quasi-legal model in meeting the challenges of twenty-first-century healthcare.

REFERENCES

Gilligan, C. (1993) *In a Different Voice: Psychological Theory and Women's Development*, 2nd edn (Cambridge, MA: Harvard University Press).

Sabat, S. R. (2001) *The Experience of Alzheimer's Disease: Life Through a Tangled Veil* (Oxford: Blackwell Publishers).

1

Toward a Feminist Ethics of Health Care

SUSAN SHERWIN

The Role of Context

Biomedical ethics, like feminist ethics, is a new, rapidly developing area of philosophic specialization. It, too, is committed to developing analyses that can offer meaningful guidance in the morally troubling situations of real life, and it shares with feminist ethics a sense of frustration with the level of abstraction and generality that characterizes most traditional philosophic work on ethics. Writers in both fields are critical of the limitations that are created when we restrict ethical analysis to the level of general principles; both perceive a need to focus on the contextual details of actual situations that morally concerned persons find problematic. The use of context is quite different in the two fields, however, and in this chapter I shall examine this difference, so that we can see what is needed to develop a feminist ethics of health care. Looking at the gaps in nonfeminist bioethics, we can see that a contextually based moral theory must maintain a level of generality that supports an analysis of gender-based power relations in its evaluations.

[Elsewhere] I have reviewed some ways in which feminists have been influenced by Carol Gilligan's (1982) claim that women are more likely than men to understand morality as consisting of caring for others and men are more likely than women to understand morality as a system of abstract, universal rules. Although intrigued by the empirical evidence of an existing gender difference in moral reasoning, many feminists remain uneasy about the normative significance of this gendered description of ethics and are unwilling to endorse an unqualified commitment to caring as a moral ideal.

In interpreting her research data, Gilligan also identifies a methodological difference in women's and men's distinctive patterns of moral reasoning. She finds that girls and women tend to evaluate ethical dilemmas in a contextualized, narrative way, looking at the particular details of a problem situation when making ethical decisions; in contrast, boys and men seem inclined to apply a general, abstract principle to the situation without paying specific attention to the unique circumstances of the case. Several feminists have found this difference in method to be a promising basis for building feminist ethics. Although still cautious of the implications of gender-specific patterns of moral reasoning, most feminists endorse including context as a central element in moral reasoning.

[. . .]

I believe, however, feminist ethicists must be more precise about the term "context." Although mainstream medical ethics also expresses a commitment to contextual ethics, it is by no means a form of feminist ethics. In reviewing the differences between feminist ethics and medical ethics, the importance of clarifying the contextual details relevant to a distinctively feminist ethical analysis will become apparent.

[. . .]

Further Areas of Similarity Between Feminist and Medical Ethics

There is substantial agreement between those who pursue feminist and medical ethics on the importance of certain kinds of contextual features. Both recognize that an ethics of actions must be supplemented by discussion of the nature of the relationships that hold between the agents performing an action and those who are affected by it. Both feminists and medical ethicists are critical of the traditional assumption – made most explicitly by contractarians but also often assumed by other sorts of theorists – that the role of ethics is to clarify the obligations that hold among individuals who are viewed as paradigmatically equal, independent, rational, and autonomous.

Feminist ethicists accept the arguments offered within the realm of "feminine" ethics, which demand that attention be paid to the interdependent, emotionally varied, unequal relationships that shape human lives. Similar claims are found in the literature of medical ethics, where it is widely recognized that the relationships that exist between physicians and their patients are far from equal (especially if the patient is very ill) and that the model of contracts negotiated by independent, rational agents does not provide a useful perspective for this sort of interaction. In particular, the disadvantaged position of the dependent patient is a major theme in the many discussions of paternalism that are found throughout the medical ethics literature. Further, many authors are sensitive to the fact that the physician–patient

relationship is not a dyad that exists in some abstract, eternal realm; it is found within overlapping networks of other relationships, which bind patients and physicians to their respective family members, other health professionals, neighbors, employers, health services administrators, and so on (for example, Hardwig 1990).

In addition, we can find parallel claims in the literatures of feminist and medical ethics of the importance of evaluating behavior in terms of its effect on the quality of relationships among persons concerned. For instance, discussions in medical ethics on the importance of telling patients the truth about their condition often refer to the effect that a discovered lie would have on the physician–patient relationship; it is frequently claimed that patients who learn that their physicians have deliberately deceived them are likely to feel especially betrayed by the violation of trust in light of their feelings of vulnerability and dependency, despite the supposedly benevolent motives that might have contributed to the deceptive behavior. Feminist theorists, for their part, note that ethics should not only be concerned with actions and relationships but also focus on questions of character and the development of attitudes of trust – and antitrust – within those relationships (see Baier 1986). For example, Sarah Hoagland (1988), Marilyn Friedman (1989), and Iris Marion Young (1989) all focus on the conditions necessary for the building of (feminist) community.

Moreover, as in feminist ethics, discussion in medical ethics often raises considerations of caring; this requirement is usually couched in the language of beneficence – an attitude that is generally assumed to be owed to patients. Medical dilemmas are sometimes discussed in terms that appear to rank sensitivity and caring ahead of applications of principle; compassion is frequently claimed to be more compelling than honesty or justice.

There seems, then, to be agreement between the two fields on a variety of concerns regarding traditional moral theory. Authors in both disciplines argue that matters of character, responsibility, and other features that affect trust are morally significant. Both reject the oversimplifying tendency of normative theorists to reduce all moral considerations to short sets of universal principles. Given their shared commitment to focusing on context in moral problem-solving, their common understanding of the ethical significance of inequality within relationships, and the tendency of some authors in both traditions to include caring values in their analyses, it might appear that medical ethics is already well on its way to being feminist. Medical ethics, however, does not display any commitment to ending oppression; thus most of the writings of contemporary medical ethics must be judged as lacking from the perspective of feminist ethics.

Feminist ethics requires that any evaluation of moral considerations attend to the power relations that structure the relevant interactions. Political analyses of the unequal power of women and men, of white people and people of color, of First World and Third World people, of the rich and the poor, of the healthy and the disabled, and so forth are central to feminist ethics. To date, that sort of analysis has been almost entirely absent from the literature of mainstream medical ethics, although the institutions in which health care is provided are deeply implicated in the maintenance of structures of oppression.

[. . .]

Other Features of a Feminist Ethics of Health Care

There are numerous other ways in which work in feminist ethics can inform and transform work in medical ethics and in which medical ethics can provide models (both good and bad) for work in feminist ethics. For instance, the literature in both feminist and medical ethics reflects an interest in questions concerning the nature and quality of particular relationships, because both feminist and medical ethicists recognize that rights and responsibilities depend upon the roles and relationships that exist among persons of differing power and status. New models of interaction within the area of health care are needed to develop a system of care that is less hierarchically structured and less focused on matters of power and control than the current institutions. Feminist explor-

ations of friendship (Code 1987) or mother–child (Held 1987a) relationships are worth pursuing as a basis of alternative models for these institutions.

A feminist ethics of health care will have other distinctive dimensions that mark its departure from the familiar mainstream approaches to medical ethics. For example, it demonstrates how the role of the patient is perceived as feminine. Patients are required to submit to medical authority and respond with gratitude for attention offered. Most recognize their vulnerability to medical power and learn the value of offering a cheerful disposition in the face of extraordinary suffering, because complaints are often met with hostility and impatience. Like those who are socially defined as subservient, patients often find themselves apologizing for the inconvenience of needing attention; most know their obligation to listen submissively to medical direction. Because feminism is occupied with redefining feminine roles, a feminist ethics of health care takes a natural interest in redefining the feminine aspects of the role of patient.

For this reason, a feminist ethics of health care includes reflection on the underlying medical views of the body. Medical practice involves the explorative study, manipulation, and modification of the body; because, under patriarchal ideology, the body is characteristically associated with the feminine, the female body is particularly subject to medical dominance. Its practitioners presume the license to probe the body for its secrets, as well as the authority to define its norms and deviations. As the contributors to *Body/Politics: Women and the Discourses of Science* (Jacobus, Keller, and Shuttleworth 1990) make clear, there are significant political and moral questions to be explored regarding the relations between medicine and the feminine body. The discourses common to medicine and science both reflect and support attitudes about the body that reinforce patriarchal forces.

Further, as Esther Frances (1990) proposes, a feminist ethics of health care should evaluate the significance of challenges to allopathic medicine with respect to the oppression of women. There are numerous critiques of the assumptions and practices of allopathic medicine and many competing visions of alternative health care practices. Many women have found some of these alternatives attractive; some seem to promise a more empowering, less hierarchical understanding of health than is found in mainstream allopathic medicine. In a feminist ethics of health care these various approaches should be explored and examined with regard to their promise for relieving some of the harms women now experience under sexism.

Like other projects in feminist ethics, a feminist ethics of health care is concerned with going beyond analysis of how women have been systematically oppressed by patriarchy; it seeks to foster agency where agency has previously been restricted by patriarchal patterns and assumptions. The agenda of traditional bioethics has been largely occupied with questions about the responsibilities of health professionals; the agenda of a feminist ethics of health care is significantly farther-reaching. It is directed also at exploring the various roles that may be open to patients and nonprofessionals in the pursuit of health and health policy. It is not sufficient to put specific moral restrictions on the behavior of health-care providers; we must also ensure that the health care delivery system is modified in appropriate ways to allow consumers to achieve their ends with respect to their own health.

A principal task of a feminist ethics of health care is to develop conceptual models for restructuring the power associated with healing, by distributing the specialized knowledge on health matters in ways that allow persons maximum control over their own health. It is important to clarify how excessive dependence can be reduced, how caring can be offered without paternalism, and how health services can be obtained within a context worthy of trust. Feminists seek to spread health information widely and foster self-help approaches to health matters. Feminist values imply that medical expertise should be viewed as a social resource, and as such, it should be held under the control of patients and their caregivers. A feminist ethics of health care suggests that the institution of medicine should be transformed from one

principally occupied with crisis management to one primarily committed to fostering health empowerment. We must, then, look at the existing structures of medicine and medical interaction when attempting to understand the details of any particular medical experience.

I have spelled out some important features of what I envision as a feminist ethics of health care, but this is not an exhaustive description. This book represents an initial step in the task of developing such an ethics, but much more work remains to be done. Others will add further dimensions. The common agenda of work characterized by the label "feminist ethics of health care" will be to provide a more comprehensive and fairer approach to medical ethics than has been evident in the literature to date.

REFERENCES

Baier, A. C. (1986) Trust and antitrust. *Ethics* 96: 231–60.

Code, L. (1987) Second persons. In Marsha Hanen and Kai Nielsen (eds.), *Science, Morality and Feminist Theory*. Supplementary volume, *Canadian Journal of Philosophy* 13: 41–56.

Frances, E. (1990) Some thoughts on the contents of Hypatia. *Hypatia* 5/3: 159–61.

Friedman, M. (1989) Feminism and modern friendship: Dislocating the community. *Ethics* 99/2: 275–90.

Gilligan, C. (1982) *In a Different Voice: Psychological Theory and Women's Moral Development* (Cambridge: Harvard University Press).

Hardwig, J. (1990) What about the family? *Hastings Center Report* 20/2: 5–10.

Held, V. (1987) Non-contractual society: A feminist view. In Marsha Hanen and Kai Nielsen (eds.), *Science, Morality and Feminist Theory*. Supplementary volume, *Canadian Journal of Philosophy* 13.

Hoagland, S. L. (1988) *Lesbian Ethics: Toward New Value* (Palo Alto, CA: Institute of Lesbian Studies).

Jacobus, M., Keller, E. F., and Shuttleworth, S. (eds.) (1990) *Body/Politics: Women and the Discourses of Science* (New York: Routledge).

Young, I. M. (1989) Polity and group difference: A critique of the ideal of universal citizenship. *Ethics* 99/2: 250–74.

2

A Deliberative Approach to Bioethics

MICHAEL PARKER

A "Rivalry of Care" Case

In their book, *The Patient in the Family*, Hilde and James Lindemann Nelson describe the case of a man whose daughter is suffering from kidney failure.[1] She is spending six hours, three times a week on a dialysis machine and the effects of this are becoming increasingly hard for her and her family to bear. She has already had one kidney transplant, which her body rejected, and her doctors are unsure whether a second would work but are willing to try if they can find a suitable donor. After some tests, the pediatrician privately tells the father that he is compatible and therefore a suitable donor.

It may seem inconceivable that a father would refuse to donate a kidney to his daughter under such circumstances. Yet he does refuse and justifies his decision on the grounds that the success of the transplant is uncertain and also on the basis of his concerns about the implications of the operation itself for him and his family. He is frightened and worried about what would happen to him and his other children if his remaining kidney were to fail. But he is ashamed to feel this way and cannot bear to refuse openly, so he asks the pediatrician to tell

the family that he is in fact not compatible. However, although sympathetic, she says she cannot lie for him and, after a silence, the father says, "OK, then I'll do it. If they knew that I was compatible but wouldn't donate my kidney, it would wreck the family."

But, why should this decision wreck the family, ask the Lindemann Nelsons? Does a father have a special obligation to donate his kidney to his daughter? What is it about families and the values that underpin them which leads to the expectation that parents will sacrifice themselves for their children (and in particular for the child who is ill)? What is it about modern patient-centered medicine that intensifies such expectations?

The case is used by the Lindemann Nelsons because they believe it suggests that there is a conflict in healthcare between two sets of value; those individualistic values that underlie patient-centered medicine and the communitarian values that sustain families and communities. They argue that modern medicine's overriding focus on the benefit of the individual patient has distorted the ways in which family members interact with one another and in particular with those who are sick. They argue that at times of stress families often adopt the individualistic values of the medical world and this leads them unintentionally to trample on the values and concerns that sustain families. It is with this tension, they suggest, that the father wrestles in the case described.

Who am I?

The claim that there are important tensions between the values of patient-centered medicine and those that sustain families and communities reflects an ongoing and important contemporary debate in bioethics (and in ethics more widely) between what have been called "individualistic" approaches and those that have come to be known as "communitarian."[2] The conflict is one that is characterized by Michael Sandel and other communitarians as one between two conceptions of what it is to be a moral subject.[3]

The communitarian analysis of the case offered by the Lindemann Nelsons urges the father to seek a resolution of his moral problem in an answer to the question "who am I?" where his identity is to be seen as informed by his membership of a community (in this case, a family) rather than through an analysis of rights[4] or a "balancing" of principles.[5] For, as Kukathas and Petit suggest:

> [For communitarians] the end of moral reasoning is not judgement but understanding and self-discovery. I ask, not "what should I be, what sort of life should I lead?" but "Who am I?" [And] to ask this question is to concern oneself first and foremost with the character of the community which constitutes one's identity.[6]

Sandel too argues that, "I [should] ask, as I deliberate, not only what I really want but who I really am, and this last question takes me beyond attention to desires alone to reflect on my identity itself."[7] At the heart of this communitarian approach to the moral, which urges us to emphasize the values which sustain families and communities over those of autonomy and patient choice, is the ontological claim that the moral world consists of fundamentally and

essentially "socially-embedded" beings who draw their identities, and their moral values, from their constitutive attachments to a "community."

Interestingly, Sandel argues that the individualist too, whose approach it is that is rejected by the Lindemann Nelsons and other communitarians as "individualistic," agrees that the question of who I am is at the core of moral deliberation.[8] In contrast to the communitarian, however, the individualist is said to conceive of the moral subject in terms of the autonomy and the free choice of the individual "free chooser," rather than in terms of a being constituted by his or her embeddedness in a constellation of social and communal values and this leads to an approach to bioethics which emphasizes the values of autonomy and patient choice over those of community and family.

The individualist argues that the value of such freedom is independently derivable by virtue of the fact that it is a necessary condition of the very possibility of the moral, and hence of the very possibility of a constellation of values at all and it is this that means that autonomy ought to "trump" other values.[9] As Sandel explains:

> For justice to be primary, certain things must be true of us. We must be creatures of a certain kind, related to human circumstance in a certain way. In particular, we must stand to our circumstance always at a certain distance, conditioned to be sure, but part of us always antecedent to any conditions. Only in this way can we view ourselves as subjects as well as objects of experience, as agents and not just instruments of the purposes we pursue.[10]

The basis of an emphasis on autonomy is thus not the ends we choose but our capacity to choose them and such capacity depends upon the free and independent nature of the subject. As Kant argues, in response to the question of what makes the moral possible, "It is nothing else than personality, i.e., the freedom and independence from the mechanism of nature regarded as a capacity of a being which is subject to special laws (pure practical laws given by its own reason)."[11] Sandel's claim, then, is that both the individualist and the communitarian seek an explanation of the moral in an answer to the question of what it means to be a moral subject, each rejecting the other on the grounds that it is incapable of providing such an explanation. I shall be going on to argue in the rest of this chapter, however, that each of these conceptions must be rejected and that this has important and far-reaching implications for the practice of bioethics, some of which I shall tease out in the final section.

Three reasons for rejecting the individual moral subject

It seems to me that the communitarian is right to reject the individualist model as conceived in this way, and the grounds for such a rejection can, I want to argue, be grouped under three headings. I have explored these arguments more fully elsewhere and, for reasons of space, I merely state them now.[12]

The first of these grounds might best be collected under the heading "The Impossibility of Moral Understanding" and draws together arguments from both philosophy and psychology which suggest that the individualist account of morality must be rejected because it is not possible to provide an explanation of the development of moral understanding from an individualistic epistemological perspective. For the very possibility of moral understanding and moral language, it is claimed, is dependent upon the social dimension of human experience. Ludwig Wittgenstein's "private language argument" is one powerful argument to this effect in which Wittgenstein argues that the very possibility of meaning and hence language depends upon the existence of standards of established social practice.[13] But this is not the only argument of this kind. Alasdair MacIntyre in *After Virtue*, for example, argues: "In so far as persons must be understood as partly individuated by their membership of traditions, the history of their lives will be embedded in the larger narrative of a historically and socially extended argument about the good life for human beings."[14]

The second group of arguments consists of those that claim, against the individualist, that

the having of moral problems and moral identity at all depends on the fact that *we are "socially embedded."* That is, it is claimed, we are all inevitably located in social, intersubjective networks from which we draw our identity and that the liberal conception of the subject as divorced from such networks inevitably comes at a price. For, as Michael Sandel writes: "To imagine a person incapable of constitutive attachments such as these is not to conceive an ideally free and rational agent, but to imagine a person wholly without character, without moral depth."[15] Perhaps the strongest proponent of this type of argument is Charles Taylor, who argues that to be a self at all is to be an essentially moral being located within what he calls "evaluative frameworks" and that such frameworks are inevitably linguistic and hence social:

> This is the sense in which one cannot be a self on one's own. I am a self only in relation to certain interlocutors: in one way in relation to those conversation partners who are essential to my achieving self-definition; in another in relation to those who are now crucial to my continuing grasp of languages of self-understanding – and, of course, these classes may overlap. A self exists only within what I call "webs of interlocution."[16]

The third group of arguments are those that attempt to describe the *unacceptable social consequences of individualism*. Communitarians sometimes argue that, historically, the over-emphasis on rights in liberal democracies has had unacceptable consequences both for societies and individuals (i.e. the breakdown of traditional structures such as the family) and for this reason should be rejected.[17]

Whilst I have my doubts about the strength of the third group of arguments in a world in which perhaps the most striking moral challenge is the oppression of individuals by communities, the combination of these arguments taken together means that communitarians are right to call for the rejection of what I have called elsewhere "overly individualistic" approaches to ethics.[18]

Three reasons for rejecting the communitarian "embedded moral subject"

It seems to me, however, that the communitarian argument for the "socially embedded subject" must itself be rejected for three sets of reason which, again for reasons of space, I shall simply state here.

First, the explanation of morality in terms of the "socially embedded self" and of "constitutive attachments" means that communitarianism is incapable of recognizing *the moral status of the individual*. Feminists, for example, have argued that while communitarianism is very good at describing the benefits of community, it says very little about the damage caused by families and communities and says nothing for those at the periphery of societies for whom we expect moral theory to have special concern. Taken to its logical conclusion, communitarianism seems capable of justifying the oppression of minorities and of the weak by the majority, of the novel by the traditional.[19] And although we might agree with the communitarians that overly individualistic approaches to ethics must be rejected, we would surely not want to reject with it that which is valuable about the individualistic approaches; namely a recognition of the moral status of the individual. For this would be to throw out the baby with the bathwater.

Secondly, and following from the above, the communitarian approach is, it is argued, incapable of providing an *explanation of social change* or of the need for the critical moral reflection, creativity, and criticism necessary for the change and development of communities. Another way of saying this is to say that communitarianism is incapable of providing an account of how the individual can come to have an effect upon the society within which they live and upon their constitutive values and relationships.[20]

Thirdly, Jürgen Habermas has argued that it is *not in fact possible to identify the shared values required by communitarians*.[21] The breakdown of shared values and traditions identified by communitarians brings into question the viability of the communitarian project itself. For, when we look around us there appear few if any candidates for the shared values upon which a communitarian New World might be built. We live in a world characterized by diversity in which candidates for the role of paradigmatic communities are revealed to be as often the sites of conflict and violence as of mutual support,[22] a world in which it is not possible to identify the kind of shared values or traditions upon which a communitarian morality might be founded.[23]

A Resolution? The Discursive Moral Subject

It seems, therefore, that both the individualist and communitarian models of ethics must be rejected. But where does this leave us? If we wish to elaborate a coherent moral theory[24] and if appeal is no longer possible either to the kind of detached, individual, rational decision-making called for by the liberal individualist or to communitarian shared values and traditions as the basis of ethical decision-making in healthcare, how are we to approach the making of ethical decisions of the kind confronting the father at the beginning of this chapter? What seems clear is that any coherent explanation of the moral will have to be one that is capable of capturing the insights of both communitarianism and individualism, whilst avoiding their weaknesses and pitfalls, and what this means is that it must be capable of capturing both the value of the individual voice and the moral status of the individual, whilst at the same time recognizing the intersubjective and social context of morality and the value of social relationships and their various manifestations.

It is worth pausing here for a moment to reflect upon the interdependent nature of the relationship between the two sets of argument I have identified for the rejection of individualism and of communitarianism. For it is an important feature of each of these arguments that such rejection is in each case put in terms of the necessity of the other to any coherent account of the moral. The argument that individualism must be rejected, for example, is based on the claim that recognition of the role of the social is a necessary element of any coherent explanation of morality. The argument for the rejection of overly social accounts, on the other hand, is phrased in terms of the necessity of a recognition of the role of the individual.

My point in juxtaposing the arguments in this way is to suggest that both the social and the individual are together necessary and it is their *combination* that makes a coherent account of the moral possible. I want further to argue that these features of our moral world are jointly and together only explicable in terms of the actual relations between people in the intersubjective contexts which constitute their everyday lives with others. For it is only here, in the intersubjective relations between people, that the community meets the individual and vice versa. It is here that morality is elaborated and here that the maintenance and the transformation of social practice occur. This is to suggest, following Harre and Shotter and other discursive psychologists, that the primary social reality is neither the individual nor the community but people in conversation and that discourse is the developmental fundamental of human experience.[25] To quote Alasdair MacIntyre: "Conversation, understood widely enough, is the form of human transactions in general."[26] This must indeed be the case, I suggest, for the reasons above and because it is through such "conversations" that we are introduced into the world of human affairs and negotiate our identity and our moral concerns. It is also here that we discover the ethical voice with which we reflect upon and change the nature of our relations to our community and other people. From this discursive perspective, it seems to me, it is possible to begin to recognize the particular value, and indeed the necessity, of the engagement of human beings in the negotiation of the meaning of their own lives and the nature of their relations with those around them, with those who constitute their communities. Hence, within a moral framework of this kind it is possible to capture, as neither individualists nor communitarians are able, both the value of communal life and the moral significance of the individual ethical voice. It is to claim that it is neither the freedom of the abstracted individual nor the emphasis of community values that ought to be given a special place in the constellation of values, but the discursive relationship between the two. It is also to claim that the discursive negotiation of meaning is the developmental fundamental of human experience and that it is this that makes the moral possible.[27]

Implications for Bioethics

What, then, are the implications of this approach for bioethics? It seems to me that there are several key features of an approach such as this and I shall attempt to outline these very briefly in conclusion.

The value of deliberation with others

First, to adopt this perspective is to argue, as I have already suggested, that the deliberative search for moral meaning is at the core of what it is to be human in a world with others. This is to locate morality and the search for moral meaning very firmly at the center of human life. To adopt this perspective therefore is to recognize the particular value of the engagement of human beings in the attempt to "make sense" of their lives and the nature of their relation with those around them. It is also to recognize, as neither individualists nor communitarians are able, both the value of communal life and the moral significance of the individual ethical voice. Whilst placing an emphasis on joint narrative, therefore, this approach nevertheless has the advantage of providing, as communitarianism does not, space for a critique of accepted or traditional values on the basis of a respect for the discursive nature of human experience. For whilst respect of this kind is capable of capturing our social embeddedness it is also capable of recognizing that individuals have a right both to be protected from, and to have a voice in, their community.

To assert the value of the discursive elaboration of the self is in many respects to follow Alasdair MacIntyre, who argues for a conception of the moral life as one that is constituted by engagement in a conversation with history and tradition in an attempt to establish the narrative unity of one's life. It is also to align oneself with Charles Taylor's claim that the identity of the self is inextricably linked to its sense of the significance and meaning of the situations it encounters in life and this is to see, as does Ronald Dworkin, life as a series of "challenges" which must be addressed.[28] The good life is at least to some extent one in which we are engaged in the attempt to make moral sense of the challenges with which we are confronted in life.

Subsidiarity and participation

Secondly, it follows from the emphasis on the value of "making sense" that ethical decisions are best made and in fact might only be capable of being made by those most closely involved, and this is to suggest that the process of making ethical decisions ought to adhere to a principle of "subsidiarity." Nevertheless, such an approach is also and perhaps primarily one that emphasizes the participation of all those who have a legitimate interest, and this means that the requirement that decisions be made by those most likely to be affected needs to be balanced against a responsibility to ensure that all who have a legitimate interest are involved. This is to suggest that decision-making in bioethics will need to take a range of different forms, from the establishing of public consensus conferences about ethical issues of widespread public or even global concern, to conversations between doctors, patients, and families, or within families themselves, about the ethical questions raised by a particular case or treatment option and in some cases, perhaps even most, this will mean that decisions will be made by the patient alone, or in collaboration with his or her doctor.

However, whilst taking a variety of forms, such forums would have to share a commitment to respecting the fundamental value of discursive involvement and hence would have to place an emphasis on both participation and subsidiarity.

Openness and truthfulness in ethical decision-making processes

Thirdly, and briefly, the emphases on the values of "making sense," "participation," and "sub-

sidiarity" all imply a requirement both for the openness of the processes of decision-making and for truthfulness in the decision-making forum. This is clearly crucial to any deliberative approach to ethics, and whilst it might be argued that such an emphasis on truthfulness might be captured by the first principle which argues for the engagement in a genuine attempt to "make sense," it seems to me that having it as a separate principle highlights the formal elements of the discursive ethical space within which "making sense" is possible.[29]

A decentralized bioethics

Finally, and perhaps most importantly, this is an argument for the democratization and decentralization of ethics. For, whilst the philosophical analysis of ethical problems and ethical theory and the elaboration of biomedical principles can be useful in creating a framework for the discussion of ethical problems, the resolution of such problems in an ethical way involves the creation and maintenance of ethical forums of the kind I have described in which those who have a legitimate interest in a case can engage jointly in the process of making moral sense of the situation. This is to argue for a genuinely participatory, democratic, and discursive bioethics, and such a perspective has, I suggest, profound and radical political implications both for the medical profession and beyond.

NOTES

1   Lindemann Nelson, H. and Lindemann Nelson, J., *The Patient in the Family* (New York: Routledge, 1995), p. 1.
2   Parker, M., *Ethics and Community in the Health Care Professions* (London: Routledge, 1999).
3   Sandel, M., *Liberalism and the Limits of Justice* (Cambridge: Cambridge University Press, 1982).
4   Lindemann Nelson and Lindemann Nelson, *The Patient in the Family*, pp. 1–30.
5   Beauchamp, T. and Childress, J., *Principles of Biomedical Ethics*, 4th edn (Oxford: Oxford University Press, 1994).
6   Kukathas, C. and Petit, P., *Rawls: A Theory of Justice and its Critics* (Cambridge: Polity, 1990), p. 106.

7   Sandel, *Liberalism*, p. 180.

8   Ibid.

9   Dworkin, R., *Taking Rights Seriously* (London: Duckworth, 1977).

10 Sandel, *Liberalism*, p. 11.

11 Kant, I., *Critique of Practical Reason*, trans. L. W. Beck (Indianapolis: Bobbs-Merrill, 1956 [1788]).

12 Parker, M., *The Growth of Understanding* (Aldershot: Avebury, 1995).

13 Wittgenstein, L., *Philosophical Investigations*, 2nd edn (Oxford: Blackwell, 1974), nn. 150–200. See also Taylor, C., *Sources of the Self* (Cambridge: Cambridge University Press, 1989); Vygotsky, L. S., *Mind in Society* (Harvard: Harvard University Press, 1978); Mead, G. H., *Mind, Self, and Society* (Chicago: 1934); Donaldson, M., *Children's Minds* (London: Fontana, 1978); MacIntyre, A., *After Virtue* (London: Duckworth, 1981), p. 197.

14 MacIntyre, *After Virtue*.

15 Sandel, *Liberalism*, p. 179.

16 Taylor, *Sources of the Self*, p. 36.

17 See, for example, many of the works by Amitai Etzioni, such as *The Spirit of Community* (New York: Crown, 1993).

18 Parker, *The Growth of Understanding* (Aldershot: Avebury, 1995).

19 Parker, M., "Communitarianism and its problems," *Cogito* 10/3 (November 1996).

20 Parker, *The Growth of Understanding*; Mendus, S., "Strangers and brothers: Liberalism, socialism and the concept of autonomy." In D. Milligan and W. Watts-Miller, *Liberalism, Citizenship and Autonomy* (Aldershot: Avebury, 1992), p. 13.

21 As indeed has Alasdair MacIntyre. See, for example, *After Virtue*.

22 Campbell, B., *The London Independent*, March 16, 1995.

23 Habermas, J., *Justification and Application: Remarks on Discourse Ethics* (Oxford: Polity, 1993).

24 I would like to thank Matti Häyry of the University of Helsinki for helping me to see that this is what I meant.

25 Harre, R. and Gillett, G., *The Discursive Mind* (London: Sage, 1994); Shotter, J., *Conversational Realities* (London: Sage, 1993).

26 MacIntyre, *After Virtue*, p. 197.

27 Parker, *The Growth of Understanding*.

28 Dworkin, R. "The foundations of liberal equality." In G. Petersen (ed.), *The Tanner Lectures on Human Values*, vol. 9 (Utah: University of Utah Press, 1988).

29 Habermas, *Justification and Application*.

3

Bodies and Persons

S. KAY TOOMBS

The doctor–patient relationship is a unique kind of relationship in that it is grounded in the patient's experience of illness. In coming to the physician, the patient seeks two things: (1) to communicate her particular experience of bodily disease; and (2) to receive assistance in dealing with the disorder – the pragmatic goal being that of healing (restoring wholeness), a goal that includes making sense of the illness experience and taking steps to re-establish a state of equilibrium and personal integrity within the context of her particular life situation. [...]

In what follows, I shall suggest that understanding "the patient's problem" requires that doctor and patient meet on the level of immediate experience – the level on which the body is lived.

The Body as the Fundamental Ground of Personhood

In the context of biomedicine, more often than not, we think of the body as a purely biophysiological organism. However, although the body is indeed such an organism, it is much more than that. The body is the fundamental ground (and expression) of the individual person. To elaborate this point it is necessary to make a distinction between the purely physical characteristics of human bodies – characteristics that can be described in terms of anatomy, physiology, and so forth – and the human experience of the body-as-it-is-lived.

The first thing to note is that the relation with one's own body is unlike any other kind of relation. I do not simply "have" a body, as I "have" a house, a car or a pet. To claim that it is "my" body is not to assert that I "own" it as I own other possessions. Nor am I "with" my body in the same manner that I am "with" my friends or my colleagues. (I cannot, for example, walk away from it, should it prove irritating to me.) Furthermore, although my body is the means by which I apprehend and interact with the world – the instrument of my actions – I do not "use" it in the same way that I use other instruments such as my computer or my telephone.

The relation with one's own body is unique in that it is an *existential* relation. I "live" or "exist" my body.[1] [...] Rather than being an object *of* the world, the *body as I live it* represents my particular point of view *on* the world. In this respect the lived body is not the objective, physiological body that can be seen by others (or examined by means of various medical technologies) but, rather, the body that is the vehicle for seeing.

Under normal circumstances the existential relation with body is taken-for-granted. We do not perceive the body as separate from the self. Indeed, the body is that which is perpetually overlooked in carrying out one's projects in the world. As I read a book, for instance, my attention is directed to the meaning of the text. I am not explicitly aware of the functioning of my eyes in focusing on the print. [...] In all my bodily involvements the lived body is given only *implicitly* as the center of reference for my world, a center which is indicated but never grasped as such.[2]

As the center of reference for my world, the lived body orients me to the world around by means of my senses and positions the world in accord with my bodily placement. [...] Additionally, the lived body is the locus of my intentions. Surrounding objects present themselves as invitations to my body's possible actions. The pen is encountered as "an instrument for writing" or as "an object to be replaced in the drawer." [...] Lived space is always encountered as functional space – that milieu within which I carry out my various activities.

In this respect the lived body is always "the-body-in-situation." Bodily acts reflect both my intentions and the concrete circumstances in which I find myself. Contained in the action of raising my arm is the intention to wave to my friend. I raise my arm *in order to* get her attention. [...] The meaning of an embodied action cannot be understood in isolation from the person who performs the action and the intention conveyed within it. [...]

As the locus of my intentions, the lived body represents the realm of my particular existential possibilities. For instance, my leg is more than a limb – it is *the possibility which I am* of standing and lecturing to my class, of walking down the steps into the back garden, of running in the park with my child. It is also *the possibility that I may become* of realizing my ambition to pursue a particular career, or of learning to dance.

[...]

The Patient's Apprehension of Illness

Recognizing the existential relation that we enjoy with our bodies provides insight into the experience of illness. In particular, it becomes clear that illness is not simply a disorder of a physical organism. In disrupting intentionality, existential possibility, and corporeal identity, bodily disorder encroaches on the many and varied facets of personhood.[3]

The perception that one is sick (and thus in need of assistance from a physician) begins with a radical change in the normal taken-for-granted existential relation with the body. Rather than being unreflectively lived, the body intrudes itself into consciousness becoming the unwilling object of one's attention. This shift in consciousness occurs when one becomes aware of alien physical sensations such as pain, fatigue, or dizziness, or an unexpected alteration in function. This change in bodily experience demands overt recognition. One must stop whatever one is doing in order explicitly to focus on the body. If I suddenly find it difficult to button my coat, my attention is immediately drawn to the ineffectiveness of my hand, the clumsiness of my fingers, and the pain in my joints. This act of bodily attentiveness also includes a search for meaning – I may conclude that this "inability to" manipulate the buttons could signify the onset of arthritis – and, further, I may fear that this condition will be constricting not only in terms of physical movement but restrictive in terms of limiting my future plans and projects.

[...]

The initial perception that the body is problematic depends upon the individual's accustomed manner of bodily being.[4] For instance, what is "normal" functioning for me as a person living with MS is quite different from the "normal" functioning of a person who does not have neurological disease. And what I perceive to be an unusual sensation worthy of medical attention may not necessarily be so judged by my friend who also has MS but who experiences her body differently.

The loss of bodily taken-for-grantedness engenders a profound threat to the self. In its most extreme form, of course, the concrete threat relates to the possibility that I may die. When the body malfunctions, one recognizes in a chilling way that the body is a physiological organism with its own nature and, more importantly, that there is a symbiotic relation between body and self. Whatever happens to *it* also necessarily happens to *me*. The experience of illness is always the experience of both "having" and "being had." I not only "have" an illness. "It" also "has" me in its clutches. Thus, bodily change engenders not only a profound sense of disunity in the lived body – a loss of wholeness characterized by alienation between body and self – but also a deep sense of loss of control.[5]

The perception of limitation and contingency that accompanies bodily disorder relates not only to the possibility of death but to the loss of existential possibility. In the context of everyday life, alien body sensations are not experienced by the patient as abstract physical symptoms indicative of a particular disease. Rather, such disorders represent the inability to engage the world in ways that are important and meaningful. A severe headache is not simply an uncomfortable sensation. It is the "inability to" concentrate on the book I am reading, or the impossibility of carrying out a personal project. [...]

Illness also encroaches on personhood in the sense that the loss of possibility directly threatens self-integrity. In our culture there is a great emphasis on the importance of "doing" rather than "being." That is a person's worth, more often than not, is judged according to his or her capacity to produce (to be useful) or the ability to achieve a certain professional status. Self-worth is assessed largely on the basis of role. In curtailing the ability to pursue plans and projects and in affecting personal relationships, bodily disorder necessarily disrupts the various roles that we occupy – father, breadwinner, student, mother. The inability to carry out one's role inevitably causes one to feel diminished in person, as well as in body.[6] [...]

Self-integrity may also be threatened when one perceives a change in body style – the familiar way of walking, talking, gesticulating, that identifies the body as peculiarly "me." Indeed, a person may decide to seek medical attention because s/he notices an altered pattern of movement such as a limp or an inexplicable change in appearance. [...]

Changes in body style are profoundly disruptive since they engender a loss of self-identity. As a person who has experienced (and continues to experience) major alterations in ways of moving and appearing, I have difficulty identifying with my body style. When I see myself on a home video and observe my disordered movements, I experience a sense of puzzlement. I catch myself wondering not so much whether the *body* projected on the screen is my body but, rather, if the *person* in the video is really *me*. At the same time, if I see older videos of myself walking, or leaning on a cane, I find it hard to recognize myself. I can no longer remember how (or who) I was when I moved like that.

Since the body represents one's self-expression to others, societal judgements with respect to body style may also threaten personal integrity. I live in a culture that places great emphasis on physical fitness, sexuality, productivity and youth – an ideal that is associated with a particular bodily physique. Consequently, there is little tolerance for physical difference or deviation from the ideal.[7] For instance, when strangers see my body, they make judgements about me *as a person*. In noting my body's incapacities, most conclude that as a person-in-a-wheelchair, I am dependent on others and unable to engage in professional activities. The negative response of others can engender a profound loss of self-esteem – a loss that is integral to the experience of bodily change.[8]

The Individual in Clinical Practice

Why is it important to understand illness in terms of lived body disruption? What are the practical implications for medical professionals? First and foremost, such understanding forcefully reminds us that clinical practice is person-centered. In comprehending and treating the illnesses of particular patients, doctors do not simply investigate malfunctioning organisms. Rather, doctors care for *embodied persons* – each one of whom is experiencing bodily change in the context of a particular life situation and from the perspective of personal meanings. *The focus of clinical interaction, and the theme of clinical dialogue, is not simply the pathology of the biological body but rather it is the particular patient's experience of the disruption in the lived body*. This is in no way to discount the importance of biomedical knowledge and the power of medical theory in the diagnosis and treatment of disease. However, it is to emphasize that in the context of clinical practice, symptoms, medical tests, diagnoses, medical procedures, and treatments are not things that happen to bodies in the abstract but rather these are profoundly personal human experiences whose meaning is different for each individual.

The clinical process is traditionally described in three distinct steps: symptom, diagnosis and therapy. In each of these the person is always present. In order to apprehend the symptom, the doctor must first comprehend the patient's description of what is wrong. As Rudebeck points out, in the reality of clinical practice doctors never meet symptoms in the abstract. The doctor "faces a human being who in her symptom presentation tries to communicate an experience, which is often quite personal since body and self are inseparable."[9] [...]

The patient's ability to communicate her experience to the doctor is, of course, influenced by many things. The most important factor is the doctor's willingness to listen. It is not hard to judge the doctor's level of interest. As many patients know from firsthand experience, and as empirical studies have shown, often the doctor controls the way the story is told, deciding what is important. (One study found that on average physicians interrupted patients eighteen seconds after the patient began to speak and patients were able to complete their statements in only 23 percent of visits.[10]) If the content of the dialogue is limited by narrowly construed questions that focus exclusively *on the impact of disease on the body*, patients "get the message" that their particular experience of disease is of little or no significance to the doctor. This "message" effectively silences the patient and prevents the doctor from fully comprehending the patient's problem.

Understanding is not only important with respect to clinical diagnosis, but also in deciding

what steps to take to ameliorate the problem. The choice of treatment cannot be determined by reference to objective clinical data alone but only by reference to the individual's values.[11] Although the doctor may consider the effects of a particular medication (or procedure) to be harmless, the patient may find the treatment too disruptive in its effects on daily life.

Understanding the patient's problem also means comprehending the meanings associated with a diagnosis of disease. Receiving a particular diagnosis changes the meaning of bodily disorder. Sometimes the change is positive (learning that the pain in one's chest is not heart disease may lessen anxiety and reduce existential threat). At other times a diagnosis, in and of itself, causes personal havoc regardless of actual bodily dysfunction. The dread diseases – cancer, AIDS, multiple sclerosis – carry with them a particularly powerful symbolic significance. The patient is forced to deal not only with overt physical symptoms but with the fears associated with the disease identification (fears that are intimately related to personal and social expectations regarding the disease). In this case the meaning of the diagnosis becomes an important factor that influences the individual's experience of illness. The only way to find out the meaning of the diagnosis is to ask the patient. In this way it may be possible for the doctor to alleviate unnecessary suffering resulting from evaluations and expectations that might be interpreted differently.[12]

Comprehending another, reaching mutual understanding, is never a simple matter. But to ignore the meaning of illness is to bypass the patient altogether and, in many instances, to lose the opportunity to heal. In the reality of clinical practice healing is more than fixing the biological body, healing is restoring, and preserving personal wholeness.

NOTES

1 Sartre, J-P., *Being and Nothingness: A Phenomenological Essay on Ontology* (New York: Pocket Books, 1956); Merleau-Ponty, M., *Phenomenology of Perception* (London: Routledge and Kegan Paul, 1962).

2 Sartre, *Being and Nothingness.*

3 Toombs, S. K., *The Meaning of Illness: A Phenomenological Account of the Different Perspectives of Physician and Patient* (Dordrecht, The Netherlands: Kluwer Academic Publishers, 1990).

4 Cassell, E. J., *Clinical Technique: Talking with Patients*, vol. 2 (Cambridge, MA: MIT Press, 1985).

5 Toombs, *The Meaning of Illness*.

6 Toombs, S. K., "Healing and incurable illness," *Humane Medicine* 11 (1995): 98–103.

7 Toombs, S. K., "Disability and the self," in T. M. Brinthaupt and R. P. Lipka (eds.), *Changing the Self: Philosophies, Techniques and Experiences* (New York: SUNY Press, 1994); Goffman, E., *Stigma: Notes on the Management of Spoiled Identity* (New Jersey: Prentice Hall, 1963).

8 Toombs, S. K., "The lived experience of disability," *Human Studies* 18 (1995): 9–23.

9 Rudebeck, C. E., "General practice and the dialogue of clinical practice: On symptoms, symptom presentation, and bodily empathy," *Scand. J. Prim. Health Care* suppl. 1 (1992): 1–87.

10 Beckman and Frankel, as quoted in C. Silberman, "The view from the patient's bed," *Health Management Quarterly* 13 (1991): 15.

11 Cassell, E. J., "The nature of suffering and the goals of medicine," *N. Eng. J. Med.* 306 (1992): 639–45.

12 Toombs, S. K., "Sufficient unto the day: A life with multiple sclerosis," in S. K. Toombs, D. Barnard, and R. A. Carson (eds.), *Chronic Illness: From Experience to Policy* (Indianapolis: Indiana University Press, 1995).

4

Alternatives to Principlism: Phenomenology, Deconstruction, Hermeneutics

GUY A. M. WIDDERSHOVEN

Introduction

Principlism can be regarded as the main paradigm in medical ethics today (Beauchamp and Childress, 1994). Medical ethics can be said to have become an autonomous discipline when the autonomy of the patient became its leading principle. Textbooks in medical ethics teach students which principles are crucial (respect for autonomy, beneficence, non-maleficence, and justice), and how to apply them to a concrete case. Yet the rise of principlism has not been uncontested. Many authors have criticized the abstract and rationalist approach embodied in the "Georgetown mantra" and have proposed alternatives.

In this chapter I will discuss some alternatives to principlism. I will argue that these alternatives are not only different from principlism, but that they also differ fundamentally from each other. In order to make my argument, I will compare the proposed alternatives with some radically different approaches in continental philosophy. I will present principlism and its alternatives by analyzing a number of comments on a well-known case: the case of

Dax Cowart (Cavalier, Covey, and Anderson, 1996; Kliever, 1989). This case shows the attraction of principlism. It has often been framed in terms of respect for autonomy versus beneficence. Yet many of the commentaries indicate discontent with this approach. They try to uncover aspects escaping a principle-based method. Therefore, the case can be used to present both principlism and its alternatives.

After a brief presentation of the case, I will first discuss the standard approach of it in terms of principles. I will show that this approach is rationalistic. Then I will examine the alternatives. Some of them focus on the patient's way of meaning-making. They are in line with the critique of the early Heidegger on rationalism. I will show that these alternatives essentially try to develop new and richer ways of problem-solving. Other alternatives try to go beyond the problem-solving approach. These alternatives can be distinguished into two strands. On the one hand, they may draw attention to the will to power involved in medical practice. On the other hand, they may emphasize the communicative nature of the doctor–patient relationship. The first are akin to the philosophy of the later Heidegger, Derrida, and Foucault; the latter can be called hermeneutic in a Gadamerian sense. I will elaborate on the differences, and argue that the hermeneutic approach is the most promising alternative to principlism.

The Dax Cowart Case

In 1973, Donald Cowart was severely injured in a gas explosion. He suffered third-degree burns over 65 percent of his body. His eyes were damaged and his hands and ears mutilated. If treatment were stopped, he would die because of wound infections. If it were continued, he would surely live. Throughout his painful treatment, Donald pleaded with his doctors and relatives to be allowed to die. Yet the doctors would not let him leave the hospital. Finally, Donald recovered. He was able to leave the hospital, and to build up a new life. He changed his name to Dax, graduated from law school, and made a successful career as a lawyer. But he always stayed indignant over the fact that the doctors had not given him the right to die.

Principlism as Rational Problem-solving

The Dax Cowart case presents us with a classical ethical dilemma. On the one hand, the physicians should respect the patient's wishes. On the other hand, they should try to do well and preserve life. Two principles are in conflict: following the principle of respect for autonomy, the physicians should let the patient die; following the principle of beneficence, they should try to keep him alive. Ethicists claim that respect for autonomy should replace medical paternalism. They present themselves as advocates of the patient's autonomy. This is illustrated by the first discussion of the case in the *Hastings Center Report* (1975). The ethicist, Tristam Engelhardt Jr., forcefully attacks medical paternalism and makes a plea for respect for the patient's autonomy. According to him, the doctors should have done what the patient asked, and let him die. "When the patient who is able to give free consent does not, the moral issue is over," he declares. The psychiatrist, R. B. White, represents the position of the physicians. He is clearly in the defense. He tries to weaken the ethicist's position, noticing that the wish of the patient might proceed from some deeper concern. However, he also concludes that in the end the doctors did not have the right to keep alive a patient who himself wanted to die.

The way in which the principle of respect for autonomy is used in the ethical debate around the Dax case is striking in two respects. In the first place, it is presupposed that it can be clearly argued when the principle is valid, and when it is not. If the patient is competent, the principle of respect for autonomy is decisive. It is clearly more important than beneficence, which only comes in when there is doubt about the patient's competence. Tristam Engelhardt Jr. does not seem to take the notion of beneficence seriously at all. By using the term "paternalism," he implicitly discredits the principle of beneficence. The same can be noticed in the discussion of the case by Childress and Campbell (in Kliever, 1989), which is certainly more subtle than Engelhardt's, but which also uses the notion of paternalism and ends up with a negative judgment of the physicians' interventions. The choice between autonomy and beneficence is thought to be clear-cut, and rationally arguable. As for Tristam Engelhardt, the choice for autonomy does not need any further consideration. Childress and Campbell are more careful, but they also claim that the priority of the principle of respect for autonomy in this case cannot be denied by any reasonable person. The problem can be rationally solved, by considering the pros and cons of the application of the principles. The conclusion is presented as valid, and it is presupposed that every rational person should agree with it.

The principle of respect for autonomy is significant in yet another way. It presupposes rational decision-making by the patient. It presents the patient as someone who takes a position by balancing options in a rational way. Thus, it implies that Dax knows the facts about his present situation and future perspectives, and rationally concludes that he values death over life in a severely handicapped condition.

Thus, the principlist approach, with its emphasis on respect for the patient's autonomy, presents ethical issues as problems to be solved by rational means. Given that patients are able to calculate what is in their best interest, it can be rationally argued that their wishes should be respected, unless the interests of others are harmed. Ethical decision-making can be enhanced by giving the patient better information about his condition and securing freedom of choice. The Dax case can be seen as problematic, in that the physicians did not respect the wishes of the patient, although he had made perfectly clear that he knew the options. In not respecting his autonomy, the physicians were morally wrong; there cannot be any doubt about it.

Or can there? Several commentators do not seem to be totally sure. They feel uncomfortable with the discussion. They do not want to take Dax's wish to die for a fact, yet they want to understand his considerations. They argue that one should get acquainted with the way in which Dax envisages his life, gives meaning to the situation he is in. They emphasize that one should not see the ethical issue as a problem that can be solved by rational argumentation. They are convinced that it can only be solved by taking into account the way in which the participants give meaning to the situation.

Phenomenology: Problem-solving Through Meaning-making

Several authors have questioned the notion of autonomy implicit in principlism. They have brought to the fore that living with illness and disease is not a matter of making informed decisions about treatment options. Someone who is ill has to place the events happening to her in the story of her life, and has to reconstruct this story in such a way that she can meaningfully integrate the new experiences into it. She has to give meaning to the situation by finding new ways of responding to it. From a phenomenological perspective, a person is *being-in-the-world*, experiencing the world before consciously making any decisions. A person understands her situation not by ration-

ally calculating alternative options, but by knowing what to do on the basis of implicit background knowledge. From this perspective, autonomy is not marked by the ability to distanciate oneself from a situation, but by the ability to take part in it, and give meaning to it. This meaning-making approach to autonomy is developed by Agich. He says: "Human action can be regarded as free if the individual agent can identify with the elements from which it flows.... Expressions of autonomy are thus enactments of who the individual is as she is becoming. The field or stage for such playing out is the social world of everyday life" (1993: 99).

In the discussion about the Dax case, this perspective turns up every now and again. A clear example is to be found in the approach of May. He draws attention to the situation that does not present itself to Dax as a rational problem, but as an existential crisis: "The patient faces, then, an existential problem...: how does one respond to one's death, to a total, comprehensive, all-penetrating, sun-blackening, oxygen-removing, flesh-charring, chilling, stilling, numbing, and isolating death?" (in Kliever, 1989: 142). The situation Dax is in, being a severely burned patient, already shows experiential aspects of death itself. Such an experience has to be integrated into one's life story, before a meaningful continuation of life is possible. The only way in which Dax seems to be able to identify with this experience is to state that he actually wants to be dead. This explains his determined will to die and his indignation over the fact that his will is not respected (see also Lauritzen, 1996).

The meaning-making approach follows the early Heidegger in focusing upon existence as being-in-the-world, interpreting the world in which one already finds oneself (Heidegger, 1975). The patient is seen as someone who has to give meaning to the situation, not by rational calculation, but by answering the situation, always already being engaged in it. Ethical issues arise when the patient is not able to give meaning to the situation. They can be solved by helping the patient to restore her relation to the situation, to identify with the situation, and thus to come to grips with it.

This approach breaks with the notion of problem-solving through uninvolved, logical reasoning. The patient cannot come to grips with her situation through logic; she will have to find new ways of experiencing. The physician cannot rationally calculate what to do; she has to understand the patient, and help her to get in touch with the situation. Still, in some ways the meaning-making approach resembles the principlist approach and shares the same ground. Both approaches define ethical issues in terms of the patient's grip on the situation. They presuppose that ethical issues can be solved by furthering the patient's autonomy. In addition, they both see the doctor's role as secondary. She should act as a counselor, enabling the patient to make her decision. Both approaches emphasize the individual process of decision-making by the patient, either through reasoning or through meaning-making. They regard ethical issues as problems that can be solved, either by furthering logical argumentation or by sustaining processes of meaning-making.

Deconstruction: Will to Power and Openness Toward Being

Both the principlist and the meaning-making approach focus upon individual problem-solving. They see ethical issues as problems that can be dealt with by enabling the patient to make a motivated choice. One may ask, however, whether such approaches are not too individualistic and instrumental regarding issues of life and death. Is Dax's case really solved when he is enabled to make an autonomous decision? Is the role of the physicians to be confined to furthering his way of mastering the situation? Can a doctor–patient relationship ever be one of uninterested attention to and support of the patient by the doctor? Does not the conflict between Dax and his physicians show that there is much more at stake? Isn't Dax entangled in a power game in which the physicians are equally involved? These questions are put on the agenda by contemporary French philosophers such as Foucault and Derrida. Following the later Heidegger, they focus on the power relationship

that is inherent in modern life in general and modern medicine in particular. Derrida (1986) refers to Nietzsche's notion of will to power; Foucault (1975) introduces the notion of disciplinary power (see also Turner, 1995).

In an essay on the Dax case, Murray (1996) brings to the fore the fact that the whole sequel of events can be characterized as a test of wills. Both Dax and the physicians try to impose their will on each other. Dax demands to be allowed to die; the doctors refuse to let him go. The resulting struggle shows a proliferation of attempts to influence the other party through the use of power. Such power is productive, in that it stresses what is at stake for each of the parties, and makes them take a stand. Dax states his case vehemently; he is forced to reiterate over and over again that he surely wants to die. The physicians insist upon him having a definite chance to live. Throughout the process, each of the parties states his case with ever more force. Because both want to control the situation, they are denied any possible doubt about the validity of their own point of view. Thus, they present themselves as completely sure about their case. As one of the doctors sums up the situation: "Here is a man who can surely survive, and yet he wishes to die." In the end, both parties have eliminated any possible doubt they might have.

According to Heidegger (1976), this process is typical of modern technology. The essence of modern technology is that it uncovers truth by challenging nature, steering it, and securing it. Modern technology has changed man. Man has become part of the challenge, and is equally mastered by the process of technology. According to Heidegger, it is useless to try and deny this historical fate. Man has become part of technology. He encounters himself everywhere in the form of technology, and therefore he can nowhere encounter himself as he really is. This, Heidegger says, is the ultimate danger. But, quoting Hölderlin, he states: "where danger is, salvation also grows." Heidegger reminds us of the relation between technology and art, which both stem from the Greek word *technē*. We cannot master our condition, since trying to become master of it, we get ever more entangled in the process of technology. We can only try to make room by becoming attentive, by listening, by opening ourselves to the lightening of being. This idea has been developed further by philosophers such as Derrida, introducing the notion of deconstruction. According to Derrida, the aim of deconstruction is to make room for the other (Derrida, 1987).

In his discussion of the Dax case, Murray gives us a glimpse of the way in which the struggle for power may be opened up, and new room for listening may be created. He describes that a turning point for Dax was reached when a medical student spent time listening to him: "Not persuading or pleading with him, not appealing to his duties as his mother's son or a child of God, not defending paternalism, just listening to him. The medical student was, himself, of course, completely powerless in the sense of institutional clout" (1996: 13). The medical student did not contest the power Dax was using (he did not argue against his plea for autonomy), nor did he strive against the power of the medical profession. He created a movement beyond the power struggle by keeping quiet and showing attention, just being there.

Still, this deconstruction story is not entirely convincing. How did the medical student succeed in bringing about a change in Dax? Could he really do this without any power, or did he make use of other means of power than the ones used by Dax and the physicians? And, more fundamentally, what change did he bring about? Did Dax really view his situation differently afterwards? How can we then explain that he remained angry with the physicians? And, finally, can we say that the situation really changed, given that the physicians were not at all involved in the process brought about by the student? Is the technological framework really questioned, or is the resulting change in Dax just an adaptation to the way in which the physicians want to master the situation (an adaptation equivalent to the one that might have taken place if the physicians had consented in letting Dax die, because they came to realize that they had to respect his autonomy)?

Hermeneutics: Understanding and Dialogue

The deconstruction approach, based upon the work of the later Heidegger, Derrida, and Foucault, is not the only route beyond the individual and instrumental approaches that are common in medical ethics. Another way can be found if we follow Gadamer (1989) in his attempt to develop a philosophical hermeneutics (see also Widdershoven, 2000). Gadamer emphasizes the importance of dialogue. In a dialogue, various perspectives on an issue are merged. None of them is taken for granted; they are put into play and become part of a process of fusion. From a hermeneutic perspective, every participant has a preconception of what is at stake. Each party stands in a tradition, which both uncovers and conceals the issue. The tradition grants access to the issue at stake and power over it. Such power is, however, not to be used against other perspectives; it should be open to any contribution from other traditions. As in Heidegger and Derrida, one should not simply try to do away with power. Power should be seen as a positive factor, opening up the issue for us. Power, however, can and should be used in such a way that the perspective of others is not repressed, but equally brought into play. Gadamer also refers to art, but in a different way from Heidegger. For Gadamer, the experience of art shows us that we can become part of a process of truth which is not controlled by us, but which encompasses us, and unites us with others. The experience of art makes concrete the process of the fusion of horizons. When we understand a work of art, we experience that our horizon is broadened, not by giving up our own viewpoint, nor by overpowering that of others, but by opening ourselves towards the view of others and thereby acquiring a new and richer view.

If we try to apply such a hermeneutic perspective to medical ethics, we have to view the medical encounter as a communicative process. This process is pervaded by the doctor's power (Katz, 1984; Brody, 1992). Medical decisions cannot be reduced to objective facts concerning the patient's condition, nor to subjective preferences of the patient. Even when the doctor really wants to do what the patient wishes, it will have to be clear that she herself will always have to interpret the patient's expressions. The doctor's power has to be acknowledged, and taken into account. The doctor has an interest in the case at hand, and views it from a certain perspective. Otherwise, communication with the patient would be impossible. According to Brody, the doctor's power should be used in such a way that it enables the patient to bring to the fore her own perspective. The doctor should use her power in order to further active participation of the patient in the decision-making process. Brody concludes:

> In short, physicians most effectively empower patients neither by reflexively disclosing nor by reflexively withholding any particular sort of information. They empower patients by creating an atmosphere that encourages participation and dialogue; by following carefully the cues provided by the patient as the dialogue unfolds; and ultimately by aiding the patient in placing the new information in the context of the patient's life experience and life story in the most meaningful, encouraging, and health-promoting way. (1992: 136)

Brody not only describes a communicative model of doctor–patient interaction; he also comments upon the Dax Cowart case (1992: 74–7). He brings to the fore that Dax is the victim of the institution's work schedule. He is regarded as a technical object, not as a person with specific wishes and desires. Even the psychiatrist who is called in to see whether Dax is competent makes him part of his work routine, rather than trying to encounter him as a person. According to Brody, there was evidently no room for a dialogue to unfold. The physicians used their power just to control Dax, not to let him bring in his own perspective.

Let us suppose, however, that a dialogue had taken place in the Dax case. What might it have looked like? It certainly would involve attention to the perspective of the patient. But this perspective would not be considered as the ultimate truth. It would, rather, be seen as something to explore, to discuss, and to change in and through

dialogue. It should become an object of discussion. In such a discussion, the physician might bring in her own considerations. But these also should not be presented as definite answers, but rather as issues to be explored.

The primary need would be time and rest, in order for all the participants to become part of the process. The process should not be governed by empty time, each person running after the other in a hurry, trying to reach rock bottom. The process should be experienced as a meaningful event, a festival in which time is experienced as *the right time* or fulfilled time (Gadamer, 1986: 42). This would require listening, not only by a medical student, but by all the parties involved, drawn together by the issue they are mutually engaged with. The result would not be a contest of power between Dax and the physicians, but a movement in which all parties feel both powerful and relaxed because their powers become united.

The process should be governed by the idea that the truth is not given beforehand, but can only be the result of communication and dialogue (Widdershoven, 2001). Both the patient and the physicians should acknowledge that they cannot be sure of what really is worthwhile pursuing as long as they see their goals as private enterprises rather than shared practices. One cannot tell what the results of a dialogue are going to be. One can only tell that the process will not be finished until all the parties are satisfied, which means that none of them regrets the decision or feels uncomfortable with it. The dialogue has not been successful as long as one of the participants (either Dax or the physicians) shows indignation about the course of action proceeding from it.

Conclusion

In an influential paper, Emanuel and Emanuel (1992) distinguish four models of the physician–patient relationship (see also Widdershoven, 1999). The first is the paternalistic model. In this, the doctor decides, acting in the patient's best interest. Here, the doctor is the guardian of the patient. The second model is the informative, or consumer model. It is based upon the autonomous choice of the patient, after being informed by the doctor. The values of the patient are considered to be given. In this model the doctor is the technical expert. The third model is the interpretive model. It aims at interpreting the patient's values and implementing the patient's selected intervention. The values of the patient are seen as inchoate and conflicting, and in need of interpretation. In this model the doctor is a counselor or adviser. The fourth model is the deliberative model. It is based upon the presupposition that the patient's values are not only in need of interpretation, but also of discussion and deliberation. The doctor is regarded as a friend or teacher. This model is the most radical. "The conception of patient autonomy is moral self-development; the patient is empowered not simply to follow unexamined preferences or examined values, but to consider, through dialogue, alternative health-related values, their worthiness and their implications for treatment" (Emanuel and Emanuel, 1992: 2222).

We can compare the approaches distinguished above with the models discussed by Emanuel and Emanuel. The principlist approach to medical ethics seems to incorporate the informative or consumer model. It presents itself as an alternative to the paternalistic model, which used to be dominant in medicine. The phenomenological approach is in line with the interpretive model, presenting the doctor as no more than a facilitator in the process of making the patient identify with the situation. The approach of the later Heidegger, Derrida, and Foucault does not fit with any of the models. This is not surprising, since they seem to leave little room for the possibility of dealing adequately with ethical issues from within the medical profession. The whole realm of medicine is governed by technical rationality; new ways of finding the truth can only be found by outsiders (such as the medical student in the Dax case). The hermeneutic approach seems to be close to the deliberative model. Both share the presupposition that values are necessarily intersubjective, and therefore the object of communication. More than the deliberative model, however, the hermeneutic approach stresses that ethics is not technical, in that it does not aim to master the situation.

Phenomenology, deconstruction, and hermeneutics can all be seen as alternatives to principlist medical ethics. The phenomenological approach, however, tends to stay within the domain of individual technical rationality, whereas the deconstruction approach wants to go beyond it in such a radical way that practitioners are not likely to have any part in it. The hermeneutic approach may offer an alternative that is neither technical nor so radical that its application would mean stepping out of medicine altogether. It seems to grant the best opportunities to overcome the limitations of current medical ethics, without having to destroy the project of medical ethics totally.

NOTE

The last version of this chapter has been written during a stay at the Oxford Institute for Ethics and Communication in Health Care Practice (ETHOX); I would like to thank Dr Tony Hope for organizing this stay, and for his useful comments on earlier drafts.

REFERENCES

Agich, G. J. (1993) *Autonomy and Long-term Care* (Oxford: Oxford University Press).

Beauchamp, T. L. and Childress, J. F. (1994) *Principles of Biomedical Ethics* (Oxford: Oxford University Press).

Brody, H. (1992) *The Healer's Power* (New Haven: Yale University Press).

Cavalier, R., Covey, P. K., and Anderson, D. (1996) *A Right to Die? The Dax Cowart Case* (London: Routledge) (CD-rom).

Derrida, J. (1986) Guter Wille zur Macht II. In P. Forget (ed.), *Text und Interpretation* (München: Fink Verlag), pp. 62–77.

Derrida, J. (1987) *Psyche. Inventions de l'autre* (Paris: Gallimard).

Emanuel, E. J. and Emanuel, L. L. (1992) Four models of the physician–patient relationship. *JAMA* 267: 2221–6.

Foucault, M. (1975) *Surveillir et punir. Naissance de la prison* (Paris: Gallimard).

Gadamer, H.-G. (1986) *The Relevance of the Beautiful* (Cambridge: Cambridge University Press).

Gadamer, H.-G. (1989) *Truth and Method* (New York: Crossroad).

Hastings Center Report (1975), vol. 5 (June): 9, 10, 47.

Heidegger, M. (1975) *Sein und Zeit* (Tübingen: Max Niemeyer Verlag).

Heidegger, M. (1976) *Die Technik und die Kehre* (Pfullingen: Günter Neske).

Katz, J. (1984) *The Silent World of Doctor and Patient* (New York: Free Press).

Kliever, L. D. (ed.) (1989) *Dax's Case* (Dallas: Southern Methodist University Press).

Lauritzen, P. (1996) Ethics and experience: The case of the curious response. *Hastings Center Report* 26/1: 6–15.

Murray, Th. H. (1996) Bioethics yesterday and tomorrow. *Medical Humanities Review* 9/2: 10–14.

Turner, B. S. (1995) *Medical Power and Social Knowledge* (London: Sage).

Widdershoven, G. A. M. (1999) Care, cure and interpersonal understanding. *Journal of Advanced Nursing* 29: 1163–9.

Widdershoven, G. A. M. (2000) The doctor–patient relationship as a Gadamerian dialogue: A response to Arnason. *Medicine, Health Care and Philosophy* 3: 25–7.

Widdershoven, G. A. M. (2001) Truth and truthtelling. In M. Parker and D. Dickenson (eds.), *The Cambridge Medical Ethics Workbook* (Cambridge: Cambridge University Press), pp. 127–30, 149–53.

5

Questions of Personal Autonomy

MORWENNA GRIFFITHS

"Autonomy" is a word that gives some difficulty to non-philosophers, while being central to the vocabulary of philosophers. In this chapter I am taking "autonomy" to mean much the same as "independence." Both terms routinely apply to the self-rule of individuals, of groups, and of states. I shall use the two words interchangeably except where I am discussing theorists who themselves use a tight definition. It is useful to have both words. "Independence" has the advantage of familiarity. "Autonomy" has the advantage that it is not so obviously related to "dependence" – it takes its meaning from the even less-used term "heteronomy" meaning "rule by others." It carries, therefore, the overtones of "liberation" and "emancipation" more obviously than "independence" does.

Autonomy is often thought to be a problem for women. It is asserted that: they haven't got it; they are frightened of it; they are insufficiently separated from their mothers; they are too reliant on the opinion of others; they are encumbered by their families; they are absorbed by caring for their husbands; they are interested in private rather than public matters; and so on and on. (I am talking about stereotypes here, not about real men and women.) In other words, autonomy is often thought to present a problem

for women because (1) it is a desirable quality and (2) women don't have it.

Philosophers have contributed to this stereotyping. To focus only on philosophy which is particularly influential in the Anglo-analytic traditions: the Kantian rational autonomous being, Rousseau's *Emile*, and the citizens of the social contract are all fathers to the contemporary understanding of the person. This is a legacy that is deeply gendered.

Kant took the exercise of autonomy to be acting rationally in the pursuit of one's own self-chosen goals. The way he develops this argument serves to exclude women, even though it appears, at first sight, to be gender-neutral. He argues that mature reason has to be developed in the public space of universal principles. Thus, rational action takes place in the public sphere. Therefore, Kant implicitly excluded women from full autonomy, since he apparently assumes that women rather than men deal with the personal, and that this is part of their nature.[1]

Rousseau, too, excludes women from his vision of man. This is particularly obvious in *Emile*, his influential book where he describes an idealized education for the young boy, Emile, and for his playmate, Sophie. Emile grows up to be rational and self-sufficient, having reveled in the "enjoyment of his natural liberty" (1956: 37) (carefully contrived as it is by his tutor) – though as an adult he is dependent on women, who have "the capacity to stimulate desires greater than can be satisfied" (p. 132). Sophie's education is to be very different from Emile's. Indeed it is essential to Emile's well-being as an autonomous adult that Sophie does not share his education; instead, she is to be "passive and weak" rather than "active and strong" like Emile (p. 131). She must learn to submit to the "hard, unceasing constraints of the proprieties . . . always to be submissive" (pp. 139–40).[2]

The citizens of the social contract are also males. This is so whether we consider Rousseau's version, or others, from Locke in the seventeenth century to Rawls in the twentieth – as Pateman (1988) shows in her thorough analysis of social contracts from a feminist perspective. In an engaging paper on the subject, Janna Thompson (1993) begins with an alternative founding story, in which women, rather than men, set out to establish a social contract: "Each of them was a mother, grandmother, or an aunt, a sister or a daughter. Most of them were several of these at once, and in connection with each identity, each had particular and sometimes conflicting responsibilities." They also traded, belonged to religious communities, and belonged to clubs. These women will make a contract founded on carrying out family responsibilities, which is very different from the usual social contract where (male) individuals are assumed to be independent and self-interested. This contract may be as one-sided as the orthodox ones, but it is very useful in pointing up their inadequacies, especially in showing how masculine their assumptions are.

In the next section, I take up this theme that the term "autonomy" can carry a different set of meanings from those of mainstream philosophy. I return to the contribution and critique of philosophy at the end of the section.

Do Women Want Personal Autonomy?

It is the argument of this section that the usual meanings ascribed to personal autonomy and

independence are inadequate to describe and explain the experience of women. Attention to that experience demonstrates that a different set of meanings for "autonomy" or "independence" are struggling to be heard. Once it is possible to hear them, it becomes possible to hear more clearly what women want – in what senses we reject, and in what senses we require autonomy. It also becomes possible to hear in what ways different groups of women (differing in their social class, nationality, or race, for instance) have different perceptions of their needs and wants for autonomy.

Many women deny that they want more independence and autonomy, if that means they should be more like a particular ideal-kind of western man: unencumbered by emotions or close personal relationships, and free of ties to the social circumstances into which he was born. Rather, they assert the value of all these things to their own lives: both the expressive life of feelings, and also social life which is rooted in ties to their family, friends, neighborhood, culture, and family history. On the other hand, women continue to want to run their own lives and to do so in their own way. In other words, they want autonomy, in the sense that autonomy means deciding for oneself.

There is an apparent paradox here. Women want autonomy: they want to decide the course of their own lives – even though this may mean that they decide to continue with precisely the situations that others may define for them as ones in which they lack autonomy. I argue that there is, in fact, no paradox, but that the apparent paradox gives us a pointer to a different set of meanings of autonomy which find it hard to be heard.

British Asian women provide a particularly clear example of women valuing their own culture while simultaneously demanding freedom to direct their own lives. Well-meaning white British have often seen the needs of Asian women as being self-sufficiency, to be achieved by escape from the extended family and its demands – as being more like white British women. Arranged marriage has been cited as an especially significant bond to burst in those Asian communities that practice it. Indeed, Asian cultural practices in general, and Muslim cultural practices in particular, are regularly described by liberals as a problem for equality, justice, and freedom for girls (Halstead, 1991; Harris, 1982; Hatem, 1989). All this is denied in the writing of British Asian girls and women, who rarely see their freedom in leaving their families and communities and the cultural practices which are part of themselves. Indeed, there is evidence that Muslim all-girls' schools, so far from being anti-feminist, can help girls both in articulating their aspirations and also in their educational achievement.[3] To leave their communities would be to deny something essential in their personal identities. They continue, nevertheless, to affirm their need to be free within family and community and to criticize specific aspects of their cultures, including specific forms of arranged marriages.[4]

Are all these women wanting to square the circle? Are we wanting to have our various cakes and to eat them too? No, there is no contradiction here, if independence – or autonomy – is the freedom to be yourself, to speak for yourself, to determine your own life. All this, in the knowledge that a worthwhile life includes cultural and social bonds, and in the knowledge that such bonds will last both during periods of relative need for the help of others and also during periods of relative responsibility to meet the needs of others.

Why does all this sound paradoxical? One reason is to be found in the power of some groups to legitimate their use of language as the proper one. There is an odd masculine logic underlying the use of words such as "independent." Indeed, both "independent" and "dependent" are very odd words. Consider who is called a dependent. It is usually assumed that dependents are women and children economically dependent on a man: he is the breadwinner. Dependents are not usually taken to be men and children dependent on a woman for housework or for emotional support. In other words, in a traditional household, when a woman and a man are both in a state of dependence, the woman is called "dependent" and the man is called "independent." Of course, it is true that the woman has the more dangerous dependence. She is making herself progressively more incapable of becoming economically independent, while he remains capable of finding emotional support and domestic help in a variety of ways.

This logic of the word "dependence" remains alive and well. In the economic climate of the late 1980s and early 1990s women increasingly became the primary "breadwinners" for the household. Their menfolk did not usually assume the other role; there is no manly "independence" attached to learning to do the domestic tasks of housework and emotional support. The men remained dependent on their women for these things, in order to keep up their "independent" masculinity. Beatrix Campbell contrasts the behavior of young men who live on run-down housing estates in the UK with that of their sisters. The young men turn to crime to assert their masculinity, while the young women turn to crime to try to keep the family together. Having described the striking difference between the crime committed by the two sexes she says, "This is not to say that boys and men are bad and girls and women are good, it is simply to repeat the obvious, that men and women do something dramatically different with their troubles" (1993: 211). That is, she says, "Crime and coercion are sustained by men. Solidarity and self-help are sustained by women. It is as stark as that" (ibid: 319).

It could be argued that solidarity and self-help are more characteristic of independence than largely symbolic assertions of gender identity. However, this is still not reflected in the use of the words. The phrase "independent woman" still refers more to someone who has broken free of family and neighborhood ties. The problem of unemployed males is still cast in terms of their being constrained to create lives for themselves within such ties, rather than as part of the wider wage-earning economy.

The same odd masculine logic is to be found in the narratives underlying popular fiction, especially where they concern the place in the story of sexual relationships. "There ain't nothing like a dame" can be sung by a group of men without any suggestion that they are dependent or vulnerable. It is true that men have complained about the seductive power of women, but even this is a limited power. A man without a woman may be sorry for himself, but he remains a whole person. A woman wanting a man is more often supposed to be in a state of need resulting from her supposed inability to function properly without one. A woman's life is supposed to revolve round a man and his children. He gives her life meaning. Popular fantasy literature bears this out. Men's thrillers are about action in which they may get a woman as a bonus. Women's romances are about getting a man. In recent popular fiction, feminist detectives have changed some of the rules. However, as Marina Warner points out in her analysis of myths of our time, mass-audience films and novels which feature powerful women depict them as deadly she-monsters who have broken free of social ties and who need to be destroyed. At the same time, video-games, films, and books underpin a vision of masculinity that is self-sufficient, self-reliant, and physically strong. Boys, she points out, are exposed "to blanket saturation in a myth of masterful, individualist independence; they're bit players training to be heroes in a narrative which can proceed only by conflict to rupture" (1994: 30–1). Reflecting on a novel by Mary Shelley, the creator of Frankenstein, Warner continues: "The hero exclaims, 'This, I thought, is power! Not to be strong of limb, hard of heart, ferocious and daring; but kind, compassionate and soft.' It's a measure of the depths of our present failure of nerve that these words sound ridiculous, embarrassing, inappropriate" (ibid: 31).

All this is as commonplace as it is extraordinary. The everyday fictional male can manage quite well on his own. He is a whole person even if he has no serious social or emotional entanglements. This is in stark contrast to the everyday fictional female, who is not really a whole person until she admits her dependency on another adult – even though everyone knows that such dependency entails looking after him. Neither of these interlocking fantasies bears much scrutiny, but they are upheld and re-inforced by the masculine logic underlying the language of dependence and independence.

The odd logic of independence and dependency is backed up by western philosophy. This is not surprising. Philosophy has been well described as a culture talking to itself.[5] Kant's view of autonomy ignores his own dependence on women. In so far as Kant notices women, he thinks that they destroy their own peculiar merits by struggling after learning, but that these merits do not include the courage to use their own understanding, as is necessary for autonomy. However, his philosophy is really directed at the rational, autonomous males of the public sphere. Rousseau spends a little more time discussing the place of women, but comes to much the same conclusions. Sophie should be a helpmeet. Rousseau admits that Emile depends on Sophie, but it is Emile who is the autonomous person. Similarly, the citizens of the social contract depend on their family life to give them opportunities to exercise their autonomy as citizens. As has been pointed out by many commentators, both these philosophers, in their different ways, require women to stay at home.

In spite of great differences between them, the two philosophers unite in the view that women should stay at home where they are meant to be, dependent on and of service to the family, while men live a so-called independent life in the rest of the world. Women who make the mistake of trying to be like men should be sharply discouraged, since society needs their distinctive (dependent, supportive) contribution. This view of the man in the public world, rational, just, and independent with a dependent woman at home providing support, is found throughout the work of social contract theorists. Even Rawls, writing in the 1970s, considered the contract to be made by male heads of household.

There are indeed competing sets of meaning for autonomy. The picture given by the philosophers is misleading. A better one (still oversimplified) can be taken from feminist theory. It is that, on the one hand, there are men who are frightened of admitting their dependency. On the other, there are women who understand that social ties give their lives meaning – give them the freedom to be themselves. However, the discourse of the males is so dominating that many women's thoughts about independence are mixed up with masculine understandings of it. So, not surprisingly, they are frightened of the loneliness that will be theirs if they look for an independence in a male world without male privileges (like wives).

But why has the women's version not taken root more robustly? Why have they not lived their understanding more boldly? Since women have been asserting their autonomy and act on those assertions, as I have argued, why are so many of us still in positions where this is so hard to do? Why does Janna Thompson's fantasy of a female social contract remain so fantastic? (Why don't women just take over?) Some of the reasons are to do with the structures of violence that support masculine ways of understanding and which constrain the possibilities of self-creation for both men and women.[6]

Structures of Violence and Personal Autonomy

The individual deciding for herself is at the center of a notion of autonomy applicable to the lives of women. This is a freedom to make yourself in recognition of the way the self is made in communities, although it is not determined by them. Thus there is a need for space for the self to be formed both in and against various communities of others, and also out of the material conditions in which it finds itself. As I argue in Griffiths (1995), a self cannot but be formed in connection with others; in love of or resistance to various social groups; among which, groupings based on gender, race, sexuality, and social class are always salient. Patricia Williams (1993) describes discovering as a small child that she was "colored" (insultingly, from her white friends) as well as Negro (as her family had told her she should be proud to be). Carolyn Steedman (1986) describes learning what members of the middle classes thought of her working-class parents.

Making oneself both in and against the community is easier if there is a variety of communities. The variety makes it easier to see first that the term "woman" (or "man" or "black" or "gay") refers to overlapping networks of constructions, and, second, that the individual can find herself within and against them. In consequence, being with others does not necessarily curb your autonomy, though having *no* others

will do so. Consider the stories of two different black women, the American lawyer Patricia Williams (1993), and the Jamaican nurse Mary Seacole (1984) (whose medical work during the Crimean War more than bears comparison with that of Florence Nightingale). Both these women's lives were constructed in groups where the majority were white, or male, or both. However, in both cases, neither tried to construct her life as if she were white or male.[7] Neither woman would condone offensive stories against themselves as black or female; nor would either woman live as their society expected black females to live.

It is a consequence of the argument that support for self-definitions as being both of and also between communities creates space for people to be autonomous. Such space is narrowed and constricted by the structures of violence which prevent people from embarking on processes of autonomous self-creation. Structures of violence support oppression by those communities that are already relatively powerful and which invoke these structures to preserve their positions. Put simply, fear keeps people in their place, as defined for them by the more powerful. The fear induced in different groups is particular to them – for instance, in young women, whether they are to be scared of being thought to be sexually active heterosexuals, lesbians, or sexless; or whether they are to be made to fear just for being black or Asian; or for having particular disabilities; or some combination of these. Sue Lees (1993) has explored one set of strictures on schoolgirls. She describes the difficulties faced by adolescent girls in British schools. There is no way that a girl can express her sexuality without taking into account the reactions of her peers. These are most obviously expressed in the terms of abuse that follow any girl who steps out of line – but the terms are different if she is white or Asian. A white girl always risks being called a slag or a lezzie, while an Asian girl is condemned for harming the family *izzat* (honor).

The fear induced in different groups is particular to them, but it is striking that the means of inducing fear are remarkably similar for all of them. It is induced through verbal and physical violence, through ridicule and condescension, or through disregard mixed with high visibility. Such fear reduces the scope for ways of living and being, from dress to the expression of affection, to the enjoyment of intellectual activities, to self-confidence, to going for a walk even. Frantz Fanon describes the difference between his being black in his home country of Martinique, and being black in France, where he emigrated in the middle of the last century. He explains the effect of the name-calling he experiences: "My body was given back to me, sprawled out, distorted, recolored, clad in mourning in that white winter day" (1986: 113). Angry, shamed, nauseous, self-contemptuous, always highly visible as "the Negro doctor," he resolves to assert himself as a "BLACK MAN" (his capitalization). Of course, biographies and autobiographies of struggle by relatively powerless people against relatively powerful ones demonstrate that, in the long term, even oppressive kinds of interaction (short of death) can be used for personal enrichment. But doing so is hard, and may only be possible for exceptional people.

Establishing autonomy is not just about equal respect and equal rights for self-sufficient individuals. It is also about human beings making themselves and being made in social webs. Therefore, a feminist politics of autonomy means responding to the changes that result in individuals working out new patterns of being in response to the various overlapping communities to which they belong. It is also about creating spaces for people to make themselves, and keeping such spaces open by reducing fear. A feminist philosophy underpinning the politics is one that reconceptualizes one of the central terms of traditional philosophy, "autonomy."

NOTES

This chapter is a shortened and re-written version of part of chapter 8 in my book, *Feminisms and the Self: The Web of Identity* (London: Routledge, 1995).

1 See Grimshaw (1986), Hill (1987), and Lloyd (1993) for some more details.
2 See Martin (1985) for a more thorough discussion.
3 See Haw (1995).

4 See Amos and Parmar (1987), Brah and Minhas (1985), and Westwood and Bhachu (1988). More fictionalized accounts are to be found in Asian Women Writers' Workshop (1988) and in Chatterjee and Islam (1990). See Bhushan (1989) on similar criticisms from within a South Asian culture.
5 I am talking about a locally specific difficulty: English has problems in this area. So does western philosophy. Not all languages and theoretical systems have such difficulties. For instance, the juxtaposition of autonomy and dependence, natural to English (and other European languages), is difficult to translate in the Philippines (Andres and Ilada Andres, 1987). Filial piety (and the dependence it represents) is central to Confucianism (Shu, 1995).
6 The phrase "structures of violence" is taken from Gayatri Spivak (1990).
7 Williams continues to construct her life like this. As the first black woman to present the Reith lectures (in 1997) she spoke *as* a black woman in her discussion of (universal) rights and the law.

REFERENCES

Amos, V. and Parmar, P. (1987) Resistances and responses: The experiences of Black girls in Britain. In M. Arnot and G. Weiner (eds.), *Gender and the Politics of Schooling* (Milton Keynes: Open University Press).

Asian Women Writers' Workshop (1988) *Right of Way* (London: Virago).

Andres and Ilada-Andres (1987) *Understanding the Filipino* (Quezon City, Philippines: New Day).

Bhushan, M. (1989) Vimochana: Women's struggles, non-violent militancy and direct action in the Indian context. *Women's Studies International Forum* 12/1.

Brah, A. and Minhas, R. (1985) Structural racism or cultural difference: Schooling for Asian girls. In G. Weiner (ed.), *Just a Bunch of Girls* (Milton Keynes: Open University Press).

Campbell, B. (1993) *Goliath: Britain's Dangerous Places* (London: Methuen).

Chatterjee, D. and Islam, R. (eds.) (1990) *Barbed Lines* (Sheffield: Bengali Women's Support Group and Yorkshire Art Circus).

Fanon, F. (1986 [1952]) *Black Skin, White Masks* (London: Pluto Press).

Griffiths, M. (1995) *Feminisms and the Self: The Web of Identity* (London: Routledge).

Grimshaw, J. (1986) *Feminist Philosophers* (Brighton: Harvester).

Halstead, M. (1991) Radical feminism, Islam and the single-sex school debate. *Gender and Education* 3/3.

Harris, J. (1982) A paradox of multicultural societies. *Journal of Philosophy of Education* 16/2.

Hatem, M. (1989) Egyptian, Levantine-Egyptian and European women 1862–1920. *Women's Studies International Forum* 12/3.

Haw, K. (1995) Why are Muslim girls more feminist in Muslim schools? In M. Griffiths and B. Troyna (eds.), *Antiracism, Culture and Social Justice* (Stoke-on-Trent: Trentham Books).

Hill, T. E. (1987) The importance of autonomy. In E. Kittay and D. Meyers (eds.), *Women and Moral Theory* (London: Rowman and Littlefield).

Lees, S. (1993) *Sugar and Spice: Sexuality and Adolescent Girls* (Harmondsworth: Penguin).

Lloyd, G. (1993) *The Man of Reason: "Male" and "Female" in Western Philosophy*, 2nd edn (London: Routledge).

Martin, J. R. (1985) *Reclaiming a Conversation* (New Haven: Yale University Press).

Pateman, C. (1988) *The Sexual Contract* (Cambridge: Polity).

Rawls, J. (1971) *A Theory of Justice* (Oxford: Oxford University Press).

Rousseau, J.-J. (1956 [1755]) *Emile*, trans. William Boyd (London: Heinemann).

Seacole, M. (1984 [1857]) *Wonderful Adventures of Mrs Seacole in Many Lands*, ed. S. Alexander and A. Dewjee (Bristol: Falling Wall Press).

Shu, Y. (1995) Reason and emotion in morality and moral education – With special reference to Taiwan. PhD thesis, University of Nottingham.

Spivak, G. (1990) *The Post-Colonial Critic: Interviews, Strategies, Dialogues*, ed. S. Harasyn (London: Routledge).

Steedman, C. (1986) *Landscape for a Good Woman: A Story of Two Lives* (London: Virago).

Thompson, J. (1993) Can social contract theory work for women? Paper given to a meeting of the Society for Women and Philosophy, Queen Mary and Westfield College, London, November.

Warner, M. (1994) *Managing Monsters: Six Myths of our Time* (London: Vintage).

Westwood, S. and Bhachu, P. (1988) *Enterprising Women: Ethnicity, Economy and Gender Relations* (London: Routledge).

Williams, P. (1993) *The Alchemy of Race and Rights* (London: Virago).

6

A Different Voice in Psychiatric Ethics

GWEN ADSHEAD

Introduction

In this chapter I will argue that the two notions of an ethic of justice and an ethic of care have particular relevance for ethical reasoning in psychiatry. Therapeutic relationships in psychiatry are based on relationships that endure over time, and are affected by the conscious and unconscious contribution of both patient and therapist (whether doctor or nurse). I will argue in this chapter that the perspective of an ethic of care is of relevance to medical as well as nursing treatment, especially in those aspects of medical practice where therapeutic relationships are themselves the vehicle of treatment. A care perspective may be of use in understanding cases of abusive practice in psychiatry. The limitations of a rights-based, or justice-based, vision alone will also be discussed.

Different Voices in Bioethics

Bioethics has been defined as "the application of reasoning in medical ethical settings" (Gillon, 1992). There are multiple theories of ethical reasoning in healthcare, including rights-based approaches, communitarian and virtue-based theories, and accounts based on relationships (Beauchamp and Childress, 1994). This last approach, drawing on the work of Carol Gilligan (1982), has not been generally applied to the field of bioethics. In relation to psychiatry, for example, the principal discourse has been one of an ethic of justice/rights, with considerable debate about the rights of vulnerable people to treatment, to be protected from coercion, and competing rights of public safety and personal freedom (Fulford and Hope, 1994).

Within psychiatry, a rights-based perspective is clearly complementary to a relationship-based perspective, and concern for rights and justice must be important in a domain where patients are made vulnerable not only by their mental illness, but also by the fact that they are vulnerable to abuse by others. However, using case examples, I will argue that ethical debates in psychiatry which focus solely on conflicts between two principles, and which set up ethical dichotomies (e.g. respect for beneficence or respect for autonomy), cannot address the complexity of the lives of individuals and the relationships in which they are embedded, both in the past and in the present. The relationships in which patients are involved contribute to their sense of enduring identity; several theorists suggest that self-identity is precipitated out of relationships with others (Brown, 1994). A rights/principles account that does not consider the patient within a matrix of relationships runs a risk of over-simplifying the patient's autonomy, and thus not doing justice (an appropriate word) to the complexity of the dilemma for this person.

Clinical Example 1: Miss A

Miss A suffered from borderline personality disorder. She had been a victim of prolonged and extensive sexual abuse in childhood from her father. Like many survivors of such abuse, she suffered from depression, and intermittent feelings of loathing toward her own body, which resulted in acts of deliberate self-harm and epi-sodes of self-starvation. She was admitted to a psychiatric hospital and over a long period of time developed a reasonable relationship with her male psychiatrist, who was concerned for her welfare.

During one admission (after a period of years), Miss A's weight began to drop so dra-matically that her doctor threatened to force-feed her in order to save her life. Miss A went to court to get an injunction to prevent him from doing so. The dilemma here for both the patient and the doctor is obvious. Respecting her au-tonomy may result in her acting so riskily to herself that she suffers harm, and dies.

It may be relevant when contemplating this dilemma to consider how force-feeding is a symbolic re-enactment of the original abuse (she was subjected to forced fellatio over a period of time). The violating of her rights as a child is likely to have left her with very par-ticular concerns about being left alone and having her rights respected even though this might be risky for herself. In assessing her, a second psychiatrist noted her ambivalence: "It's my way of coping...the only way for me to survive is to hurt myself."

A further aspect to consider in contemplating this dilemma is the issue of Miss A's self-concept in her attitudes of herself toward her-self (Attanucci, 1988). Her own ambivalence about herself ("I don't matter...I do matter") is mirrored in the attitudes of staff, who alter-natively saw her as incompetent to care for herself and needing to be force-fed, or as ma-nipulative and trying to bully them. The rela-tionship between herself and her parents seems to have been replicated in a relationship that she had with the care team, some of whom saw her vulnerability, some of whom saw her manipula-tion, and some of whom were considering action toward her which she was going to experience as abusive.

The legal position focused on her compe-tence to make decisions and refuse help. The arguments will not be rehearsed here (see Fen-nell, 1996). I am suggesting that looking at the past relationships between Miss A and the staff might give another voice to the debate; for example, by offering supervision sessions to the staff in which they can explore their reac-tions to her. Understanding the feelings of staff confronted by Miss A's suffering could help to reduce the tension between them. It might also have reduced the staff's capacity to act in an abusive way toward her, and also reduced her need to act in a way that others find threa-tening.

Miss A herself could also be offered individ-ual time to explore her feelings about the staff. On a rights/principles perspective, or even a utilitarian analysis, there is clearly still some tension between her view of what was right for her, and the staff's. A broader view of her welfare, which included thinking about her past and present relationships with caretakers, might understand the dilemma as part of the concern that abused adults have about their control over their own bodies. By supporting her at these times, when she was at her most self-destructive, it might be more possible to understand her self-destruction (and thus her ethical conflict with staff) as a response to her own previous experiences of abuse.

Clinical Example 2: Miss B

Miss B seeks psychotherapy for depression. She recalls, in her therapy, a history of abuse and neglect, especially from her mother, with whom she is still in contact. Miss B becomes very dependent on her therapist, who responds warmly and empathically, partly with a wish to make a reparative measure for all the previous neglect and grief. At Miss B's request, the therapy sessions become more frequent, and take place outside the clinic, because "it feels too impersonal and frightening there."

Miss B and the therapist become closer, and one day during a stormy session the therapist offers physical comfort in the form of a hug, which then turns into an embrace. Miss B and her therapist become lovers; the therapy sessions continue. But the therapist becomes anxious at the way the turn of events has taken, and abruptly terminates therapy. Miss B takes an overdose and threatens to kill her therapist.

This case (based on several similar cases) shows how the relationship between the therapist and the patient is crucial to an understanding of how an ethical principle (that of not exploiting a patient) was violated. It also provides an example of how a principles approach alone cannot do justice to the complexity of the management of this case.

The principles approach would argue that the principles of beneficence and non-maleficence were breached. The therapist might counter with the argument that she did as the patient wished by ending the therapy sessions, by responding to the embrace, and that the patient consented to become sexually involved with her. To this it might be counter-argued that Miss B was not competent to exercise her autonomy to make that kind of decision. One might also argue that Miss B was harmed by the therapist's failure to maintain boundaries, even though she had requested that they be breached; and Miss B is also wronged because she is treated as a means to the therapist's pleasure.

What is then set up is a conflict between the therapist's understanding of Miss B's autonomy, and her vision of professional beneficence. Miss B's own view is in danger of being lost, and is to some extent replaced by the therapist's own view of what has been going on. The relationship between them has changed, and with it, the therapeutic perspective that is part of the duty of care. There seems to be no way out of the dilemma, except to conclude that there

should be an absolute bar to sexual contact between therapist and patient.

Although, practically, this conclusion is probably a good one, the justification for such a conclusion does not lie in either a rights/principles perspective, nor in an analysis of harms and wrongs. A relational perspective may shed light on the situation, and offer more justification for absolute proscription of such behavior. Looking at it from a relational perspective, we may try and understand how the therapist may have mistaken her personal feelings of wanting to respond to Miss B's neediness as a professional duty. There is no duty on healthcare professionals to make up for past injuries; healthcare professionals can offer care, but not reparation. The therapist may well be encouraged to ask herself why she feels the need to make reparation for past wrongs and whether, indeed, that is possible or even desirable.

This question raises another: of what the duty/ies of a therapist should be. Care and containment of feelings are the bare minimum that a patient can expect. Care and containment reflect a parental stance, where the therapist cares for the feelings of the patient and contains the anxiety about feelings of vulnerability and dependence, which many patients feel. Care and containment also includes attention to the therapist's own feelings. In this case, the therapist may not have taken seriously her own attachment to the patient, or the patient's to her. Requests for increased contact, especially those away from the clinic, suggest a wish for a close relationship out of the professional sphere, and could have been understood as such.

Sexual relationships (ideally) take place between equals, and involve a level of mutuality that differs from parental relationships, which recognize the importance of power differentials. A shift in the nature of the relationship, from professional to sexual, means that there is a shift in the management of power relationships within the therapeutic setting. The feelings of the therapist may complicate the feelings of the patient, and make it difficult for work to proceed. It arguably also gives the patient an extra problem to contend with: that of the therapist's feelings.

Thus a sexual relationship between patient and therapist has undesirable and potentially harmful consequences for the patient, and prevents the therapist from carrying out her professional duties. Rather than justifying a ban on therapist–patient sexual contact from an absolutist position (as suggested by the Hippocratic Oath), a relational perspective, including attention to both professional duties of care and patient rights, can offer a more coherent justification for prohibiting therapist–patient sexual relationships.

Such a perspective may also offer a way forward in managing the aftermath of such an event. A professional response would be to look at the relationship between the two parties and reflect on the way the therapist is feeling, if not with the patient, then with a supervisor. In such cases it is common for the therapist to be quite aware that she is doing something "wrong," but she could be unable to think about it. Thinking about how one "should" behave in the context of an ongoing connection is the very substance of a notion of the duty of care. Management of psychiatric cases therefore includes attention to the relationship between the therapist and the patient; helping the patient to understand her needs, and the therapist to understand how her own relational needs may have caused her to come to take action which was ethically unjustifiable.

Clinical Example 3: Mr C

One of the limitations of a rights-based or a principles approach rests on the definition of autonomy. Rights-based accounts of autonomy provide a rather static atomistic picture of autonomy, which allows little flexibility and disallows the importance of connections between persons (Christman, 1988). This type of account has several limitations, especially for those persons where autonomy is developing or held in a matrix of dependent relationships. Examples of this include children, people with head injuries, dementia, and chronic conditions that affect identity (see Agich, 1990, 1992, 1993). Some recent research has suggested that the level of development of self-identity is reflected in the use of a care perspective in moral reasoning (Skoe and Marcia, 1991).

What is needed is a more complex notion of autonomy within a relationship; a synthesis and dynamic of independence and dependence. The reality is that most of us, but especially those who are made vulnerable by physical or mental disability, actually need connections with others in order to act freely. The case of Mr C demonstrates the impact of physical disability on psychological autonomy; and also the importance of family relationships when making assessments of harms and benefits.

Mr C was maimed by a truck at the age of 10, leaving him disabled and requiring help. His disability, which still persists some 10 years later, provides a caring role for his mother in their home. Mr C seems completely passive, allowing her to do for him tasks that he is well able to do physically. He is also ambivalent about going out and socializing, expressing concerns about others' response to his disability. His mother supports him in his reluctance and suggests that it is too difficult for him to go out. Attempts to increase his opportunities for socialization (money for taxis, identification of peer groups) are met with verbal aggression by his mother and benign sabotage on the part of the patient. The young man's family appears to be connected together by his disability so that attempts to rehabilitate him out of the house, which would indeed do him "some good," seem to cause distress within the family system.

The psychiatrist is asked to assess the level of help he needs, both physically and financially. She feels that Mr C needs both less and more than he is asking for. His passivity seems problematic, but active interventions to motivate him may actually do him harm, in the sense that they disarrange a complex family dynamic. Changing that family dynamic requires a subtle assessment of harms and benefits, and an understanding of the relationships between all members of the family. A less subtle analysis of harms and benefits, which focused on only the young man's physical context and not his contextual one, may lead to difficulties and clinical failure. Such failures are not uncommon, particularly in the area of psychiatric care in the community; and may reflect the lack of training which clinicians receive, both about the scope and nature of their ethical duties, and the nature of relationships between people (Carse, 1991).

Discussion

Psychiatry and relationships

There are many types of healthcare relationships within medicine, and not all are equivalent in terms of time, mutuality, and complexity. The relationship between an orthopaedic surgeon and his patient may be quite different to that between the same patient and his GP. The relationship may change if their contact is prolonged (as is not uncommon with GPs), or it may be affected by the patient's condition. The surgeon may have a different relationship with a cancer sufferer than with a patient whose fracture has mended and will be seen only intermittently after a brief stay in hospital. In fact, it is often one of the complaints made by patients that they "just" get to "know" a clinician, when their clinical connection is broken; usually by discharge, or by rotation of staff.

All this may not matter very much if the condition is short-lived and does not seriously threaten the patient's independence or self-esteem. If, however, the condition is likely to be life-long, wide-ranging in terms of its effects, and to cause substantial disability, then this will result in a very different system of relationships between the patient and his carers. To have his needs met, he and they will have to negotiate; and to this end, he and they will have to get to know each other well over a long period of time. During this time, a relationship will form, which will impose duties and responsibilities on both parties. Feelings also arise on both sides of these relationships, which affect the perceptions of responsibilities and are an important aspect of any empathic connection between carers and patients.

A broader contextual vision of psychiatric illness addresses the impact of the illness on a patient's relationships, both towards himself and with his carers. This is true for both the major mental illnesses, such as the psychotic disorders, including schizophrenia or manic depression illness, and the neurotic disorders, where external reality perception is preserved. In psychotic disorders, where reality is impaired and patients may experience perceptual abnormalities such as hallucinations, or suffer from persistent distorted irrational beliefs such as delusions, then relationships between patients and their carers may be profoundly affected by these symptoms. Patients can be dangerous to their carers because of them. High levels of expressed emotion by relatives may cause deterioration of the patient's mental state or a relapse from a healthy state. Delusions of being possessed or invaded by external forces may also have profound effects upon one's view of one's self and self-identity.

However, it is perhaps in the field of neurotic disorders that the issue of relationships becomes most prominent. Healthy relationships appear to be important for normal adult mental health, in so far as they may protect against mental illness. People suffering from neurotic depression or anxiety (such as Miss B) frequently describe failures in relationships as their presenting problem. Both depression and anxiety encourage people to withdraw from relationships, which increases a sense of isolation and anxiety. It is perhaps of relevance that the absence of a confiding relationship, or the presence of an abusive relationship, is an actual risk factor for depression in adult women (Brown and Harris, 1978; Mullen et al., 1990). It is for this reason that Miss B may have been harmed by the failure of the therapeutic relationship; she may also have been wronged, in so far as the therapist failed to respect her identity as a patient and used her as a means of (possibly unconscious) gratification.

The importance of relationships is even clearer in relation to the so-called "personality disorders" (such as Miss A). The conceptual status of these disorders has long been debated, particularly whether they can be considered "illnesses." What is clear is that their essential feature lies in an inability to make and sustain relationships. For example, a significant feature of antisocial personality disorder is an increased capacity to be detached from other people and the lack of empathy in connection with others (American Psychiatric Association, 1994). One of the defining criteria of "borderline personality disorder" is instability of relationships, which are characterized by intense positive attachments followed by quick rejections and fluctuating attachments (ibid).

Therefore, the therapeutic relationships within psychiatry are important in a number of ways. First, the patient and their psychiatrist (and/or GP) are likely to be involved in a developing relationship over time, where the psychiatrist has to manage the patient's dependence, while at the same time facilitating his independence. Secondly, the illness itself may have profound influence on the relationship that the patient forms with his doctor, with his other carers, and with those important to him. Thirdly, the ability to form relationships may be affected by the illness. Lastly, the contribution of the psychiatrist is just as important to the relationship as any other aspect of treatment. This is particularly true in the context of those specifically psychotherapeutic relationships, where there is a high degree of dependence on the therapist which is developed by a regular meeting over a long period of time. The psychiatrist contributes either by having a direct impact on the patient, so that changes in the psychiatrist can actually have an effect upon the mental health of the patients (Persaud and Meux, 1994); or indirectly by the effect of her feelings on therapeutic decision-making.

Conclusion: Four Principles and Psychiatric Relationships

The three cases outlined above (drawn from real cases, but not based on any individual patient) show the complexity of relationships that have to be considered in the management of ethical dilemmas that affect psychiatric patients. Miss A's case highlights how an ethical dilemma may be understood in terms of the relationships between a patient and the multidisciplinary team. Miss B's case shows how the relationship with an individual therapist can become complex over time, and thus generate ethical tensions that were not there at the start of treatment. Mr C's case demonstrates how difficult it can be to delineate harms and benefits in the case of patients who are chronically dependent on others; and where their interests may have a direct bearing on the interests of the patient. Such cases are common in psychiatric care, involving both out-patients and in-patients, be-

cause patients are often dependent on others for help and support over long periods of time, and because relationships with staff are at the core of any psychiatric treatment program.

"Bare" principlism, which addresses ethical dilemmas in psychiatry only in terms of competing principles (such as beneficence versus autonomy), might not do justice to the complexity of the relationships and feelings that may be involved between the psychiatrist and the patient, and between the patient and his family. Too strong an emphasis on competing principles may cause clinicians caught up in ethical dilemmas to ignore important relationships in the patient's life which are ethically significant (Jinnet-Sack, 1993).

Traditional approaches to the principle of respect for autonomy are a good example of the way in which principlism may be an insufficient approach to ethical dilemmas in psychiatric and psychotherapeutic relationships. In such cases, patients may be not only physically but psychologically dependent on others, and their personal identity is embedded in a matrix of caring relationships. Respect for autonomy and, more generally, respect for persons is crucial in psychiatry, because of patients' vulnerability to coercion (what Christman (1988) describes as R-autonomy); nevertheless, the setting-up of artificial competitions between varying types of rights is unlikely to be able to explicate what degree of autonomy the patient actually has, or the extent to which it can be exercised (Agich, 1990, 1992, 1993).

The issue of respect for justice also needs careful consideration in relation to psychiatric patients. Real concerns about the abuse of psychiatric patients led to an undoubtedly valuable trend toward deinstitutionalization and an emphasis on individual human rights (Szasz, 1974). Nevertheless, the lack of services, care, and the presence of stigma in the community has meant that patients could sometimes be abandoned with their autonomy respected; "dying with their rights on" as one commentator put it. Such outcomes seem to suggest an understanding of justice as having an "all or nothing" quality. It also sees justice in an adversarial form, where A is pitted against B. In cases where A is a dependent member of the same society as B, and where A and B are not as different as they may seem, then a more complex analysis is needed.

It may be that more communitarian approaches to justice, which emphasize relationships with one another and consensus views within a community, may help to reduce setting-up the interest of the patient against the interest of the community in quite the dichotomous way that the law and civil rights movements sometimes see it. However, there are real tensions, for which there are no easy solutions, particularly in that sphere of psychiatry where patients may be actively dangerous because of their disabilities. Sutton (1997) describes the difficulties presented by adolescent patients with mental health problems, whose autonomy is not only interconnected but also developing.

Principles theory needs to be supplemented, developed, and enriched by other perspectives, including the ethic of care (Pellegrino, 1994; Robertson, 1996). This would appear to be particularly true in the practice of psychiatry and psychotherapy. This approach is also likely to have some value in other settings where patients suffer from long-term disabilities, and where relationships with others are both a significant part of their problem and part of the approach to treatment.

REFERENCES

Agich, G. (1990) Reassessing autonomy in long-term care. *Hastings Center Report* 20/6: 12–17.

Agich, G. (1992) Chronic Illness and freedom. In R. Carson, D. Barnard, and K. Toombs (eds.), *Chronic Illness and the Humanities* (Indianapolis: Indiana University Press).

Agich, G. (1993) Actual autonomy and long-term care decision-making. In L. McCullough and N. Wilson (eds.), *Ethical and Conceptual Issues in Long-term Care Decision-making* (Baltimore, MD: Johns Hopkins University Press).

American Psychiatric Association (1994) *Diagnostic and Statistical Manual*, Version IV (Washington, DC: American Psychiatric Press).

Attanucci, J. (1988) In whose terms: A new perspective on self, role, and relationship. In C. Gilligan et al. (eds.), *Mapping the Moral Domain* (Cambridge, MA: Harvard University Press).

Beauchamp, T. and Childress, J. (1994) *Principles of Biomedical Ethics* (Oxford: Oxford University Press, 4th edn).

Brown, D. (1994) Self-development through subjective interaction: A fresh look at ego training in action. In D. Brown and L. Zinkin (eds.), *The Psyche and the Social World* (London: Routledge).

Brown, G. and Harris, T. (1978) *The Social Origins of Depression* (London: Tavistock).

Carse, A. L. (1991) The "voice of care": Implications for bioethical education. *Journal of Medicine and Philosophy* 16: 5–28.

Christman, J. (1988) Constructing the inner citadel: Recent work on the concept of autonomy. *Ethics*: 109–24.

Fennell, P. (1996) *Treatment Without Consent* (London: Routledge).

Fulford, K. W. M. and Hope, A. (1994) Psychiatric ethics: A bioethical ugly duckling? In R. Gillon (ed.), *Principles of Health Care Ethics* (Chichester: John Wiley).

Gilligan, C. (1982) *In a Different Voice: Psychological Theory and Women's Development* (Cambridge: Cambridge University Press).

Gillon, R. (1992) Editorial: Caring, men and women, nurses and doctors and health care ethics. *Journal of Medical Ethics* 18: 171–2.

Jinnet-Sack, S. (1993) Autonomy in the company of others. In A. Grubb (ed.), *Choices and Decisions in Health Care* (Chichester: John Wiley).

Mullen, P. (1990) The long-term influence of childhood sexual abuse on mental health of victims. *Journal of Forensic Psychiatry* 1: 13–34.

Pellegrino, E. (1994) The four principles and the doctor–patient relationship: The need for a better linkage. In R. Gillon (ed.), *Principles of Health Care Ethics* (Chichester: John Wiley).

Persaud, R. D. and Meux, C. (1994) The psychopathology of authority and its loss: The effect on a ward of losing a consultant psychiatrist. *British Journal of Medical Psychology* 67: 1–11.

Robertson, D. (1996) Ethical theory, ethnography and differences between doctors and nurses in approaches to patient care. *Journal of Medical Ethics* 22: 292–9.

Skoe, E. and Marcia, J. (1991) A measure of care-based morality and its relation to ego identity. *Merrill Palmer Quarterly* 37: 289–304.

Sutton, A. (1997) Authority, autonomy, responsibility and authorisation: With specific reference to adolescent mental health practice. *Journal of Medical Ethics* 23: 26–31.

Szasz, T. (1974) *The Myth of Mental Illness* (New York: Harper Row).

7

Can There Be an Ethics of Care?

PETER ALLMARK

Introduction

The idea of an ethics based around the concepts of care and caring is one that has gained currency in the last ten years. [...] Amongst nurse theorists the idea of an ethics of caring is especially popular. Nursing has long sought to gain an identity separate from medicine and some writers hope that care may be the key to finding this identity.[1] 'Caring' ethics has roots in the work of Gilligan.[2] The key idea is that the detached, impartial observer ideal of morality, characteristic of ethics since the enlightenment, is flawed and inappropriate, particularly for women. In its place is recommended an approach stressing involvement in the situation, with an attitude of care for others also involved. As such, the importance of relations between people in their practical reasoning is highlighted rather than the more common approach stressing abstract principles.

I shall attempt to establish three points:

1. As described by its proponents, caring ethics is hopelessly vague. It lacks both normative and descriptive content.
2. This vagueness is due to an inadequate analysis of 'care', and thus of the source of any moral meaning which may attach to the term and its cognates. 'Caring' ethicists take the fact that care-related terms are used to express moral judgement to imply that care is itself a good, or the good. This inference is both invalid and false.
3. When care-related terms are used to express a moral judgement (for instance, to criticise someone as 'uncaring') the source of that judgement is not in the fact of care or its absence. Rather it is in what the person cares about and in how they express that care. 'Caring' ethicists can tell us nothing of the 'what' and the 'how' which underlie the judgement.

'Caring' Ethics

'Caring' ethics developed from discussions in the field of moral development theory. A key writer in this field was Kohlberg[3] who, by use of interviews in which moral dilemmas were presented, particularly to children, developed a stages theory of moral development.

Kohlberg suggested there were various levels of moral development from a form of primitive egoism as an infant, to a supreme objectivity, a level which few achieved. Blum characterises the ethical theory underlying this view as 'impartialism', the view that ethics is based upon impartiality, impersonality, universal principle, and formal rationality. This 'dominant conception' of morality is reflected in utilitarianism and Kantianism which both, despite their differences, incorporate impartialism. Impartialism is seen also in the 'principles' approach used widely in bioethics.[4]

Gilligan said that in her various studies she began to discern 'another voice' from that of impartialism (or the ethics of justice as she termed it). This voice was often heard from women or girls, although Gilligan was at pains to point out that this was a statistical tendency, not an empirical necessity.[5]

Kohlberg had interpreted the different way in which many, particularly girls, tended to approach problems as suggesting that they had 'arrested' at a certain stage. Given the right challenges they might be able to see beyond relationships to a more universal plane, although boys might do this more easily.

Gilligan pointed to girls' refusal to take decisions out of context, their desire to avoid conflict, and to their emphasis on the relationships between the protagonists in these dilemmas. She claimed that what girls were showing was not a lower level of ethical reasoning, but a different one. Where boys might use the language of the ethics of justice (impartialism), girls tended to use the language of the ethics of care. At times Gilligan appears to suggest that both are legitimate approaches which complement each other. At other times there is the impression that she believes the ethics of care to be superior. This is certainly the view of some of the writers who have appeared in her wake, such as Noddings.[6] The idea that 'caring' ethics can be complementary to other approaches is suggested by Gillon[7] and Dillon.[8]

Whilst the details of the 'caring ethics' seem obscure, one gets a flavour of what is meant from the various writers in the field. Blum lists what he sees as some of the differences between 'impartialism' and the ethics of care.[9]

1.   The care approach is particularised. It does not abstract from the particular situation and attempt to see, for example, which principles are operative, or what is the ethical framework. Gilligan and Noddings have both criticised Gandhi for his 'blind willingness to sacrifice people to truth', that is, some form of abstract truth. In practice this unwillingness of 'caring' ethicists to acknowledge the importance of abstract ideals has some disturbing consequences, which are discussed below.

2.   The care approach is involved. It does not see the person making moral decisions as a radically autonomous, self-legislating individual. Rather she is tied to others. Autonomy is not seen as some kind of ideal. Involvement with the person on whom one acts draws on capacities of love, care, empathy, comparison and sensitivity. This dimension of moral understanding is ignored by the impartialist approach.

3.   For the care approach, moral reasoning does not involve rationality alone, but an intertwining of emotion, cognition and action. Noddings quotes Hume, with approval.[10] It seems that for both, 'Reason is, and ought only to be the slave of the passions'.[11]

4.   The care approach is not concerned with universalistic right action. Gilligan talked instead of situationally based responses based upon 'cognizance of interdependence'.[12]

5.   Kohlberg's ultimate concern is with morality itself, whereas Gilligan's is with the relations between people ('relational ethics').

Problems with the Ethics of Care

1.   There is a vagueness about the approach which manifests itself in a disturbing lack of content. This is clear in the discussion of problematic situations given by Noddings. She gives an example of a mother whose son is at a school which has a rule that any absence must be due to illness or bereavement.[13] Other absences are punished. Her son needs permission to do something away from school on a regular basis which she considers worthwhile. She therefore writes regular letters saying her son is ill. Noddings believes that the 'masculine' ethics would have to justify this deception. For example, it might put someone under an obligation to try to change the stupid rule. The 'feminine' approach

is unconcerned with this debate. The mother remains faithful as 'one-caring' (Noddings's compound noun for someone who cares behaviourally and emotionally for another, 'the cared-for'). For Noddings, this is an example of how caring ethics will not put principle over person. The question which arises is, how far will 'one-caring' go?

This question arises more acutely when Noddings discusses an example developed in critiques of utilitarianism.[14] In essence the situation is one where someone is forced to choose between killing one innocent person, or allowing several innocent people to be killed by an evil person. Noddings suggests that the one-caring might try to kill the innocent person but that 'as I reach toward him, I feel the life, and fear, and trust, and hope...emanating from him'. She suggests then that the 'one-caring' could not kill. But what if she felt the life, fear and so on emanating from the others? Perhaps then she would kill.

In a later example[15] Noddings suggests that 'one-caring' might fight for the bigoted white people one grew up with if it 'came to the crunch' in a civil-rights-type war. Noddings does try to suggest that there would be limits beyond which one would not go, if, for example, the person one cared for became involved in setting up concentration camps.[16] However, it is hard to conceive how 'care' sets any limits or what rationale lies behind them.

2. Noddings suggests that the feeling that one must care (which she terms an 'ethical ideal') has its source in 'natural' caring experienced when young. Putnam points out that this obscures more than it illuminates.[17] It is clear that there are other things, such as hate and jealousy, which are 'natural' in relationships. It is not obvious why we should choose caring as our ideal, and commit ourselves to it rather than to, say, revenge.

3. Noddings's description of the development of an ethical ideal on the basis of memories of caring which we inevitably recall as good has another difficulty. It is not caring we recall as good, but good caring. It would be perfectly possible to remember caring, particularly as a child, which left one smothered and stifled. To reply that this is not *true* care would be simply to move the problem along. What one would be

saying then is that one inevitably recalls the care which was good as good. This is obvious and unhelpful.

4. The key problem is that the ethics of care approach assumes that caring is good, or the good, whereas the source of our moral approval of care and caring comes from outside the fact of care itself. To show this we must look at care and caring in more detail.

Care and Caring

The words 'care' and 'caring' are used frequently, and in differing ways and contexts. As a noun, care can mean a worry or anxiety. It can mean some form of state institution, as in 'put someone into care'. It can be adjectivally amended, as in intensive care, coronary care, community care and so forth. As verbs, 'I care', and 'I care for...' convey slightly different meanings. The first tends to suggest a meaning where the attitude of care is primary, the second a meaning where the action of care is primary. 'I am caring' suggests a judgement about the sort of person one is.

Whilst 'care' and 'caring' seem to be used in a wide variety of ways they do seem to be linked to each other.

The key link in all these notions seems to be that of emotional attachment. I shall term this the 'core definition' of care. There are two aspects, cognitive and emotional.[18]

Cognitive When someone cares about something they see that thing as of concern, interest or value to them. To care about something is to believe it to be good, or constitutive of a good, or the good.

Emotional The attachment of care is betrayed by a whole set of emotions and emotional dispositions. The emotions may include anger or sorrow at what one cares about being treated unfairly or unjustly (or damaged if it is an object), pity or compassion if it is hurt or fails to thrive, joy or contentment if it does thrive. It should be emphasised that no one emotion is conveyed by care. It is also clear that the phrase allows for degrees, as in 'I care a lot' and 'I do care but...'.

Someone might make the following objections to this core definition. First, it could be objected that someone could believe something to be a good, but at the same time not care about it. This is not a problem for the core definition. All that one may infer from this definition is that whatever one cares about, one perceives to be a good (or constitutive of a good and so on). One cannot infer that whatever one perceives to be good, one cares about. This does not present a problem for the argument presented here.

Second, it could be objected that the cognitive element is not a necessary part of care. This objection might be divided into two forms. (i) People care about things they believe to be bad, hence they care about pollution or nuclear war. (ii) People care about, and actively pursue things they believe to be bad, hence they smoke, eat cream cakes or whatever.

Let us look at these respectively. (i) The use of the term care in such cases is still linked to cognition. People care about pollution because it threatens what they care about. It is permissible to say one cares about the things which threaten what one cares about, this does not break the link with the core definition. (ii) This is a case of confused cognition, not of emotion and cognition in conflict. People both care about their health and about things which are bad for their health. It is not necessary for the core definition of care that people's cognitive valuings be in good order.

And thirdly, it could be objected that the emotional element is not a necessary part of care. (Call this (iii).) (iii) There are people who cognitively value things, but who do not have the emotional reactions related to those things that permit us to talk as we normally talk of people as 'caring'. We may all have some such 'things', sick relatives, projects we have tired of and so on. However, someone whose life consisted only of such cares would approach psychopathy. It is necessary for the argument here only that *most* care involves cognitive and emotional elements, and that other usages are derived from this core meaning. In these cases people behave *as if* they care.

One last objection (iv) might be that neither the emotional nor cognitive element is required in care. Thus people care about things they believe to be trivial, or about things about which they have barely thought at all. (iv) This might be seen in the use of the term 'care for', as in 'do you care for blackcurrants?' If someone were to affirm this, but never chose to eat them when they were available, only enjoying them by accident, and felt no sense of loss if blackcurrants were wiped off the face of the earth by a blight then it might be said that the term 'care' had been applied without any cognitive or emotional element. However, this seems most unlikely. If someone says they care for something then one would expect it to be manifest, or potentially manifest, in their behaviour. If it is not, then it seems the term has not been applied appropriately.

It is important to stress that care is not *behind* our emotions. Rather, it is made up of cognitive judgement and an array of emotions and potential emotions. If we care about something then we shall feel, and be disposed to feel, certain emotions in relation to that thing.

Emotions, desires and actions are closely linked. Anger involves a desire for revenge, pity involves a desire to relieve distress, love, a desire to nurture, protect and so on. Desires are linked to our chosen action, so that when we care about something we shall behave, and be disposed to behave, in certain ways towards that thing.

It might be objected that there are things we choose to do which are not based upon caring about anything, upon emotional attachments to anything. This seems to be true although not commonplace. Sometimes our life is guided by unthinking habit, and sometimes it may be directed by a momentary whim. Nonetheless, it would be almost impossible to live one's life without quite a large set of things about which one cares (in the core sense) to varying degrees. Without these, as Frankfurt suggests, one's life would be a sequence of events which one made no attempt to fashion; one would have no preferences.[19]

The core sense of care does not, in itself, carry any moral connotations. People prefer to do all sorts of bad things; in so doing they are aiming at what they perceive as some good, something they care about. However, from the writers in the 'ethics of care' tradition it is clear that, where care and its various cognates are used, often a moral judgement is being made, for example when we talk of a 'caring person'.

How is it that we can describe, for example, the failure of someone to prime a bomb as careless, but would rarely (or never) describe someone who succeeds in such a venture as caring? If we examine the times that care-related terms do imply a moral judgement we can see that it has nothing to do with the presence or absence of care in itself.

Careless/Careful

Take the term 'careless'. This is a word applied to actions or to someone who habitually performs such actions (including speech and omissions). It conveys a sense of clumsiness, but there is rather more to it than this. Consider the following examples:

1. A woman leaves a pair of sunglasses on the bed. Her husband sits on, and breaks, them. The way we describe the two actors' actions depends on various factors. For the husband to be termed 'careless' his action must be culpable. If the sunglasses were hidden by the sheets then his action is blamefree. Even if the husband were habitually clumsy he might not be termed careless. It is possible to be clumsy, but not careless; one might describe someone with Parkinson's disease in this way. Culpability is crucial to the use of this term.

The description of the wife's action depends, in part, on her reaction. If she is not upset (the sunglasses were very old, and not much use) then her action is not careless. If she is unmoved but the glasses were new and expensive then she might be termed careless, the implication being that she ought to care. She may also be termed uncaring (see below). Whether or not the glasses are valuable, if she *is* upset then her action may be termed careless.

2. Blum describes two mothers watching their children playing in the park.[20] One perceives that the game is becoming too rough and that a form of intervention is required, the other does not. Both mothers would describe themselves as caring about their children, but one is careless.

It seems that the term 'careless' may apply if and only if: (a) The action is chosen; (b) Something, or someone is damaged, or could easily have been damaged as a result of that action (including omissions), and either (c) The agent is emotionally hurt by the damage, or would have been, had it occurred, or (d) The agent should, or should be disposed to, be hurt by such damage.

Type (c) is probably the more common usage of the term. It suggests a failing in an individual, that the person lacks the sensitivity and skill to protect the things she/he cares about in her/his chosen actions. The person's care is not sufficiently manifest.

The mother in the example who does not see the need for intervention may be extremely upset by any injury to her child, but her disposition to be upset by such things is not matched by a disposition to act in such a way as to avoid such injuries happening. In such a case it might be said that she does not care as much as the other mother, or that her actions do not match her care.

Is this a moral failing? It is worth saying that one might use the term 'careless' of someone who does not make his/her care sufficiently manifest, even if what he/she cares about is reprehensible. Hence our terrorist who failed to turn on the time-switch of a bomb may be termed (fortuitously) careless.

The ethics of care suggests that the qualities needed to make one's care manifest, such as sensitivity, skill and attentiveness, are moral qualities. But once it is seen that the things we care about may be morally neutral or wrong, then the same must be true of the qualities needed to make these cares manifest.

On the other hand, if someone has the 'right' cares, ie, cares about the 'right' things, then his/her lack of ability to manifest these, say to nurture and protect, may be seen as a moral failing. Thus, in the second example, sensitivity, skill and attentiveness are qualities it is reasonable to ask of the mother. If she has failed to develop these then it does show a type of moral failing. However, the mere development of these qualities alone does not ensure morally praiseworthy action. Furthermore, it is far from clear that the moral failing is lack of care. It might be, say, laziness.

Mutatis mutandis someone who is 'careful' has the sensitivity and skill to protect and nurture the things they care about. What is clear from the bomber example is that it may not be desirable that someone has these qualities.

Uncaring/Caring

'Careless' type (d) suggests a different type of failing. It is closer to what we might more usually term 'uncaring'. If, in the first example, the glasses had been a gift from the husband, and he is upset by the breakage, then the woman's action is as likely to be called uncaring as careless. In the second example, if the mother had been unmoved by damage to her child then she would certainly be called uncaring. The temptation might be to think that 'uncaring' is appropriately used only where someone is hurt directly and the agent is unmoved, but this is not so. Damage to the environment may be termed careless (if one is moved, having done the damage) or uncaring (if one is not).

Uncaring applies if: One does not care (in the core sense) about things for which one should care.

Whenever the term is applied, a moral failing is implied. Someone who is uncaring lacks compassion, kindness, charity and so on. There are huge numbers of things about which we are uncaring, in a sense, but the term applies in its moral sense only when we are uncaring towards things to which we should be caring. With the term careless, a failing is being implied, but not always the same sort as when the term uncaring is used.

Mutatis mutandis a caring person is not someone who cares indiscriminately. She is someone who cares in the core sense about the things she ought to care about, and to the right degree. If called upon this will be manifest in action, in fact the person will have acquired the epithet on the basis of her actions. Such a person is kind, unselfish, charitable, compassionate and so on. It is this sort of use which is implied in phrases such as 'nurse's care', or 'using a condom shows that you care'.

Conclusion

We are now in a position to see what is at the root of the problems with 'caring' ethics. Almost all of us care, in the core sense, about different things to different degrees. Without such cares our lives would be directionless and psychopathic. However, the fact that we care does not make us 'caring' in the sense that the term is used when it conveys moral approval. For someone to be 'caring' at least two additional components are required.

First, the person must care about the right things, have the right set of values, as we might say. Hence someone who lovingly tends his allotment or racing pigeons, but neglects his family, is not a 'caring' person.

Second, the person must care in the right way, have sensitivity and skill. Hence, the 'non-interventionist' mother in the park example could not be called 'caring'.

The ethics of care says that we should care, that caring is a moral quality and that we should encourage conditions which create care. What it means is that we should care about the right things in the right way and encourage the required qualities. But by focusing on care as a moral quality in itself, something it is not, the ethics of care can tell us nothing of what those right things are.

It does seem to tell us something of the second component. It tells us that the sensitivity and skill needed to nurture and protect the things one cares about are moral qualities. However, a 'good' torturer has these qualities; you need to be sensitive to people's needs in order to deprive them of them. Once it is seen that what we care about may be morally neutral or wrong it can be seen also that so may be such required or attendant qualities.

Thus I conclude there can be no 'caring' ethics. What we care about is morally important,[21] the fact that we care *per se* is not.

NOTES

1 Benner, P., *From Novice to Expert* (Menlo Park, California: Addison-Wesley, 1984).

2 Gilligan, C., *In a Different Voice* (London: Harvard University Press, 1982).

3 Described in Blum, L., 'Gilligan and Kohlberg: Implications for moral theory', *Ethics* 98 (1988): 472–91.

4 For example, Beauchamp, T., Childress, J., *Principles of Biomedical Ethics* (New York: Oxford University Press, 1989).

5 See Gilligan, *In a Different Voice*, p. 2.

6 Noddings, N., *Caring: A Feminine Approach to Ethics and Moral Education* (Berkeley: University of California Press, 1984).

7 Gillon, R., 'Caring, men and women, nurses and doctors, and health care ethics', *Journal of Medical Ethics* 18 (1992): 171–2.

8 Dillon, R., 'Respect and care: toward moral integration', *Canadian Journal of Philosophy* 22/1 (1996): 105–31.

9 See Blum, 'Gilligan and Kohlberg', pp. 474–9.

10 See Noddings, *Caring*, p. 79.

11 Hume, D., cited in Macintyre, A., *A Short History of Ethics* (London: Routledge and Kegan Paul, 1991), p. 169.

12 See Gilligan, *In a Different Voice*, p. 147.

13 See Noddings, *Caring*, p. 56.

14 Ibid, p. 105.

15 Ibid, p. 110.

16 Ibid, p. 111.

17 Putnam, D., 'Relational ethics and virtue theory', *Metaphilosophy* 22 (1991): 231–8.

18 See also Griffin, A., 'A philosophical analysis of caring', *Journal of Advanced Nursing* 8 (1983): 289–95.

19 Frankfurt, H., 'The importance of what we care about', *Synthese* 53 (1982): 257–72.

20 See Blum, 'Gilligan and Kohlberg', p. 485.

21 Macintyre, A., 'Comments on Frankfurt', *Synthese* 53 (1982): 291–4.

8

The Literary Nature of Ethical Inquiry

TOD CHAMBERS

[. . .]
If there is any strongly held article of faith within their discipline, it is that bioethicists deal with the Aristotelian messy "real world" and that academic philosophers spend their time in a Platonic domain of unclouded abstraction. Bioethicists confront actual cases; academic philosophers contemplate imagined ones.
[. . .]
Yet for the ethicist to present the data received from real life situations, he or she must present those events in a narrative; a story must be constructed. Every telling of a story – real or imagined – encompasses a series of choices about what will be revealed, what will be privileged, and what will be concealed; there are no artless narrations. All stories are shaped by a particular teller for a particular purpose, for all narratives are infected by their situatedness. Consequently the ethics case, even though it may be based on a real life event, is mediated and thereby interpreted through narrative discourse. [. . .] In what follows, I demonstrate this through examining one particular feature of narrative discourse, point of view. Through an examination of how different narrative perspectives are constructed, I show that cases even in the hands of good bioethicists tend to be theory-driven and partial in the same manner as those of academic philosophers.

From the Clinician's Point of View

Terrence Ackerman and Carson Strong, in the preface to *A Casebook of Medical Ethics*, explicitly state that almost all the cases in their textbook are derived from their experience in the clinical setting and are "accurate accounts of actual cases." All of the cases, save three, "were typically encountered during clinical rounds or special consultations" and were "discussed extensively" with the health care team. [. . .] These assertions suggest their interest in establishing a personal relationship to the cases they are telling much in the same way Clifford Geertz argues that ethnographers have traditionally striven to establish authorial presence or what he terms "signature."[1] According to Geertz, ethnographers wish their readers to know in no uncertain terms that they were "there," and by establishing their signature to the descriptions, they convince their readers of the accuracy of these accounts of strange worlds. [. . .]

Ackerman and Strong maintain a consistent narrative form throughout their textbook, and beyond a richness of medical and psychosocial details, their style of presentation is similar to many case presentations in medical ethics. Look at the beginning of the first case in their collection.

M. J., a sixty-year-old man, was admitted to the psychiatric ward of the Veterans Administration hospital after he threatened to kill himself and his wife with a hunting rifle. The incident followed almost two years of increasing physical and mental difficulties. The patient had suffered continually from depression and often contemplated suicide. He admitted to sleep disturbance (early-morning awakening), loss of interest in outside activities, absence of sexual interest, and problems with concentration and memory. He also had a variety of nonspecific physical complaints (such as "weakness in the legs") and considerable loss of appetite.

Formerly, the patient had been happily married for thirty-five years. He also had a good relationship with his only child, a thirty-three-year-old son who lived in the same town. He reported no special problems in childhood or adolescence and has never had a problem with alcohol or drugs. However, his mother was treated for depression and later died in a mental hospital, possibly by suicide. His brother has also been treated for depression.

[. . .]

The opening of this ethics case story is written in the style of medical case histories as physicians, residents, and students present them at morning reports and grand rounds presentations and in patient discharge summaries. Ackerman and Strong provide more background information and explanation of clinical definitions and procedures than a clinical presentation would. Their case presentation, on the whole, however, appropriates many of the defining traits of medical storytelling: plot, passive constructions, and clinical linguistic features.[2] Note how Ackerman and Strong plot this case by beginning with M. J.'s "presentation" to the psychiatric ward and, following a description of his "present complaints," they move into the

past to describe what led up to the current condition: "Formerly, the patient had been happily married for thirty-five years." For the physician the plot of the story is determined by diagnostic concerns,[3] and Ackerman and Strong take their plot structure for this ethics case from medicine. They do not tell the patient's story, nor do they tell their story, that is, the ethicist's story; instead they tell the physician's story. [. . .]

Many of the linguistic features in Ackerman and Strong's text are intelligible only within the context of clinical medicine. The narrative can "make sense" only if one already shares with the narrator assumptions about how an ill person should be viewed. A story, like every other act of communication, is an act of collaboration, for information must be shared between the teller and the audience. Without these shared cultural norms, the narrative would be incomprehensible. The first sentence, "M. J., a sixty-year-old man, was admitted to the psychiatric ward of the Veterans Administration hospital after he threatened to kill himself and his wife with a hunting rifle," identifies this man through the clinical gaze. First it identifies him by his initials (rather than by name or pseudonym). The reader is also told M. J.'s age and sex, and then the verb "was admitted" indicates the first action performed on this individual. Unlike writers who wish to depict a character who has some event occur to him or her, Ackerman and Strong "present" a patient. They also use the contrasting signs of "admission/ denial," a characteristic binary split within medical discourse: "He admitted to sleep disturbance" and is said to have "reported no special problems in childhood." All of these linguistic features are borrowed from the way a clinician views a patient.

When describing actions taken upon this patient, Ackerman and Strong primarily use the passive voice. Similarly within the hospital performance of presenting patients to other physicians the passive voice becomes a covert code of insidership, of a shared viewpoint. The patient is the one acted upon but the subject of the sentence is an implied, and sometimes explicit, "we." Yet this is an ethics case not a medical case; its teller is not a physician but two ethicists. As a result the use of passive construction acts as a secondary sign, communicating that the ethicist is one of the implied agents. [...] In each of the three aspects of their narration – plot, language, and passive verb constructions – Ackerman and Strong adopt the clinician's voice and thereby the clinician's authority. They are not quoting a case presentation but in effect writing it themselves, assuming a clinician's presentational style and particular viewpoint in telling about an ethical problem.

[...]

This point of view reflects the role ethicists have had within medicine, sometimes putting on white coats, acting as consultants, working up ethical problems, and writing chart notes with moral prescriptions. Ackerman and Strong's style of presentation nevertheless raises questions of the degree to which one can rhetorically appropriate the point of view of another while remaining critical of that other's perspective.

From the Observer's Point of View

Baruch Brody in *Life and Death Decision Making* supports his argument for a pluralistic approach to ethical dilemmas through an analysis of forty ethics cases.[4] Like Ackerman and Strong, he establishes his signature to these cases in a preface. Brody contends that his cases "are composites drawn from several hundred real cases I have encountered in teaching rounds and/or consultations," and although none of these "real" cases "corresponds exactly" to the facts in his written cases, all the facts are "drawn from a real case." Moreover, his accounts of the medical team's arguments "are drawn from arguments actually offered by sensitive and talented clinicians in several hundred real cases." Brody specifies that he was there in a professional capacity. [...] Yet determining Brody's exact relationship to the participants in the cases is substantially more difficult than for Ackerman and Strong. His presentation of case 11: " 'I want to see again before I die': Accepting appropriate risks," for example, uses a different point of view from Ackerman and Strong. Brody separates the "facts" from the "questions," which as he notes in his preface are usually the "arguments presented by the team."

FACTS   Mrs. K is a 69-year-old woman diagnosed as having adenocarcinoma of the lungs. Surgery to remove the primary tumor was ruled out because of a local lymph node involvement. She received radiotherapy both for her lung disease and for more recent metastases to the brain. She then became blind. [*sic*] probably because of optic nerve compression as a result of her metastatic disease. Everyone is amazed that she is still alive, but no one believes that she has much longer to live. She is very depressed, more by blindness than by her impending death, and she won't attempt to learn any skills. All she keeps asking is whether or not she can be operated on to remove the local compressing masses so that she can see again. Her husband supports this request. A social worker has spent a fair amount of time working with them, explaining that the surgeons don't wish to operate in light of her very short life expectancy and the uncertainty of success of this difficult surgery and that Mrs. K would do better to learn certain elementary skills so that she can make the best of the time left to her. She and her husband refuse to accept his idea. She says that she wants to see again. He says that all he cares about is that she can have her chance to see, and he is very angry at the surgeons for refusing to operate.

QUESTIONS   Some people see Mrs. K as being very depressed by her blindness and impending death and insisting on surgery to correct her sight as a way to avoid dealing with the thought of dying blind. Others argue that there is insufficient evidence of depression to challenge the judgment of competency. They insist that those who challenge her competency are doing so simply as a way of not agreeing to her wishes. ...Everyone has a great deal of pity and compassion for this woman, who is dying blind, and her loving husband, who wants at least some of her wishes to be fulfilled. (p. 136)

Although in the preface Brody acknowledges that he was present in these cases, that like

Ackerman and Strong he was "there," the reader has difficulty situating him in the flow of the events. In the first sentence he suggests that he has also adopted the clinician's viewpoint ("Mrs. K is a 69-year-old woman diagnosed as having adenocarcinoma of the lungs") and afterward maintains many of the traits of medical discourse as well as its plot structure. In the next two sentences Brody uses the passive voice, "Surgery . . . was ruled out," and "She received radiotherapy." Then he makes an observation that would ordinarily be out of place in a clinical case presentation: "Everyone is amazed that she is still alive, but no one believes that she has much longer to live." [. . .]

In his telling of the events, Brody is an invisible observer, a secret sharer, who gathers all the "facts" and listens to all the voices. His position and participation in the events seems not to affect his description. He hears not only the clinician's perspective, but also "observes" the social worker spending time with the family "working with them, explaining that the surgeons don't wish to operate." And finally Brody records, "She says that she wants to see again. He says that all he cares about is that she can have her chance to see, and he is very angry at the surgeons for refusing to operate." This case is not told from the clinician's point of view, nor the social worker's, nor the patient's. Even with Brody's explanation that this is a composite of several cases, it must strike the reader as odd that Brody has chosen not to place himself in the case. [. . .]

Boris Uspensky has categorized this type of literary point of view as a "sequential survey" in which "the narrator's viewpoint moves sequentially from one character to another and from one detail to another, and the reader is given the task of piecing together the separate descriptions into one coherent picture."[5] Uspensky compares this style of viewpoint to a film presentation in which the reader receives a montage of scenes. Similarly Brody's narration delivers fragments of different perspectives that the reader must patch together, and there is no single perspective that holds the narrative together. [. . .]

These stylistic features reflect Brody's interest in a pluralistic approach that "accepts the legitimacy of a wide variety of very different moral appeals" (p. 9). Confronted with often equally compelling arguments, Brody argues against approaches that provide a hierarchy of values or that attempt to provide a contextual scale for moral conflicts, similar to the priority and balancing approaches discussed by Ackerman and Strong. Advocating a process of judgment in which "We look at the various appeals and their significance, and then we judge what we ought to do" (p. 77), Brody acknowledges the inherent messiness in which this may leave moral decisions. He asserts, however, that bringing into focus the various conflicting values is "the most a moral theory can provide" (p. 79).

Brody thus narrates his ethics cases from the point of view of an impartial observer who can judge the various appeals. This textual point of view, then, is consistent with the moral perspective that Brody advances. Although involved in the cases, Brody recalls the narrative through external focalization, that is, as an uninvolved observer. The reader of Brody's narrative sees the problem through the perspective of a supposedly unbiased judge who regards the various conflicting appeals. The viewpoint of the narrator is not "natural," but one that Brody has chosen and constructed and one that supports the way he wishes the reader to see and evaluate the questions.

From the Protagonist's Point of View

I was alone, waiting for the start of an ethics case conference in an all-purpose room of the Child Development Center. I remember that the cement block walls of the 1960s vintage building were painted with a stark yellow (they must have wanted it to look like sunshine, to cheer up the handicapped, I said to myself). Feeling very much the displaced, I was in the grip of wondering whether the gray molded plastic chair would really continue to support me, when the pediatric resident, who would be presenting the case – and whom I will call Dr. McDonough – arrived and started telling me the following story while we waited for the other committee members.

"The patient is 21 years old," he said, "is the size of a 7-year-old, and has the mental age of a 2- to $2\frac{1}{2}$ -year-old."[6]

The opening of Warren Reich's "The Case of the White Oaks Boy" in his article "Caring for Life in the First of It: Moral Paradigms for Perinatal and Neonatal Ethics" is startling when one compares it with the cases presented thus far. Here is an instance of an ethicist who situates himself in relation to the events narrated, yet in Reich's tale the use of "I" has just as much rhetorical force as the narrative viewpoints of the clinician and the observer presented above. The first sentence radically locates the ethicist as the teller – "I was alone" – and the reader knows whose expression this is.[7] [...] When the physician arrives on the scene, he breaks Reich's reminiscences with a cold clinical presentation: " 'The patient is 21 years.' " In Ackerman and Strong's style, this would be the first sentence of the ethics case presentation, and it would not have quotation marks around it. [...] The physician tells him of a patient whose quality of life they are unable to determine. Unlike Brody, Reich indicates that he plays a role in gathering information:

> Itchy to shift attention elsewhere, I asked my conversation partner: "Dr. McDonough, what was this patient like? How did he strike you? What did you think of him?" McDonough, his face now transformed by curiosity and amazement, told me what I (as a nonphysician) regard as the "real story" inside the case history.
>   He said: "Michael is a very strange individual. He shows unusual behavior. I'll never forget him – how he seems to be capable of just three things."

In this, Reich maintains the status of an outsider or one who seems unconcerned with the details of clinical evaluation. Reich knows that there is a "real story" to be found, and it is not the case history but someone inside it.
  [...]
In contrast to Brody's sequential viewpoint, the unity of the "White Oaks Boy" narration is

achieved through the protagonist's perspective, that is, the ethicist's point of view. [...] Just as Reich gets "inside" the case history in his conversation with the clinician to find the "real story," he gets inside Michael to see the "real person." Is it surprising that the method that Reich advocates in understanding this case is an "experiential" ethics? According to Reich one should begin "with a perception and interpretation of values related to moral experience – that are conveyed through life experiences, narratives, images, models known from behavior sciences, etc." (p. 283). He proposes an ethic based on response to an "Other" rather than on abstract moral reasoning. By sensitively penetrating the inner world of patients, an ethicist, he believes, can determine how to respond to their needs. Reich's choice of a case that uses the first-person voice makes sense in view of his phenomenological orientation. It persuades the reader of the success of such an ethical position because he has provided an account that reveals a point of "experiential" epiphany.

Reading the Case

In "Caring for Life in the First of It," Reich arrives at his support for an "experiential" approach after he has attempted to apply other, more traditional, paradigms in medical ethics. He is dissatisfied with each of these approaches for they do not truly provide aid in resolving the moral problem of his case. Tellingly, Reich comments that the "thrust" of his "experiential" method is "to break the preoccupation of ethics with reasoning stemming from the ethical analyst's point of view ... and recenter ethics on the stranger, by allowing his or her story to refocus our vision, and expose the relativity of our own orientation to what is meaningful" (p. 285). Yet could the reader be persuaded of this argument against the previous paradigms and for this particular revisioning if Reich had used the case presentation – with its narrative point of view – of Ackerman and Strong? Similarly could Brody have used Reich's radically subjective first-person account for a pluralistic ethics that requires the evaluation of conflicting moral appeals? Could Ackerman and Strong be as persuasive on behalf of a balancing approach using Brody's external focalization?

In each instance the preferred means of resolving the ethical problem is embedded within the rhetoric of the narrative. Bioethics is deemed an applied discipline primarily because it attempts to ground moral theory in the real world, yet the discipline has remained generally unmindful of the fact that it encounters the real world as it is mediated through narrative. [. . .]

If there is no unbiased point of view to use when presenting an ethics case, how should these ethicists have written the cases in a manner that would encourage a critical reading? It is not as important to find directions for writing ethics cases as for reading them. For the question of how one should write an ethics case implies that there exists some technique that will construct cases that are innocent of a way of seeing the world. I have examined the issue of points of view taken within ethics cases, but this same analysis needs to be carried out in terms of the other constructed features of bioethics cases, such as character, plot, structure, conventions, and dialogue. What needs to be discovered is not some innocuous way to write cases but a series of readings of ethics cases that uncovers the rhetorical force of the case. If cases are the data for bioethics, we must come to understand how our data are rhetorically shaped, not so we can write an unbiased case but so that we can see the manner in which the case's presentation attempts to thwart us. What I propose is that we do not so much need thicker or richer cases as we do more sophisticated readings of cases. Reading cases with attention to their fictional qualities, that is, their constructedness, in turn reveals how dilemmas are framed in ways that conceal as well as reveal other ways of seeing. To ignore the narrative characteristics that the bioethics case shares with fiction is to confuse representation with the thing it represents – to mistake the story with the reality – and thus to miss the theory in the case.

of this paper and for providing such useful suggestions.

1   Clifford Geertz, *Works and Lives* (Stanford: Stanford University Press, 1988), p. 9.

2   I am deriving these concepts and their meaning within clinical case presentations from the following sources: Kathryn Montgomery Hunter, *Doctors' Stories: The Narrative Structure of Medical Knowledge* (Princeton: Princeton University Press, 1991); William J. Donnelly, "Medical language as symptom: Doctor talk in teaching hospitals," *Perspectives in Biology and Medicine* 30 (1986): 81–94; Renée R. Anspach, "Notes on the sociology of medical discourse: The language of case presentation," *Journal of Health and Social Behavior* (1988): 357–75; David Mintz, "What's in a word: The distancing function of language in medicine," *Journal of Medical Humanities* 13 (1992): 223–33.

3   See Hunter, *Doctors' Stories.*

4   Baruch A. Brody, *Life and Death Decision Making* (New York: Oxford University Press, 1988), p. vi.

5   Boris Uspensky, *A Poetics of Composition* (Berkeley: University of California Press, 1973), p. 60.

6   Warren Thomas Reich, "Caring for life in the first of it: Moral paradigms for perinatal and neonatal ethics," *Seminars in Perinatology* 11 (1987): 279.

7   An important issue concerning "authorship" should be noted, however. Reich's employment of the first person leads the reader to assume that the author of the case and of the philosophical perspective are one and the same, and the reader also assumes that this establishment of signature through the first person indicates that this is a "real" case drawn from Reich's experiences. Yet Reich does not explicitly claim that he is the author of the case, and he treats this narrative in his analysis as if it were given to him by someone else. By doing so, Reich suggests that the case is brute data, objective, empirical, and distant from the philosophy. The reader, however, is given clear signs in the story that, like Reich, the narrator is an ethicist. For an analysis of the various forms of implied authors and narrators, see Wayne C. Booth, *The Rhetoric of Fiction* (Chicago: University of Chicago Press, 1968).

NOTES

I wish to thank Kathryn Montgomery Hunter, Douglas Reifler, William Donnelly, Anne Hunsaker Hawkins, and Ann Stanford for reading earlier drafts

9

Two Theories of Modernity

CHARLES TAYLOR

There seem to be at large in our culture two ways of understanding the rise of modernity. They are in effect two different "takes" on what makes our contemporary society different from its forebears. In one take, [which I will call the "cultural" perspective,] we can look on the difference between present-day society and, say, that of medieval Europe as analogous to the difference between medieval Europe and China or India. In other words, we can think of the difference as one between civilizations, each with their own culture.

Or alternatively, we can see the change from earlier centuries to today as involving something like "development," as the demise of a "traditional" society and the rise of the "modern." And in this perspective, which seems to be the dominant one, things look rather different. [... As an "acultural" experience, this] conceives of modernity as the growth of reason, defined in various ways: as the growth of scientific consciousness, or the development of a secular outlook, or the rise of instrumental rationality, or an ever-clearer distinction between fact-finding and evaluation. Or else modernity might be accounted for in terms of social, as well as intellectual changes: the transformations, including the intellectual ones, are seen

as coming about as a result of increased mobility, concentration of populations, industrialization, or the like. In all these cases, modernity is conceived as a set of transformations that any and every culture can go through – and that all will probably be forced to undergo.

[...]

Acultural explanations of modernity in terms of "reason" seem to be the most popular. And even the "social" explanations tend to invoke reason as well, since the social transformations, like mobility and industrialization, are thought to bring about intellectual and spiritual changes because they shake people loose from old habits and beliefs – in, for example, religion or traditional morality – which then become unsustainable because they have no independent rational grounding in the way the beliefs of modernity – in, for example, individualism or instrumental reason – are assumed to have.

But, one might object, how about the widespread and popular *negative* theories of modernity, those that see it not as gain but as loss or decline? [...] Instead of seeing the transformations as the unfolding of capacities, negative theories have often interpreted them as falling prey to dangers. [...] Modernity is characterized by the loss of the horizon; by a loss of roots;

by the hubris that denies human limits and denies our dependence on history or God, which places unlimited confidence in the powers of frail human reason; by a trivializing self-indulgence which has no stomach for the heroic dimension of life, and so on.

The overwhelming weight of interpretation in our culture, positive and negative, tends to assume that all societies will take the same path, for good or ill. [. . .] Is this bad? I think it is. In order to see why, we have to bring out a bit more clearly what these theories foreground and what they tend to screen out.

Acultural theories tend to describe the transition in terms of a loss of traditional beliefs and allegiances. This may be seen as coming about as a result of institutional changes: for example, mobility and urbanization erode the beliefs and reference points of static rural society. Or the loss may be supposed to arise from the increasing operation of modern scientific reason. The change may be positively valued – or it may be judged a disaster by those for whom the traditional reference points were valuable and scientific reason too narrow. But all these theories concur in describing the process: old views and loyalties are eroded. Old horizons are washed away, in Nietzsche's image. The sea of faith recedes, following Matthew Arnold. This stanza from his "Dover Beach" captures this perspective:

The Sea of Faith
Was once, too, at the full, and round earth's
    shore
Lay like the folds of a bright girdle furled.
But now I only hear
Its melancholy, long, withdrawing roar,
Retreating, to the breath
Of the night-wind, down the vast edges
    drear
And naked shingles of the world.

The tone here is one of regret and nostalgia. But the underlying image of eroded faith could serve just as well for an upbeat story of the progress of triumphant scientific reason. From one point of view, humanity has shed a lot of false and harmful myths. From another, it has lost touch with crucial spiritual realities. But in either case, the change is seen as a loss of belief.

What emerges comes about through this loss. The upbeat story cherishes the dominance of an empirical-scientific approach to knowledge claims, of individualism, negative freedom, instrumental rationality. But these come to the fore because they are what we humans "normally" value, once we are no longer impeded or blinded by false or superstitious beliefs and the stultifying modes of life that accompany them. Once myth and error are dissipated, these are the only games in town. The empirical approach is the only valid way of acquiring knowledge, and this becomes evident as soon as we free ourselves from the thraldom of a false metaphysics. Increasing recourse to instrumental rationality allows us to get more and more of what we want, and we were only ever deterred from this by unfounded injunctions to limit ourselves. Individualism is the normal fruit of human self-regard absent the illusory claims of God, the Chain of Being, or the sacred order of society.

In other words, we moderns behave as we do because we have "come to see" that certain claims were false – or on the negative reading, because we have lost from view certain perennial truths. What this view reads out of the picture is the possibility that Western modernity might be powered by its own positive visions of the good, that is, by one constellation of such visions among available others, rather than by the only viable set left after the old myths and legends have been exploded. It screens out whatever there might be of a specific moral direction to Western modernity, beyond what is dictated by the general form of human life itself, once old error is shown up (or old truth forgotten). For example, people behave as individuals, because that's what they "naturally" do when no longer held in by the old religions, metaphysics, and customs, though this may be seen as a glorious liberation, or a purblind enmiring in egoism, depending on our perspective. What it cannot be seen as is a novel form of moral self-understanding, not definable simply by the negation of what preceded it.

Otherwise put, what gets screened out is the possibility that Western modernity might be sustained by its own original spiritual vision, that is, not one generated simply and inescapably out of the transition.

[...] In one way, it is quite understandable when we reflect that we Westerners have been living the transition to modernity for some centuries out of the civilization we used to call Christendom. It is hard to live through a change of this moment without being partisan, and in this spirit we quite naturally reach for explanations that are immediately evaluative, on one side or the other. Now nothing stamps the change as more unproblematically right than the account that we have "come to see" through certain falsehoods, just as the explanation that we have come to forget important truths brands it as unquestionably wrong. [...] This is partly because an immediately evaluative explanation (on the right side) is more satisfying – we tend to want to glorify modernity, or vilify it.

[...]

So what, if anything, is bad about this? Two things. First, I think Western modernity *is* in part based on an original moral outlook. This is not to say that our account of it in terms of our "coming to see" certain things is wholly wrong. On the contrary: post-seventeenth-century natural science has a validity, and the accompanying technology an efficacy, that we have established. And all societies are sooner or later forced to acquire this efficacy, or be dominated by others (and hence have it imposed on them anyway). [...] But science itself has grown in the West in close symbiosis with a certain culture in the sense I'm using that term here, namely, a constellation of understandings of person, nature, society, and the good.

[...]

We all too easily imagine that people have always seen themselves as we do, in respect, for example, of dichotomies like inward/outward. And we thus utterly miss the role these new understandings have played in the rise of Western modernity. [...] [This] distorts and impoverishes our understanding of ourselves, both through misclassification (the Enlightenment package error), and through too narrow a focus. But its effects on our understanding of other cultures is even more devastating. The belief that modernity comes from one single universally applicable operation imposes a falsely uniform pattern on the multiple encounters of non-Western cultures with the exigencies of sci-

ence, technology, and industrialization. As long as we are bemused by the Enlightenment package, we will believe that they all *have* to undergo a range of cultural changes drawn from our experience – such as "secularization" or the growth of atomistic forms of self-identification. As long as we leave our own notions of identity unexamined, so long will we fail to see how theirs differ, and how this difference crucially conditions the way in which they integrate the truly universal features of "modernity."

Moreover, the view that modernity arises through the dissipation of certain unsupported religious and metaphysical beliefs seems to imply that the paths of different civilizations are bound to converge. As they lose their traditional illusions, they will come together on the "rationally grounded" outlook that has resisted the challenge. The march of modernity will end up making all cultures look the same. This means, of course, that we expect they will end up looking like us.

[...]

So the view from Dover Beach foreshortens our understanding of Western modernity. But it also gives us a false and distorted perspective on the transition. It makes us read the rise of modernity in terms of the dissipation of certain beliefs, either as its major cause ("rational" explanations), or as inevitable concomitant ("social" explanations). What is beyond the horizon on Dover Beach is the possibility that what mainly differentiates us from our forebears is not so much our explicit beliefs as what I want to call the background understanding against which our beliefs are formulated.

[...]

The notion is that our explicit beliefs about our world and ourselves are held against a background of unformulated (and perhaps in part unformulable) understandings, in relation to which these beliefs make the sense they do. These understandings take a variety of forms, and range over a number of matters. In one dimension, the background incorporates matters that *could* be formulated as beliefs, but aren't functioning as such in our world (and couldn't *all* function as such because of their unlimited extent). To take Wittgenstein's example from *On Certainty*, I don't normally have a *belief* that the world didn't start only five minutes ago, but the whole way I inquire into things treats the world as being there since time out of mind.[1] Similarly, I don't usually have the belief that a huge pit hasn't been dug in front of my door, but I treat the world that way as I emerge in the morning to go to work. In my ways of dealing with things is incorporated the background understanding that the world is stable and has been there a long time.

In other dimensions, I have this kind of understanding of myself as an agent with certain powers, of myself as an agent among other agents, on certain, only partly explicit footings with them. And I want to add: an agent moving in certain kinds of social spaces, with a sense of how both I and these spaces inhabit time, a sense of how both I and they relate to the cosmos and to God or whatever I recognize as the source(s) of good.

[...]

Now if this is true, then we can see how inadequate and misleading acultural accounts can be. In my sense of this term, these are explanations of Western modernity that see it not as one culture among others, but rather as what emerges when any "traditional" culture is put through certain (rational or social) changes. On this view, modernity is not specifically Western, even though it may have started in the West. It is rather that form of life toward which all cultures converge, as they go through, one after another, substantially the same changes. These may be seen primarily in "intellectual" terms, as the growth of rationality and science; or primarily in "social" terms, as the development of certain institutions and practices: a market economy, or rationalized forms of administration. But in either case, the changes are partly understood in terms of the loss of traditional beliefs, either because they are undermined by the growth of reason, or because they are marginalized by institutional change.

Even the social explanations assume that these beliefs suffer from a lack of rational justification, since the solvent effect of social change is held to lie in the fact that it disturbs old patterns that made it possible to hold on to these earlier beliefs in spite of their lack of rational grounding. For instance, the continu-

ance of a static, agricultural way of life, largely at the mercy of the vagaries of climate, supposedly makes certain religious beliefs look plausible, which lose their hold once humans see what it is to take their fate in their own hands through industrial development. Or a largely immobile society leads individuals to see their fate as bound up closely with that of their neighbors, and inhibits the growth of an individualism that naturally flourishes once these constricting limits are lifted.

The acultural theory tends to see the process of modernity as involving among other things the shucking off of beliefs and ways that don't have much rational justification, leaving us with an outlook many of whose elements can be seen more as hard, residual facts: that we are individuals (that is, beings whose behavior is ultimately to be explained as individuals), living in profane time, who have to extract what we need to live from nature, and whom it behooves therefore to be maximally instrumentally rational, without allowing ourselves to be diverted from this goal by the metaphysical and religious beliefs that held our forefathers back.[2] Instrumental rationality commands a scientific attitude to nature and human life.

The Homogeneity of Kernel Truths

At the heart of the acultural approach is the view that modernity involves our "coming to see" certain kernel truths about the human condition, those I have just adverted to. There is some justification for talking of our "coming to see" the truth when we consider the revolution of natural science that begins in the seventeenth century. But the mistake of the acultural approach is to lump all the supposed kernel truths about human life into the same package, as though they were all endorsed equally by "science," on a par, say, with particle physics.[3]

I have been arguing that this is a crucial mistake. It misrepresents our forebears, and it distorts the process of transition from them to us. In particular, seeing the change as the decline of certain *beliefs* covers up the great differences in background understanding and in the social imaginary of different ages. More, it involves a sort of ethnocentrism of the present. Since human beings always do hold their explicit beliefs against a background and in the context of an imaginary, failure to notice the difference amounts to the unwitting attribution to them of our own. This is the classic ethnocentric projection.

This projection gives support to the implicit Whiggism of the acultural theory, whereby moderns have "come to see" the kernel truths. If you think of premoderns as operating with the same background understanding of human beings as moderns, namely, as instrumental individuals, and you code their understandings of God, cosmos, and multidimensional time as "beliefs" held against this background, then these beliefs do indeed appear as arbitrary and lacking in justification, and it is not surprising that the social changes dislodged them.

[...]

From a standpoint immured within any culture, other cultures look weird. No doubt we would look strange – as well as blasphemous and licentious – to our medieval ancestors. But there is a particularly high cost in self-misunderstanding that attaches to the ethnocentrism of the modern. The kernel truths of the acultural theory incorporate an often unreflective methodological individualism, and a belief in the omnicompetence of natural science. Impelled by the latter, its protagonists are frequently tempted to cast our "coming to see" the kernel truths as a sort of "discovery" in science. But the discoveries of natural science are of "neutral" facts, that is, truths that are "value-free," on which value may be subsequently placed by human beings, but which themselves are devoid of moral significance. Belonging to the range of such "natural" facts is that we are individuals, impelled to operate by instrumental reason, maximizing our advantage when we are not deterred from doing so by unfounded belief.[4]

Selves, Society, and the Good

Now this hides from view two important connections. First, the way in which our implicit understanding of ourselves as agents always places us in certain relations to others. Because of the very nature of the human condition – that

we can only define ourselves in exchange with others, those who bring us up, and those whose society we come to see as constitutive of our identity – our self-understanding always places us among others. The placements differ greatly, and understanding these differences and their change is the stuff of history.

[...] [is] closely tied up with the rise of modern "individualism." The account I would like to offer would have us see the rise of this new individual identity as inextricably linked to the new understandings of time and society. [...] By contrast, a widespread alternative view sees individualism as involving a completely self-referential identity; one in which agents are first of all aware of and focused on themselves, and only subsequently discover a need for, and determine their relations to, others. [...] Modern "individualism" is coterminous with, indeed, is defined by a new understanding of our placement among others, one that gives an important place to common action in profane time, and hence to the idea of consensually founded unions, which receives influential formulation in the myth of an original state of nature and a social contract. Individualism is not just a withdrawal from society, but a reconception of what human society can be. To think of it as pure withdrawal is to confuse individualism, which is always a moral ideal, with the anomie of breakdown.

[...]

The very idea of an individual who might become aware of himself, and then only subsequently, or at least independently, determine what importance others have for him and what he will accept as good, belongs to [...] fantasy. Once we recognize that our explicit thoughts only can be entertained against a background sense of who and where we are in the world and among others and in moral space, we can see that we can never be without some relation to the crucial reference points I enumerated above: world, others, time, the good. This relation can, indeed, be transformed as we move from one culture or age to another, but it cannot just fall away. We cannot be without *some* sense of our moral situation, *some* sense of our connectedness to others.

[...]

NOTES

1 Ludwig Wittgenstein, *On Certainty* (Oxford: Blackwell, 1977), paragraphs 260 ff.
2 This development of instrumental rationality is what is frequently described as "secularization." See, for instance, Gabriel Almond and G. Bingham Powell, *Comparative Politics: A Developmental Approach* (Boston: Little Brown, 1966), pp. 24–5: "A village chief in a tribal society operates largely with a given set of goals and a given set of means of attaining these goals which have grown up and been hallowed by custom. The secularization of culture is the process whereby traditional orientations and attitudes give way to more dynamic decision-making processes involving the gathering of information, the evaluation of information, the laying out of alternative courses of action, the selection of a given action from among those possible courses, and the means whereby one tests whether or not a given course of action is producing the consequences which were intended." And later: "The emergence of a pragmatic, empirical orientation is one component of the secularization process" (p. 58).
3 Even Ernest Gellner, who is light years of sophistication away from the crudities of Almond and Powell, puts himself in the acultural camp, for all his interesting insights into modernity as a new constellation. He does this by linking what I am calling the supposed "kernel truths" with what he calls "cognitive advance," in a single package. The modern constellation unchained science, and that in his view seems to confer the same epistemic status on the whole package. "Specialization, atomization, instrumental rationality, independence of fact and value, growth and provisionality of knowledge are all linked with each other." See *Plough, Sword and Book* (Chicago: University of Chicago Press, 1988), p. 122.
4 Thus Gellner includes "independence of fact and value" in his package, along with "growth and provisionality of knowledge."

Part II

Staying Well: Screening and Preventive Medicine

Introduction

The rise (and rise) of genetics as an area of bioethical controversy has tended to highlight the "high-tech," "sci-fi" sorts of genetic issue: cloning, "designer babies," and the like, which have become something of a media fixation. In keeping with the spirit of this book, however, we begin Part II with a much more everyday but no less momentous issue, that of what counts as success in genetic counseling. Ruth Chadwick's chapter alerts us to the risk that (at least in a context where abortion is fully legalized) success may come to be measured in terms of terminations of "defective" fetuses. Not only does this raise disability-rights issues, one might note; it cannot be said to be patient-centered or non-prescriptive. Termination is not necessarily success in the woman's terms, one might think: merely avoidance of what she sees as a greater evil. An alternative approach is to measure success in terms of workload, but although this approach works up to a point, it too is a managerial rather than a patient-centered measure. Yet in the context of evidence-based medicine, with its concomitant call for greater efficiency in healthcare, it seems that we cannot avoid positing some measure of success: what sort of measure is compatible with patient autonomy? In answering this question, we need to remember that "if the outcome measure is found unacceptable, it is not just this that has to be argued against, but also the political philosophy that underpins both it and a certain interpretation of autonomy." Chadwick adds, "I would argue further that it *should* be argued against precisely because it does distort the meaning of autonomy for the purpose of denying public responsibility for those in need."

The next chapter, "The Genetic Underclass," by Jay Rayner, is a journalistic exposé of misuses of genetic information by insurance companies which deny cover to people who are presently "well." We include it not so much because of the ethical issues involved, but because of the challenge of the term "well" and the notion of health promotion which these practices entail. As an example, Rayner takes the possibility of mapping the genetic basis for hypertrophic cardiomyopathy, or primary heart disease. Genetic screening would alert vulnerable members of the population to their condition before sudden, premature death; on the other hand, undergoing a genetic test voluntarily (perhaps as opposed to mass screening) might rule "victims" out for life insurance. Yet precisely because they have been diagnosed, individuals and families with known genetic mutations actually pose less of a threat to insurance company figures, since the actuarial risk is known. Furthermore, one might add, these people are not ill, and all of us suffer from several potentially fatal genetic mutations. Does this mean that we are all ill? Does the concept of health have to be reinterpreted as "well up to a point" or "not yet dying of one's genetic malfunctions"? If we are all potentially an underclass, with one genetic weakness or another, does the concept of a genetic underclass itself make any sense? Rayner himself does not consider these wider issues, but the notion of genetic underclass which he introduces has since been picked up and analyzed in terms of its broader meaning for health and health promotion.

Another unexpected aspect of genetic screening and testing is the way in which they may threaten the notion of individual informed consent. In the case and analysis presented by Donna Dickenson in "Ethical Issues in Precancer Testing," a son and daughter gave "consent" (though probably not legally valid consent in the UK, where no one can consent on behalf of an incompetent adult) to submitting their elderly father, "Henry," to the linked marker test for Huntington's disease. "When the family gave their consent to having Henry tested," Dickenson notes, "the son and daughter, at least, were also consenting to a certain level of torment about their own genetic status." Do they now have an obligation to know their own status, or can it be rational not to want to know? Dickenson argues that the "or" should be "although": it may be rational not to want to know, but it cannot be ethical. She offers a further analysis of the extent to which the Huntington's situation, with its near 100 percent level of certainty, can offer insight into the ethical dilemmas raised by ethical screening for precancerous conditions, where much greater uncertainty is involved.

In chapter 13, "Eugenics and Public Health in American History," Martin Pernick argues that eugenics had a much greater influence on American public health programs than is usually admitted. However, within the eugenics movement of the early twentieth century there was widespread disagreement over the meaning of improvement in the population gene pool, the content of what could be included under heredity, the methods by which heredity should be improved, and the rightful locus of authority to decide the other questions. The eugenics movement is now notorious for such sentiments, cited by Pernick, as "in prolonging the lives of defectives we are tampering with the function of the social kidneys." As well as being seen as socially maleficent, it is also pilloried for its scientific inaccuracy. But although eugenicists are generally attacked for failing to accept the germ theory of disease, many accepted the theory while continuing to insist that resistance to infectious disease had a genetic basis. (In the wake of the *Moore* case, concerning the commercial exploitation of a man with unusually powerful T-cells which confer a genetically based immunity to disease, we may well wonder whether the distinction between the gene and germ models of disease causation is so watertight after all.) Pernick concludes by considering a theme that recurs throughout this volume, the connection between healthcare and human values: "The problem, then, was not that past health sciences *had* values, but that they had *bad* values." Yet can we be sure that this is the correct conclusion from the fact that the eugenicists' values, together with those of some early public health promoters, would be anathema today? One major difference is precisely that we now recognize the importance of values, that we no longer believe – as did Helen Keller, ironically enough – that a jury of objective scientists and doctors could decide which learning-disabled infants should be allowed to die, since "their findings would be free from the prejudice and inaccuracy of untrained observation."

Julian Savulescu's short first-person account, "Parental Choice? Letter from a Doctor as a Dad," examines the risks and benefits of antenatal testing from the viewpoint of two parents who are both medical practitioners, and who describe themselves as at the risk-averse end of the spectrum. Having medical qualifications and knowing something about the evidence of risk levels in amniocentesis and ultrasound does not actually make the decision about what testing to accept any easier; if anything, it seems to make it more difficult. Nor do the parents' medical backgrounds cut a great deal of ice with obstetricians, who are uncompromisingly committed to two "truths": that there is no risk in ultrasound and that ultrasound helps the mother to bond with the fetus. At the end the parents feel that they have "let the child down," although there is no fetal anomaly. This account pairs well with a later one in this collection, Joanna Richards's "But Didn't You Have the Tests?", in Part V.

Finally, in "Do We Really Want to Know the Odds?", David Runciman sums up the complex interrelationship between "objective" risk indicators and the values we attach to them. Analogizing from our attitudes to car and air travel to our attitudes toward medical risks, Runciman argues that even if the probability of death is lower, "we tend to be most frightened of those things that we don't experience very often . . . and of those things that when they go wrong, go wrong irreparably." Because we fly less often than we drive, and because there are rarely survivors of an air as opposed to a car crash, we find flying more frightening than driving a car – an activity that also gives us some illusory sense that we can control what happens to us, which we cannot do in a plane. Runciman notes: "The same applies to illness. The habitual killers that strike on the widest scale are also the ones that have an infrastructure of medical care built around them, so that the risks are at least shrouded in the prospect of recovery." This contamination of objective probabilities by the values we attach to the outcomes will radically undermine any health promotion attempt to teach people what the "real" risks are. As Runciman puts it: "people don't choose the lives they lead according to their understanding of risk; in the end, they choose their understanding of risk according to the lives they lead."

READING GUIDE

The complex relationship between risk and rationality is considered in chapter 3 of Donna Dickenson, *Moral Luck in Medical Ethics and Practical Politics* (Aldershot: Gower, 1991); 2nd edn forthcoming as *Luck and Risk in Medical Ethics* (Cambridge: Polity).

There are a number of sources on what is called in philosophy the problem of induction: the difficulty of generalizing from empirical data to a conclusion that cannot be disproved. Besides the well-known works of Karl Popper, other sources, concerned more with the parallels in theory of probability, include: L. Jonathan Cohen, *The Probable and the Provable* (Oxford: Clarendon Press, 1977); Bruno de Finetti, *The Theory of Probability* (Chichester: John Wiley, 1974); and Charles Nesson's very interesting problem case in "Reasonable doubt and permissible inference: The value of complexity," *Harvard Law Review* (1979), v. 92, pp. 1187–225. How well patients understand probabilities communicated to them about forthcoming interventions is evaluated in a survey of 30 cardiac patients by George Robinson and Avraham Merar, "Informed Consent: Recall by patients tested postoperatively," in Samuel Gorovitz et al. (eds.), *Moral Problems in Medicine* (Englewood Cliffs, NJ: Prentice-Hall, 2nd edn).

10

What Counts as Success in Genetic Counselling?

RUTH F. CHADWICK

The question of what counts as a successful outcome of genetics counselling has recently become critical because of increasing calls for efficiency in health care. Angus Clarke in the *Lancet* has drawn attention to this trend and to the possibility of a desire, coming from management, to measure the efficiency of a medical genetics unit in terms of the number of terminations performed as a result of genetics counselling.[1] His additional concern is that a medical genetics unit might be assessed in terms of its contribution to a national eugenics policy. He suggests instead that efficiency could be measured in terms of workload.

What is Genetic Counselling?

Much turns on what genetics counselling is. Clarke is anxious to distinguish counselling from advice. He writes that whereas advice is a 'prescriptive activity, often subtly authoritarian', genetics counselling is 'informative, supportive and "enabling".'[2] It supports people in reaching their own decisions.

'Genetics counselling' I take to include the following kinds of activity: (a) advising adults, pre-conception, of the probability of their con-ceiving a child suffering from a genetic disorder; (b) advising adults, post-conception, and as a result of some method of fetal screening, as to whether or not a fetus is suffering from a genetic disorder; (c) alerting them to the options open to them.

This account, I think, avoids any suggestion that genetics counselling involves telling people what option they ought to choose. It is not, however, intended to be an exhaustive account of what genetics counsellors do. It omits, for example, the notion of counselling as helping people to live with the consequences of genetic disorders and of their decisions.

So how can we judge its success?

Medical Audit and Number of Terminations

The pressures towards a termination measure are obvious: such an approach would give an outcome that could be measured in numerical terms. Further, the number of terminations could be translated into a figure representing the expected financial saving to the health service of the amount of money that would have been needed to provide care for a child with a genetic disorder.

It may be that we feel an intuitive repugnance towards accepting such a measure of success for a medical genetics service, but we need to look at whether there are any good arguments for opposing it. It will be argued by some that the aim of any medical service ought not to be the termination of life, but this argument will not do here if it is accepted that offering terminations is one acceptable response to the finding of genetic disease. I shall not argue this here. For the purposes of this chapter I shall assume that there are at least some cases in which termination is a morally acceptable outcome.

Clarke's objection to the use of this particular outcome measure is that it would put 'subtle – and possibly less than subtle – pressure upon clinicians to maximise the rate of terminations for "costly" disorders'[3] by, for example, persuading possibly reluctant couples to choose termination.

There is clearly a risk of undesirable consequences for the client–counsellor relationship of using the particular outcome measure outlined. However, there is a further, logical point. There is a contradiction between the proposed outcome measure and the above account of genetic counselling, in terms of facilitating choice.

This was in accordance with respecting the autonomy of clients, respecting their right to choose. If the measure of success is in terms of one particular decision about outcome, how can this be compatible with the autonomy model of health care?

The contradiction only exists if the belief in the value of the autonomy model and the belief in the value of one particular outcome measure are held simultaneously. Perhaps those who put forward the outcome measure do not themselves subscribe to the autonomy model and are suggesting that it itself has to give way.

Interestingly, though, the outcome measure proposal comes from the same stable, politically speaking, as belief in autonomy as a political value. The drive towards what is described as a more efficient health service goes hand in hand with the purported upholding of consumer choice, underpinned by an expressed belief in the value of autonomy.

I have argued in another context[4] that this political ideology in fact distorts the concept of autonomy; that a value whose rationale is to support the freedom of choice of the individual against the power of government and professionals has been brought into the service of the promotion of self-reliance. Being autonomous, rather than meaning self-determining, comes to mean standing on your own two feet, so that a rationalisation is provided for cutting services while apparently upholding freedom of choice, even though in fact the cuts diminish choice.

How does this apply in the present context? I am suggesting that in order to see if there is any contradiction between the advocating of the outcome measure and the upholding of the autonomy model, it is necessary to look at the meaning of autonomy involved. While there may be a contradiction between a belief in freedom of choice and measuring outcomes in terms of one particular decision, the same does not apply if what is valued under the name of autonomy is self-reliance. Both advocate less dependence on public funding for those suffering from genetic disorders.

This makes it clear that if the outcome measure is found unacceptable, it is not just this that has to be argued against, but also the political philosophy that underpins both it and a certain interpretation of autonomy. I would argue further that it *should* be argued against precisely because it does distort the meaning of autonomy for the purpose of denying public responsibility for those in need.

Eugenics

If not the number of terminations, then what? Clarke suggests a workload audit.[5] While a satisfactory workload may be a necessary condition of a service's being successful, however, it is not sufficient. It is necessary to know not just how much work is being done but whether that work is meeting objectives, and those objectives need to be specified. Clarke is anxious to avoid the suggestion that what a medical genetics unit is about is eugenics. He asks, 'Are we concerned with the "genetic health" of the population, of the race? Or are we instead concerned with the concrete individual or family sitting in front of us now, and with providing information and support for them'?[6]

Clarke recognises, rightly, that there is no necessary contradiction here. To decide that one's objectives are concerned with the genetic health of the population is not incompatible with a decision to achieve that by means which show respect and concern for individual clients. But he is worried that conflicts of interest may arise.

The supposed conflict of interest again arises from the worry that if government takes an interest in the genetic health of the population, there may be pressure on individuals to make certain sorts of reproductive decisions.

There are, also, quite widespread fears about potential undesirable longer term consequences of advances in genetic-screening programmes, such as job discrimination against people who are thought to have undesirable genes. Now discrimination on the basis of genes alone is as unjustifiable as discrimination on the basis of race or sex, and must be argued against on the same grounds. Nothing follows from this, however, about the desirability or otherwise of a medical genetics unit being concerned with the incidence of genetic disease in the population as a whole. There are reasons for wanting to reduce the incidence of genetic disease and these are connected with the consequences of genetic diseases for their sufferers.

In fact if medical geneticists do not hold views of this nature, it is difficult to see how they can justify their service, unless they *do* fall into the trap of arguing in terms of money-saving, in the way outlined above.

In an influential article, Bernard Williams drew a distinction between internal and external goals of an activity.[7] An internal goal is one to which the activity is logically connected; an external goal is one to which the activity is only contingently linked. As a matter of logic the goal of a medical genetics service must be connected in some way with the incidence of genetic disease, whether this is expressed in a negative way, in terms of a reduction in the incidence of genetic disease, or in a positive way, in terms of promotion of genetic health. The very fact that geneticists think it desirable to offer their service to individuals shows that

there is at least a presumption that it is undesirable to suffer from genetic disease and that means should be offered of avoiding it.

The concern that Clarke has about its being seen as a eugenics service arises from a confusion about ends and means. The worry arises from the possibility that clinicians will be given targets to fulfil in accordance with a national eugenics policy. He says:

> our funding might depend upon 'units of handicap prevented', which might pressurise parents into screening programmes and then into unwanted terminations with the active collusion of clinical geneticists anxious about their budgets. Such targets could well be set at local level, by district managers, whose overlords could then truthfully deny the existence of a national eugenic policy.[8]

In this scenario not only patient autonomy but also clinical autonomy has given way. In order to restore it, arguments must be found against this threat. What I am suggesting is that it is incorrect to do this by arguing against eugenics as such. In fact Clarke himself says: 'There certainly is a role for public health genetics'.[9] I would go further and suggest that there is a logical connection between a genetics counselling service and public health genetics (the latter being a term with fewer negative associations than eugenics).

But the fact that the genetic health of the population is an objective does not license *any* means whatever towards it, such as pressurising people to make particular choices.

Reproductive Autonomy

A possible objection to the above would be to argue that autonomy, in particular reproductive autonomy, is itself the outcome sought. In other words, the aim of the service is the facilitation of reproductive choice. But then the question arises – why *these* choices? What about sex choice? Should terminations be offered, on autonomy grounds, to parents who want only male children? Clarke himself says 'no' to choices of blue-eyed girls.[10]

There is an important difference between saying that an objective must be pursued by means compatible with autonomy, and saying that autonomy is itself the objective. The goals of the service set limits to the options available.

The autonomy model tells us who should be allowed to choose, not what the objectives should be. The objectives operate within the constraints set by autonomy. It is difficult to conceive of circumstances in which the potential benefit of pressurising a woman into a termination would outweigh the potential harm to her, and to the clinician/client relationship.

Outcomes

What, then, is the measure of a successful outcome? If what is important is autonomous decision-making then what would be required would be some measure of the extent to which individuals feel that they have been helped by the service. Clarke mentions the importance of client satisfaction.[11] One way of measuring this would be a questionnaire to establish the extent to which clients are satisfied. But it has been argued that autonomous decision-making itself cannot be the only criterion of success. If implications for genetic health are important, how can that be measured? A questionnaire would need to elicit the kind of considerations that influenced decision-making, not with a view to measuring success in terms of decisions made, but in order to measure the extent of awareness, brought about by genetics counselling, of factors relevant to genetic disease.

The fact that it has been argued that genetics counsellors must have an eye to the genetic health of the population does, however, raise a question about the extent and nature of the information that can and should be provided. Although it might be argued that the counsellor can convey impartial factual information it is not clear that this is the case. The decisions that people will have to make involve questions about the worthwhileness of lives that future people will live, and whether or not it can be said to be better that someone should not be born. These are philosophical questions. How can individuals be provided with the necessary information to make such choices? Should they be acquainted with the latest moves in the philosophical debate about the value of life?

It might be argued that this would not strictly speaking be *genetics* counselling. It is consistent with what has been argued here, however, that if there *is* concern for genetic health at a national level, and attempts to set national targets, then this information itself should be provided. This might be seen as 'pressurising', but it is arguably preferable to keeping such a policy secret and dressing up a service as promoting individual choice when in fact there are constraints on the choices on offer.

Conclusion

I have argued as follows:

1. An outcome measure for a medical genetics unit that equates success with the number of terminations performed is incompatible with the autonomy model of health care. The latter, and not the former, should be retained.
2. A concern for eugenics, however, is not incompatible with the autonomy model. The one relates to objectives; the other to means. Autonomy should not itself be seen as the objective because in fact there are reasons for limiting choice in this area.
3. The autonomy model tells us who should be allowed to choose but does not tell us what the objectives should be.
4. Given the specified objectives it is arguable that the kind of information conveyed in counselling should include what they are, beyond the immediate context of the individual client. Success consists in individuals making choices in the light of relevant genetic information. A suitable outcome measure would be a questionnaire measuring satisfaction with the service and the reasons given for choice.

NOTES

1   Clarke, A., 'Genetics, ethics and audit', *Lancet* 335 (1990): 1145–7.

2 Ibid, p. 1146.

3 Ibid.

4 Chadwick, R. and Russell, J., 'Hospital discharge of frail elderly people: Social and ethical considerations', *Ageing and Society* 9 (1989): 277–95.

5 Clarke, 'Genetics, ethics and audit', p. 1147.

6 Clarke, A., 'Genetics in medicine: Ethical implications'. Paper presented to the Galton Institute symposium held in London, 22 Sept 1989.

7 Williams, B., 'The idea of equality', in *Problems of the Self* (Cambridge: Cambridge University Press, 1973). Williams does not himself use the 'internal–external' language.

8 Clarke, 'Genetics, ethics and audit', p. 1147.

9 Ibid.

10 Ibid, p. 1146.

11 Ibid, p. 1147.

11

The Genetic Underclass

JAY RAYNER

Science can tell me a lot about my heart. It can tell me what it is doing right now; it can tell me why it is doing it. Science may even be able to tell me what my heart will do in the future. Imagine, for example, that I suffer from primary heart disease, or cardiomyopathy (CM). Until a few years ago, the majority of the one in 10,000 people affected by the most common form – hypertrophic cardiomyopathy, in which the muscle bulks up – discovered they had it only when their heart stopped and they dropped dead. Which is to say they probably never knew anything about it at all. CM is what kills those apparently healthy athletes who keel over on sports fields.

But it needn't kill me. Not immediately, anyway. Because we now live in the age of the Human Genome Project, an international effort to map every one of the body's thousands of genes – the code that defines our hereditary characteristics – and through it we have learned an awful lot about CM. Primarily, we have learned that it is a genetic condition, passed down the family tree from parent to child and on again. [. . .]

Knowing this is a Good Thing. Through genetics, doctors can make a pre-clinical diagnosis. They can catch CM before the major symptom strikes – which, as we know, is sudden, premature death. Avoiding that has to be a Good Thing. They can prescribe drugs, or implant pacemakers, or give advice on lifestyle – all of which should help. So if I turn out to have CM, the science of genetics will have made my life a whole lot easier.

Unless I want to insure it. And if I wanted a mortgage I would have little choice but to do so; no finance company will lend you money on a property unless it has a guaranteed way of getting it all back should you die. But as Carolyn Biro of the Cardiomyopathy Association found, genetic conditions and mortgages do not make happy bedfellows. Her organisation, which represents about 1,000 families affected by the condition, wrote to 20 insurance companies, asking them if they would deal with people who had hypertrophic cardiomyopathy. 'Either they said they wouldn't,' she says, 'or they just didn't reply.'

The problem lies with the £22 billion life insurance industry's natural obsession with risk. When you take out life insurance, contracting with a company to pay a monthly premium in return for them paying out a large lump sum on your death, they want to have some idea of how much longer you are going to live. [. . .]

Until now, the information has been de-cidedly sketchy. Insurers knew if someone smoked or not. They knew if you were male or female. They knew what you did for a living. And that was about it. But the advent of genetic testing has promised to change everything. Now the risk assessors can know if you have the gene for CM or tuberous sclerosis or breast cancer. And then they can refuse to insure you. All too often, that's exactly what they are doing. While the medical fraternity is doing its best to create solutions to rarefied problems, the insur-ance men are doing their best to create a genetic underclass.

[. . .]

Wendy Watson's case is a good example of how lack of understanding puts people at risk of being unfairly discriminated against because of their genes. Three years ago, she became the first woman in Britain to have a full double mastectomy as a preventative measure against hereditary breast cancer. Nine women in her immediate family had died of the disease, and even before scientists had identified the gene, she had concluded that in her case it was an inherited condition – and a killer. Shortly after the operation, she was proved right. The gene was discovered and she tested positive.

About 5 per cent of breast cancer cases in Britain are believed to be gene-related. Before the operation, Wendy had about a 90 per cent chance of developing cancer. Now her doctors tell her the chances are negligible, indeed lower than the one-in-12 risk for women who don't carry the gene. Even though she had life insur-ance already, we asked Wendy to apply to a number of companies for £90,000 cover. While Scottish Widows said it was happy to provide the cover at no extra cost, Norwich Union said it thought it would have to charge her more but wanted to put the case before its medical committee.

To confuse matters further, Wendy's 14-year-old daughter Rebecca would definitely be able to get life insurance at standard rates, even though she has a 50 per cent chance of having the gene and thus almost the same chance of developing the disease. The insurance com-panies will never know anything about this. Any insurance form will simply ask Rebecca if

her mother has suffered from cancer, to which she can honestly answer no. Because she has not been tested for the gene, she need make no mention of the great likelihood that she carries it. Statistically, Rebecca will be one of the worst risks – but she will come out as a perfect client because insurers know so little about genetics.

'They don't really understand these things at all,' says Wendy, 'and I don't think they should be altering people's premiums on the basis of so little information.'

The Watsons are fortunate, however. Wendy obtained her life insurance before she was diag-nosed, and her daughter can now do likewise. Mick Newing was not so lucky. He is a classic example of someone thrust unfairly into the genetic underclass. Like another one in 10,000 of the population, Mick – a 39-year-old indus-trial cleaner from Barnstaple – is affected by a genetic condition called tuberous sclerosis (TS). Sufferers have growths on the brain (and other organs) which calcify with age and become hard or sclerotic. Because it affects the brain, the symptoms can be very severe, ranging from epileptic fits to major learning difficulties, as well as heart and kidney problems. It can also reduce life expectancy.

But the emphasis here must be on the word 'can', a distinction that seems to have eluded the insurance industry. More than 50 per cent of people with TS are intellectually normal and lead perfectly ordinary lives; their only symp-tom is a slight skin rash. That is all Mick suffers from. 'I suppose I had a sense of having some-thing as a kid,' he says, 'but I wasn't sure what. It was just a case of doctors having a look at me and concluding that whatever I had wasn't too serious. Basically, they were right.'

Mick only discovered he had TS when his son Matthew was born five years ago and suffered a number of fits soon after birth. It didn't take long for doctors to work out that Mick had the condition as well, and that he had passed it on to Matthew. The genetic mutation started with Mick himself and affects no other members of his family.

Like many people, he only thought about getting life insurance when he became a parent for the first time. 'I applied to Allied Dunbar but they turned me down flat,' he says. 'I then tried other places but they rejected me, too, because I had to declare on the form that Allied Dunbar had turned me down.' His insurance broker later told him that one company had a simple policy of not covering anybody with the condition. 'It's ludicrous. I'm not on any medication; I'm not mentally affected; I've been driving since I was 18 and I've never had a claim. I suppose I'm getting over it now, but at the time the refusals made me feel like I was a prisoner of the disease and that nobody would touch me. The insurance companies need to be seriously educated.'

He is attempting to get an endowment mortgage which requires life cover and has been advised by his doctors to appeal to the same company if it turns him down the first time, rather than trying to move on to another. It was a strategy that worked for Alec Garrett, a 27-year-old interior landscape gardener from Strathclyde, whose experience shows just how far a little education can go. Like Mick, his TS symptoms are very slight. He has a facial rash and suffered one epileptic fit in 1988. Since then he has been on medication and has experienced no others.

'The moment I applied for life insurance, the brokers turned me down,' he says. 'They refused it without even looking into my condition. They just wrote me off.' His broker was apologetic, as well he might be. He had met a healthy man with a perfectly normal life expectancy – and his company had turned him down. Alec decided to take them on, going for medicals, consulting professors of medicine, gathering the evidence. The insurance company had played judge and jury. In turn, Alec became the defence barrister representing his own body. He fought to prove that, however TS might affect some people, he was innocent of major medical dysfunction. He won.

'All the evidence was presented to them, and from refusing me for one specific kind of insurance cover they went to telling me I was eligible for any kind of insurance cover I wanted – and at no extra cost.'

The key, according to insurance man Russell Veitch, is learning to play the system. Not that it always works. Veitch is an insurance man who cannot get himself insured. Three years ago his brother Christopher stuttered to an early death through cardiomyopathy, finally succumbing to the disease while awaiting a heart transplant, the most radical kind of treatment there is for the condition. Shortly afterwards the whole family went through a raft of tests, culminating in genetic testing as part of the research work at St George's Hospital. The results were a classic example of root and branch genetic disease.

As well as Christopher, Russell has two other brothers. All of them carry the gene. All four of his nieces and nephews have it, as does one of his own sons. All have symptoms of one form or another, and a number are on medication. 'So far I've managed to get my son and my two nieces covered for life insurance, but I can't do anything about myself,' he says. 'Basically, if I can get them to an insurer young enough, the company accepts it. My son was 18 when I got him insured, so it was OK. If they were taking medication, it was a problem; if they weren't, it wasn't.'

The key, he says, is to give the companies as much information as possible. 'But there's still a limit to what I can do,' he adds, 'and personally I don't understand the mindset of the insurance companies. The protocols vary enormously from one firm to another. It really is quite a shock to find yourself uninsurable.'

The irony is that a family like Russell's may be less of a risk – not more – specifically because they have been diagnosed. As with all the families under the supervision of the team at St George's, their condition is constantly monitored through regular health screening. So far, the doctors have picked up three kinds of cancers (in early, treatable stages) among their patients, which almost certainly would have killed them long before cardiomyopathy kicked in. The same is true with any genetic condition where a diagnosis has occurred. That individual is going to be far more health-conscious than the thousands of others clogging up the actuarial tables with their strokes and heart disease, simply because they have a clear and distinct understanding of personal health risk.

[. . .]

Unsurprisingly the insurance industry has refused to be pinned down on its plans, but at least accepts that the question of genetic testing needs to be addressed. In 1995, Spencer Leigh, chief underwriter for Royal Life in Liverpool, submitted a paper to the Institute of Actuaries in London called 'The Freedom to Underwrite'. It is a jolly document, each chapter headed by a quote from a Bob Dylan or Leonard Cohen song about just how much of a bummer life can be. While it does not represent the official position of the industry, it certainly puts forward the view of a large cross-section of it.

Leigh argues that it is reasonable for insurers to take an interest in the results of genetic tests already taken, a position with which few would disagree. Insurance is about assessing risk, and anything that helps companies do that has to be acceptable. Leigh, however, goes on to claim that the industry is more than competent to use such information. 'From a theoretical viewpoint, and assuming [insurance] offices act responsibly, we are invariably right. This is not arrogance because, looked at objectively, anybody would have to concede the arguments... Life offices employ eminent consultant physicians as chief medical officers, and so they have access to the best medical advice.' But even the most eminent doctors can disagree on this whole issue.

Whether genetic testing will become a fundamental part of insurance depends on social attitudes. 'If genetic tests become a regular and acceptable routine which people regard as part of a regular health check, they could become part of the underwriting process. If not, then it is unlikely that the underwriters will call for genetic testing except to clarify the position on a person with an already identified problem.' Next he takes up Massow's scenario: 'Think of the people who have favourable genetic tests,' he writes. 'Would they not want to use this information to obtain standard terms, or even to request discounts? They might object strongly to not being allowed to use this information to obtain more favourable rates.'

[...]

The Human Genome Project promises a glorious future. The more we know about our genes and the diseases carried by them, the more we can do to cure ourselves. At some point the science should make us all healthier, happier people. But that really is only in the future and, like the past, the future is another country. For the time being, diagnosis is far ahead of treatment and so long as this remains the case, thousands of people will find themselves discriminated against every year. They will be forced to become an underclass – not by their own fecklessness, or even by that of their parents, but by a mutation on a gene which may have occurred generations before they were even conceived.

12

Ethical Issues in Pre-Cancer Testing: The Parallel with Huntington's Disease

DONNA L. DICKENSON

Genetic testing and screening for susceptibility to various forms of cancer raise ethical issues about consent, confidentiality, the professional–patient relationship, and duties of care toward third parties, such as family members. The questions are both broad – because they cover so many core areas of medical ethics – and frustrating – because genetic knowledge for cancer remains imperfect. In this chapter I want to do two things that may alleviate some of the frustration. First, I want to look primarily at one set of ethical questions out of the many that arise: decisions about whether genetically susceptible individuals should have children. The ethical debate about pre-cancer testing and screening, at least in the West,[1] has so far largely centered on the affected individual's right to know, together with the confidentiality of that information. In practical terms this may be understandable, given the conflicting interests of those tested and their employers, health providers, and insurers. But an equally pressing issue is the decision whether or not to have children, if testing reveals a strong familial tendency towards breast, bowel, or any of the other cancers that are thought to have a genetic component. Is it morally wrong to transmit the risk to the next generation? I will be drawing on a case study from UK clinical practice, about "Peter" – a young man whose father tested positive for Huntington's disease shortly before his death. But Peter did not want to know his own genetic status, although he and his wife had young children and were considering having more.

I shall thus suggest that we can gain a better grip on the issues involved in pre-cancer testing by looking at genetic testing for quite a different condition. This is the second way of making the ethical issues in pre-cancer testing less frustrating. There, the imprecision that marks genetic testing at the pre-cancer level is replaced by something much more akin to black and white. What we have in the case of Huntington's disease is a small population of at-risk individuals – compared with an enormous population at risk for one form of cancer or another – whose probability of developing the disease is accurately predictable with a low error rate mutation test – compared to much fuzzier probabilities in the case of cancer. By using Huntington's disease as an extreme limit of questions about risk, benefit, and certainty of the testing procedure, we can suggest parallels that may help us to predict with greater clarity the ethical issues which will arise as pre-cancer testing and screening become more sophisticated. Because Huntington's disease is an autosomal dominant condition, because the condition is not multi-factorial, and because the test procedure is very accurate, the issues about testing for Huntington's disease are less confused, although no less troubling, than those for pre-cancer testing.

Let us take these differences one by one, together with their ethical impact:

1. The *risk of genetic transmission* from affected individual to child is 50 percent for Huntington's disease, a far higher correlation than for any cancers. In a philosophical utilitarian calculus, at least, it is more wrong to choose to have children if you have a condition with a high probability of affecting the next generation than if your condition has only a slight chance of being transmitted. This is particularly true *if high probability of transmitting the condition* combines with *low probability of curing the disease* once it has been transmitted. A progressive disease of the central nervous system, Huntington's most commonly manifests itself in middle age, with death occurring inexorably between 15 and 20 years later. Although genetic transplantation techniques may eventually offer some promise, at the time of writing the disease was effectively incurable.

2. *Single-factor* conditions such as Huntington's disease are *simpler to predict*. No other risks, such as environmental factors, enter the equation: if you have the genetic mutation on chromosome 4, you will definitely develop Huntington's disease, although the exact time of onset is less predictable. The converse is that at present there is nothing that the affected person can do to prevent the disease. So there is arguably no benefit in knowing your genetic status, and possibly a great deal of anguish. The ethical question then becomes whether it is wrong for healthcare professionals to impart adverse information about genetic status – even if someone consents to be tested.[2]

3. There are effectively *no false positives or false negatives* in the testing procedure for Huntington's disease. The single genetic mutation for the condition can now be identified with

great predictive accuracy in a test involving numbers of repeats of the gene, isolated in March 1993. As of 1995, the screening procedure had been tested on approximately 4,000 patients, amassing a record of very few false results. The ethical effect of this unusually great degree of certainty is two-edged. Clinicians do not run the risk of falsely worrying a patient who will not develop the condition, but they cannot offer hope either: any positive is a true positive. Even asking someone to come for testing alerts them to the possibility that something is wrong: in that sense the patient is not consenting entirely of their own free will to being given the information about their genetic status.[3] And if disclosure of an unfavorable genetic status takes away all hope, clinicians in some cultures might be unwilling to test at all. For example, in rural Italy preservation of the cancer patient's tranquillity is more important to family and doctors alike than is the full knowledge and control that Northern Europeans and Americans value.[4] We must be cautious about generalizing from what has been called the western "autonomy-control narrative."[5]

So now, the "Peter" case study, taken from a large UK psychiatric teaching hospital.[6] Peter's 73-year-old father, "Henry," had been diagnosed with atypical Alzheimer's disease, but his symptoms were still not fully explained. The family history, however, included a number of other members who had manifested jerky movements or dementia late in life. Henry's clinical team decided to request permission from his family to use the newly available genetic test for Huntington's disease, which revealed a positive result.[7] But after Henry's death ten days later, it became clear that neither his wife "Mary," his son "Peter," nor his daughter "Ann" had fully understood the implications for themselves and other family members of giving their consent to testing Henry. Henry's wife Mary wanted to test everyone in the family immediately: the four grandchildren, in addition to the son and daughter. Peter, himself a healthcare worker, was determined that he did not want to know his genetic status – to the doctors' dismay, since Peter had two young children and was of an age to father more. Henry's daughter Ann wanted to be tested immediately, without any genetic counseling. She was glad that the issue had been brought out into the open; Peter wished he had never been told.

This case raises unusual issues about ownership of information and informed consent. When the family gave their consent to have Henry tested, the son and daughter, at least, were also consenting to a certain level of torment about their own genetic status. Even more important, the case raises important questions about rationality and the possession of full information. Philosophers have tended to associate rationality with possession of full information,[8] and autonomy with an instrumental model of rationality, one about using reason to satisfy preferences. Arguments in favor of informed consent in turn rest on autonomy and rationality: a rational autonomous individual wants to know as much as possible before making treatment decisions. The usual dynamic in medical ethics has been the demand for more information from the patient, against paternalistic secrecy from the clinician. So, again, this case looks odd. Here we have clinicians who want the (prospective) patient, Peter, to know his genetic status – but Peter doesn't want to know.

Is it *irrational* for Peter not to want to know whether he has inherited the gene for Huntington's disease? Is it *unethical* not to want to know? The archetypically rational individual wants information for instrumental purposes, in order to act so as to produce the best possible outcome, avoiding mistakes deriving from inadequate reflection.[9] But if Peter does carry the Huntington's disease genetic mutation, there are no mistakes to avoid and no treatment decisions to make: there is simply no possible treatment. In a twist on the notion of rationality as possession of full information, it might well be rational for Peter not to want to know. Let us assume he does carry the genetic mutation, and that he will begin to develop symptoms within ten years. Perhaps the best possible outcome, given that the disease will progress inexorably once it begins, is for him to enjoy ten years' comparative peace of mind beforehand. But can Peter really return to an innocent state of total ignorance? He does not consent to be tested

himself, but, at the time he consented to have his father tested, he knew that the results would affect the entire family. It now seems hypocritical of him to maintain that ignorance would be bliss. This is particularly true because Peter and his wife "Beth" could well have more children. Peter's ignorance is not going to be Beth's bliss. So far, he has kept the true cause of Henry's death and the ensuing family debate from her. But she needs to know, before she undergoes another pregnancy, whether she is bearing a child who may die of Huntington's disease. Peter and Beth's existing children may not need to know their genetic status yet, but the couple need to know Peter's risk level in order to plan as best they can for their individual and collective futures.

The issue is not the particular level of risk; it is who has a right to know. Because Beth has rights in the matter too, Peter's secrecy would be just as wrong even if his risk of developing a fatal disease were less than 50 percent, or if the chances of recovery were higher than nil. Another way of putting the issue is this: to whom does Peter owe a duty? Philosophers have discussed the problem of future generations in terms of what duties we owe to hypothetical individuals – when it is difficult enough to spell out our duties to those in the land of the living. But in this case, it seems plausible that Peter can even have duties to those descendents whom he will not have, whose birth Peter and Beth will want to prevent if Peter does carry the gene. Yet this is primarily Peter's duty; the clinical team does not have the duty to divulge his genetic status, on his behalf, any more than your failure to give to charity gives me the duty to take the wallet out of your pocket and hand it over to Oxfam.

All this is instructive for pre-cancer testing and screening. Although genetic information is normally seen as belonging solely to the affected individual, and therefore as subject to stringent confidentiality even from other family members, it is family property in a way that other medical data are not.[10] By definition, as germ-line data, genetic information concerns other generations, other family members: it is about them too. But their rights are enforceable vis à vis other family members, not clinicians. It is Peter who has the duty to inform Beth, not the doctors. He cannot avoid this duty by saying that he does not know his own genetic status; he ought to want to know it, in order to fulfill his duties toward his wife and prospective children. Although he may be acting rationally in not wanting to know, he is not acting ethically.

This conclusion imposes strong obligations on Peter, but it might be criticized for imposing few on the doctors. On the other hand, it does not absolve clinicians who let how much to inform depend on the level of risk.[11] The implications about risk and rights are strenuous; the right to know does not vary with the level of risk. Beth would have had just as great a claim to know Peter's genetic status, given the possibility of future pregnancies, if there were only a 1 percent risk of transmission to the next generation, not 50 percent. And the legitimate claims of others should make clinicians less troubled about whether it is right to impart adverse genetic information to family members who might be affected. Those individuals' rights to sensitive communication and skillful counseling remain important;[12] but they do not extend to the right not to know, when exercise of that right is likely to harm others.

NOTES

1 For an alternative approach stressing family ramifications which may be more typical of non-western views, see Hoshino, K., "Bioethical concerns with rights of patients receiving genetic tests." Paper delivered at the UICC Symposium on Familial Cancer and Prevention, Kobe, Japan, May 14, 1997.

2 However, one study indicates that there is no greater psychological morbidity for patients informed that they have tested positive for the Huntington's marker than for those who were told they had a negative status. But there is already a high prevalence of affective psychological disorders in persons at risk for Huntington's disease. See Brandt, J., "Ethical considerations in genetic testing: An empirical study of presymptomatic

diagnosis of Huntington's disease," in K. W. M. Fulford, G. Gillett, and J. Soskice (eds.), Medicine and Moral Reasoning (Cambridge: Cambridge University Press, 1994).

3 Elgesem, D., "Patient rights and the management of personal information." Paper given at the sixth workshop of the European Biomedical Ethics Practitioner Education project, Naantali, Finland, September 6, 1996.

4 Gordon, D. R. and Paci, E., "Disclosure practices and cultural narratives: Understanding concealment and silence around cancer in Tuscany, Italy," Social Science and Medicine (November 1995).

5 Ibid. Blackhall et al. found that Korean Americans and Mexican Americans were significantly less likely than European Americans and African Americans to value patient autonomy and rights in relation to disclosure of a terminal diagnosis and ongoing care decisions. They also felt that the family should be the main decision-making authority about the use of life support, and that it should not be up to the individual patient. (Blackhall, L. J. et al., "Ethnicity and attitudes toward patient autonomy," JAMA 274/10 (1995): 820–5.)

6 First published in Dickenson, D., "Carriers of genetic disorder and the right to have children," Acta Geneticae Medicae et Gemellologiae 44: (1995): 75–80.

7 Although next of kin have no right in English law to give or withhold consent to treatment, the clinicians felt obliged to consult the family because Henry's competence fluctuated.

8 Brandt, R., A Theory of the Good and the Right (Oxford: Clarendon Press, 1979), p. 10.

9 Ibid, p. 153.

10 For a similar argument about gametes, see Dickenson, D., "Procuring gametes for research and therapy: the case for unisex altruism," Journal of Medical Ethics 23/2 (1997): 93–5.

11 As is legitimate in United Kingdom consent doctrine: Sidaway v. Board of Governors of the Bethlem Royal Hospital and Maudsley Hospital [1985] AC 871 1 All ER 643, HL.

12 Chadwick, R., "What counts as success in genetic counselling?" Journal of Medical Ethics 19 (1993): 43–6.

13

Eugenics and Public Health in American History

MARTIN S. PERNICK

Introduction

Supporters of eugenics, the powerful early 20th-century movement for improving human heredity, often attacked that era's dramatic improvements in public health and medicine for preserving the lives of people they considered hereditarily unfit.[1] However, American public health and eugenics had much in common as well. [...]

Like such other turn-of-the-century catchwords as *progressivism* and *efficiency*, the term *eugenics* encompassed a large and shifting constellation of meanings. The term was first popularized by Charles Darwin's cousin Sir Francis Galton, who defined it as the science of improving heredity. American eugenicists sponsored a diverse range of activities, including statistically sophisticated analyses of disease inheritance, "better baby contests" modeled on rural livestock shows, forced sterilization of criminals and the retarded, selective ethnic restrictions on immigration, and even euthanasia for those deemed unfit to live.[2] These and other programs were seen as eugenic because they all aimed at improving human heredity. But that common denominator also allowed many divergent responses to such key questions as

- What does "improvement" mean?
- What does "heredity" mean?
- By what methods should heredity be improved?
- Who has the authority to answer the other questions?

Disputes over these issues produced very different competing concepts of eugenics[3] and its relationship to public health.

Eugenics vs Public Health

Many eugenicists regarded disease as nature's way of weeding out the unfit. Charles Davenport, America's foremost eugenic scientist, warned in 1915, "The artificial preservation of those whom the operation of natural agencies tends to eliminate...may conceivably destroy the race." He considered it "anti-social" to "unduly restrict the operation of what is one of Nature's greatest racial blessings – death."[4]

His comments exemplified the close kinship between eugenics and earlier Social Darwinist and Malthusian attacks on public health and social welfare programs, a link that remained powerful throughout the history of eugenics.

A speaker at the 1914 National Conference on Race Betterment, the first major American eugenics conference, explained that "death is the normal process of elimination in the social organism, and . . . in prolonging the lives of defectives we are tampering with the functioning of the social kidneys."[5] A speaker at the last such American meeting, the Third International Congress on Eugenics in New York in 1932, echoed the same view: "The growth of sanitation, hygiene, and State medicine . . . attempts to secure an ever-increasing survival rate for the least competent types. . . . This interference with Natural Selection [is] disastrous."[6] Leading eugenics popularizer Michael Guyer summarized the argument: "[O]ur improved methods of sanitation and care of the sick . . . so eased the rigors of . . . *natural selection* that decadent stocks . . . are increasing relatively faster than normal stocks."[7]

A second point of contention between public health and eugenics concerned the role of heredity in infectious diseases. Public health officials generally attributed the era's unprecedented decline in infections to the success of new preventive techniques based on bacteriology and immunology, from water filtration to vaccinations. In the case of tuberculosis, bacteriologists took particular pride in having disproved earlier beliefs that the disease was inherited.[8] Yet many eugenicists continued to claim that infections, from tuberculosis to syphilis to infant diarrheas, *were* hereditary.

Historians often ridicule such claims as an unscientific repudiation of the germ theory.[9] However, the struggle between eugenics and public health for jurisdiction over infectious diseases cannot be dismissed that simply. Eugenicists accepted that germs were necessary to cause infections, but they believed that hereditary resistance was the best way to cure and prevent them. One speaker told the Third International Congress, "It has been known for a good while that . . . infections are caused by germ invasions, [but] it needs to be remembered that in most cases medical science is wholly impotent to cure a disease without the aid of the . . . resistance of the individual, and the degree . . . of such resistance is inborn and hereditary."[10] Such arguments were one side of a debate between eugenics and bacteriology concerning which science offered the best techniques for fighting infections. Each side could appeal to both science and logic.

Rivalries such as this one were increasingly characteristic of early 20th-century health sciences. The competition between microbiology and eugenics, like the era's many other similar disputes, was triggered by the emergence of professional specialization. [. . .] Such controversies constituted both a struggle for professional power and a substantive contest over incompatible values fostered by the emergence of separate specialty professional cultures.

Early 20th-century health scientists and Progressive Era social reformers expected specialization to be simply an efficient division of labor. So long as each social or medical specialty followed the same supposedly objective scientific method, each would produce complementary solutions. This faith in the harmonious efficiency of scientific specialization was a central feature of Progressive Era medicine and social reform. But to the extent that differing subjective interests and values proved intrinsic to both medical science and social policy, specialization resulted in competition, not complementarity. The conflict between eugenics and public health resulted in large part from the different values, interests, and methods fostered by two competing medical specialties.[11]

Yet at a deeper level, such conflicts were exacerbated, ironically, by a basic value the opponents shared: the faith that their common allegiance to the scientific method would eliminate such subjective sources of disagreement. To the extent that each side believed in the objective validity of its own science's methods, opposing conclusions could only be attributed to the opponents' bad science or bad faith.

Eugenic Affinities with Public Health

[. . .]

Public health agencies and eugenics organizations often overlapped in goals and methods, programs, and personnel. Many public health institutions included eugenics in their official duties. [. . .] Likewise, eugenic institutions actively promoted nongenetic programs for general health. [...]

This overlap in organizations resulted from important underlying similarities in values and ideas. Thus, many eugenics supporters rejected the claim that disease selectively killed the "unfit." They argued that hereditary resistance to disease was not a sign of overall genetic superiority and insisted that some highly advantageous traits were actually correlated with heightened susceptibility to particular diseases. The 1912 American translation of a book by Socialist eugenicist and child welfare pioneer Sigmund Engel attacked the "ultra-Darwinian" view that spontaneous infant mortality was beneficial, noting that the leading childhood diseases killed the fit and the unfit alike.[12] E. Blanche Sterling, a child hygiene worker for the Public Health Service, reminded the Third International Congress that "in laying so much stress on the fact that we are saving the unfit, the fact that we are also saving the fit seems to have been forgotten.... Very superior stock...may have no immunity to certain serious diseases and it is our privilege to aid in preserving such strains."[13] These views were especially common among women social reformers and child health advocates, for whom eugenics meant not simply "good genes" but "better babies."[14] This debate over whether disease deaths were dysgenic combined scientific and value issues. The unresolved empirical questions included whether disease resistance was hereditary and whether any such hereditary resistance was positively or negatively correlated with other desirable traits. The value issues included which hereditary traits were judged to be beneficial and which traits should be valued most if disease susceptibility turned out to be correlated with something good, such as intelligence.

In addition, regardless of whether disease aided natural selection, many eugenicists opposed relying on nature's slow, cruel mechanism of Darwinian evolution. They considered eugenics to mean "artificial selection," the active intentional control of reproduction to achieve nature's goals by more efficient means. Pioneer eugenic popularizers Paul Popenoe and John Harvey Kellogg explained to the 1914 Race Betterment Conference that the death of

"weaklings" constituted "Nature's way, the old method of natural selection." However, nature's methods were inefficient and inhumane; natural selection therefore "must be supplanted" by eugenic selection.[15] Thus, eugenics and public health could cooperate instead of competing. Public health could continue to prevent the deaths of the unfit so long as eugenics prevented the unfit from passing on their defects.

[...]

Convergence of Genes and Germs

Such arguments show that, even in the hotly contested arena of infection control, eugenics and public health could converge as well as compete. For a variety of reasons that illustrate how the meanings of both eugenics and public health were shaped by the interrelation of science and culture, eugenics sometimes was defined to include antibacterial measures.

First, it was widely believed that some of the damage done to people by infections could be biologically inherited by their descendants. In the 19th century, such beliefs had been based on the Lamarckian view that acquired traits could become hereditary. Thus, reform-minded 19th-century eugenicists urged the adoption of public health measures to prevent epidemics from becoming hereditary and to produce health improvements that might themselves be inherited. Such ideas retained support well into the early 20th century.[16]

By the 1910s, however, scientists generally accepted August Weismann's opposite hypothesis – that environmentally caused changes in the body could not cause corresponding changes in the hereditary "germ plasm." Yet even Weismann's disciples believed that some infections were "germ poisons" that could damage the germ plasm in ways that could be inherited. In this view, catching malaria or typhoid did not cause your children to inherit those specific diseases, but the high fevers they produced might cause other kinds of birth defects that would be passed on. The scientific reasoning had changed, but the practical conclusion remained the same: that fighting infections could help reduce hereditary disease as well.

Germs and genes also were seen as specific, reductionist causes of disease, more technical and less subjective than the broad array of personal and social conditions previously blamed for causing bad health. Progressive Era health reformers still sought to change individual behavior and social conditions, but both germs and genes provided precise targets for these reform efforts, thus making them seem more objective and efficient.[17]

Second, broad linguistic and cultural associations linked heredity and contagion. Infections were caused by germs; inheritance was governed by germ plasm. In both cases, "germs" meant microscopic seeds. Both types of germs enabled disease to propagate and grow, to spread contamination from the bodies of the diseased to the healthy. The association was strengthened by the identification of blood as a medium of infection for diseases such as malaria, and by the introduction of blood tests for infections from typhoid to syphilis. Blood, the age-old metaphor for heredity, became identified as a vehicle for infection as well. Having "bad blood" meant you were contaminated and contaminating, whether the specific agent was a germ or the germ plasm.[18]

Eugenics could even be expanded to include not just germ fighting but virtually all of public health. While eugenics aimed at improving heredity, the meaning of *heredity* could reach far beyond genetics. In both common usage and some scientific literature, calling a trait "hereditary" meant that "you got it from your parents," regardless of whether "it" was transmitted by genes or germs, precepts or probate. The Public Health Service film *The Science of Life* defined a man's heredity as "what he receives from his ancestors."[19]

This expansive definition was based not on wrong science but on broader moral concerns. Attributing something to heredity meant holding the parents morally responsible for having caused it, not necessarily specifying the technical mechanism through which parental responsibility operated. By this definition of heredity, *eugenics* meant not just having good genes but also being a good parent, raising good children, or promoting good health for future generations.[20] This version of eugenics was virtually synonymous with public health.

The similarities between infection and heredity also led to parallels in the methods of disease prevention adopted by public health and eugenics. Eugenicists urged the "segregation" of defectives in institutions, isolating them from society and from members of the opposite sex to prevent their reproduction and the consequent spread of hereditary disease. Such eugenic segregation directly echoed the centuries-old effort to stop the spread of infections through quarantine. The term *segregation* itself first was used medically in the mid-19th century to mean "selective isolation" or "quarantine."[21] Infectious germs and bad germ plasm could also be stopped from spreading by a new method called sterilization. In both eugenics and bacteriology, to *sterilize* meant to eliminate the agents that reproduced disease.[22]

[. . .]

The goals of early 20th-century public health and eugenics also converged to promise the permanent eradication of disease rather than just the reduction of morbidity. Such a thorough and lasting elimination of illness now seemed attainable owing to new concepts in both bacteriology and genetics. Although the similarities between them were not much noted then or since, August Weismann's theory of heredity and Louis Pasteur's view of infection each implied that disease could be not just reduced but eradicated. Both Weismann's rejection of Lamarckian inheritance and Pasteur's refutation of the spontaneous generation of microbes were presented as demonstrations that diseases could not be spawned anew by a bad environment but could only come from specific preexisting seeds. Thus, if all disease germs and all defective germ plasm could be completely wiped out, the diseases they caused would become extinct and could never return. Pasteur and Weismann each made permanent disease eradication seem possible, enabling both eugenics and public health to promise "final solutions" to both infectious and hereditary diseases.[23]

Eugenics is notorious today for having promoted bigoted concepts of illness, in which race, class, ethnic, religious, and sexual prejudices determined who was defined as unfit. Eugenics leaders regularly portrayed African Americans and Native Americans as loathsome, disease-doomed races.[24] Eugenicists also routinely ranked the genetic worth of various European "races." Harvey Wiley summed up what he alleged to be the overwhelming eugenic consensus when he told the readers of *Good Housekeeping* in 1922, "[I]t is universally acknowledged that descendants of the Scotch and Irish Presbyterians . . . have always shown themselves to be a superior people."[25] J. G. Wilson, a Public Health Service doctor in charge of examining immigrants on New York's Ellis Island, wrote in the 1913 *Popular Science Monthly*, "[T]he Jews are a highly inbred and psychopathically inclined race" whose defects are "almost entirely due to heredity." That Jews disagreed with his diagnosis simply confirmed its validity: "The general paranoid attitude of the race is shown in an almost universal tendency to fail to appreciate the point of view of the one who opposes them."[26]

But eugenics was not unique among the health sciences in diagnosing social outcasts as diseased. Medical justifications for racial slavery predated Darwin and Galton, and even in its heyday, eugenics had no monopoly on scientific racism. Bacteriology, not just genetics, was also commonly used to label other races as diseased.[27] Both eugenics and microbiology contributed to the assumptions about racial epidemiology that shaped the Public Health Service's decision to use African-American men for the Tuskegee study of untreated syphilis.[28]

By emphasizing heredity as the engine of human progress, eugenics expanded the medical importance of ancestry and race. But the identification of which specific races were good or bad was not intrinsic to eugenics. Instead, these diagnoses medicalized broader cultural biases. The specific values that shaped eugenic definitions of disease reflected the eugenicists' primarily White, native, middle-class, professional backgrounds, characteristics they shared with many other professionals, including many public health officials.[29]

Past and Present

Cultural values thus deeply influenced past eugenics and public health proponents in their definitions of disease and their responses to it.

The point is not that, in the benighted past, pure genetics or bacteriology were corrupted by extraneous social concerns. Rather, this history provides some particularly vivid examples of how cultural values have been integral to every effort to define and fight disease. Past eugenics and public health included values most thoughtful people now consider anathema. The problem, then, was not that past health sciences *had* values, but that they had *bad* values.

Racism and other social prejudices became part of both eugenics and public health in the past, not just because these values were prevalent among health professionals, but because health professionals convinced themselves that their sciences were purely objective. Helen Keller, the famed blind and deaf advocate for the disabled, captured the power of this faith when she urged letting doctors select which mentally impaired infants to let die. "A jury of physicians considering the case of an idiot would be exact and scientific. Their findings would be free from the prejudice and inaccuracy of untrained observation."[30] This widely shared faith in objectivity did not succeed in eliminating subjective values from medicine, but it did serve to delegitimate the openly political and ethical debate that is necessary if a culture is to assess its value judgments intelligently.

In pointing out that there were similarities as well as differences between eugenics and public health, this [chapter] refutes two comforting but simplistic notions: that eugenics was uniquely value laden, unscientific, and prejudiced; and that any science that is valid and well-intentioned can have nothing in common with eugenics. Some of what was done in the name of eugenics was also done in the name of infection control and public health. Eugenics was not an isolated movement whose significance is confined to the histories of genetics and pseudoscience. It is an important and cautionary part of past public health and of general medical history as well.[31]

However, historical similarities are not moral equivalents. Their intertwined past certainly does not mean that public health was "as bad" as eugenics or that human genetics is "as good" as public health today. Past similarities between eugenics and public health serve as an alarm clock for all the health sciences, not as a lullaby for genetics.

NOTES

Support was provided by the National Library of Medicine, the National Endowment for the Humanities, the Spencer Foundation, the Burroughs Wellcome Fund, and the University of Michigan. An earlier version of this [chapter] was presented in a series of lectures on the history of public health at the University of Michigan School of Public Health, Ann Arbor, February 19, 1997. Susan Reverby and the editors of this issue provided helpful advice. The seeds were planted in conversations with Barbara Gutmann Rosenkrantz.

1 Today, terms such as *unfit* or *defective* are pejorative and offensive. However, early 20th-century eugenicists considered them to be objective technical diagnoses. At that time, simply using such terms did not necessarily indicate intentional conscious hostility. Nevertheless, this paper argues that, despite this belief in their objectivity, these labels were inherently value based. These terms are used here not to endorse but to understand the values implicit in them and the claims for their objectivity.

2 The forgotten story of eugenic euthanasia in America is documented in Martin S. Pernick, *The Black Stork: Eugenics and the Death of "Defective" Babies in American Medicine and Motion Pictures since 1915* (New York, NY: Oxford University Press, 1996). See also Francis Galton, "Eugenics: Its definition, scope, and aims," in *Essays in Eugenics* (New York: Garland Press, 1985 [1909]), p. 35.

3 The literature on eugenics is vast. For an introduction to American eugenics, see Diane Paul, *Controlling Human Heredity 1865 to the Present* (Atlantic Highlands, NJ: Humanities Press, 1996). To place America in a comparative context, see Daniel Kevles, *In the Name of Eugenics* (New York: Knopf, 1985).

4 Charles Davenport, quoted in "Was the doctor right?" *Independent*, January 3, 1916: 23. See also *A Decade of Progress in Eugenics: Scientific Papers of the Third International Congress of Eugenics* (Baltimore, MD: Williams and Wilkins, 1934), pp. 196, 289–93, 300–13; and Pernick, *Black Stork*, pp. 84, 113.

5 Leon J. Cole, quoting G. Chatterton-Hill, National Conference on Race Betterment, *Proceedings* 1 (1914): 503.

6 Cora B. S. Hodson, "Contra-Selection in England," in *Decade of Progress*, p. 373.

7 Michael Guyer, *Being Well-Born* (Indianapolis, IN: Bobbs-Merrill, 1927), p. 414.

8 For an example of how public health became focused on germ fighting, see Charles V. Chapin, "Dirt, disease, and the health officer," *Public Health: Papers and Reports Presented at the Annual Meeting of the American Public Health Association* 28 (1902): 296–9; and Rene Dubos and Jean Dubos, *The White Plague: Tuberculosis, Man and Society* (London, England: Victor Gollancz, 1953), chs. 4 and 9.

9 For typical examples, see Kevles, *Name of Eugenics*, pp. 57, 100; Mark Haller, *Eugenics* (New Brunswick, NJ: Rutgers University Press, 1963), pp. 141–3.

10 C. G. Campbell in *Decade of Progress*, p. 291. See also *Eugenics in Race and State: Scientific Papers of the Second International Congress of Eugenics* (Baltimore, MD: Williams and Wilkins, 1923), pp. 300–1; and Dubos and Dubos, *White Plague*. Until the mid-1930s, antimicrobial drugs for internal use were available clinically only for malaria, diphtheria, and syphilis.

11 This paragraph paraphrases and summarizes the argument in Pernick, *Black Stork*, pp. 111–14.

12 Sigmund Engel, *The Elements of Child-Protection*, trans. Eden Paul (New York: Macmillan, 1912), p. 47. While Engel regarded *natural* infant mortality as dysgenic, he strongly supported actively killing those who were medically diagnosed as unfit to live (pp. 257–8).

13 *Decade of Progress*, pp. 344–5. Disease could selectively influence reproduction not only by killing its victims but also by making them infertile. This was one important reason why venereal diseases were the infections that most particularly concerned eugenicists. Some regarded disease-induced sterility as a valuable form of natural selection, but others found the process too unselective and considered the overall decline in fertility caused by infectious sterility to be a form of "race suicide."

14 Richard Meckel, *Save the Babies: American Public Health Reform and the Prevention of Infant Mortality* (Baltimore, MD: Johns Hopkins University Press, 1990); Edward J. Larson, *Sex, Race, and Science: Eugenics in the Deep South* (Baltimore, MD: Johns Hopkins University Press, 1995), pp. 72–3, 85–90, 131–3; Pernick, *Black Stork*, pp. 53–4, 109–11. See also Renate Bridenthal, Atina Grossmann, and Marion Kaplan, *When Biology Became Destiny: Women*

in Weimar and Nazi Germany (New York: Monthly Review Press, 1984).

15   The quotes are from Popenoe, Race Betterment Conference, *Proceedings* 1 (1914), addendum p. 61. For the similar views of Kellogg, see pp. 89–90.

16   Charles Rosenberg, "The bitter fruit: Heredity, disease, and social thought," in *No Other Gods* (Baltimore, MD: Johns Hopkins University Press, 1976), pp. 89–97. See also Adrian Desmond, *The Politics of Evolution* (Chicago, IL: University of Chicago, 1989). For 20th-century Lamarckian eugenics, see Aldred Scott Warthin, *Creed of a Biologist* (New York: PB Hoeber, 1930), p. 18; Pernick, *Black Stork*, p. 206 n. 15.

       However, not all Lamarckians were so optimistic. Many believed that the longer a trait had been transmitted, the longer it took for environmental influences to change it. Since the advances of civilization were more recent than the primitive aspects of human nature, changes in heredity were much more likely to produce atavistic degeneration than progress. Lamarckian pessimists were likely to believe that selective breeding was the only practical way to guarantee improvements in heredity.

17   *Eugenics in Race and State*, pp. 309, 346–7; Allan Brandt, *No Magic Bullet* (New York: Oxford University Press, 1985), pp. 14–15. For related insights into the influence of evolution and Social Darwinist ideas on constructions of the germ theory, see Nancy Tomes, "American attitudes toward the germ theory of disease," *Journal of the History of Medicine and Allied Sciences* 52 (January 1997): esp. 37–40.

18   This paragraph paraphrases points made in Pernick, *Black Stork*, p. 52. For related points, see Keith Wailoo, *Drawing Blood: Technology and Disease Identity in Twentieth-Century America* (Baltimore, MD: Johns Hopkins University Press, 1997); and Mary Douglas, *Purity and Danger: An Analysis of Concepts of Pollution and Danger* (New York: Praeger, 1966).

19   *Science of Life*, reel 90.26. See also Martin S. Pernick, "Sex education films, US government," *Isis* 84 (1993): 766–8.

20   This paragraph paraphrases Pernick, *Black Stork*, pp. 52–3. On the link between etiology and moral responsibility in public health, see Sylvia Tesh, *Hidden Arguments: Political Ideology and Disease Prevention Policy* (New Brunswick, NJ: Rutgers University Press, 1988).

21   Charles S. Bacon, "The race problem," *Medicine* [Detroit] 9 (1903): 341, exemplifies how racial

segregation, both of Native Americans on reservations and of African Americans, was also supported by eugenicists for similar reasons. Racial segregation was intended both to prevent contamination of the White population through miscegenation and to encourage natural selection to eliminate these allegedly defective populations.

       John P. Radford, "Sterilization versus segregation: Control of the 'feebleminded' 1900–1938," *Social Science and Medicine* 33 (1991): 449–59; *Oxford English Dictionary*, "Segregation," quoting A. Bryson in 1849. On quarantine, see Howard Markel, *Quarantine! East European Jewish Immigrants and the New York City Epidemics of 1892* (Baltimore, MD: Johns Hopkins University Press, 1997); Alan M. Kraut, *Silent Travelers: Germs, Genes and the Immigrant Menace* (New York: Basic Books, 1994). For a typical link between quarantine and eugenics, see *Physical Culture* 21 (January 1909): 50.

22   On eugenic sterilization, see Philip R. Reilly, *The Surgical Solution: A History of Involuntary Sterilization in the United States* (Baltimore, MD: Johns Hopkins University Press, 1991).

23   For a brief history of early infectious disease eradication efforts, see Fred L. Soper, "Rehabilitation of the eradication concept in prevention of communicable disease," *Public Health Reports* 80 (1965): 855–69. For American eugenic enthusiasm for a "final solution" to disease problems, see Harry Haiselden in *Chicago American*, December 30, 1915, magazine page; and similar concepts of Irving Fisher in Race Betterment Conference, *Proceedings* 2 (1915): 64.

       Both Pasteur and Weismann extended Rudolf Virchow's 1858 doctrine that all cells come from other cells.

24   Bacon, "The race problem," p. 341. In addition to n. 3 above, see especially Larson, *Sex, Race, and Science*; Kenneth L. Ludmerer, *Genetics and American Society* (Baltimore, MD: Johns Hopkins University Press, 1972); and Haller, *Eugenics*.

25   Harvey Wiley, "The rights of the unborn," *Good Housekeeping* (October 1922): 32.

26   J. G. Wilson, "A study in Jewish psychopathology," *Popular Science Monthly* 82 (1913): 265, 271.

27   Markel, *Quarantine!*; Kraut, *Silent Travelers*. For Nazi images of Jews as infectious germs, see Lucy Dawidowicz, *The War against the Jews, 1933–1945* (New York: Holt, Rinehart and Winston, 1975), pp. 21, 25, 41, 54; Robert Proctor, *Racial Hygiene: Medicine under the*

Nazis (Cambridge, MA: Harvard University Press, 1988), pp. 194–202.

28   Allan Brandt, "Racism and research: The case of the Tuskegee syphilis study," in *Sickness and Health in America*, ed. Judith Leavitt and Ronald Numbers, 2nd edn (Madison, WI: University of Wisconsin Press, 1985), pp. 331–43; James Jones, *Bad Blood: The Tuskegee Syphilis Experiment* (New York: Free Press, 1981).

29   For specific illustrations, see Pernick, *Black Stork*, ch. 3, esp. pp. 56–75 and 80.

30   Helen Keller, "Physicians' juries for defective babies," *The New Republic* (December 18, 1915): 173–4. See also Pernick, *Black Stork*, pp. 78–80, 97–9, 111–14.

31   Pernick, *Black Stork*, pp. 175–6.

14

Parental Choice? Letter from a Doctor as a Dad

JULIAN SAVULESCU

When my wife became pregnant, what we both wanted, for ourselves, was a normal baby. We are both doctors and have an unromantic view of what it would be like to have a disabled child. We have seen how bringing up handicapped children can wreck lives. And, quite independently, we very strongly wanted not to have a disabled child.[1]

Our first thought concerned the risks and benefits of ultrasound scanning. We tried to gather as much information as time allowed. We talked to friends who were obstetricians, read medical journals and consumer information. Good-quality information was hard to find. We had heard of one study that had associated repeated ultrasound scanning with low birth weight and others that had associated it with learning difficulties at school. There were also concerns about increasing doses of new high-resolution machines. However, it was difficult to draw firm conclusions from the available evidence about the risks involved and how much ultrasound was necessary. We were alarmed to find that adequate studies simply had not been done to show that ultrasound was safe.

Our doctors were less concerned about the possible adverse effects of ultrasound. One friend offered to do an ultrasound at 8 weeks.

"It's great to see the baby," he said. "It helps bonding and reassures you that all this is worthwhile." "But will it make any difference to the outcome?" we asked. "Will we still need another one at 20 weeks to pick up abnormalities?" "Yes, you will need another one at 20 weeks."

We decided to follow something like Pascal's principle: if the potential harm of ultrasound scanning was very great, we should try to do whatever we could to avoid our baby being exposed to it, even if that harm was unlikely.[2] We chose not to subject our baby to ultrasound for the sake of our own reassurance.

Our next major decision then loomed: whether or not to have an amniocentesis. Because of our strong aversion to having a handicapped child, we had always assumed that we *would* have an amniocentesis, which was necessary to pick up chromosomal abnormalities. However, our view changed once we discovered the facts. Amniocentesis had about a 1/400 chance of picking up a major abnormality. It was also associated with about a 1/100 chance of spontaneous abortion. So it was roughly four times more likely that we would abort a normal child through this test than we would pick up an abnormal child. There was also a small chance the amniocentesis might result in an infection that would damage our baby.

We inquired into the alternatives. One option available then in England was a blood test at 15–18 weeks: the triple test. This could be coupled with a new test not routinely available, called nuchal thickness assessment. This test requires an ultrasound at around 12 weeks and estimates the thickness of the skin on the back of the neck. These tests together can pick up Down's syndrome and other abnormalities. When we asked about the sensitivity of these two tests compared to amniocentesis, we were told that they were a good alternative. How good? No one seemed able to tell us.

We decided not to have an amniocentesis, despite the words of caution from our medical friends ("It's better to abort a normal child and have another one than to have a child with Down's syndrome," one of our friends, a surgeon, said.) But we had committed our baby to an ultrasound, and this worried us. Was it really necessary? We were never sure.

The next important test was the anomaly scan at 20 weeks, which picks up some major physical abnormalities. This involves another ultrasound. When we arrived for the scan, we were surprised to find three doctors in the ultrasound cubicle. The obstetrician performing the scan, an expert at ultrasound scanning, informed us that another doctor in training would perform the scan and he would check the results. The third doctor was observing. The obstetrician then devoted his full attention to a computer in the corner of the room. My wife and I exchanged anxious glances and after several minutes I said, "We would prefer it, Dr X, if you did the ultrasound. We are concerned to minimize our child's exposure to radiation. We have private health insurance and are quite prepared to pay ourselves." The obstetrician then began flipping through my wife's medical notes, obviously wondering who these difficult patients were. (My wife was consultant anaesthetist to one of the chief obstetricians in the hospital, who was managing her pregnancy.) "But there is no risk from ultrasound scanning," he said. "We are aware of one study associating multiple scans with low birth weight and subtle neurological abnormalities," I replied. "That study is flawed methodologically. I will check the scan myself. Are you happy with that?" I asked my wife if she was happy with that. She wasn't, but acceded in order to break the deadlock.

We left that day, deflated. We had so looked forward to seeing our baby alive and healthy, and doing things just right. We had asserted ourselves more than many other patients could have done, and we were better informed. But we still felt that we should have pushed harder for what we believed in. We felt we had let our child down.

We will never know if the choices we made had an effect on our child. Most people don't know or don't care about such small possibilities. Doctors reassure us, but on the basis of present information, they can't know. We wanted to do what was best for our child. Of course, if we had only wanted this, we would have had only those tests that were necessary to detect abnormalities that were so severe that they made life not worth living (perhaps one ultrasound scan). We were also motivated to have a normal baby.

My wife and I are at one end of the spectrum: we are very risk-averse. We are also very well informed, members of the medical profession, and assertive. Yet we had great difficulty in getting information to determine which antenatal tests best achieved what we valued. More importantly, we had great difficulty in getting these values to impact on practice.

NOTES

1 Some of our friends and family for whom we have the highest respect have disabilities. It is a separate issue how we love and care for those people who exist now with disabilities – we didn't want to have a child with a disability if we could have one without.

2 The French philosopher, Pascal, argued that we have more to lose if we do *not* believe in God and we are wrong (eternal torment), than we have to lose if we *do* believe in God and we are wrong (living a life according to religious observance). So, we ought to believe that God exists (Pascal, *Pensées*, Fragment 223), even if the chance that God does exist is very small. When harm is great and avoidable, we should go to considerable lengths to avoid it.

15

Do We Really Want to Know the Odds?

DAVID RUNCIMAN

In September 1996 Sir Kenneth Calman, the then Chief Medical Officer for England, decided that it was time we all started to get things in perspective. His department had just published proposals for a system which would rate the risks attached to new drugs and other medical procedures in order to let us know exactly how likely, or unlikely, it is that we will be killed by them. The idea was to educate patients and doctors about the real risks involved in the periodic health scares to which we seem increasingly prone. He wanted us to know that compared to the risks we run every day there is usually nothing to worry about.

The new system would translate the words that are trotted out in times of crisis into figures we can all understand, and compare them to risks we all know about. The scale would run from "high" (a more than one in 100 chance of pulling the short straw in a given year, as is the case with certain hereditary diseases), to "moderate" (one in 100 to one in 1,000; steady smoking), to "low" (one in 1,000 to one in 10,000; death on the roads); to "very low" (one in 10,000 to one in 100,000; death on the railways or in the air), to, ultimately, "negligible" (less than one in 1,000,000; killed by lightning, winning the lottery, contracting

CJD from eating beef). Armed with these stats, the hope is that we will become a little safer from ourselves.

It is an admirable project. There is only one flaw – it assumes that people respond rationally to risk when the real facts are spelt out for them. The evidence, unfortunately, suggests otherwise. We are just as hopeless at getting things in perspective when it comes to the dangers that we know about as we are when the dangers spring unbidden from the murky depths of medical science. We all recognise that it is statistically more dangerous to drive than it is to fly, but that doesn't stop us from worrying incessantly about the safer option. The fact is that when it comes to chance, our fears have little or nothing to do with the actual prospects of a given event coming to pass. And this is true even when we ought to know better.

Instead of worrying about the probability of something happening, we tend to base our worries on our imaginative response to the event itself. We don't usually think so much about what *ought* to happen according to the laws of chance as we do about what it would be like *if it did* happen. To us. And as a result, we tend to dwell on precisely those events which give us the most to dwell on, the ones that are most out of the ordinary, unpredictable, extreme. We are drawn to dwell on the unexpected. Which is another way of saying that we choose to worry about just those things which are the least likely to happen anyway.

Take driving, for example, a "low" risk activity according to Sir Kenneth's scale, and one about which few people experience undue concern. The chances of any one of us being killed by a car this year are about one in 8,000. Truly, it is not a lot, if you think about the amount of driving we do, and about what a crowd of 8,000 looks like (think of what a queue of 80 people looks like), only one of whom is going to be chosen. But it is astronomical if couched in the terms of other activities further down the scale. Between 80 and 90 people are killed each week on Britain's roads. This is roughly the equivalent of one Hillsborough disaster every seven days. Or one medium-sized plane crash.

The reason that we can happily deal with this level of automotive carnage is that we encounter it in manageable chunks. After all, we see a great deal of cars but relatively little of their fatal consequences. Our experience of air travel is exactly the opposite. Most of us don't do it very often, but we know all about it when it goes wrong. What's more, flying, unlike driving, is something that we don't on the whole do for ourselves. The risks seem exaggerated because we are powerless to counteract them, having put ourselves wholly in someone else's hands. And what is true of flying is equally true of most forms of medicine. We tend to be most frightened of those things that we don't experience very often, and part of the reason we don't experience them very often is that we have to get someone else to do them for us. It's a vicious circle, and probability has got nothing to do with it.

We are also disproportionately scared of those things that when they go wrong, go wrong irreparably. The news of a plane crash brings to mind one invariable idea, involving a lot of screaming followed by certain and imminent death on a large scale and in unforeseen company, the details of which are always unimaginable but also somehow predictable. A car crash, by contrast, can be anything you want it to be, from a minor scrape to a murderous pile-up, and nothing about the frequency with which the latter occurs can dampen our instinctive sense that it is possible we will walk away unscathed.

The same applies to illness. The habitual killers that strike on the widest scale are also the ones that have an infrastructure of medical care built around them, so that the risks are at least shrouded in the prospect of recovery. It is the unheralded and untreatable killer, like mad cow disease, which induces morbid panic attacks, because however "negligible" the risks, there is no way to think the "what if" question and expect to come out smiling on the other side.

If this bias works to conceal the real risks that we have of encountering accidental death, it works even harder when it comes to those activities that carry with them dangers that only develop over time. Smoking, which rates as a "moderate" risk on Sir Kenneth's scale, rates as a monumental risk on any other scale you care to mention. It is often said, particularly to schoolchildren, that no one would dream of taking a flight if they were told that their chances of survival were the same as those of a moderate smoker.

But this is really beside the point (no one would take a flight if they thought it would take them 30 years to discover whether they had made it). Much more relevant is the thought that no one would smoke at all, not even if smoking carried the same low risks that attach to flying, once the dangers came to be perceived in the same way. Even, say, if only one cigarette in every 10 million produced by the tobacco companies was marked death, and all the others were perfectly safe, making smoking a much less risky activity than it is now, very few people would relish the chances they were taking on a pack a day. When danger accumulates in a steady drip, drip, drip we can ignore it. It is only when we can see the caprice of chance for what it is that we start to run scared. And then almost nothing will reassure us.

The tobacco companies know this, which is why they are so keen to keep our perceptions of risk as they are. In an advertising campaign [in the mid-1990s], it was pointed out that the risks associated with passive smoking were no greater than those associated with a one-digestive-biscuit-a-day habit. Perhaps this ought to be enough to put some people off eating digestive biscuits. But the cigarette manufacturers are aware that their livelihood depends on persuading enough people that smoking is no different from the unavoidable risks they take for granted in the course of their everyday lives.

This is the problem that faces anyone who tries to rationalise and re-order our responses to risk: the quality of the danger always counts for more than the quantity. We can know all the figures in the world, have them all neatly set out for us on easy-to-read labels, but everything will still depend on the ways in which we choose to imagine disaster to strike.

You could say that flying was no more dangerous than eating biscuits (and you would probably be right) but no one would listen, because the imaginative leap is just too great. That is the thing about probability, as Sir Kenneth will surely discover: people don't choose the lives they lead according to their understanding of risk; in the end, they choose their understanding of risk according to the lives that they lead.

Part III

Falling Ill

Introduction

The structure and rationale of this volume, particularly its concentration on first-person accounts and literature, is premised on the value of experience, like the theoretical accounts in Part I. Although the bulk of this book is arranged by stages of the clinical encounter, Part I is not. Instead, the selections there take the patient-centered approach of this volume to a more conceptual level. Each of the authors represented in Part I offered a reinterpretation of "canonical" bioethics. What unites these new conceptualizations, as we argue in the Introduction to this volume, is a focus on individual perspectives rather than a priori principles. This is also what unites the selections in the remainder of the book, as can readily be seen here in Part III, "Falling Ill."

The a priori principles of autonomy, beneficence, non-maleficence, and justice have the apparent advantage of providing an objective, formal method of rational decision-making. Most importantly, they appear to allow us to reduce the great bustle and confusion of the typical clinical situation into a commensurable comparison, with a common standard. It has been said that "Commensuration is essentially a method for discarding information in order to make decision-making easier by ignoring aspects of the problem that cannot be translated to the common metric. Principlism is a form of commensuration, although not as pure a form as money or utility, and not as commensurable as some critics would like." (Evans, 2000: 32).

It is not the role of this book as a whole to offer a sustained critique of principlism: others have done that more effectively (e.g. Clouser and Gert, 1990). What we do want is to suggest that we view the function of this volume as restoring information that should *not* be discarded or ignored: particularly, experience relating to patients' narratives and lived bodily experience. It is the focus on narrative, bodies, discourse, and the patient's voice which unites the selections in the book as a whole.

The focus on lived experience means that we, as editors, have been heavily committed to using first-person accounts. One particular story, with which Part III begins, is used as a linking thread throughout the remainder of the book. It is the account by the poet Jenny Lewis of her breast cancer and mastectomy, as told in her mythologized account in verse, *When I Became an Amazon*. Lewis intersperses the story of her own illness and recovery with an imaginary tale of an Amazon warrior-priestess, connecting her personal suffering to a wider epic, heroic tradition. Rarely have heroes been conceived as women, although recent feminist scholarship has reclaimed the heroic "quest" narrative and applied it to the task of "writing a woman's life" (Heilbrun, 1988; Dickenson, 1993). Lewis takes the image of the deliberately one-breasted Amazon as her own, reclaiming her mutilation. The first poem from the selections we have chosen, entitled "Premonition," describes Lewis's first encounter with her Amazon alter ego, and with her cancer.

Chapter 17 also forms one of a series within the book, although it is a more conventionally "academic" article, one commissioned for this volume. "Emotional Disturbance: Philip and Lucy," by Priscilla Alderson and Chris Goodey, looks at a type of illness that is less easily categorized *as* an illness, with a clear diagnosis and treatment options – that is, emotional and behavioral disturbance. As Alderson and Goodey put the paradox, "'How does the pattern of falling ill, having treatment and recovering fit children and teenagers who are diagnosed as emotionally disturbed? A vital part of this pattern is assumed to be that patients see themselves as ill, and they want to recover and co-operate with their treatment. Yet a usual symptom of emotional and behavioral disturbance (EBD) is refusal to agree and co-operate with adults" – including co-operation in diagnosis and treatment. To take the paradox to the extreme, what if the diagnosis of behavioral disturbance is merely a social construction, and not an illness at all? This possibility would arise from an extension of the arguments of the anti-psychiatry movement, led by authors such as Thomas Szasz (1960 and 1987). What distinguishes Alderson and Goodey's work from that of Szasz is that it centers on the concrete narrative of two young people diagnosed with emotional and behavioral disorder. In other words, their three chapters in the story of Philip and Lucy – the second in Part VI, and the final one in Part VII – illustrate this book's commitment to lived experience and narrative.

The American philosopher Kay Toombs, who herself has multiple sclerosis, writes, in "Healing and Incurable Illness," of the dislocation from one's body which occurs in diagnosis. In Toombs's words: "In our culture, incurable illness almost invariably engenders a profound sense of loss of wholeness, which includes feelings of bodily alienation, a transformation in the familiar world, a change in the significance of time, a disruption in social relations, and a profound loss of self-esteem." Cherished assumptions of personal invulnerability fall away before the experience of both "having" and "being had by" a terminal illness. A phenomenological approach which sees the embodied self as constructing meaning problematically from its surroundings, rather than a liberal approach which sees the patient as "owning" the body, is more likely to help people with chronic illness to repair their narratives.

Toombs's piece leads naturally into chapter 19, Howard Brody's canonical piece, "My Story is Broken: Can You Help Me Fix It?" Subtitled "Medical Ethics and the Joint Construction of Narrative," Brody's chapter looks to joint construction of meaning and narrative as a form of power-sharing in the doctor–patient relationship. The doctor's power, either to heal or to obstruct healing, traditionally rests on his or her superior expertise; but the patient is probably the expert on his or her own story. Furthermore, listening to the patient is therapeutic in itself, as is helping him or her to construct a meaningful understanding of what is going on. As Brody points out: "In Western culture people are used to the idea of gaining mastery or control over events by being able to tell a coherent story about them. Thus, listening carefully to the patient's story begins the process of healing at the symbolic level." One could take Brody's argument further. If this process can be begun at the time of diagnosis, at the moment of "falling ill," it may assist healing in the sense of cure; if that form of healing is impossible, a sense of control during the dying trajectory is a form of patient power, too.

Chapter 20, by Mike Jackson and Bill Fulford, "Spiritual Experience and Psychopathology," uses patient narratives to argue that pathological psychosis is to be diagnosed not by "objective" clinical criteria alone, but by the manner in which possibly psychotic phenomena are embedded in the values and beliefs of the person concerned. Using the example of a man with religious "delusions," the authors look to the person and his values rather than the symptoms alone, concluding that he is actually functioning well, not badly. Chapter 21, "The Occurrence of High Levels of Acute Behavioral Distress in Children and Adolescents Undergoing Routine Venipunctures," is another primarily "clinical" article, because it actually illustrates exactly how clinicians need to, and can, take into account the patient's own interpretation of what appears a routine clinical encounter: venipuncture. As the authors G. Bennett Humphry et al. note, research on children's reactions to venipuncture is sparse, as is research on children's perception of pain more generally. Essentially, taking the child's interpretation into account as a large factor in his or her perception of the pain, the authors emphasize that "it is not only the pain but also the anticipation of pain that contribute to the complexity of the phenomenon. The procedure is an inevitable invasion of the child's psychological and physical space, and there is the threat that the child will lose control." These themes of control and psychological/physical space have occurred elsewhere in Part III, most notably in the articles by Brody and Toombs.

The final chapter in Part III, "Benjamin's Story," by Eric Kodish, tells the story of a 10-year-old boy with a bone sarcoma and metastasis to the lungs. Benjamin was an active football player, and while he was old enough to focus primarily on clearing up his "lung spots," the clinicians were uncertain how to break the news that although his "spots" were getting better, his leg tumor was growing and would require an amputation. "How do you prepare a 10-year-old for an amputation? In the old days, the answer was probably: 'You don't.' Just do the procedure, and deal with the consequences when the child wakes up and discovers that his leg is missing. Now, with our progressive attitudes and emphasis on honesty with children, I suppose the answer is more like: 'You can't, but you do the best you can.'" Honesty takes its toll on the clinician, however. After Benjamin dies, his hospital friend Martin, a boy of the same age whose prognosis is uncertain, grieves for his friend and is clearly distressed that the same thing might happen to him. Kodish reassures him that he is going to be all right, although he knows this is less than honest. "As I said these words, I could feel the relief go through his body. Perhaps I even felt

it in my own." The physician's need for control during the dying trajectory is also a factor which must be taken into account.

REFERENCES

Clouser, K. D. and Gert, B. (1990) A critique of principlism. *Journal of Medicine and Philosophy* 15: 219–36.

Dickenson, D. (1993) *Margaret Fuller: Writing a Woman's Life* (Basingstoke: Macmillan).

Evans, J. H. (2000) A sociological account of the growth of principlism. *Hastings Center Report* 30: 31–8.

Heilbrun, C. G. (1988) *Writing a Woman's Life* (New York and London: W. H. Norton).

Szasz, T. S. (1960) The myth of mental illness. *American Psychologist* 15: 113–18.

Szasz, T. S. (1987) *Insanity: The Idea and its Consequences* (New York: John Wiley and Sons).

READING GUIDE

For a similar commitment to use of first-person accounts, making the text accessible to the general reader, see Donna Dickenson, Malcolm Johnson, and Jeanne Samson Katz (eds.), *Death, Dying and Bereavement*, 2nd edn (London: Sage, 2000). Narratives of illness by children and young people have also been at the center of Priscilla Alderson's work: see her *Choosing for Children* (Oxford: Oxford University Press, 1990) and *Children's Consent to Surgery* (Milton Keynes: Open University Press, 1993).

Kay Toombs has further developed her interest in a phenomenological, embodied understanding of selfhood and illness in *The Meaning of Illness: A Phenomenological Account of the Different Perspectives of Doctor and Patient* (Dordrecht: Kluwer, 1992). Bill Fulford identifies the importance of loss of agency in the primary experience of illness in chapter 5 of his *Moral Theory and Medical Practice* (Cambridge: Cambridge University Press, 1989). Howard Brody's more political focus, on narrative and power in the doctor–patient relationship, is comprehensively detailed and beautifully argued in *The Healer's Power* (New Haven and London: Yale University Press, 1992). The book is a further development of Brody's assertion in his chapter in this volume that "The critical goal of medical ethics should be to enhance the physician's use of power against the disease on the side of the patient and minimize any temptation or opportunity to use power to the patient's detriment."

16

Premonition
10th March, 1985

JENNY LEWIS

You found it first –
That night you touched me
with nerve endings like your finest paintbrush
sending a wash of sunrise through me,
flooding with luminous brilliance the misty
landscapes I never dreamt existed –

the love I felt before seemed dim
as candlelight beside those deep webs
of radiance, showing me peaceful contours
lit by intense morning and evening colours
like falls of silk over mountains.

Only you have met the warrior-priestess
in me, at once your primeval lover
and arch enemy – she stands by our side
in battle helping us draw up lines
for the next hundred thousand millennia.

She made me see – it wasn't how much
you loved me that mattered,
but how much love
you showed me I was capable of.
That was your gift – why you alone
could come inside the inner sanctum.

Later you told me what your lips
had found already, and kissing my breast
goodbye, you held me to your body
to block out the darkness of centuries;
but by daylight you had left and I was
bitterly alone – that night you touched me.

17

Emotional Disturbance: Philip and Lucy

PRISCILLA ALDERSON AND CHRIS GOODEY

How does the pattern of falling ill, having treatment, and recovering fit children and teenagers who are diagnosed as emotionally disturbed? A vital part of this pattern is assumed to be that patients see themselves as ill, and they want to recover and cooperate with their treatment.[1] Yet a usual symptom of emotional and behavioral disturbance (EBD) is refusal to agree and cooperate with adults. The experiences of Philip in East City and Lucy in West County illustrate the difficulties of treating EBD as a form of clinical illness with a clear diagnosis, treatment, and cure. Their lives also illustrate the contrasting treatments which they and many of their peers have, depending on where they live.[2] This chapter considers the first stage, falling ill, and later chapters (47 and 60) will consider negotiating a treatment plan and getting well.

Philip in East City

When Philip was 7 years old, his mother left home and he and his brother were going to be put into care. His father gave up work in order to look after his sons; they became homeless and lived in bed and breakfast for a while. Philip had bowel problems; his father remembered: "He

was in and out of hospital for tests but it didn't get any better." Philip would "go for little walks," as his father put it, and be brought back by the police. He was in trouble at school for "throwing books, pushing chairs over, screaming and things like that." Furthermore:

> He could only concentrate on something for about five minutes, then he'd want to go and do something else. He couldn't sit and listen to a story – it was too boring for him. . . . He wanted to do something else . . . and because he wasn't getting it he was losing his temper, ranting and raving. . . . If someone was having a go at him, he just shut down in a little world of his own. I didn't know anything was wrong.

Philip spent five months out of school waiting for a statement of special educational need (SEN); then he went to an EBD school.

Lucy in West County

Lucy lives on a council estate on the edge of an affluent village. Blinds are closed on all the windows in Lucy's house so that the neighbors cannot look in. Lucy was first interviewed when she was 13 years old. When the interviewer arrived, her parents spoke at length about their own problems, and then about Lucy's problems. After an hour, when the interviewer asked to see Lucy, her parents were surprised at the request and called her from her bedroom where she spends most of her time. When she was 5 years old, Lucy was referred to a school for deaf children for moderate learning difficulties (MLD). When she was 7, her younger stepbrother went into care and she started boarding. Her parents showed her SEN statements, which record that she has good hearing and "normal ability."

Mother: She's had operations since she was 3 years old, grommets five or six times, adenoids out twice [*sic*] then they done a brain scan on her this year, and they're telling me she's not deaf and she never has been, it's more –

Father: – her brain –

Mother: – her brain, it's not functioning....She got to this stage where if she didn't understand she'd say "pardon?" and people would think there was something wrong in there.

Lucy went on to another MLD school at the age of 11. Her mother said Lucy had "set her heart on going to a midstream school [*sic*], she calls that a proper school." Lucy enjoyed talking, and confirmed her father's earlier account.

Lucy: I like computers. We've got a Nimbus, yes it's quite good.

Interviewer: Do the teachers know how to use them?

Lucy: [shakes her head.] All they know is they've got a computer in their office. Mr Green knows how to use that, but the Nimbus, even, like the boys they don't know how to put them in.

Interviewer: They have to call you to do it? [Lucy nods.] And you know how to? [She nods.] Where did you learn?

Lucy: At me other school, we had a Nimbus at me other school.

Despite remembering computers from the school she left two years earlier, Lucy accepted her parents' repeated emphasis on her limitations.

Mother: She's got a good long term memory, but she hasn't got a short term memory. If I ask her "What did you have for lunch at school?" she can't remember.

Lucy: I can't remember what I have for lunch.

Mother: And I have to watch her all the time, or she'd just wander off and get lost, she wouldn't understand.

Lucy: I'd just wander off.

Mother: So I can't ever let her out of my sight.

Father: She's not getting any activities like other children. All she's got is her bedroom. She'd rather be out with the other girls.

Mother: She wants to be out and she can't understand why I won't let her. I can't trust her, even the head teacher told me there is no way I can let Lucy out to play....Lucy's taken to lying and the lying's getting worse.

Father: Like at school she says she gets picked on....

Mother: She said the teachers wouldn't let her go to the toilet and she started wetting. We had that for nine months. I think she didn't like it at that school....

Father: It used to be a borstal school for bad boys, then it changed to children with bad habits....

Mother: And Lucy's got in with them and now she's being like them.

While in her bedroom, Lucy was playing tunes on her keyboard by ear, and teaching herself to type, but her parents continued to emphasize her failings and her assessment two years earlier of having a "mental age of 7."

Mother: She wanders off. She wouldn't be able to catch a bus home, plus she's too familiar with adults and she would go off. She's easily tempted. It doesn't matter how much you drum it in. Like crossing the road, even at school, they have to grab her or she's gone, things, you know, that a 7-year-old would ...

Father: She's picked up every day by bus for school.

Interviewer: And does she mind that?

Mother: Er ye-es and no. I don't really know. I don't think she wants to upset the house. I have terrible trouble getting her to tell me what's wrong. . . . But she knows it's the only way and the only place she can go to.

Father: She doesn't like the school.

Interviewer: Might you have tried an ordinary school?

Mother: She's too backward.

Lucy's parents emphasized her need for constant attendance, and that the school did not guard her carefully enough, as she had once run away and found her way home, 20 miles on two trains and two buses, a remarkable feat for someone who had always traveled by car or the school bus. Lucy's parents complained that her attendance allowance had been reduced. They had "battled" to have it increased again and kept saying it was essential to watch Lucy constantly. Her mother criticized Lucy's teachers, but also sympathized with them.

Mother: She was a lovely child. Her key worker is not satisfied that she's in the right school because her behavioral problems have got worse. I mean I love her but sometimes I really don't like her, 'cos you just can't talk to her. She's so moody all the time.

Father: Making signs behind your back and –

Mother: – I know – a 13-year-old being a teenager, they probably all do it – but it's even worse being her, and if it's because she's really unhappy. . . . I think it sort of came out that she thought we'd put her in there [junior boarding school] just to get rid of her. But there was nothing else we could do. . . . But there's always one bad apple, and Lucy's got in with them and now she's being like them. She had a behavioral problem but now she's got a nasty behavioral problem. She was the only girl in the class and she's been stabbed, had bricks thrown at her, she's had

Father: – scissors in her eye nearly –

Mother: – her coat put down the toilet –

Father: – still can't get the money for that, we're fighting that –

Mother: – and I think she's getting worse and worse [explains how she thought the problem was mainly with the teachers, and then how she happened to visit the school]. And Lucy didn't see me, I was standing in a corner, and she [Lucy] was right verballing somebody and it was a teacher and [heavy irony and outrage] it was lovely, and if I'd ever heard her – she's never done it here – I'd have washed her mouth out with soap. I couldn't believe it. When she saw me, she stood back and I said, "I'm amazed. I'm really disappointed in you and I want nothing more to do with you," and I just walked out. . . . I apologized to the head teacher, and I said, "I thought you were picking on her and I've seen it for myself now, so how do we get about sorting it out?" She said, "She'll settle down in time," but it's getting worse.

Father: She might just as well be at home for what she's learning at school.

Is EBD an Illness?

Experts agree that it is hard to define and distinguish between a mental health problem and normality.[3] One (subjective) measure is whether behavior appears to be reasonable. Philip's father saw rationality in Philip's behavior at infant school as not unreasonable reactions to unskillful teachers. Philip had not had an easy life, and his father believed that he needed to be respected rather than harassed. In order to understand anyone's behavior it has to be seen in context; even making a cup of tea looks crazy if you do not understand the rationale. Lucy's mother expected her to be irrational, so was angry when she swore at school, without considering possible provocation or Lucy's possible frustration and even despair at not being heard. During research visits to that school, teachers were observed to tease, goad, and bore the pupils who also harassed one another. Students were trapped in a double bind when all their responses, however reasonable, were taken as further evidence of disturbance.[4] To the interviewer, Lucy appeared to be remarkably patient, at home and school, about her extremely lonely, restricted life. She might have been "putting on an act," but if she was capable at times of behaving so well, it seemed strange to emphasize her negative sides instead of encouraging her positive ones.

EBD special schools places are increasing partly because of medical referrals.[5] Doctors contribute to SEN statements, and EBD is constructed on a medical model: the problem/illness is in the child or *is* the child, who needs to be assessed and diagnosed, and "specially" treated to achieve a cure. When a problem is social rather than biological, a constant emphasis on difficulties can create and exaggerate them. Lucy's "symptoms" were contradictory (does she really have a poor memory?), and their origins and nature were uncertain (is she deaf, or confused, or trying to protect herself by not hearing the negative stream of reproaches?), so that "progress," "treatment," and "cure" also cannot be clearly defined. Assessments can become self-fulfilling prophesies: believing that Lucy "has a mental age of 7," her parents infantilize her in a way many 3-year-olds would not accept. She is disabled by being forced to accept restrictions which make her look incapable. Her parents have financial rewards by stressing her "disability" which they would lose if Lucy were seen to improve. The illness model, by isolating the problem inside the child and ignoring the context, denies how "falling ill" with EBD is not simply a response to a disturbing situation, it can be produced, exacerbated, and perpetuated by the situation.[6] It is highly questionable whether EBD is an illness that is no one's fault, deliberate naughtiness, or a distressed or even reasonable response to disturbing situations in which young people are placed through no fault of their own.

NOTES

1 Parsons, T., *The Social System* (London: Routledge, 1951).

2 See Alderson, P. and Goodey, C., *Enabling Education: Experiences in Special and Ordinary Schools* (London: Tufnell Press, 1998). Our research study about disabled and disturbed pupils' views and experiences "What kind of school is best for me?" 1994–7 was conducted in two contrasting local education authorities (LEAs). East City has an inclusive policy and most disabled children attend mixed-ability-range classes in mainstream coeducational, multi-racial, comprehensive schools; only one of the original eight special schools remains open and it is in a transitional stage. East City, unlike most "inner city" areas, entirely lacks middle-class housing pockets, and there is no clear consensus that some schools are better than others. In West County, there are 13 LEA special schools and units, besides further special schools run by voluntary organizations; the mainstream secondary schools are grammar or high (secondary modern) schools, mostly single-sex, with pupils who are almost all white. There are also 23 private schools in the area. In West County, school uniforms symbolize sharp and wide divisions between pupils, as statements of class, income, and officially assessed ability. We observed daily activities in 22 schools and interviewed 45 pupils with physical, sensory, emotional, or learning difficulties, and also their parents, teachers, and classroom assistants, governors, councilors, and LEA staff. The students were aged from 7 to 17.

3 House of Commons Health Committee, *Child and Adolescent Mental Health Services* (London: HMSO, 1997).

4 Watzlavic, P., Beavin, J., and Jackson, D., *Pragmatics of Human Communication* (New York: W. W. Norton and Co., 1967).

5 Norwich, B., *Segregation and Inclusion; English LEA Statistics* (Bristol: Centre for Studies on Inclusive Education, 1994).

6 Laing, R. and Esterson, A., *Sanity, Madness and the Family*, 2nd edn (Harmondsworth: Penguin, 1973); Clough, P. and Barton, L., *Making Difficulties: Research and the Construction of SEN* (London: Paul Chapman, 1995); Barnes, C. and Oliver, M., "Disability rights: Rhetoric and reality in the UK," *Disability and Society* 10: 111–16.

18

Healing and Incurable Illness

S. KAY TOOMBS

As a person living with a progressively debilitating disease I have thought a great deal about healing and incurable illness. In 1973, at the age of thirty, I was diagnosed with multiple sclerosis (MS). Since that time I have struggled with the loss of wholeness – the experience of disunity and alienation – that accompanies incurable disease in the context of Western medicine and Western (and more particularly) North American culture. In this chapter I suggest that thinking carefully about the dynamic relation between body/mind/world/self/others, as it plays itself out against the background of personal and cultural meanings, not only provides insight into the experience of loss of wholeness but also provides invaluable clues with respect to healing – that is, the process of restoring and preserving a sense of personal harmony that does not depend upon the integrity of the physical body.

My reflections on meaning and wholeness have grown out of my life experience. Over the years this illness has affected my ability to see, feel, move, stand, sit, walk, control my bowels and bladder, and to maintain my balance. Some abilities, such as sensing the position of a limb, I have lost abruptly and then slowly regained. Some, such as clear vision in one or the other eye, I have lost and regained numerous times. Other physical capacities have disappeared and never returned; for example, I can no longer walk because I am unable to lift my legs. Progression toward the inability to walk has been gradual. I now use a manual wheelchair and battery-operated scooter for mobility.

In the midst of this life journey I began graduate studies in philosophy. I became interested in the work of such thinkers as Husserl, Merleau-Ponty, Sartre and Schutz, all of whom focus their attention on the way in which we experience the world and constitute meaning. This philosophic interest has caused me to think deeply about the ways in which we experience our bodies differently in health and illness, the transformations that occur in space and time, the changed relation with surrounding objects, the existential significance of differing types of disability, and so forth.[1] However, this interest is not a purely academic exercise. I am convinced that such reflections have implications not only for medical practice and the care of sick persons but for the way in which we, as individuals, respond to the existential challenges posed by illness, disability and death.

In the course of my work I have become increasingly aware that the prevailing Western biomedical model of disease – a model that focuses almost exclusively on the "objective" pathophysiology of the disease state – captures little, if anything, of the global experience of disorder that is the patient's illness. In a profound way, this model not only separates the disease from the person, who lives it in all its messy particularity, but also splits mind-consciousness from body, and thus does not take into account the dynamic relation between our bodies, our sense of self, our involvements with the surrounding world, our relations with others, our experience of space and time, and the emotional dimension of bodily being. Yet it is the disruption of this web of interrelationships that precipitates the sense of alienation that is felt so intensely in incurable disease.

The Impact of the Diagnosis

Personal unity shatters vividly at the moment one receives a definitive diagnosis of incurable illness. Suddenly all one's taken-for-granted assumptions about the world are transformed. In that instant one recognizes that nothing will ever be (or can ever be) the same again. Every patient can recall that moment in exquisite detail. It is imprinted on the mind – the marker of a transition from one way of being to another. Even though it is more than 20 years since I received my diagnosis, I can tell you what day of the week it was, what month, what clothes I was wearing, and repeat almost verbatim the words used by the neurosurgeon. Also I can remember wishing fervently that I could go back a few moments in time because I recognized that my life had changed in a fundamental way. From that point on I would be a person living with multiple sclerosis.

Diagnoses mean much more to patients than simply the identification of a particular disease state. The dread diseases – cancer, AIDS, multiple sclerosis, heart disease – carry with them a particularly powerful symbolic significance. In receiving such a diagnosis, one is forced to deal not only with the physical symptoms of the illness, as well as the profound uncertainty that accompanies it, but – as importantly – to

confront the personal and cultural meanings associated with the disorder. The stigma that accompany diseases such as AIDS and cancer, as well as the negative stereotypes associated with physical disability, immediately set one apart from others and contribute to a profound sense of aloneness. One is faced not only with the question "What does this illness mean for *me* now and in the future?" but, as importantly, "What does this illness mean for me in my relation with others?" These questions must be addressed again and again.

Bodily Alienation

A diagnosis of incurable illness immediately alienates one from one's body. When in good health, we take our bodies for granted. Normally we act in the world through the medium of our bodies in an unreflective fashion. We speak, see, hear, move unthinkingly – paying little attention to our physical capacities. Illness destroys this taken-for-grantedness. With pain, loss of function, change in appearance, the body intrudes itself into consciousness, becoming the unwelcome focus of one's attention. Rather than being that which is routinely overlooked, the body is felt as an insistent presence that remains always at the fringes of consciousness. This forced attention to body is disruptive and profoundly threatening.

It is threatening in the sense that it forces one to recognize the symbiotic relation between body and self. I don't just have a body, as I "have" a house, a car or a dog. In a fundamental way I *am* my body. Whatever happens to *it* also necessarily happens to *me*. (If I recognized nothing else when I received the diagnosis of MS, I recognized that whatever was going on in the deep recesses of my central nervous system – albeit unseen, unfelt, unstoppable – threatened totally to disrupt my existence.) The experience of illness is always the experience of both "having" and "being had." I not only "have" an illness, it also "has" me. Although we can, and do, objectify our bodies, we do not immediately say or think with reference to ourselves in sickness, "My body has cancer, my body is going to die."

The most cherished assumption we hold is that of personal indestructibility. In our culture this primordial sense of personal invulnerability is bolstered by unrealistic expectations about the power of science to control nature and the ability of medicine to intervene and to "fix" bodily malfunction. To discover, in the context of Western medicine, that one's body cannot be "fixed" is to experience a most extraordinary sense of loss of control, of powerlessness, of helplessness. This feeling is intensified by the fact that the predominant focus of Western medicine is on acute illness with a corresponding emphasis on cure of disease. Thus, incurably ill patients feel abandoned by the medical profession – a feeling that is intensified when health professionals withdraw in the face of failure to eradicate disease. If healing is to be achieved, it is vital that patients feel they are not "medically" alone, that they have not been abandoned as "incurable" and, therefore, beyond help. What patients need most is someone to accompany, to be with them on the life journey that is their illness. This is especially true as they come to grips with the reality that cure is not a possibility. Although health professionals do not (and cannot) have all the answers, they are in a unique position to be present as patients confront the most profound existential questions.

Advances in medical technology also increase the patient's perception of loss of control. In a culture that views death primarily as a failure of medical science (rather than as an inevitable aspect of being human) there is enormous pressure to prevent death at almost any cost. Consequently, as patients, we find ourselves terrified not only by medicine's impotence to cure our disease but also by medicine's power to keep us alive. The bodily threat to the self is accentuated by the fear that medical technology may be used to keep my body functioning long after my integrity as a person has been destroyed. This fear is at least one of the factors that fuels the debate on legalizing assisted suicide. As paradoxical as this may seem, the option of assisted suicide can provide some sense of control over a desperately threatening future. When they embrace the notion of assisted suicide, what patients fear most is not death itself but rather a process of dying (or living) that robs them of dignity and personal integrity.

As someone who lives with progressive neurologic disease, my greatest fear is not death; rather, I am most afraid that eventually the inevitable progression of my disease will leave me dependent for my every need on the assistance of strangers who do not care about me. One of the most powerful acts of healing is that of assuring sick persons that they will always be worthy of care regardless of the degradation of illness. Such an assurance goes a long way towards ameliorating the bodily threat to the self.

The sense of alienation from one's body is also experienced in illness as the profound loss of possibility. My body is not simply a physiologic organism, it is the vehicle through which I interact with others and the means by which I carry out my various projects in the world. For instance my leg is more than a limb, it is the possibility (which I have) of walking, running, playing tennis or the possibility (that I may become) of learning to rock climb, of pursuing certain professional activities, or of strolling in the park with my child. The significance of a particular existential loss is different for each individual, and the loss of possibility may have different meanings for the same individual at different times. Suffering is always related to personal meanings and to the context of a particular life.

The Change in the Familiar World

The loss of possibility inherent in the body forces us to recognize the dynamic relation between our bodies and the surrounding world. In our culture we tend to think in terms of dualisms – subject–object, body–mind, body–self, body–world. However, we are not simply bodily beings: we are beings-in-the-world. Loss of wholeness is experienced in a multitude of ways as dis-ability – the inability to interact with and engage the world in ways that are meaningful to us. Pain or nausea are not just uncomfortable sensations, they are the impossibility of giving undivided attention to my spouse or carrying out an important project. Additionally, physical debility transforms our taken-for-granted relation with familiar objects. For instance, a flight of stairs that formerly was unnoticed presents itself as an overt challenge to the body, an obstacle to be avoided or viewed with dismay.

The familiar world also changes when spatial dimensions shift. What was once experienced as "near" (the bathroom, the next-door neighbor's house, the office) is now experienced as "far." When I could walk, the distance from my office to the classroom (about 30 yards) was unremarkable. As my mobility decreased, the office appeared "near" to the classroom on the way to the lecture, but "far" from it on the return journey. Now, if I were deprived of my wheelchair, the distance to traverse would appear immense. The answer to the question "Is it too far?" bears no relation to objective measurement of distance. For me, it depends upon what is between here and there. Are there obstacles preventing access with the wheelchair? Is the terrain suitable for my scooter? It also depends upon physical stamina, level of fatigue, and even the will to make the trip. The world may shrink to the confines of the sick person's house or to the boundaries of one's room. This spatial transformation can be a source of great suffering because it denotes the shrinking of meaningful involvements in the world. Also, the progressive dwindling of space has personal meaning because it represents different stages of illness.

Space has emotional import in another sense. We not only act in space, we dwell in space. We all have places that are particularly significant to us – the beach we walk along together, the bed in which we share our most intimate moments, the garden that gives us a sense of peace. Just as a piece of music evokes a flashback to a time and place, so a physical space can evoke a deep and profound meaning in us. Illness may engender a transformation, or loss, of these most precious spaces. Achieving a renewed sense of harmony means learning to dwell differently in the intimate spaces of our lives.

In spite of our cultural tendency to separate the physical from the emotional, we not only act in the world, we feel the world. We know this well in moments of grief and intense happiness

when the world is transformed for us. Indeed, at those moments, we find it hard to comprehend that for others the world seems unchanged. The emotional significance of space varies according to personal meanings and the context of a particular life. While spaces such as a hospital room or a bed in the intensive-care unit evoke a sense of dread in patients and their loved ones, these spaces have a quite different meaning for health professionals.

It is important for caregivers to pay attention to the emotional aspect of space – to ask not only "How are you doing in everyday life?" but "How do things feel?" Knowing how the world feels to the individual (exceedingly effortful, demeaning, frightening) allows one to change the meaning of worldly involvement. If a patient senses the surrounding world as overtly restrictive, for instance, strategies can be developed to open up space. These could be as simple as encouraging the use of aids such as a walker or wheelchair, or they could involve exploring innovative ways to transform the experience of being in space. I am thinking here of possibilities such as meditating, listening to music, expanding horizons through immersion in literature or art.

The Significance of Time

A most important aspect of illness is a change in the significance of time. In our culture we think of time as a series of more or less discrete moments along a time line of past, present and future. With the prospect of increasing debility, the future assumes an inherently problematic and threatening character. So pervasive is this threat that the future engulfs the present. An uncertain or dire prognosis may cause the sick person to start living as if already incapacitated or as if death is imminent. For instance, a survey carried out at the MS clinic at the University of Western Ontario, London, Ont., suggested that simply receiving a diagnosis of MS was equivalent to moderate disability, regardless of the actual degree of physical impairment.[2] In the face of overwhelming uncertainty, it is hard to resist the natural impulse to project one's thoughts into a dreaded future. One is preoccupied with what may happen or with the significance of a present symptom for one's future prognosis. Since one cannot deal with what has not yet happened, fear is increased and the future appears unmanageable.

Time may also be disrupted in that pain and debility in the present moment demand complete attention. In this event the present assumes an enduring and inescapable quality. One longs for a future time when all this will be over. The present is not a time to be lived but rather a period to "get through." At the same time, however, the longed for future is extremely tenuous.

Alternatively, one may be tempted to cling tenaciously to the past. The knowledge that I will never again be the way I was (because of a change in my body or an alteration of physical function) concretely reminds me that a certain way of bodily being, and the way of life that accompanied it, is over. Invariably this loss must be confronted again and again in light of increasing physical or mental debility.

Perhaps the greatest challenge to living fully in the present relates to the significance of the future. Normally we act in the present in light of anticipations that are to come – more or less specific goals relating to future possibilities. This taken-for-granted future disappears. One can think only of the things one will be unable to do, the personal relationships that will never be, the projects that will never come to fruition.

Societal and cultural meanings exacerbate this experienced loss of possibility. In our culture, for the most part, we are future-oriented. We act now in light of projected goals and plans. We work toward achieving future aims, future rewards. The metaphor for a purposeful life is that of the journey, the goal being to reach a more or less predetermined destination. This metaphor is understood in terms of motion – getting from here to there. In such a futuristic goal-oriented society we are, so to speak, always on an interstate highway focused on the quickest and most efficient way to get to our destination. We are not much interested in, let alone aware of, the actual process of journeying. If and when we reach a projected destination, more often than not we immediately set our sights on another one.

This emphasis on future-directedness causes us consistently (on a daily basis) to miss the value and importance of the present moment. The present is valuable only insofar as it contributes to the future. Consequently, when we are confronted with the actual loss of our own future, we experience a profound feeling that life in the present has no meaning.

If healing is to be achieved, patients have to learn to live fully in the present moment – neither preoccupied by dread for the future, frozen in the act of trying to recapture the past, nor overwhelmed by the everyday demands of debilitating illness and paralyzed by the experience of uncertainty. In our goal-oriented society, this means deliberately changing our perspective on the relation between present and future, as well as paying attention to the ways in which the meanings of past and future invade the present.

With respect to future threat it is essential that caregivers ask patients what their particular anxieties are. Once concrete fears have been identified, specific strategies can be developed to deal with them. This gives patients a certain amount of control and allows them to focus their energies on the business of living, rather than the process of dying. Nevertheless, as Anatole Broyard noted in his book, *Intoxicated By My Illness*, "there is a time of the night between midnight and dawn when people despair."[3] If one is to remain intact in the face of progressively debilitating illness, one has to refuse to go where the imagination insistently calls. In those hours when I am most often beset by the terrors of the future, I have learned to say: "I will not go to that place. I will think only of now. Of this day. Of this moment. Of what I have. Of what gives me joy." It is an act of will. Like many others, I cannot look the possibilities of the future fully in the face and remain intact. A concrete way to initiate the process of healing is to develop ways of focusing the mind in the present moment.

Living fully in the present means letting go of the past. However, letting go of the past is necessarily an ongoing process. Changes in physical appearance and functional capacity provide reminders of the continuing transformation from one way of being to another. In this respect, a vital aspect of care is the chronicling of loss. What sick persons seek is a genuine recognition that what is happening to them is significant not just in medical but in existential terms.

Balancing Coexistence and Distancing From Illness

Achieving harmony in the face of illness means learning to live with bodily disorder as a permanent way of being. Consequently, one has to balance between the need to coexist with, and distance oneself from, one's own body. With respect to coexistence, the shock and realization that I am in a symbiotic relation with my body can provide the impetus to become involved with, and take responsibility for, one's body. In this sense I am motivated to reclaim the body that I am, especially since I recognize I cannot hand it over to medical science to be "fixed" and returned to me in good working order.

Becoming attuned to one's body is beneficial, not just in terms of physiologic effects but in reducing the sense of bodily alienation. The act of taking the body back gives one a sense of control. In addition, mastering new ways of being-in-the-world, such as learning successfully to negotiate space in a wheelchair, is an empowering experience that changes the significance of bodily disorder.

With a cultural perspective that equates health with complete physical well-being, the prevailing emphasis in Western medicine on cure of disease ill prepares us for the task of living with sickness and death. We tend to believe that no amount of pain or debility is acceptable. Consequently, in illness we spend a great deal of energy and emotion fighting pain and rejecting our changing bodies – rather than attempting to live with them. An alternative perspective that may help us in this regard is that of practitioners such as Dr Jon Kabat-Zinn at the University of Massachusetts Medical Center, Worcester, Massachusetts. He provides his patients with rigorous and systematic training in "mindfulness" – a form of meditation that moves the explicit focus towards the body, and into the pain, rather than away from it.[4]

Distancing oneself from one's body can also help to change meanings. As a person with neurologic disease, I know well the feelings of shame, disgust and self-loathing that invariably accompany indignities such as loss of bowel and bladder control. If patients can learn to separate feelings from bodily functions, to view the "mess" of sickness dispassionately, they are less likely to feel degraded by illness.

Humour can play a transformative role in counteracting negative feelings such as shame, anger, frustration and disgust. The ability to laugh at oneself and the absurdity of one's situation makes life bearable even in the direst of circumstances. It is a concrete way to "de-fuse" emotionally painful circumstances. Often others find humour to be an inappropriate response – an indication that patients and their families are denying the seriousness of the situation. However, humour is not necessarily inappropriate. Indeed, it is an integral aspect of joyful living. Distancing from the body can also be achieved by deliberately focusing outwards, engaging in activities that take up one's concentration – reading, working, listening to music, pursuing hobbies. The goal is to dis-place the body as an unwelcome and insistent presence.

The Threat to the Self

In incurable illness the threat to the self at its deepest and most profound level is, of course, the existential threat of non-being. However, loss of self-integrity is also intimately related to cultural meanings regarding illness, disability and death. A formidable barrier to the preservation of self-esteem is the emphasis in our culture on the importance of "doing" as opposed to "being." More often than not, a person's worth is judged according to his or her capacity to produce or on the ability to achieve a certain professional status. The emphasis on productivity, the accumulation of material goods or the achievement of a certain status, focuses our attention outward on our involvements, our impact on the world. Such a stance is active, controlling and (above all) oriented toward the future. Consequently, as activities become circumscribed, as roles inevitably change and as the future disappears, this cultural emphasis on the importance of "doing" directly contributes to a sense of diminished self-worth.

Moreover, the cultural emphasis on self-reliance and the ideal of autonomy makes it particularly hard to request and accept assistance from others. Dependence on others is perceived as weakness. There is a strong cultural message that we should be able to look after ourselves, make our own decisions, run our own lives. Issues of dependence and interdependence intrude upon even the most intimate relationships. Serious illness necessarily changes our roles as wife, lover, friend, parent, breadwinner. Incurable disease is never simply a disorder that affects a particular stricken individual, it strikes equally at family members and other intimates.

Cultural attitudes towards death and sickness also contribute to loss of self-esteem. Ours is a culture obsessed with physical fitness, sexuality and youth. There is the clear assumption that physical incapacity and wholeness are incompatible. This assumption overtly manifests itself in social perceptions of disability. When strangers look at me, what they see is the wheelchair. They make the immediate judgement that my quality of life is diminished and that my situation is an essentially negative and unhappy one. In the first place, since my mobility is limited, others conclude that my intellect is likewise affected. For instance, in my presence strangers invariably address questions to my companion and refer to me in the third person. "Where would *she* like to sit? Does *she* want us to move this chair?" (When we travel through airports my husband is usually asked: "Can *she* walk at all?" We now have a standard response. He says: "No, but *she* can talk!")

If healing is to be achieved it is vital that we recognize the extent to which cultural, as well as personal, meanings contribute to suffering and weaken the resolve to live well in spite of illness. For example, in my own situation, preserving self-integrity means deliberately ignoring cultural meanings with respect to disability – choosing to construe my wheelchair as an "instrument of freedom" rather than as a "symbol of disability." This is not simply a matter of semantics. If individuals feel ashamed to use devices such as wheelchairs, they will not do so. (This is also true with respect to an individual's willingness to take medications, undergo treatment, or even seek professional help.) An important aspect of care is assuring individuals that illness and disability do not denigrate self-worth. This means assisting them to change the significance of preconceived cultural and personal meanings.

The Importance of Choice

Recognizing that one always has the capacity and opportunity to make meaningful choices (even though such choices may be severely circumscribed) is essential for the task of preserving self-integrity (healing). As Viktor Frankl has so eloquently noted, even in the most difficult circumstances, everything can be taken away from a person except for "the last of human freedoms" – the freedom to choose how to react to any given circumstances.[5] This is no empty freedom. It allows one to assume responsibility for the things one can change, while accepting the fact that there are circumstances that will always be beyond one's control. The freedom to choose one's way is not merely some sort of abstract, contemplative activity. It involves many aspects of living with illness. Concrete and individual choices can be made with respect to such issues as pain control, types of medication, treatment options, and when to engage and when to forego certain types of care.

Hope

The possibility and necessity for choice is an integral part of the dynamics of hope. For those with incurable illness the choice between hope and despair is a choice that must be made not once but every day. Hope cannot primarily be related to cure of disease. Nevertheless, to be seriously and incurably ill is not to be hope-less. Hope relates, rather, to the ability to face forthrightly and with courage whatever comes one's way. Hope is tempered with flexibility, a willingness to remain open to the possibilities of different ways of being-in-the-world. In this respect, hope is bolstered by the affirmation of others, the knowledge that one is not in this alone and will not be alone in the future.

Summary

In our culture, incurable illness almost invariably engenders a profound sense of loss of wholeness, which includes feelings of bodily alienation, a transformation in the familiar world, a change in the significance of time, a disruption in social relations, and a profound loss of self-esteem. Understanding these various facets of loss of wholeness can provide important insights into ways to initiate the process of healing – a process that enables individuals to attain a sense of personal unity and harmony despite physical debility.

NOTES

1 Toombs, S. K., *The Meaning of Illness: A Phenomenologic Account of the Different Perspectives of Physician and Patient* (Dordrecht, Germany: Kluwer, 1992).
2 Ebers, G. C., Survey, University of Western Ontario, London, Ont.
3 Broyard, A., *Intoxicated By My Illness* (New York: Potter, 1992), p. 66.
4 Kabat-Zinn, J., *Full Catastrophe Living: Using the Wisdom of Your Body and Mind to Face Stress, Pain and Illness* (New York: Dell, 1990).
5 Frankl, V., *Man's Search For Meaning: An Introduction to Logotherapy* (New York: Simon and Schuster, 1974).

19

"My Story Is Broken; Can You Help Me Fix It?" Medical Ethics and the Joint Construction of Narrative

HOWARD BRODY

[. . .] Ideally, the physician–patient relationship should be both ethically sound and therapeutically effective. Constructing certain sorts of narratives within that relationship attaches meaning to the patient's illness experience in a way that enhances the healing potential of the encounter. Moreover, when narratives are jointly constructed, power is shared between physician and patient, and the sharing of power constitutes an important ethical safeguard within the relationship.

The Meaning of Illness and the Patient's Story

Physicians have known, at least since the time of Hippocrates, that the mental, emotional, and symbolic aspects of the physician–patient encounter can ameliorate (or worsen) disease every bit as much as the specific medications and other treatments the physician employs. Modern research into the placebo response has amply documented the power of symbolic healing.[1]

Although the concept of *symbolic healing* is vague, a careful review of the literature allows a more precise identification of its operating components. These may be roughly subdivided as explanatory system, care and compassion, and mastery and control. As a general rule, patients will be more inclined to get better when they are provided with satisfactory explanations for what bothers them, sense care and concern among those around them, and are helped to achieve a sense of mastery or control over their illness and its symptoms.[2] Patients will become worse when the illness remains mysterious and frightening, when they sense social isolation and lack of support, and when the illness is accompanied by a feeling of helplessness. These components can in turn be broken down into further subdivisions for more detailed empirical study.[3]

The physician who listens carefully to the patient's story of the illness lays the groundwork for all the important dimensions of symbolic healing. It is the patient's story of the illness – the way the patient has tried to organize, and hence to make sense of, the various manifestations of disease within the context of his own life – that displays the meaning the patient has attached to the illness experience before his contact with the physician. The physician can hardly offer a more satisfying explanation for the illness unless she has first heard out the patient, because the patient will not recognize the new explanation as being about *his own* illness unless he knows that he has been listened to initially. Being willing to listen to the patient's story – which oftentimes family and friends have dismissed with impatience – sets a tone of care and compassion for the physician–patient relationship. Finally, in Western culture people are used to the idea of gaining mastery or control over events by being able to tell a coherent story about them. Thus, listening carefully to the patient's story begins the process of healing at the symbolic level.

It might be argued that healing at the symbolic level is a poor substitute for the scientific application of medical therapy to a properly diagnosed disease state. But symbolic healing as just described is totally congruent with a proper scientific approach to medical diagnosis and therapy, properly understood. George L. Engel, in a highly important paper on this subject, has noted that the beginning of all science is the careful, reproducible gathering of data.[4] In the case of illness, the patient's history is the major source of data, since one cannot really perform an appropriate physical exam, or order the appropriate laboratory tests and x-rays, unless one has been guided by the patient's description of his own symptoms. But taking an accurate history is far more difficult than it might first appear. The patient must be in a particular state of alert, thoughtful candor in order to describe the course of the illness clearly and accurately and to be willing to expose all of his innermost thoughts and feelings to the physician's gaze. This state, in turn, entails a particular sort of curious, compassionate, and supportive style of interviewing on the physician's part. If care is not taken from the beginning to set the proper tone for the medical interview, the physician will never gather the scientific data necessary to make an appropriate diagnosis. (She might as well go into the laboratory and try to study slides through a dirty microscope lens.)

Given the very short time available for most physician–patient encounters, one might well wonder how an accurate history could ever be taken and how the patient could ever be healed. It would appear that hours, if not days, of careful conversation and negotiation would be necessary to create exactly the right setting for the scientifically valid medical interview. Engel shrewdly observed that doctor and patient are aided by some deep emotional drives, which one could almost attribute to the biological makeup of human beings. On the physician's side, there is a deeply rooted "need to know" – the physician's scientific curiosity is aroused by the patient, and the mystery of the illness is there to be solved. On the patient's side is an equally deep "need to be known" – as if the patient senses that by allowing the physician to understand his disease, he will in turn be healed, by the symbolic route, as well as by whatever specific remedies the physician might apply. The complementarity of these basic drives means that the physician who genuinely appreciates the power of medical interviewing and history taking can begin to elicit scientifically valid information within a few minutes of the start of the encounter. Unfortunately, as Engel and others have noted, this is no longer the norm in modern medical practice. Much more common is the physician who interrupts the patient, who begins early on to ask closed-ended and overly technical questions, and who in a variety of ways guarantees that she will hear apparently useful bits of information but will never hear the patient's story of the illness.

Intriguing support for Engel's recommendations comes from studies conducted by family physicians at the University of Western Ontario. These physicians considered a variety of common presenting symptoms that patients bring to their family physicians; the investigators asked what characteristics of medical care would best predict the patient's report of relief of symptoms after a given interval (ranging from one month to one year). Virtually all technical aspects of care, including adequacy of history and physical exam, types of laboratory investigations, and drugs ordered, failed to correlate with improvement of symptoms. The single most important predictor of relief of symptoms was the report of the patient that he had had a chance to discuss the problem fully with the physician at an early visit and that the physician had come to an understanding of the problem that was basically identical to the patient's own.[5] Other studies have shown that agreement between physician and patient about the nature of the presenting problem is closely linked to a good outcome.[6] In other words, the patient who feels *listened to* in the first encounter with the physician is far more likely to show a positive response to treatment.

It therefore appears that the physician, depending upon how well she listens to the patient and what sort of atmosphere she creates in the interview, has substantial power to alter the patient's health status for better or for worse. How the physician uses that power is an important ethical question for medicine.

Patients, Physicians, and Power

John Ladd has commented that the central ethical problem in medicine is the responsible use of the physician's power.[7] However, the term *power* has not been a favorite with philosophers investigating the ethical principles underlying medical practice. I have argued elsewhere that there are some special benefits to be gained from looking explicitly at power issues in medicine and putting the term *power* back into the vocabulary of medical ethics.[8]

In most relationships marked by a power disparity between the parties, an obvious resolution is to equalize the power, either by empowering the weaker party or by taking away some of the power of the stronger. Indeed, the ethical principle of respect for the patient's autonomy might seem superficially to accomplish precisely that, thereby explaining the popularity of this principle in discussions of medical ethics in the last two decades. But on deeper analysis, any simple approach to equalizing power, particularly by removing power from the physician's side of the equation, runs into serious problems. Most important is the fact that patients, given the choice, do not seek the help of relatively powerless physicians. Patients seek out the most powerful physicians and want very much for the physician to use that power on their behalf. This behavior occurs despite the fact that pa-

tients, at some level, inevitably fear the physician's power and realize that there are a number of ways in which it can be used against them.

The same scalpel that can cut out a diseased organ or a tumor may nick a vital artery or nerve. The same medication that can heal may cause toxic side effects. As I argued above, the physician's words can promote healing or can increase the patient's suffering. There is simply no handy dividing line between the helpful and the hurtful uses of the tools the physician possesses. And, of course, the physician is seldom consciously malicious in those circumstances where the tools are misused and where the patient suffers harm as a result of the physician's exercise of power.

The critical goal of medical ethics should be to enhance the physician's use of power against the disease on the side of the patient and minimize any temptation or opportunity to use power to the patient's detriment. What this goal means in practice often requires a careful analysis of the case at hand. (I contend that a relationship based on power tends to favor casuistic and virtue-based approaches to medical ethics and to look somewhat askance at approaches that are heavily dependent on ethical principles.) Still, some general guidelines can be given. One obvious safeguard of the patient, which still avoids interfering with the physician's power to eliminate disease and promote health, is a genuine sharing of power in the physician–patient relationship. [. . .]

It is immediately apparent that symbolic healing, as described in the previous section, and a shared-power model of the physician–patient relationship have many features in common. Giving the patient an adequate explanation for the illness certainly allows the patient to participate more actively in medical care. Demonstrating care and compassion may give the patient the reassurance that he needs to participate in this way. Finally, instilling a sense of mastery or control is vital if the patient is truly to feel empowered and to take specific actions that will promote health and ameliorate symptoms. When symbolic healing is construed in an appropriately broad fashion, it is seen to enhance an ethical physician–patient relationship, and vice versa.

Symbolic healing is closely tied to the meaning of the illness experience for the patient, which in turn is tied closely to the story that the patient tells in an effort to make sense of the illness. The next question is how the shared-power model and the symbolic-healing model can be combined to suggest an optimal approach to the patient's story.

The Joint Construction of Narrative

To summarize the argument thus far, the physician who hopes to heal and to relieve suffering ought to attend as seriously to the patient's story of the illness experience as to the purely bodily manifestations of disease. (Put more accurately, the physician should approach a deeper inquiry into bodily processes through the vehicle of the patient's story.) And the physician should approach the story in a way that encourages the ultimate goal of shared power: making the patient a more active participant in his medical care.

Something more must be said here about the difference between curing and healing. Eric J. Cassell has argued eloquently that today's medicine is usually better at curing than healing and ironically may increase suffering even as it cures, or tries to cure.[9] At the heart of suffering is a feeling that what ought to be whole is being split apart. This feeling may be experienced as a split between one's self and one's malfunctioning body or as an isolation of the self from the human community. Suffering cannot be relieved, however elegant a cure one performs, unless the patient's subjective sense of split and isolation has been assuaged. Almost always, this assuagement requires a sense of reattachment to the human community from which the patient, through illness, has felt cut off. The physician is the human ambassador who most often and most directly can reach out and reestablish this sense of human connection. Her willingness to listen to the patient's story may be the first step in this process. (Until this point, the patient may have felt, "People are unwilling to listen to my story; it either bores them or frightens them.")

Taking the patient's story seriously begins at the very start of the interview, with the natural question of why the patient is seeking help from the physician. Sometimes this is totally obvious, as when the patient needs a piece of paper to be signed in order to go back to work or to get married. But very often in general medical practice, it is not totally clear at the outset why the patient has sought help at that particular time. (Merely reporting a backache or a headache or a cough does not really explain the visit, as it has been well documented that for every patient in the physician's office, there are three or four people walking around with equally severe backaches, headaches, and coughs who have not even thought of seeking medical attention.) The physician who takes stories seriously will, in any case where there is any mystery about the patient's reason for seeking help, adopt as a working hypothesis that the patient is asking a question like the following: "Something is happening to me that seems abnormal, and either I cannot think of a story that will explain it, or the only story I can think of is very frightening. Can you help me to tell a better story, one that will cause me less distress, about this experience?" If this formulation seems overly wordy, a shorter form of the patient's possible plea to the physician might be, "My story is broken; can you help me fix it?"

This question may seem at first a highly unusual way of characterizing the patient's request of the physician. It is unlikely that any patient in Western society, without a good deal of guidance, would articulate his concerns in this way. Nevertheless, this question has the virtue of clarifying an important task that the physician and patient must engage in together. This task is a major part of all good doctor–patient encounters, but it usually happens under the table, because the traditional way of looking at that encounter focuses so heavily on history taking, physical examination, diagnosis, and treatment. I have labeled this task the *joint construction of narrative*.

The joint construction of narrative is a complex task that consists of many elements. Its complexity may be illustrated by an example that may at first seem trivial but that is, for this very reason, a valuable glimpse of some of the important features of everyday practice.

The patient consults the physician because of a cough that has been going on for several days. The physician's careful interview elicits, along with the usual description of symptoms, the fact that the patient's aunt recently nearly died of pneumonia and the patient is worried that he might have pneumonia also. The physician reassures the patient, after an appropriate examination, that he does not have pneumonia and that the cough is probably related to postnasal drip. The physician recommends a vaporizer and other simple home remedies to try to relieve the nasal congestion that is thought to be the basis for the cough.

One important element of the joint construction of narrative is that the patient is fully involved throughout the process. The physician does not hand the new narrative "postnasal drip" instead of "pneumonia" to the patient in the way that the traditional physician hands out a prescription at the end of the visit. There is an ongoing, partly nonverbal give-and-take as the physician listens carefully, throws out a few tentative comments, and modifies her approach depending upon how the patient responds to her initial offers of advice, explanation, and reassurance. If the patient indicates acceptance and relief, the physician moves quickly to complete her account of what is bothering the patient and what should be done about it. If any of these comments produce a raised eyebrow or other evidence of questioning or resistance, the physician will stop at that point and explore much more fully what the patient might be thinking.

The involvement of the patient is critical in the next element of the joint construction of narrative, which is that the narrative must be meaningful *from the patient's point of view*. To explain an episode of illness, it must be the sort of story that the patient has grown to expect. If, in my example, the patient feels as if the origin of the cough must be in his chest, he is unlikely to accept the explanation that nasal congestion is the cause. Moreover, the patient has to accept that the story is truly *about him*. If the physician listens carefully to his account and performs an appropriate physical exam, the patient is likely to believe this story. If the physician seems rushed and does not perform an exam that the patient feels is sufficient, then the story will not seem to be a story of the *patient's* illness, but rather a stock story that the physician simply took off the shelf and will use for all other patients who show up with a cough that week.[10]

Another important element is that the story must be biomedically sound. The patient sought the physician because the physician represents the vast powers of medical science; the physician engages in a fundamental fraud if the story offered to explain the illness is not congruent with appropriate scientific thought. In my example, the patient might be greatly relieved by being told that the physician thinks an antibiotic is required and that it will surely cure any pneumonia that might be present. But if an antibiotic is not truly indicated, the physician ought not to construct such a narrative simply to please the patient.

Another critical element in the joint construction of narrative is that the new story ought to promote the healing action that the physician and patient agree ought to be carried out. If the best way to get over a cough caused by postnasal drip is to use a vaporizer and to drink more fluids, an ideal story of the illness will show how these measures actually play a role in producing an improvement in the symptoms. For the patient to be as highly motivated as possible to carry out the practices in question, he must see the practices themselves as efficacious and must envision himself actually doing those things. Such a shift in outlook involves both the explanatory system and the patient's sense of mastery or control (empowerment) over the illness.

A final element is that the new narrative must facilitate either the patient's getting on with his life story or his modifying it as required by the illness. In my example, the patient can go about his usual projects and routines in a day or so and need not significantly postpone or replace any of his cherished goals in life because of this cough. The new narrative account of the illness is aimed at getting the patient back into this frame of thinking as quickly as possible. This result would not have occurred, for example, if the physician had not elicited the fear about the patient's aunt and had not offered adequate reassurance. Instead of a healthy patient going about his business in a few days, this encounter might have produced a worried patient who is continually asking himself whether the doctor missed something important and whether he can safely resume his usual activities.

In most encounters in general medicine, this sort of reassurance is the appropriate outcome, as long as the physician has taken the time to find out what really is worrying the patient. Occasionally, however, a serious disease will be diagnosed, and then the construction of narrative becomes much more difficult and taxing. The patient must then begin the task of reconstructing the story of the rest of his life to take into account this new disease and the limitations it will impose upon his activities; he must go through a grieving process for the loss of the old life plans and goals that the disease has rendered now out of reach. In that event, the joint construction of narrative obviously requires much greater skill and sensitivity on the physician's part, and the construction occurs over an extended period, not in one encounter.

The joint construction of narrative, as just described, is not a new recommendation for physician–patient interaction. Good physicians have generally done this as a matter of course. But they have done this because it seemed instinctively like the right thing to do, not because anyone taught them to, and still less because anyone had carried out detailed research to show how each element could be performed optimally. The point of listing the various elements in the joint construction of narrative is to suggest that this task will be performed much better if more attention is paid to it explicitly. This attention, in turn, requires that one take very seriously the notion of story or narrative in medicine, which will not occur if one thinks that medicine is about biomedical abnormalities rather than about what the patient is thinking.

Taking narrative seriously will require increased attention to spoken as well as unspoken communication between physician and patient. The metaphors employed by each will require much more careful scrutiny. The rituals of the encounter will require explicit study. To the committed advocate of a purely biomedical model, it will seem as if scientific physicians are being asked to embrace precisely those aspects of "good bedside manner" that have usually been

associated with quacks – people who were forced to employ as pleasing a manner as possible because they lacked any *scientific* tools for healing – rather than with legitimate physicians.

Is this conscious employment of ritual, metaphor, and storytelling not insincere, fraudulent, or manipulative? The answer will lie both in the physician's assessment of the scientific evidence that supports the efficacy of symbolic modes of healing and in the physician's attitude toward this behavior. It might well be that the narrative approach will degenerate into a shallow pose if it is employed merely as a tool in the interview, in the way that one might use, for example, an alcoholism-screening questionnaire. Or the approach might represent a sincere attempt on the physician's part to *develop over time into a certain sort of person* – a healing sort of person – for whom the primary focus of attention is outward, toward the experience and suffering of the patient, and not inward, toward the physician's own preconceived agenda. As Warren Thomas Reich has argued, the litmus test of the sincerity of this approach will be the extent to which the physician becomes vulnerable to a compassionate and empathic experience of the patient's suffering.[11] That is, when "narrative interviewing" is used as an impersonal tool, the patient's experience of suffering (and the patient) are kept at a safe distance, and the patient is likely to feel this. When a narrative approach is used in the way advocated in this essay, both physician and patient feel that the physician is open and vulnerable to the patient's experience of suffering.

The notion that one is trying over time to develop into a special sort of person and that one is willing to open oneself to being changed by experiencing the suffering of others proves finally that the physician has accepted a suitably humble status in the power hierarchy of the physician–patient relationship. The physician has not abandoned the very powerful scientific armamentarium for which the patient initially sought her assistance. But neither has the physician used that armamentarium as a prop to protect herself from any possible feelings of powerlessness as she confronts the patient's experience. To the biomedically oriented physician, any such sense of powerlessness is threatening and unseemly, so that the physician emphasizes the importance of objective detachment. The "narrative physician" knows that sometimes objective detachment is both necessary and comforting to the patient but sometimes a compassionate vulnerability is required. The choice between them is dictated by what is necessary to empower the patient in the face of the illness, rather than what will make the physician *feel* powerful. Mastering this approach to patient care requires an understanding that sometimes what *seems* to be an admission of powerlessness actually makes the physician *more* powerful in terms of being able genuinely to help the patient.

[...]

Patients have always emerged from an encounter with a physician bearing a new story about the nature and significance of their illnesses. Sensitive physicians have generally seen to it that the new story bears the stamp of a particular patient's unique individuality and that the patient himself has been involved in constructing the story. Scientific medicine has made great strides by ignoring this level of storytelling and by focusing instead on quite different stories, at the organic, cellular, and molecular levels, to explain how medicine works. For a complete understanding of medical activity, the question of how physicians and patients can best construct stories about illness must be returned to the center stage of medical inquiry. This is an inquiry to which both scientific investigators and humanities scholars can contribute significantly, with the outcome being an enhanced healing ability for modern medical practice.

NOTES

1   The most comprehensive overview of placebo research and theory is Leonard White, Bernard Tursky, and Gary E. Schwartz (eds.), *Placebo: Theory, Research, and Mechanisms* (New York: Guilford, 1985). See also Howard Brody, *Placebos and the Philosophy of Medicine: Clinical, Conceptual, and Ethical Issues* (Chicago: University of Chicago Press, 1980). This research documents at great length that the bodily changes produced by placebo responses and related mechanisms are real and measurable. Thus, the term *symbolic*

healing, as used in this [chapter], refers to those aspects of the physician–patient encounter that bring about measurable bodily responses; the term is not intended to suggest that the responses themselves are imaginary or fleeting.

2   For further discussion of what I have termed the *meaning model*, see Howard Brody and David B. Waters, "Diagnosis is treatment," *Journal of Family Practice* 10 (March 1980): 445–9; Howard Brody, "The placebo response. Part 1: Exploring the myths" and "The placebo response. Part 2: Use in clinical practice," *Drug Therapy* 16 (July 1986): 106–18, 119–31, respectively; and Howard Brody, "The symbolic power of the modern personal physician: The placebo response under challenge," *Journal of Drug Issues* 18 (Winter 1988): 149–61. Other very influential treatments are Arthur Kleinman, *The Illness Narratives: Suffering, Healing, and The Human Condition* (New York: Basic Books, 1988), and Barbara F. Sharf, "Patient–physician communication as interpersonal rhetoric: A narrative approach," *Health Communication* 2 (1990): 217–31.

3   See Dennis H. Novack, "Therapeutic aspects of the clinical encounter," *Journal of General Internal Medicine* 2 (September–October 1987): 346–55.

4   George L. Engel, "How much longer must medicine's science be bound by a seventeenth-century world view?" in *The Task of Medicine: Dialogue at Wickenburg*, ed. Kerr L. White (Menlo Park, CA: Henry J. Kaiser Family Foundation, 1988), pp. 113–36.

5   Martin J. Bass et al., "The physician's actions and the outcome of illness in family practice," *Journal of Family Practice* 23 (July 1986): 43–7, and Martin J. Bass et al., "Predictors of outcome in headache patients presenting to family physicians – A one-year prospective study," *Headache* 26 (June 1986): 285–94.

6   See, for example, Barbara Starfield et al., "The influence of patient–practitioner agreement on outcome of care," *American Journal of Public Health* 71 (February 1981): 127–31.

7   John Ladd, "Medical ethics: Who knows best?" *Lancet* ii (22 November 1980): 1127–9.

8   Howard Brody, *The Healer's Power* (New Haven, CN: Yale University Press, 1992).

9   Eric J. Cassell, "The nature of suffering and the goals of medicine," *New England Journal of Medicine* 306 (18 March 1982): 639–45.

10   This discussion makes it appear as if a few simple moves on the physician's part will assure that the patient accepts the meaning that the

physician feels is the best explanation of the symptom. Of course, the real world is not so simple: sometimes a protracted process of negotiation is required for physician and patient to arrive together at a satisfactory meaning (assuming that the patient doesn't simply go out shopping for a more agreeable physician). One case of my own comes to mind in which the negotiation as to whether a recurring problem with eye pain and double vision meant "undiagnosed brain tumor, like my mother had" or "emotional stress triggered by unresolved grief over your mother's death" lasted for several years and had not finally been resolved when the patient moved to another state.

11   Warren Thomas Reich, "Speaking of suffering: A moral account of compassion," *Soundings* 72 (Spring 1989): 83–108.

20

Spiritual Experience and Psychopathology

MIKE JACKSON AND K. W. M. FULFORD

Introduction

This [chapter] explores some of the conceptual and practical implications of the finding that phenomena which in a medical context would probably be diagnosed as psychotic *symptoms* may occur in the context of non-pathological, and indeed essentially benign, spiritual experiences.

The existence of non-pathological psychotic experiences of this kind (we will call them "psychotic *phenomena*" as distinct from "psychotic *symptoms*") was a key finding in a study carried out by one of us (MJ) at the Alister Hardy Research Centre (AHRC) in Oxford (Jackson 1991, 1997 and forthcoming). The interpretation of this finding, as pointing to the central importance of human values in psychiatric diagnosis, draws on the philosophical work by the second author (KWMF) on the hidden values embedded in all areas of medical disease classification (Fulford, 1989, 2nd edn forthcoming).

In the present [chapter], (1) the background to the study is described briefly in relation to earlier work on the possible links between spiritual experience and psychopathology; (2) some of the psychotic phenomena identified are illustrated with three detailed case histories; (3) the

significance of these phenomena is reviewed for our understanding respectively of psychopathology, of diagnostic syndromes, and of the concept of mental illness; and (4) some of the practical implications of the study for clinical work and research in psychiatry are indicated.

Background

It has long been recognized that there are similarities between spiritual and psychotic experiences. William James (1902), for example, argued that "in delusional insanity, paranoia as they sometimes call it, we may have a kind of diabolical mysticism, a sort of religious mysticism turned upside down" (p. 426). Other commentators have noted a wide variety of phenomena, such as time distortion, synesthesias, loss of self-object boundaries and the transition from a state of conflict and anxiety to one of sudden "understanding," all of which are reported in both spiritual and psychotic experiences (Buckley, 1981; Watson, 1982; Wapnick, 1969; and Wootton and Allen, 1983).

Yet the similarities notwithstanding, the distinction between these two kinds of experience can be crucially important. *Spiritual* experiences, whether welcome or unwelcome, and whether or not they are psychotic in form, have nothing (directly) to do with medicine (Fulford, 1996a). It would be quite wrong, then, to "treat" spiritual psychotic experiences with neuroleptic drugs, just as it is quite wrong to "treat" political dissidents as though they were ill (Fulford, Smirnoff, and Snow, 1993). Pathological psychotic experiences, on the other hand, or psychotic *symptoms*, are by definition a proper object of medical treatment, sometimes even against the wishes of the person concerned. Hence it would be both negligent and, as Wing (1978) put it, morally "repellent," to leave untreated someone who is genuinely ill (p. 244).

The Study

The current study was made possible in part by the opportunity offered by the Alister Hardy Research Centre in Oxford to use their uniquely extensive data base of more than five thousand contemporary accounts of spiritual experience. With access to such a large and diverse pool of subjects, it was possible to select test cases strategically. As already emphasized, this approach was not designed to explore in a general way the relationship between spiritual experience and psychotic illness. It was intended, rather, to focus specifically on issues arising in the area of overlap between them, a key purpose of the study being to decide whether, in fact, psychotic phenomena can occur in the context of benign spiritual experiences, and if so, to explain the significance of this occurrence.

Methods

Cases were selected from the 1,000 most recent accounts received by the AHRC (covering the period 1984–9). A semi-structured interview was developed, covering the participant's background and history, the context, phenomenology and effects of their spiritual experiences, and the interpretations which they and others placed on them. Tape-recorded interviews were conducted in the participants' homes and subsequently transcribed. These lasted between

two and four hours. The purpose of the study was explained at the start of the interview. It was made clear that the interviewer, being a representative of a research organization concerned with spiritual experience, was sympathetic to the spiritual significance for the interviewees of their experiences.

Fifteen individuals were contacted with a request for an interview,[1] and nine interviews were eventually conducted, of which three are reported here. One of these ("Simon") was entirely self-selected, in that he simply arrived at the Research Centre during the study.

Overview of results

The original study (Jackson, 1991) included a comparison of five subjects selected as above (the "undiagnosed group") with five who had recovered from major psychoses but nonetheless interpreted their experiences in strongly spiritual terms (the "diagnosed group").

Far from being phenomenologically distinct, therefore, what was perhaps most striking about the two groups was the extent of their phenomenological similarities. Even in this highly selected sample, it should be said that there were certain overall differences of degree between the experiences described by the diagnosed and undiagnosed subjects. None of the differences was decisive, though, and the question remains whether in an individual case the distinction between spiritual experience and psychopathology can be made solely in terms of traditional diagnostic methods as set out in standard psychiatric texts. We return to this question after describing three cases in detail.[2]

1.   Simon

Simon (40) was a senior black American professional from a middle–class Baptist family. Before the main period of his spiritual experiences, he reported sporadic, relatively unremarkable, psychic experiences. These had led him to seek the guidance of a professional "seer," with whom he occasionally consulted on major life events and decisions.

Around four years before the first interview, his hitherto successful career was threatened by legal action from his colleagues. Although he claimed to be innocent, mounting a defense would be expensive and hazardous. He responded to this crisis by praying at a small altar which he set up in his front room. After an emotional evening's "outpouring," he discovered that the candle wax had left a "seal" (or "sun") on several consecutive pages of his Bible, covering certain letters and words. He described his experiences thus. "*I got up and I saw the seal that was in my father's Bible and I called X and I said, 'You know, something remarkable is going on over here.' I think the beauty of it was the specificity by which the sun burned through. It was ... in my mind, a clever play on words.*" Although the marked words and letters had no explicit meaning, Simon interpreted this event as a direct communication from God, which signified that he had a special purpose or mission. This belief meets the PSE definition of a *Primary Delusion*, in that it was "based on sensory experiences," and involved him "suddenly becoming convinced that a particular set of events had a special meaning" (PSE symptom 82).[3]

From this time on, Simon received a complex series of "revelations" largely conveyed through the images left in melted candle wax. He carried photos of these, which left most observers unimpressed, but were, for him, clearly representations of biblical symbols, particularly from the book of Revelations (the bull, the twenty-four elders, the ark of the covenant, etc.). His interpretations of them, moreover, would be consistent with *Delusions of Grandiose Ability* (PSE symptom 76): they signified that "*I am the living son of David ... and I'm also a relative of Ishmael, and ... of Joseph.*" He was also the "*captain of the guard of Israel.*" He found this role carried awesome responsibilities: "*Sometimes I'm saying – O my God, why did you choose me, and there's no answer to that.*" His special status had the effect of "*Increasing my own inward sense, wisdom, understanding, and endurance*" which would "*allow me to do whatever is required in terms of bringing whatever message it is that God wants me to bring.*"

The PSE (symptom 78) defines *Religious Delusions* as "both a religious identification on the part of a subject and an explanation in religious terms of other abnormal experiences." This clearly applies to Simon's central beliefs, which he expressed with full conviction: "*The truths that are up in that room are the truths that have been spoken of for 4,000 years.*" When confronted with skepticism, he commented: "*I don't get upset, because I know within myself, what I know.*"

His central belief was highly systematized, in that he interpreted much of his ongoing experience in terms of it. His colleagues were agents of Satan, trying to thwart him, and his career successes were evidence of God's special favor. Relatively trivial obstacles which he encountered in daily life – such as having a cold at the time of the interview – were satanically motivated trials of purpose.

He also described experiences of *Inserted Thoughts* (PSE symptom 55), using the following evocative simile: "*If you're sitting and watching television, and then somebody turns on the vacuum cleaner, and the TV goes on the fritz, it's like that*"/ "*the things that come are not the things that I have been thinking about.... They kind of short circuit the brain, and bring their message.*" In the course of these experiences he had both heard God's voice and seen "prophetic" visions.

Simon had no *insight*, in the sense (defined in the PSE, symptom 104) that he considered his mental processes to be completely normal. He had told various friends and ministers about them, and believed that "*No one really thought I was crazy because ... they've known me all my life ... and I think God would not permit it, to be honest with you.*" However, he was careful to conceal what was happening from his colleagues, as he recognized that they would perceive it as suspect.

While his beliefs were clearly sub-culturally influenced, they were "further elaborated ... so that other members of the sub-group might well recognize them as abnormal" (PSE symptom 83: *Sub-culturally influenced delusions*). Indeed, Simon was puzzled by the way in which certain of the ministers he had consulted drew attention to their messianic overtones. He had "*stopped talking to some of the ministers*" and he commented that "*people want to take it away from me, and say 'I'm glad that you don't see it as something especially for you.'... They'll try and dismiss me out of the equation, which I find fascinating."*

Diagnostically, Simon's experiences, if assumed to be pathological, might suggest schizophrenia (on the basis of thought insertion and a primary delusion). Alternatively, the presence of a well systematized set of delusions, in the absence of prominent hallucinations, might suggest a DSM-IIIR diagnosis of delusional disorder. However, as far as Simon was concerned, his revelations had been entirely beneficial in his life. He claimed that they gave him the conviction to contest and win the lawsuit against him, and more generally to succeed as a high-achieving black person in a predominantly white, racist context. He had high self-esteem, firm moral convictions, and a strong sense of purpose in life. His beliefs then, whilst unusual in content, and psychotic in form, were essentially affirming, and if anything increased rather than detracted from his ability to function effectively.

A year after the initial interview he made contact again. He reported that in the interval his career had flourished and that he had successfully set up a new charitably oriented institution. His revelations had continued; indeed they had increased in frequency and scope. He confided that his mission involved unifying "true Christianity" (a *"return to the ancient ways of the worship of the Lord"*) and "true Islam." He had plans to announce himself live on TV but was waiting for the right signs.

2. Sara

Sara (aged 43) was a pastoral worker from a middle-class, Christian family. She had trained as a secretary and worked for a large industrial company. In her early thirties, she went through a period of untreated depression after discovering that she could not have children. This abated when she received accelerated promotion into middle management. Her initial experience occurred at a time when she was beginning to question her level of commitment to her career. She was waiting at a traffic light on her way to work, when *"I heard a voice say 'Sara, this is Jesus. When are you coming to work for me?' And*

my first reaction was, I honestly thought it was my brother hidden in the back of the car....I thought he was having me on. I turned round to look and there was nobody there. I turned back and thought 'He's put a tape in the car' because it was so real and there was nothing there. Then I heard it again...I knew beyond any shadow of a doubt who it was and I also thought to myself 'You must be joking. I'm not giving up my management career. On your bike, sunshine! No way.'"

In the PSE this would be classified as a psychotic or *True Hallucination* because the voice is experienced as coming from outside the mind (PSE symptom 65). Moreover, consistently with a diagnosis of schizophrenia, it is not affectively bound (i.e., the content is not a direct reflection of the subject's mood) and it is in the first person (i.e., it is addressing the subject). For Sara this occurrence marked the beginning of a sequence of frequent experiences of *"God's voice,"* giving her detailed instructions and information: for example, in a library she heard *"fourth shelf down, third book along, page 170."* She had compiled these experiences into a book on the workings of the kingdom of heaven.

Over the four years between the onset of her experiences and the interview, the "voice" became increasingly internal and less prominent: *"In the first five months it was ultra clear because I couldn't hear anything else, but God doesn't take your free will away....It was just that he'd turned his own volume up, if you like. When you equalize the volumes I can listen to Him or I can do my own thing. Most of the time I'm clear but not always."* At the time of the interview, she still heard *"that little voice"* but had learned to distinguish it reliably from *"outside voices"*: *"There is total inner stillness, inner peace and silence and it's as if there's something inside me, but that's where it communicates and moves. I can feel it. I can't explain it but I can feel it."*

Sara believed that through God's intervention she had acquired various paranormal capabilities. The dominant paranormal element in her subsequent experiences was synchronicity: *"the co-ordinating...at the right time in life, the right books, the right references and the right people and the right courses. The information being given to me."* She also described numerous experiences involving telepathy, precognition, healing and communication with the dead, together with corroborating evidence. These often involved visual imagery which she described as *"picture language inside me."* She interpreted her experiences as a divine calling: *"For some reason I have been asked to be a specialist in this and I know an awful lot more than many people and priests come and talk to me about it and other people in that field."* According to the PSE, these beliefs involve *Delusions of Grandiose Ability* (symptom 76, "subject thinks he is chosen by some power . . . for a special mission or purpose, because of his unusual talents. He thinks he is able to read people's thoughts. . . ."): and *Religious Delusions* (symptom 78, as described above for Simon). They were expressed with full conviction (she "knew" rather than believed), and she claimed to be unconcerned about skeptical interpretations: *"You can't convince people unless they want to look. I don't care if they are skeptical."*

The onset of these experiences precipitated a period of intense conflict for Sara, during which she was *"terrified of going mad,"* and eventually sought the counsel of her minister. *"He thought I was having a religious wobbler at first and said 'Don't give up your management career.' But he gradually realized that it wasn't, it was something solid, not a schizophrenic breakdown."* He gave her a number of well-grounded reasons why he decided that her experiences were authentic: *"I was behaving rationally, coping with my job, making decisions, talking to my husband about the fact that I needed to leave work . . . making sensible arrangements about changing my life, and because I wasn't showing any phobias, paranoias or whatever."*

From her perspective, and apparently that of her priest, Sara's experiences were firmly embedded in mainstream Christian (Anglican) doctrine. However, other cases in the AHRC archive describe considerably less open-minded responses from clergy to less unusual experiences, including, in some cases, the suggestion that the confidant was in need of psychiatric help. As we discuss in the concluding section of this [chapter], it is interesting to speculate how Sara's experiences would have developed had she met with a less validating response from her priest.

At the time of the interview Sara was living a fulfilling and altruistic life. This involved working as a counselor and as a spiritual director to Anglican priests. As a member of the university chaplaincy pastoral team, she was also running a prayer group. Her experiences, if delusional and hallucinatory, were overwhelmingly positive in their content and fruits: *"It has always enhanced my life; it's brought a great deal to other people and it is benign; it is co-operative; it is loving; it helps me see the beauty of nature; hear the beauty of music; understand myself and others; reach out to others; begin to grasp something about ultimate reality and the way the universe is. It never torments me or taunts me; it teases me lovingly sometimes. . . . If I'm mad, so be it, but this is the most real thing I've ever known."*

3.   Sean

Sean was a 53-year-old life insurance salesman from a middle-class background. He had a "very basic" education in a secondary modern school. Apart from a brief period of involvement with an evangelical Christian group in his youth, he had been a "militant atheist" for most of his life until the onset of his spiritual experiences.

At the time, he was in a financial crisis due to unemployment, and strongly suspected that he had multiple sclerosis. He was "worried sick" about this as he walked his dog through some local fields, when he *"heard words not of my choice, but like another voice within me saying my name – 'Sean, none of this matters, you will always have what you need.'"* The voice then "instructed" him about the ephemeral nature of mundane reality and the need for an attitude of acceptance rather than resistance towards events. When he reached the road, *"my own thoughts started to come back"* and *"all the worry lifted."*

This and other voices continued to speak to Sean at length *"almost daily"* for about nine months, and then less frequently, on subjects related to the nature of the cosmic order and the practical consequences of this for him. He was clear that it was an internal voice, *"like coming through a headset."* But he was equally certain that it was not his own voice: "*it was not my voice, not my sound of voice.... Everything was so simply said and yet directly to the point. The meaning was there with few words and...not clever words but a phraseology that I wouldn't normally use.*" He gave a number of examples of what he had heard, for example: "*This is the beginning of things. Have no worries because ...you are living in a timed existence now. That will pass, and this is the beginning of eternity.... We are all part of one another. Our intelligence is all linked.*" He believed his communicants (who referred to themselves as "we") were from a "higher" level of the cosmic hierarchy. He referred to them as the CIA (Central Intelligence Agency). He believed that they knew a lot about subjects he had no opinions on and could answer questions that he put to them. This included confirming that he did indeed have multiple sclerosis, while reassuring him that he would still be able to function sufficiently well for his needs.

Sean's experiences, understood as psychopathology, fall somewhere between *Thought Insertion* (PSE symptom 55) and *Auditory Pseudohallucinations* (PSE symptom 65). The PSE defines thought insertion as follows: "the essence of the symptom is that the subject experiences thoughts *which are not his own* intruding into his mind" (emphasis in original). It notes that "auditory pseudohallucinations (voices experienced as being within the mind) may be very difficult to distinguish (from thought insertion), since sometimes the subject is unable to say whether the experience is a voice or a thought. In such cases rate both symptoms as present." This would apply to Sean, who described his experiences as both voices and thoughts. Initially, these were involuntary and uninvited, but he quickly began to seek them out, returning to the same site, and looking for "*contact.*"

In his original letter to the AHRC, Sean wrote: "*It is fascinating to find I'm not on my own in this. I have naturally queried my own sanity, and generally don't discuss it.... When I saw that article...it was not only interesting but a great relief to find I'm not cracking up after all!*" In the interview he said: "*I know me, I ain't no loony, I don't go and do crazy things. I lead a perfectly*

normal, respectable type of life, not because I have to but because it suits me....I am definitely sure ...that I am open to hear things that most people aren't.*" Finally, he said that he did not feel that a doctor would be competent to judge whether his experiences were real, although he would be worried about other people's reactions to a doctor's opinion. "*I just simply don't want anyone to know I'm a loony if I am.*"

As far as he was concerned, his experiences were completely separate from his cultural background. Although they involved universal religious themes, the only religion he had encountered previously was relatively fundamentalist Christianity, which he regarded as irrelevant to his experiences. He had never discussed his experience with anyone before the interview except, briefly, with his wife. She thought he was joking and he didn't raise the subject again.

Sean was emphatic that his experiences had a profound and entirely positive effect in his life. When they started, he was in a state of hopeless despair, and the voice marked a turning point for him. "*It turned me upside down in many ways. It altered my views completely.... [I] live life now as far as I can by what I'm learning.*" He felt that it had helped him to cope with his difficulties, including multiple sclerosis, in an effective but effortless and relaxed way. "*I think I have support and guidance, so nothing in this world can worry me.*" At the time of the interview, he no longer heard the voices in the same concrete way, although he still felt that he was "*guided.*"

Overview of cases

Collectively, these cases involve a number of psychotic phenomena, including a primary delusion (Simon), religious delusions (Simon and Sara), delusions of grandiose ability (Simon and Sara), thought insertion (Simon and Sean), auditory pseudohallucination (Sean), and auditory hallucinations (Sara and Sean). These phenomena, however, occurred in the context of experiences which, *prima facie*, were not pathological. On the contrary, the experiences were of a kind which appeared to the subjects themselves and to others to be spiritual in nature and benign in their effects.

Interpretation of findings

The three cases described here, taken together with the larger study from which they were drawn, suggest, contrary to the canons of medical-scientific psychopathology, that genuinely pathological experiences (symptoms of mental *illness*) cannot be defined merely by their form and content alone. Instead, value judgments, as to whether these experiences are good or bad experiences, are essential. Such judgments, it is important to add, are not sufficient to mark out pathology,[4] but they are at least necessary.

This interpretation is contentious. Yet in the case of psychotic experiences, which are at the heart of traditional conceptions of mental disorder, the importance of values in psychiatric diagnosis is evident (though not always recognized for what it is) in the very classifications of disorder on which the medical-scientific model of psychiatry depends. Thus, in both the DSM IIIR and DSM IV (American Psychiatric Association, 1987 and 1994), for instance, though not in the earlier DSM III (American Psychiatric Association, 1980) or the current ICD 10 (World Health Organization, 1992), a diagnosis of schizophrenia requires, not only the presence of first rank (or certain other) symptoms, but also that these "[lead to] a deterioration in life functioning," that is, functioning in employment, in relationships and so forth. There are certainly practical problems about deciding what should count as "deterioration." But we can see at least that this inescapably involves value judgments. Had Sara's voices led her into a minority sect, for example, rather than to her local church, or perhaps into the life of an ascetic hermit, we might have been less inclined to regard them as benign. We might have had a similar reaction had Simon lost his court case. This is not to say that such value judgments would be justified, of course. It is rather to indicate that the distinction between spiritual experience and psychopathology, even in the terms of the DSM-IIIR's own criteria, turns not just on objective scientific facts (the basis of genuine "diseases" according to the medical model, Boorse, 1975), but on value judgments. We return to this in the next subsection.

Conclusions: Implications for Clinical Work

That psychotic phenomena may be spiritual as well as pathological, and that the distinction turns in part (though crucially) on value judgments, has profound implications for clinical work in psychiatry.

In the first place, it reinforces the view increasingly expressed by authors from a number of disciplines, that greater attention should be paid to the spiritual aspects of the experiences and beliefs of psychiatric patients (Cox, 1996). Psychiatric assessment routinely covers many highly sensitive areas, from suicidal feelings to sexual history; but the nearest approach to spiritual experience is a routine question in the mental state examination about "odd" experiences or beliefs. So clear a bias in psychiatric assessment may well reflect the concerns of psychiatry to be identified with a "down-to-earth" scientific view of their discipline, a view which, surely mistakenly (Sims, 1994), often takes itself to be antithetical to the religious world view. But one important practical implication of the present study is to underline, if underlining were needed, the fact that however uncomfortably spiritual experience is felt to fit alongside the scientific self-image of psychiatry, psychiatrists can no longer afford to neglect the spiritual aspects of their patients' lives.

The present study underlines this point both in a general way and also specifically in relation to the importance of the values and beliefs of the patient. This is increasingly well recognized in relation to treatment. It is reflected, for example, in the movement in bioethics toward patient-autonomy in treatment choice. This in turn reflects the central role of communication skills (Hope, Fulford, and Yates, 1996). In relation specifically to psychotic disorders, it leads to a cognitive problem-solving model, described in detail by one of us elsewhere (Jackson, 1997).

In relation to diagnosis, though, the importance of values is more contentious. For many, it seems to undermine the status of medical science (Boorse, 1975). Yet there are clear pointers from a number of disciplines that in diagnosis, too, psychiatrists can no longer ignore their patients' values and beliefs – from philosophy (Fulford, 1989: ch. 11; Sadler, Schwartz, and Wiggins, 1994; see also Radden, 1994, Wallace, 1993, and others on the value-laden nature of criteria of rationality); but also from cross-cultural psychiatry and from social science (Cox, 1996).

The present study adds to these pointers by showing that the patient's values and beliefs are important, not just to diagnostic assessment in general, but to the diagnosis of particular psychiatric symptoms, including, in particular, the psychotic symptoms (delusions, hallucinations and disorders of thought) at the heart of traditional psychopathology.

NOTES

1   The selection criteria for the cases were:

1.   Report of a significant period of intense experience, explained in religious or paranormal terms by the respondent, and assessed as possibly involving delusions or hallucinations as defined in the Glossary to the Present State Examination (Wing, Cooper, and Sartorius, 1974).

2.   Apparent absence of functional deficits, as indicated by lack of psychiatric involvement and evidence of positive social adjustment.

3.   Geographical proximity to the research center.

2   In the following cases, the symptomatology of reported experiences is described by reference to the diagnostic criteria defined in traditional descriptive psychopathology, drawing especially on one of the most widely used standardized diagnostic tools, the Present State Examination, or PSE (Wing, Cooper, and Sartorius, 1974).

3   References to PSE symptom numbers are all as in Wing, Cooper, and Sartorius, 1974.

4   This point is explored fully in the original paper. This also includes a detailed analysis of the significance of these cases for psychopathology.

REFERENCES

American Psychiatric Association (1980) *Diagnostic and Statistical Manual of Mental Disorders* (3rd edn) (Washington: American Psychiatric Association).

American Psychiatric Association (1987) *Diagnostic and Statistical Manual of Mental Disorders* (3rd edn, rev.) (Washington: American Psychiatric Association).

American Psychiatric Association (1994) *Diagnostic and Statistical Manual of Mental Disorders* (4th edn) (Washington: American Psychiatric Association).

Boorse, C. (1975) On the distinction between disease and illness. *Philosophy and Public Affairs* 5: 49–68.

Buckley, P. (1981) Mystical experience and schizophrenia. *Schizophrenia Bulletin* 7: 516–21.

Cox, J. L. (1996) Psychiatry and religion: Sociocultural aspects. In D. Bhugra (ed.), *Religion and Psychiatry: Context, Consensus and Controversies* (New York: Routledge).

Fulford, K. W. M. (1989) *Moral Theory and Medical Practice* (Cambridge: Cambridge University Press).

Fulford, K. W. M., Smirnoff, A. Y. U., and Snow, E. (1993) Concepts of disease and the abuse of psychiatry in the USSR. *British Journal of Psychiatry* 162: 801–10.

Hope, T., Fulford, K. W. M., and Yates, A. (1996) *The Oxford Practice Skills Course: Ethics, Law and Communication Skills in Health Care Education* (Oxford: Oxford University Press).

Jackson, M. C. (1991) A study of the relationship between psychotic and religious experience. Ph.D. thesis. University of Oxford.

Jackson, M. C. (1997) Benign schizotypy? The case of spiritual experience. In G. S. Claridge (ed.), *Schizotypy: Relations to illness and health* (Oxford: Oxford University Press).

Jackson, M. C. (forthcoming) Psychotic and spiritual experience. A case comparison study. *British Journal of Medical Psychology*.

James, W. (1902) *The Varieties of Religious Experience*. (New York: Longmans).

Radden, J. (1994) Recent criticisms of psychiatric nosology: A review. *Philosophy, Psychiatry and Psychology* 1: 193–200.

Sadler, J. Z., Wiggins, O. P., and Schwartz, M. A. (1994) *Philosophical Perspectives on Psychiatric Diagnostic Classification* (Baltimore: Johns Hopkins University Press).

Sims, A. (1994) "Psyche"-spirit as well as mind? *British Journal of Psychiatry* 165: 441–6.

Wallace, K. (1993) Reconstructing judgment: Emotion and moral judgment. *Hypatia* 8: 61–83.

Wapnick, K. (1969) Mysticism and schizophrenia. *Journal of Transpersonal Psychology* 1: 49–68.

Watson, J. P. (1982) Aspects of personal meaning in schizophrenia. In E. Sheperd and J. P. Watson (eds.), *Personal Meanings* (London: John Wiley).

Wing, J. K. (1978) *Reasoning About Madness* (Oxford: Oxford University Press).

Wing, J. K., Cooper, J. E., and Sartorius, N. (1974) *Measurement and Classification of Psychiatric Symptoms* (Cambridge: Cambridge University Press).

Wootton, R. J. and Allen, D. F. (1983) Dramatic religious conversion and schizophrenic decompensation. *Journal of Religion and Health* 22: 212–320.

World Health Organisation (1992) *The ICD-10 Classification of Mental and Behavioural Disorders: Clinical Descriptions and Diagnostic Guidelines* (Geneva: World Health Organisation).

21

The Occurrence of High Levels of Acute Behavioral Distress in Children and Adolescents Undergoing Routine Venipunctures

G. BENNETT HUMPHREY, CHRIS M. J. BOON, G. F. E. CHIQUIT VAN LINDEN VAN DEN HEUVELL, AND HARRY B. M. VAN DE WIEL

Children fear needles and the pain they inflict.[1] It is therefore surprising that research on pain caused by needles in children is "sparse," to quote Schechter.[2] The problem is not only the lack of research but also misconceptions about pain in children. Despite adequate documentation of the problem in the previous decade, children are still undertreated for pain.[3] Although research on pain may be developing slowly, at least attention is being directed to the subject.[4]

Acute pain is a complex phenomenon.[5] For all invasive medical procedures, it is not only the pain but also the anticipation of pain that contribute to the complexity of this phenomenon. The procedure is an inevitable invasion of the child's psychological and physical space, and there is the threat that the child will lose control. All of these factors collaborate to make the event both painful and stressful. For this interwoven complexity, we prefer to use, as others have, the more inclusive term distress to describe this phenomenon.[6]

[...]

Although dramatic procedures such as surgery, bone marrow aspirations, and lumbar punctures have been subjected to both assessment and interventions studies,[7] very little research has been done on routine venipunctures.[8]

[...]

Methods

Patients

We studied 223 different children and adolescents from the inpatient service. None of them was critically ill or mentally retarded. Prior to the venipuncture, none of the subjects received premedication or specific psychological interventions. Our protocol (including the method of informed consent) was reviewed and approved by the Medical Ethics Committee in Grorungen (the Dutch equivalent of the institutional review board), and then submitted for national and international review before the research began. All venipunctures were ordered by the responsible physician. The blood tests were required for patient care, and none were ordered just to provide data for this study. The parents were informed about the study by a poster that hung in each department. Parents could withdraw their child from the study at any time. This type of study does not require written informed consent in the Netherlands.

The number of patients per year of age, and the sex distribution of our subjects for three different age groups, are included in figure 21.1 and table 21.1. The vast majority of patients had experienced at least 20 or more venipunctures (mean = 40), and none were experiencing their first or even their third to fifth venipuncture. Neither physicians nor students drew blood. Due to hospital visitation rules, the lack of rooming-in facilities, and the time of day, parents were not present in the vast majority of cases (> 90 %). [...] During the venipuncture the phlebotomist and the nurse provided emotional support and gave age-appropriate information to the patient.

Distress measurements

Using a trained observer, we measured distress by a behavioral observation scale that we developed (Groningen Distress Scale, GDS). The GDS is modeled in part on the behavioral subscale for distress of the Behavioral Approach/Avoidance and Distress Scale.[9] The latter was developed for evaluation of bone marrow aspiration. [...] The GDS has five defined levels: 1, calm; 2, timid/nervous; 3, serious distress but still under control; 4, severe distress with loss of control; 5, panic. Three behavioral categories (crying, muscle tension, and breathing) are evaluated separately prior to the assignment of

a subject to one of the five GDS levels of distress. The assessment of behavioral distress was designed to be a helpful guide for scoring the subject's level of distress.

This study was aimed at the occurrence of high levels of distress and not on the duration of such distress. Therefore, time sampling was not used, and only the highest level of distress was recorded within each of two periods of observation: distress period one (D1), the preparatory phase, and distress period two (D2), the actual venipuncture. [...]

Procedure

All venipunctures were scheduled in the morning (8:00 to 10:00). The trained observers met the phlebotomist in the laboratory and accompanied that individual to the child's room. Observation of the preparatory phase (D1) began with the moment of first contact (verbal or visual) and ended with the beginning of the actual venipuncture which was the beginning of the second phase (D2). The second phase ended with the withdrawal of the needle from the arm. After an age-appropriate explanation of the VAS, the patient was asked to fill in the two VASs (VASp and VASn) for the actual venipuncture (D2). After leaving the child the phlebotomist was asked to make a global assessment of the distress the subject experienced during preparation (D1). In this way, the phlebotomist was not distracted from the actual venipuncture during D2.

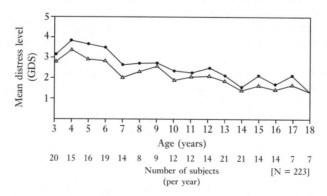

Figure 21.1 The mean distress score (GDS) recorded for both the preparatory phase (D1) (△—△) and the actual venipuncture phase (D2) (●—●) for each year of life. The regression equation for D2 on age is: $-0.135 \times$ (age in years) $+ 3.92$ ($r = .55, r^2 = .30, P < .0001$).

Results

Measurement of behavioral distress

[...]

A very high correlation was noted between the recorded distress level (GDS) during the preparatory phase (D1) and the actual puncture (D2) ($r = .87$, $P < .001$) and as seen in figure 21.1. For the majority of patients the level of distress observed during the preparatory phase (D1) was the same as that observed during the actual venipuncture (D2). The next most common pattern recorded was an increase by one level of distress observed during the actual venipuncture (D2). Very few patients were observed to increase their initial (D1) level of distress by two levels or dropped one level during the actual venipuncture (data not shown).

Distress in relation to the factors age and gender

There was a very strong relationship between age and observed distress (see figure 21.1). Ten patients panicked during the actual venipuncture. Nine of these were in the youngest age group, and the other patient was in the middle age group. None of the patients in the younger age group had a distress level of one during the actual venipuncture. Furthermore, 83 percent of the youngest age group but only 27.5 percent of the oldest age group had a score of 3 or more recorded during actual venipuncture. An analysis of the mean GDS observed during the actual venipuncture (D2) per age group for gender revealed a very significant main effect for age but not for gender (see table 21.1). There was no interactive effect of age and gender.

[...]

Discussion

The main finding was that a large percentage of subjects experienced a high level of distress and that age but not gender correlate with distress associated with routine venipunctures. It is not

Table 21.1 The mean distress score – GDS/ D2* per age group for gender

Age, y	Mean distress score (number of subjects in each group)†		
	Boys	Girls	Total
2½ to 6	3.49 (45)	3.32 (25)	3.43 (70)
7 to 11	2.54 (35)	2.60 (20)	2.56 (55)‡
12 to 19	1.82 (45)	2.09 (53)	1.97 (98)‡

*GDS/D2 = Groningen Distress Scale recorded during the second (2) period of observation, the actual venipuncture.

† Results of a two-way analysis of variance on group means: main effect of age, F is 48.14, $P < .001$; main effect of gender, F is 0.499, $P = $ NS; interaction effect of age × gender, F is 1.054, $P = $ NS.

‡ Results for total age groups 7 to 11 and 12 to 19 years. Effect of age group on GDS: F is 13.57, $P < .001$.

surprising that younger children experience more distress. Our findings are in agreement with those of Fradet et al.[10] These investigators also studied venipunctures in pediatric subjects. The main difference is that in their protocol a parent was always present and even participated in the study by predicting how the child would react. In our hospital inpatient department, routine early morning venipunctures are generally performed when the vast majority of parents are not present. The opposite is true in our outpatient department. The presence of a parent during a procedure is an important variable.[11] Research on whether the presence of a parent increases, decreases, or does not influence the distress of the child is mixed.[12] Our study supports the conclusion of Fradet et al.[13] that age and not gender is an important factor in defining risk groups and that venipunctures induce distress in a large number of children.

The GDS distress level observed during the preparatory phase (D1) was an excellent predictor of the GDS distress level observed during the second phase, the actual venipuncture. The former may therefore be thought of as anticipatory distress. This concept of anticipatory distress may be important in developing intervention strategies. Recent research by Halperin et al.[14] has evaluated a topical anesthetic cream used to decrease the pain children experience from venipunctures and other procedures. [...] A significant decrease in pain was observed.

[...]

It is a point of discussion as to what level of distress should be called unacceptable. We are of the opinion that distress levels 4 and 5 represent unacceptable distress because of the "loss of control." The description of unacceptable distress was thought to be too strong for level 3, but we do feel that this still represents significant distress. Thus we choose to refer to levels of 3 or greater as high levels of distress. From the patient's point of view, all needle procedures are unacceptable. In more than 20 years of practice in pediatric oncology clinics in the United States, one of us (G.B.H.) can recall only one child who volunteered to undergo an extra needle procedure to gain the small toy that is so commonly given to patients as a reward after a needle procedure.

Finally, it was remarkable that some pediatricians did not regard this research as being necessary, claiming that a venipuncture is only a "minor procedure." There is now a recent brief report that suggests that repeated painful procedure in neonates may result in abnormal development.[15] Other factors could also contribute to this observation, and it is not known if such would be the case in older children.

We now feel that we can use the GDS to identify patients experiencing high levels of distress. The study has been useful to convince hospital staff that intervention is necessary. The experimental interventions in which the GDS will be used for evaluations are under development. If successful interventions are produced, the long-term benefits for the child's psychological development of these interventions remain to be seen. The development of successful interventions should also benefit the hospital staff and parents.

NOTES

This work was supported by the Dutch Cancer Society (NKB), the Foundation Children Cancer Groningen (SKOG), and the Domino Foundation. The authors would like to thank: Dr. Sandy Jackson for scientific involvement and help in coordinating the students who participated in this project; Marguerite Koeneman, Jean Houwing, Petra Davidse, Jeanine Bourgonjen, Els Weier, and Marike Eelhart for help in collecting the data; Anneke Johnson and Beatrix Gauw for preparation of the manuscript, and Lodewijk Martijn from the medical illustration department.

1   Eland, J. M. and Anderson, J. E., "The experience of pain in children," in Jacox, A. (ed.), *Pain: A Source Book for Nurses and Other Health Professionals* (Boston: Little Brown and Co., 1977), pp. 453–73; Kassowitz, K. E., "Psychodynamic reactions of children to the use of hypodermic needles," *J. Dis. Child.* 95 (1958): 253–7; Fassler, D. and Wallace, N., "Children's fear of needles," *Clin. Pediatr.* 21 (1982): 59–60.

2   Schechter, N. L., "Preface: Acute pain in children," *Pediatr. Clin. North Am.* 36 (1989): xi–xii.

3   Schechter, N. L., Allen, P. A., and Hanson, K., "Status of pediatric pain control: A comparison of hospital analgesic usage in children and adults," *Pediatrics* 77: 11–15; Beyer, Je., De Good, D. E., Ashley, L. C., et al., "Patterns of post-operative analgesic use with adults and children following cardiac surgery," *Pain* 17 (1983): 17–81; Schechter, N. L., "The undertreatment of pain in children: An overview," *Pediatr. Clin. North Am.* 36 (1989): 781–94.

4   McGrath, P. A., "Evaluating a child's pain," *J. Pain Sym. Management* 4 (1989): 198–214; Lloyd-Thomas, A. R., "Pain management in pediatric patients," *Br./Anaesth.* 64 (1990): 85–104; Schechter, N. L., Altman, A., and Weisman, S. (eds.), "Report of the consensus conference on the management of pain in childhood cancer," *Pediatrics* 86 (suppl) (1990): 813–34.

5   Abu-Saad, H., "Assessing children's responses to pain," *Pain* 19 (1984): 163–71.

6   Jay, S. M., Ozolins, M., Elliott, C., et al., "Assessment of children's distress during painful medical procedures," *Health Psychol.* 2 (1983): 133–48; Katz, E. R., Kellerman, J., and Siegel, S., "Behavioral distress in children undergoing medical procedures: Developmental considerations," *Consult. Clin. Psychol.* 48 (1980): 356–65.

7   Jay et al., "Assessment of children's distress"; Katz et al., "Behavioral distress in children undergoing medical procedures"; Jay, S. M and Elliott, C. H., "Psychological interventions for pain in pediatric cancer patients," in Humphrey, G. B. et al. (eds.), *Adrenal and Endocrine Tumors in Children* (Boston: Martinus Nijhoff Publishers, 1983), pp. 123–54;

Wolfer, J. A. and Visintainer, M. A., "Pre-hospital psychological preparation for tonsillectomy patients: Effects on children's and parents' adjustments," *Pediatrics* 64 (1979): 646–55.

8   Halperin, D. L., Koren, G., Attias, D., et al., "Topical skin anesthesia for venous, subcutaneous drug reservoir and lumbar punctures in children," *Pediatric* 84 (1989): 281–4; Fradet, C., McGrath, P. J., Kay, J., et al., "A prospective survey of reactions to blood tests by children and adolescents," *Pain* 40 (1990): 53–60.

9   Jay, S. M., Katz, E. R., Elliott, C. H., and Siegel, S. E., "Cognitive behavioral pharmacologic intervention for children's distress during painful medical procedures," *J. Child. Clin. Psychol.* 55 (1987): 860–5.

10   Fradet et al., "A prospective survey of reactions."

11   Jay and Elliott, "Psychological interventions."

12   Ibid.

13   Fradet et al., "A prospective survey of reactions."

14   Halperin et al., "Topical skin anesthesia."

15   Grunau, R. V. E., Whitefield, M. F., Petrie, J. H., and Fryer, L., "Somatization at 4.5 years of age in preterm children and controls as a function of family factors, mother–child interaction, child temperament and pain sensitivity at 3 years of age," *Pain Sym. Management* 6 (1991): 146 (abstract).

22

Benjamin's Story

ERIC D. KODISH

From the beginning, I knew it would be a difficult case. Benjamin was a 10-year-old who loved football. When his left leg began to hurt after Halloween, he and his parents thought it was a football injury. As the part of his leg right above the kneecap became more swollen, they wondered what kind of tackle could cause so much pain and swelling without clear memory of the play. A week before Thanksgiving, someone ordered an X-ray.

I am a pediatric oncologist, and I met Benjamin a couple of days later. The X-ray showed a destructive tumor growing out from his left distal femur, and he came into the hospital to have a biopsy. From looking at the film, it was hard to imagine this would be anything but a cancerous bone tumor. Even worse, the CT scan of Benjamin's chest showed several nodules of tumor spread to his lungs. When the biopsy came back showing osteogenic sarcoma, I sat down to tell Benjamin's parents. While all patients with this type of cancer need chemotherapy because malignant cells might be lurking in the lungs, the prognosis for those with visible lung disease at the time of diagnosis is considerably worse. I tried to be honest, telling his parents this information while maintaining some hope of cure. I empha-

sized the fact that Benjamin might have a terrific response to chemotherapy. While I suspected that he would need an amputation in several months, I decided not to talk about this during the first meeting. Benjamin's parents didn't ask. Like all the parents that I have told, they were devastated by the news.

When we told Benjamin himself, he was also worried. He immediately focused on the "spots in his lungs," and wanted us to give him medicine to make them go away. We started his treatment and hoped for a good response. Benjamin spent most of the next few months in the hospital. When his blood counts were good, we gave him chemotherapy. When he finished, he went home for a couple of days and then developed fevers, mouth sores, and low blood counts from our treatment. He would be back in the hospital until his counts recovered and then begin another cycle of chemotherapy. His experience was in this way typical of children receiving intensive treatment for cancer.

Ten years old is a funny age. Benjamin seemed to understand how sick he was, and he desperately wanted to get better. While he often acted mature beyond his years, there were also times when he seemed to regress. I would walk into his hospital room and find him curled up in bed, practically attached to his father, sucking on his thumb. One time, when his white blood count was low from chemotherapy, he sucked his thumb so hard that he developed a skin infection. But it seemed to give him comfort in the midst of great suffering, so we didn't try to break him of the habit.

The tumor in his leg grew, while the "spots" in his lungs seemed to go away. Four months after I met him, Benjamin had an amputation of his left leg. How do you prepare a 10-year-old for an amputation? In the old days, the answer was probably: "You don't." Just do the procedure, and deal with the consequences when the child wakes up and discovers that his leg is missing. Now, with our progressive attitudes and emphasis on honesty with children, I suppose the answer is more like: "You can't, but you do the best you can." This was our approach with Benjamin. Having been trained in more recent years, I felt compelled to be honest with Benjamin. Although the word "surgery" triggered an intense shower of tears during a previous discussion, I felt strongly that we had to tell Benjamin about the amputation. His parents asked that I minimize discussion of this topic prior to the operation, and we compromised with a plan to speak to him all together. We talked about the need to remove the tumor, emphasized the positive (his lung metastases were getting better), and described the inevitable phantom pain that follows amputation. We also introduced him to a teenage boy who had the same tumor and went through treatment and amputation four years ago. He showed Benjamin his prosthesis, and tried to show him that life can go on.

A couple of weeks after Benjamin's amputation, another 10-year-old boy named Martin came to the hospital. He had been having severe headaches for several months, and more recently had trouble with vomiting and balance. The head CT showed a tumor in the posterior fossa, and the neurosurgeon operated. He removed a medulloblastoma from Martin's brain, and Martin met Benjamin as they both recovered from surgery.

These two boys became good friends, as did their families. Their times in the hospital often overlapped, and they would request room assignments together. Benjamin and his family taught the new patient much about what to expect from cancer treatment, everything from who the good nurses and doctors were to finding the best pizza in Little Italy near the hospital.

Benjamin seemed to adjust well to life without his leg, but soon his hearing started to fail. One of the most important drugs used to treat osteogenic sarcoma is cisplatinum, a toxin that is well known to cause hearing loss. This poor boy had lost his leg and was losing his hearing, struggling against the odds with a disease likely to kill him anyway. The pathologists examined the leg that was removed and saw too many healthy cancer cells that had been untouched by our chemotherapy. And, sure enough, a month after his amputation the lung nodules seemed to be growing back. We hoped that this was because of the necessary delay after surgery and quickly gave Benjamin more chemo, but the progression of his tumor was relentless.

I began to prepare his parents for the worst, telling them how dismal things looked and at the same time outlining other treatment options. In teaching clinical ethics, we like to use the cliché: "Just because you can do something doesn't mean you should do something." Although I don't question the wisdom of this thinking, such restraint is very hard to implement in practice. His parents wanted to try different chemotherapy, and this made sense to me. I just did not want to see him suffer, and his parents agreed that we needed to keep that foremost in our minds.

The new chemotherapy did make him quite sick, but Benjamin's chest CT looked better after a couple of cycles of the drugs. Although his insurance company would not pay for hearing aids, we located a charitable foundation willing to support the cost. Since no patient with osteosarcoma that remains in the lungs has any chance of cure, we asked a surgeon to evaluate Benjamin and his scans. The surgeon agreed that removing the residual tumor made sense even though it meant putting Benjamin through another major operation. Again, we told Benjamin he needed surgery, and explained our reasons in a way this 10-year-old could understand. He quickly agreed to go ahead with the operation, hopeful that removing those "spots" from his lungs would make him better.

The surgeon planned to render Benjamin "tumor-free" in two stages, operating first on his left lung and later on his right. The lesions on the left side were located in a more accessible part of the lung, and the surgery was figured to be safer. We planned on one cycle of chemotherapy between procedures, with the second operation about one month later. The first operation went well, but the pathologist reported more bad news. Not only was the tumor removed from Benjamin's left lung completely viable, but a microscopic focus of cancer was identified in what appeared to be the normal lung. This meant that there was more tumor than we could identify on the CT scan, and that our chemotherapy was not as effective as we had hoped. Given this news, and the severe postoperative pain Benjamin suffered after his first lung operation, I began to think twice about the second operation. It was time to talk to Benjamin and his parents again, with more bad news. The challenge of mixing honesty with hope for cure was becoming ever more difficult.

When Benjamin and his parents got this bad news, it was Martin and his parents who provided comfort. While I could give very little hope, Martin and his parents rallied to support their friends and urged them to keep their spirits up. Benjamin's parents decided he should travel to New York and enroll on an experimental study of a new class of anti-cancer drug. The plan would be for his father to accompany him, while his mother stayed home with his sisters. While I worried about the emotional impact of this decision on Benjamin's family, and the geographic fragmentation of the family unit at this most stressful of times, I realized that this was a decision they had to

make as a family. I worked with the doctors in New York to set up a smooth transition of care, and asked both the family and doctors to keep me informed. I also had an explicit discussion with the doctor in New York about the end of Benjamin's life; I asked her to look closely for any early signs of deterioration so that he could be flown home at the end.

After a few weeks of experimental treatment, things did begin to go badly. Benjamin developed low blood pressure and trouble with breathing. The doctors in New York stabilized him and sent him home, where he was reunited with his mother and sisters. He smiled and seemed to feel better, but then began to have trouble breathing again. Benjamin went to sleep and never woke up. He died in the hospital three days after returning home.

Several weeks before Benjamin's death, Martin had an MRI of the brain. Near the original site of his tumor, we saw an area that looked like a recurrence. Martin went back to the operating room around the same time that Benjamin was returning from New York, and had a biopsy of this area. Fortunately, the pathologist reported that the abnormality was only scar tissue. When I saw Martin and his parents in the oncology clinic after Benjamin's death, we talked about Benjamin and his family. It was clear to me that Martin and his parents were grieving the loss of a friend, but worried at the same time about Martin's own cancer. My own need for complete honesty and commitment to avoid false promises finally broke down. I put my arm around Martin and told him: "I know you are scared that what happened to Benjamin might happen to you. Please, Martin, try not to worry. You are going to be alright." As I said these words, I could feel the relief go through his body. Perhaps I even felt it in my own.

Part IV

First Contact

Introduction

First contact, coming as it does between awareness that there is a problem (our stage of "Falling Ill") and diagnosis ("Deciding What the Problem Is"), is pivotal in the clinical encounter. Yet it has been relatively neglected by biomedicine and bioethics alike: there is little literature, remarkably, even on the communication skills involved (see Reading Guide for some important exceptions).

The neglect of first contact directly reflects the fact-centered medical model, which, as we noted in the Introduction to this volume, lies behind not only biomedicine but also the dominant quasi-legal development of modern bioethics. In the medical model, first contact, where it is identified at all, is, merely, an event: it is a *condition precedent* for the deployment of the professional's skills of diagnosis and treatment, skills which, although requiring regulation by medical law and ethics, are, essentially, technical in nature. In a healthcare (fact + value) model, by contrast, first contact, wherever in the clinical encounter it comes, is an action: it is an action of "making contact," defined not by facts of spatial and temporal location, but by the intentions of those concerned and by the meanings they bring to it. Thus we hear, in the poem that introduces Part IV, that Jenny Lewis's doctor, although taking time to tell her that her breast cancer is fatal, "all that technical data so patiently explained," nonetheless fails to make contact: "he turned his head away to avoid my eyes."

First contact, understood in this way, as a pivotal action rather than a pivotal event, draws together and distills all the themes of healthcare ethics described in the Introduction to this book (and summarized in table I.1, p. 2). First, as to the aims of ethics, regulation, at least as it reflects particular values, has no obvious prima facie role. This is evident in Emilio Mordini's insightful analysis of the issues of confidentiality in child psychotherapy in chapter 24. We have already drawn attention to the paradox that increasingly stringent regulations on confidentiality, aimed at improving practice, are in some areas making matters worse (see Introduction; also Fulford, 2001; Osborn, 1999). Mordini's account explains this paradox, at least for his particular client group. Central to maintaining confidentiality in child psychotherapy, he argues, is defining for each child their particular "private sphere." That "which on no account should be spread abroad," in the original Hippocratic phrase, is therefore highly individual (Bloch et al., 1999). But more than this, Mordini continues, the therapy itself should become part of the child's private sphere. This requires trust. And regulation is the enemy of trust (Baier, 1996).

The ethicist, nonetheless, though now as a partner rather than a regulator, still has much to contribute – perhaps uniquely so at this stage in the clinical encounter, given that first contact, as a meaningful action, is defined in part by values. In terms of healthcare ethics, then, this is a headline example of the way in which we need to extend the scope of application of bioethics beyond a narrow focus on treatment, as in quasi-legal ethics, to encompass every stage of the clinical encounter. In the case of first contact, moreover, it is clear that this is true of secondary care, with which quasi-legal ethics has been mainly concerned, as much as of primary care. The inclusion of mental health in the 1967 Abortion Act (in England and Wales), as Naomi Pfeffer argues in chapter 32, "gave doctors greater scope in making covert moral, as opposed to technical, decisions about women's suitability as mothers." And subsequent technological advances, notably in the area of assisted conception, have "enormously extend(ed) obstetricians' authority over women during pregnancy."

Showing values for what they are, taking them out of the closet as it were (Fulford, 1994), is a key function of ethical reasoning in healthcare ethics. As we noted in the Introduction to this volume, this is especially important where the value judgments concerned are disguised as "technical judgments." In chapter 26, Tony Hope, David Spriggings, and Roger Crisp provide a striking example of this in their discussion on that notorious treatment chart euphemism "not clinically indicated." Behind this scientific sounding phrase, they argue, lie at least two kinds of value judgment: that treatment for the patient is not in his or her best interests; or that the required resources would be better used elsewhere.

Hope et al.'s chapter is a paradigm of the value of analytic philosophy in ethical reasoning in healthcare ethics: besides exposing the hidden value judgments, they describe five theories of the concept of need which may be helpful in exploring the space of values, as we

called it in the volume Introduction, opened up by issues of resource allocation. Continental philosophy, with its narrative focus on meanings and the intentional structure of action, may be even more effective in exposing the nature of first contact. Perri Klass's vivid vignettes of her life as a medical student, described in chapter 28, show how ethical, as well as technical, barriers may shut out the patient. "I was," she says, "congratulating myself on my ability to escape the doctor's perspective . . . [but] was in fact as caught up in my own performance as any of [theirs]." This Sartrean "bad faith," like the more transparent professional rivalry described in Perri Klass's second vignette in chapter 30, blocked all contact with "the patient." Far from being at the center of the clinical encounter, the baby in Klass's "Baby Poop" and the elderly Mr Rachmaninoff in her "Power Plays" drop out of the story altogether.

Philosophical ethics, then, whether analytic or continental, may be powerfully employed in ethical reasoning in healthcare. As we described in the volume Introduction, though, it has to be combined with empirical methods of inquiry – clinical, psychological, social scientific, etc. – if it is to be used to reach ethical conclusions. This is a key respect in which it differs from the substantive uses of ethical reasoning in quasi-legal ethics. Substantive ethical reasoning aims to draw conclusions, paradigmatically in the form of codes, regulations, and other prescriptions. Analytic ethics, to the contrary, while it may help to clarify the issues, and to this modest extent may contribute to the resolution of ethical problems, is, in itself, ethically neutral. As in other areas of theory, then, such as mathematics, content must be added to form, data to concept, if conclusions bearing on concrete issues are to be drawn.

Among empirical methods, the value of well-designed surveys in ethics is illustrated by Leslie Blackhall et al.'s study, "Ethnicity and Attitudes Toward Patient Autonomy," in chapter 29. Originally published in *JAMA* (the *Journal of the American Medical Association*), their study showed that a majority of both European and African Americans believed, consistently with the standard line in bioethics, that a patient should be told if their prognosis is terminal, and that the patient (rather than the family) should make decisions about end-of-life issues, such as when life support should be withdrawn. Korean Americans and Mexican Americans, however, flatly contradicted the standard line. A majority of these two groups believed that a patient should not be told a fatal prognosis; that the family, by contrast, should be told; and that the family, rather than the patient, should make end-of-life decisions.

Blackhall et al. conclude that we should broaden "our view of autonomy so that respect for persons includes respect for the cultural values they bring with them to the decision-making process." The Egyptian psychiatrist and ethicist, Ahmed Okasha, has made a similar point in a European and North African context (Okasha, 2000). Cultural embedding of identity may also be important clinically, in the management of trauma for example (Bracken, forthcoming). Such observations have a wider significance, however. They show that personal identity itself, and hence the action of "making contact," is in some cultures less individualist than "western" bioethics has tended to assume. Personal identity, indeed, as the Oxford philosopher and psychiatrist, Rom Harré (1998), has argued, is not a "given." It is, rather, built up through processes of discursive (meaningful) exchange largely borne by the culturally distinctive grammars of personal pronoun and other terms of address (Harré, 1998). First contact, then, in cultures in which identity itself is less personal and more family- and community-based, may involve engagement as much with the patient's cultural group as with the patient him- or herself.

Our values, however, individual or cultural, are not always worn on our sleeves. Hence, besides surveys and other ways of assessing explicit values, deeper methods of inquiry may be important in supplying crucial content for ethical reasoning in healthcare. Joan Raffael-Leff's account, "The Kinder Egg" (ch. 31), illustrates the potential of psychoanalysis as one such method. In this area, Raffael-Leff says, "paradoxes abound." New conception technologies have been a blessing for many otherwise infertile couples. But these same technologies, through the choices they have

opened up, are eroding traditional notions of identity and kinship. Thus, making contact, for example, with a woman who is seeking a termination after a three-year struggle to conceive requires going beyond the surface structure of her desires and beliefs. The paradox in this woman's overt motivations points to a deeper level of engagement as a necessary (though of course not in itself sufficient) condition for making genuine contact with her.

The outputs from analytic ethical reasoning, combined with empirical methods, are not ethical rules, conventionally understood, but improved clinical skills, notably of communication. This is why communication skills, as we put it in the volume Introduction, have a substantive rather than merely executive role in healthcare ethics. The danger with communication skills, however, is that instead of making contact possible, they become mechanical and manipulative, and, hence, a barrier to genuine engagement.

This danger can be offset by appropriate training, in particular by separating learning from doing, viz. by separating the acquisition of a new skill (which has to be a self-conscious process) from deploying it in practice for real (which should not be self-conscious – see Reading Guide). It can also be offset by an understanding of communication skills which goes beyond the important (but nonetheless limited) emphasis on technique to be found in most textbooks. Guy Widdershoven's concept of "style," described in chapter 25 and derived from the work of the French philosopher Maurice Merleau-Ponty, is helpful here. Individual communications, he points out, are made meaningful by a pattern of action; "the style or pattern is the whole which makes the action intelligible." He describes three distinct styles in the doctor–patient relationship, of which only the third ("dialogical") amounts to the "mutual engagement" of genuine contact.

Styles of communication, importantly in Merleau-Ponty's formulation, and further offsetting the dangers of self-consciously manipulative uses of communication skills, are not primarily verbal. They are expressed through sedimented "bodily habits" of which we are not

normally aware. Contrary, therefore, to the rationalism of the medical model, the meaningful
action of contact is made as much through the
body as the mind. (Merleau-Ponty indeed
rejected this dualism altogether.) But it is this
rationalist medical model, we have argued, that
lies behind much of our thinking not only in
biomedicine but also in bioethics. It is not, then,
after all, paradoxical, as Patricia Alderson suggests in chapter 27, in her account of the importance of body language in communicating
with children, that this "tends to be denigrated
and mistrusted [not only] in science and philosophy [but], paradoxically, even in medicine
and medical ethics."

First contact, then, illustrates, in each of the
above respects, the importance of strengthening
the healthcare strand in ethical reasoning to
balance up the quasi-legal approach. First contact shows the importance of a fact+value
model of medicine, of aiming for partnership
rather than policing between ethicists and clinicians, of recognizing the impact of values alongside facts at all stages of the clinical encounter, of
combining analytic ethical reasoning with empirical methods in tackling ethical problems,
and, above all, of the substantive role of communication skills in a clinical problem-solving
approach to ethical reasoning in healthcare.

There is more, though. For first contact
makes clear, as perhaps no other stage of the
clinical encounter can do, that far from meaningful actions becoming less important in
healthcare with future advances in medical science, as the fact-centered medical model suggests, they will become more important. This is
because, as we have several times noted, scientific advances themselves are driving healthcare
into areas in which the critical clinical issues are
not, centrally, scientific in nature, but concerned with the desires, wishes, beliefs, motivations, and so on, of real people. As one of
Raphael-Leff's patients put it, she was being
"impelled *by technology* into new social relationships without understanding the consequences"
(emphasis added). Science is our ally in healthcare. But absent the humanities, and our first
contact will be, like Patricia Eakins's wistful
encounter with a dead mother in chapter 33,
not with a real but with a remembered person.

REFERENCES

Baier, A. (1996) *Moral Prejudices: Essays on Ethics*
(Cambridge, MA: Harvard University Press).
Bloch, S., Chodoff, P., and Green, S. A. (eds.) (1999)
Psychiatric Ethics, 3rd edn (Oxford: Oxford Uni-
versity Press), pp. 511–31, appendix. This includes
a number of recent codes as well as the Hippocratic
Oath.
Bracken, P. (forthcoming) *Meaning and Trauma in the
Post-Modern Age: Heidegger and a New Direction
for Psychiatry* (London: Whurr Publishers).
Fulford, K. W. M. (1994) Closet logics: hidden
conceptual elements in the DSM and ICD
classifications of mental disorders. In J. Z. Sadler,
O. P. Wiggins, and M. A. Schwartz (eds.), *Philo-
sophical Perspectives on Psychiatric Diagnostic Classification* (Baltimore: Johns Hopkins University
Press).
Fulford, K. W. M. (2001) The paradoxes of confi-
dentiality. A philosophical introduction. In C. Cordess (ed.), *Confidentiality and Medical Practice*
(London: Jessica Kingsley Publishers).
Harré, R. (1998) *The Singular Self* (London and LA:
Sage).
Okasha, A. (2000) Ethics of psychiatric practice: Consent, compulsion and confidentiality. *Current Opinion in Psychiatry* 13: 693–8.
Osborn, D. (1999) Research and ethics: leaving exclusion behind. *Current Opinion in Psychiatry* 12/5:
601–4.

READING GUIDE

Observational studies of the communication aspects
of the initial contact between patient and healthcare
professionals are included in Dulmen, A. M. van,
Verhaak, P. F. M., and Bilo, H. J. G. (1997) Shifts
in doctor–patient communication during a series of
outpatient consultations in non-insulin-dependent
diabetes mellitus, *Patient Educational Counselling* 30:
227–37, and in Van den Brink-Muinen, A., Verhaak,
P. F. M., Bensing, J. M., Bahrs, O., Deveugele, M.,
Gask, L., Mead, N., Leiva-Fernandez, F., Messerli-
Rohrbach, V., Oppizzi, L., Peltenburg, M., and
Perez, A. (1999) *The Eurocommunication Study: An
International Comparative Study in Six European
Countries on Doctor–Patient Communication in General
Practice* (Utrecht: NIVEL). The relationship between
ethical and communication aspects of healthcare has
traditionally been considered mainly in the literature
on patient-centered care: see, for example, Pendleton,
D., Schofield, T., Tate, P., and Havelock, P. (1984)

The Consultation: An Approach to Learning and Teaching (Oxford: Oxford University Press); also Bensing, J. (2000) Bridging the gap: The separate worlds of evidence-based medicine and patient-centered medicine, *Patient Educational Counselling* 39/1: 17–25; and Fulford, K. W. M. (1995) Concepts of disease and the meaning of patient-centered care, in K. W. M. Fulford, S. Ersser, and T. Hope (eds.), *Essential Practice in Patient-Centred Care* (Oxford: Blackwell Science), ch. 1. An integrated course, bringing together ethics, law, and communication skills in a clinical problem-solving approach to ethics education for medical students, is described in T. Hope, K. W. M. Fulford, and A. Yates (eds.), *The Oxford Practice Skills Course: Ethics, Law and Communication Skills in Health Care Education* (Oxford: Oxford University Press, 1996). An extension of this approach in psychiatric ethics is described in chapters 2 and 9 of Donna Dickenson and Bill Fulford, *In Two Minds: A Casebook of Psychiatric Ethics* (Oxford: Oxford University Press, 2000). A valuable collection of essays on ethics and the new reproductive technologies, which figure in several of our readings in Part IV, is Ruth F. Chadwick's *Ethics: Reproduction and Genetic Control* (London and New York: Routledge, 1987; paperback, 1990). Cross-cultural aspects of medical ethics are explored in a wide-ranging collection of readings edited by Robert M. Veatch in *Cross Cultural Perspectives in Medical Ethics* (Boston, MA: Jones and Bartlett Publishers, 1989). Naom J. Zohar's *Alternatives in Jewish Bioethics* (Albany, NY: State University of New York Press, 1997) gives an in-depth and insightful account of the issues arising at the interface between "western" moral philosophy and the Jewish tradition of Halakha (legal/moral discourse) in contemporary bioethics. Also by Robert Veatch (as author) is a two-volume analysis, richly illustrated with many case histories, of ethical aspects, in *The Patient Physician Relation* (Bloomington and Indianapolis, IN: Indiana University Press, 1991); vol. 2, *The Patient as Partner*, includes a chapter called "The Physician as Stranger." As in many other areas, psychiatry provides a window on good cross-cultural practice for medicine generally: see, for example, several chapters in Kamaldeep Bhui and Dele Olajide's *Mental Health Service Provision for a Multi-Cultural Society* (London: W. B. Saunders Ltd, 1999).

23

Doctor
20th March, 1985

JENNY LEWIS

As he talks his hands jump in and out
of his pockets, square hands,
brave with the exact science
of mending faulty instruments.
(And the pain of his knife
is like violin strings breaking.)

His white coat gives him immunity
against our germs, and griefs –
our women's longings for love, babies
and healthy breast tissue.

All we want is the right answer.
Pecking after facts, ignorant as hens,
eyes small with hope, only half digesting
what he says. All that technical data
so patiently explained, falls before us
in a sombre harvest to be winnowed blindly
for the magic words – 'non fatal'.

But instead he tells me I am the one in twelve.
He cannot say how long I have to live
until the results of further tests come.

To the eleven others life is more benign.
They touch his hand, weeping with gratitude.
Then he turns his head away to avoid my eyes
which plead 'save me'.

And people come with unwanted gifts
of comfort and pity.

24

Confidentiality in Child Psychiatry

EMILIO MORDINI

Introduction

The idea of confidentiality is articulated in almost all codes of professional ethics. Confidentiality is "present when one person discloses information to another, whether through words or an examination, and the person to whom the information is disclosed pledges not to divulge that information to a third party without the confider's permission. In schematic terms, information I is confidential if and only if A discloses I to B, and B pledges to refrain from disclosing I to any other party C without A's consent. By definition, confidential information is both private and voluntarily imparted in confidence and trust" (Beauchamp and Childress, 1994: 420). Confidentiality therefore implies:

- the existence of two different domains, or spheres, or realms: the public and the private;
- the definition of boundaries between these two spheres;
- the voluntary infringement of these boundaries according to some rules known and accepted by the actors in a contract.

The debate in child psychiatry has focused above all on the last point, i.e., voluntariness.

It has been argued in fact that children are not competent enough to give their consent, or to establish a therapeutic contract which may include some rules concerning confidentiality. However, some previous problems should be solved before facing the issue of competence. In this chapter I am going to deal with the definition of the child's private sphere. Ultimately, my argument will be that there are different degrees of privacy in childhood and that we need to respect all of them, though in different manners.

Public and Private

In medicine we deal with information about the patient's life, body, and state of health. In our societies this kind of information is supposed to be largely part of the private sphere (while, say, information on one's education is public). Of course there may be exceptions: for example, information about the body of an athlete, such as his or her weight, is, in general, public. It has also been argued that persons who are candidates for high political positions are not entitled to keep their medical records secret. However, generally speaking, medical information concerns the private domain. Doctors are therefore entitled to have access to this information under rules involved in the medical contract. In particular, doctors must

- use this information for the patient's benefit;
- not cause any harm to the patient by means of the information obtained for therapeutic reasons;
- not reveal to any third party (even other members of the same family, who are inherently part of the patient's private sphere) any piece of medical information if it was not explicitly authorized by the patient.

However, doctors are not expected to keep secrets from other medical doctors. Medical information is, in fact, public, even if only amongst doctors. This implies many interesting consequences. It has been said that the medical secret is more of a ritual, the mark of an interdict, than a true secret (Beauchamp and Childress, 1994). Moreover, exceptions to the patient's absolute right to confidentiality have always been recognized. These exceptions most often occur when the professional must also address society's right (or need) to know. In the current medical scenario, information is no longer shared among providers and consumers. Third- and fourth-party entities are involved more and more. As a consequence, rather than discussing confidentiality, it would be better to speak of the patient's right to control sources and flow of information. It means that the question that we should address is not: "Who, when, and why is entitled to breach confidentiality?" but "How can the patient control the information flow concerning him- or herself?" (Rodotà, 1996).

As far as the private/public distinction in childhood is concerned, we face two very different perspectives. From the first perspective, only adults possess a public sphere (or, better, have access to the public sphere), since only adults are truly subject to the law. According to this view, there is no point trying to define a child's private space; children are *part* of an adult's private sphere but they have no right themselves to privacy, because their privacy belongs to an adult. For example, in any medical context a child's feeling of modesty is not respected, and the child is examined by the doctor in front of his or her parents. This is a typical example of infringement of the child's privacy, based on the assumption that there is no true privacy to defend since the child's body is actually *part of* the parents' private sphere.

From the second perspective, any human, qua human, possesses privacy, whatever their age. The distinction between public and private concerns children not because they are possessed by an adult, but because they possess both a private and a public sphere of their own. In fact, in modern western societies children as well as adults are subject to the law; they have some public obligations (e.g., to attend school, to undergo medical preventive measures such as vaccinations), and they are entitled to certain civil rights (e.g., they cannot be battered, they can express their wishes if their parents seek a divorce). The mere fact that these obligations and rights are very often guaranteed by an adult (parent, guardian, judge, or anybody else) does not imply that they are not obligations and rights of the children themselves.

In child psychiatry we deal with several secrets. The first is the secret of childhood itself. Childhood is something of a mystery for adults. In western culture – from Dionysus to the child Jesus – people have felt that an inner, sacred secret is kept in the first ages of life. The image of the "divine child" has always been taken as a symbol of temporal renewal, of cyclic regeneration (for example, Christmas coincides with an old pagan feast devoted to the sun).

It is very important that the doctor does not disclose this secret of childhood, namely that he or she does not expose the child's internal world with the aim of turning it into a "normal" adult mental world. Child psychiatrists should be careful not to confuse the child's use of multiple and non-Aristotelian logic, fantasies, and dreams with psychological symptoms. In particular, good psychotherapy should help the child to confront his or her mental contents with reality, without impairing the richness of his or her mental life.

A second group of secrets that we have to face in child psychiatry concerns family secrets. It has been said that all families are built on secrets. From a therapeutic perspective, family secrets are those that a child should learn to understand. For example, a child might need to understand that his or her father feels a sense of inadequacy toward his wife and for this reason tends to react aggressively to certain remarks.

However, it is important to note that not all family secrets are purely emotional, i.e. concerning relationships within the family. Sometimes there are true secrets (previous divorces, abortions, cases of abuse, petty offences, or even crimes committed by one or both members of the parental couple). Sometimes these secrets directly concern the child (e.g., the child was conceived for economic reasons, or the child was not wanted and the mother attempted an abortion, or the child is given the same name as a previous dead sibling). In all these cases it might turn out that the therapist comes to know the secret through both or one of the parents. Since the information is confidential, is the doctor entitled to disclose it to the child? Usually, psychotherapists can maneuver in such a way that the child may come to understand the secret (or that part of the secret that really matters for the treatment) without explicitly breaking the parents' confidentiality.

A third group of secrets directly concerns the child. Each child has his or her own inner mental, emotional, and private life. Even if each family can be considered as a system, the child is also an individual with secrets – information that he or she needs to communicate to the doctor but which the child does not want others to know. Here the matter is rather simple, since it does not differ from general medical practice. To respect a child's privacy is an ethical commitment for every therapist. In particular, there are no clinical reasons to disclose information to parents without the child's informed consent, as has been stated in the *Principles of Practice of Child Psychiatry* adopted by the American Academy of Child Psychiatry Code of Ethics.[1]

A fourth group of secrets concerns the child–therapist relationship. These are the secrets of the treatment, things that happen and are told during psychotherapy sessions. Very often, parents feel jealous of these secrets and try to unravel them. Since these are secrets shared between the child and the therapist, it is they who should decide together whether and when to disclose them to the child's parents or other third parties. It is important to emphasize that the mentally disturbed child often comes from an intrusive family, where he or she lacks privacy. One of the goals of therapy should be that of creating a child's private sphere. The therapy in itself should become part of child privacy, and the psychiatrist should defend the therapy from any external intrusion.

One last point should be considered. When we talk about families, we are not speaking only of the traditional family but, more and more, of new kinds of families: step-families, reconstructed families, single-parent families, families made by homosexual couples. This poses new ethical questions, since children/family structures have changed. For instance, to what extent does a step-parent have the right to participate in a child's life? Is a child with a single parent entitled to know the reason why his or her father/mother divorced or was never married in the first place?

Generally speaking, questions posed by new family structures imply the need to define the persons who are part of a child's private sphere. In the past, the private sphere and the family used to coincide, but it is no longer possible to conclude that persons have a deep relationship simply because they belong to the same family. Perhaps, in an era of social changes such as the present, we need to give an operational definition of "private relationships" which avoids any legal and bureaucratic definition based on formal family structures.

Even if it is clear that further discussion is needed to clarify the issue of confidentiality in child psychiatry, some conclusions can be drawn all the same. First of all, it is unquestionable that a child, as a patient, carries the same rights as an adult. As a consequence, those guarantees given by most ethical and medical codes on confidentiality in the doctor–patient relationship also have force in relation to childhood. In no case should children be less well protected than adults, for example in epidemiological studies, and anonymity should be respected in publishing clinical cases as far as possible.

Second, in child psychiatry the relationship with the child's family is critical: parents and relatives are not always the right people to be informed about what the child told the therapist in confidence. Moreover, a serious problem arises when one tries to define the boundaries of the child's private sphere. Even if the child is definitely entitled to the same right to privacy as an adult, it is more difficult to understand the complex nature of the child's privacy. It implies that we cannot be sure about what is felt by the child as belonging to his or her privacy and what is not. Third, beyond any juridical formalism, it is recommended always to obtain the child's consent before any disclosure of information and to respect his or her will to keep communications confidential, except where there are very relevant clinical or legal reasons. Even in these cases, doctor should always try to negotiate the child's consent before any breach of confidentiality.

NOTE

1   "A child or adolescent and the family may expect the Child Psychiatrist to [...] protect specific confidences of the child or adolescent and the parents or guardians and other involved, unless this course would involve untenable risks or jeopardise care-taking responsability" (*Am. Academ. Child. Psych.* May 16, 1982).

REFERENCES

Beauchamp, T. L. and Childress, J. F. (1994) *Principles of Medical Ethics* (New York: Oxford University Press).
Rodotà, S. (1996) *Tecnologie e Diritti* (Bologna: Il Mulino).

25

Diagnostic Styles in Clinical Relationships

GUY A. M. WIDDERSHOVEN AND WIES WEIJTS

Introduction

The concept of style is usually applied to artistic products and artistic movements. It may, however, be used more generally, indicating a pattern of thought or a pattern of action. Within philosophy of science, for instance, both Fleck (1935) and Hacking (1985, 1990) analyze scientific development in terms of style. In this chapter we will apply the notion of style to medical practice.

The chapter consists of three parts. First, we will go into the concept of style, referring to phenomenology and hermeneutics. Next, we will distinguish three diagnostic styles. Following the classical parallel between the physician investigating a sick person and the detective investigating a crime, we will draw examples from detective novels (see also Oderwald and Sebus, 1991). In the third section we will interpret three cases, stemming from a study on doctor–patient interaction in gynaecological practice.

Style as Meaningful Pattern of Action

Merleau-Ponty describes the relation between body and world as a process of meaning-making (Merleau-Ponty, 1945). According to Merleau-Ponty, bodily movements are not caused by external stimuli, they are motivated by phenomena in the life-world. The meaningful relation between body and world can be regarded as a dialogue. In a dialogue a question elicits an answer without determining the latter. The question gives the conversation a certain direction. The meaning of the question, however, is specified in the sequel of the communication.

Human action presupposes that people live in a familiar world. The familiarity of the world is founded in our bodily habits. The process of habituation makes individual actions part of a larger pattern. This pattern may be called a *style* (Merleau-Ponty, 1945: 197). Action can be explained by referring to the style it is characteristic of. The style or pattern is the whole which makes the action intelligible. The style creates a unity which makes various actions akin, although they are all different. Like different paintings within an artistic movement, different actions within a pattern are similar but not identical. They all express the style in their own, unique way (Merleau-Ponty, 1968: 63).

By virtue of their style, different actions may be recognized as expressions of the same person. The concept of style also implies a relation between individual actions and collective events. An individual acquires a specific pattern of action in communication with others, in very much the same way as a painter acquires his style within an artistic movement, interacting with the style of others.

The relation between action and style may be further clarified with the help of philosophical hermeneutics. From a hermeneutic perspective, this relation is a *hermeneutic circle*, since the action is an expression of the style, which in its turn is modified by its instantiations (Gadamer, 1960). In the action the general principle is applied to the specific situation, in very much the same way a judge applies the general law in a specific case. The law is modified, which does not mean that it is made invalid, but that its validity is further specified. By virtue of its style, each action is at once general (in that it follows a general rule) and particular (in that it is a particular instantiation of the rule). This is recognized by the early hermeneutic philosopher Schleiermacher, who stresses that style combines rule and individuality (Schleiermacher, 1977; cf. Frank, 1980: 28–32).

Three Diagnostic Styles

One of the central elements of medicine is diagnosis. A physician has to be able to see what's wrong with the patient, and to find an adequate treatment. Each diagnosis is individual, in that every physician will act in her own specific way, depending on the concrete situation. It is, however, possible to discern patterns in various diagnostic procedures, or diagnostic styles.

The rationalist style: Poirot

The first diagnostic style may be called rationalist. This style exemplifies a rationalist way of meaning-making. A doctor who behaves in this way relies heavily on deduction and combination. He tries to deduce what's wrong by combining the facts so that they match. Reality is thought to be ordered and intelligible. For every problem, there exists one specific cause and one good solution. Since diseases have a specific cause, they can be explained.

The attitude that characterizes this diagnostic style may be described as distanced and superior. In the process of diagnosis, the patient is seen first and for all as a source of information. In the second place she is regarded as a person who may either cooperate or be a hindrance. The rationalist style thus has a specific interpersonal character. The doctor is the central actor and the patient plays a complementary role. The doctor consciously directs the process of investigation, aiming at specific results. The patient either follows or tries to get away, without really knowing, in both cases, where the road leads to.

From a rhetorical perspective, this style is based on the presupposition that there is one truth, which can be seen if one uses the right method. Because it is linked up with the notion of objective truth, the rationalist style implies power. It is also oppressive, in that it pushes away everything that is ambiguous or contingent. Everything has to follow the pattern of causal events.

A good example of the rationalist style can be found in the detective novels by Agatha Christie. Hercule Poirot can be seen as the personification of the investigator of the rationalist type. No problem is proof against his intellect. Although it may take some time, eventually the mystery is unraveled by an analysis of the situation and a combination of the facts. In a typical Poirot case there is a master plan, which has to be discovered. Everything is part of the scheme; there is no detail that does not fit. In *Ten Little Indians*, for example, the murderer has planned all of the "executions" beforehand, leaving nothing to chance. In every Poirot story there is only one solution to the riddle, although there may be several factors involved, as can be seen in *Murder on the Orient Express*, where it turns out that the victim is killed not by one, but by all of the suspects. The world in which Poirot operates is extremely well ordered and totally intelligible; it only requires an ordered and intelligent mind to see through the apparent chaos.

The relativist style: William of Baskerville

The second diagnostic style may be called relativist. In this approach, there is no one method guaranteeing the right solution. A problem can be regarded from various perspectives, each following its own logic. Facts are not given, they are in need of interpretation. Diseases never have one sole cause. One can tell various stories about a disease, each following a different story-line and having a different plot. A doctor applying a relativist style acknowledges that there is always a variety of perspectives. He knows that reality is open to more than one interpretation and that it is impossible to say that one solution is definitely better than another one.

The attitude of a doctor acting in a relativist style can be described as detached. He is aware of the fact that there are several perspectives, each with its own value. He knows that his perspective can only be presented as one among many. This creates a certain distance between doctor and patient, not out of superiority (as in the rationalist style), but of reticence. If the patient does not comply, this is not regarded as irrationality on the patient's side, but as a sign of a divergent interpretation of the situation. The interpersonal relation is one of two parties competing on an equal basis.

The relativist style has a specific rhetorical force. Objectivity is no longer relevant. This may seem to weaken the position of the doctor, but it also gives some strength. The doctor may acknowledge that he does not know the exact truth, but then neither does the patient. By stressing that objectivity does not exist, the doctor may counteract claims made by the patient. Furthermore, the doctor may emphasize that he is more experienced than the patient, and more subtle in judging the situation. Thus, the doctor can try to persuade the patient that his perspective is more promising. This strategy may be just as convincing as claiming that one has the right method to find the truth.

A good example of the relativist style can be found in the novel *The Name of the Rose* by Umberto Eco. William of Baskerville, the principal figure in the novel, certainly is a good detective. His investigations are, however, very different from those of Poirot. The book starts with what seems to be a fine example of deduction in the rationalist style, when William is able to infer that the monks he encounters are looking for a valuable horse. Later on, however,

William explicitly states that his success was dependent on his ability to make the monks believe that he was clever, and that he just as easily might have failed in doing so. Thus, his success depended not on deduction, but on argumentation. In the monastery William is confronted with a series of crimes. He tries to make sense of what happens by looking for a pattern that may explain every crime. In the end, however, he realizes that there was no pattern behind the various murders. The master plan, which might explain all events, was not there – or better: there was a person who had tried to make such a plan, but who was unable to keep things under control. William discovers the murderers not by reconstructing their ingenious plans (they are either non-existent or ineffective), but by following his own line of reasoning and by arguing with everybody who opposed his ideas. In the end it is hard to say whether he has succeeded or failed. He has succeeded in so far as the various murderers are discovered. He has failed, however, in that the monastery, of which he had to protect the good name, becomes an object of scandal and is physically destroyed.

The dialogical style: Maigret

The third diagnostic style may be called dialogical. As in the relativist style, it is acknowledged that objectivity does not exist. None of the participants can claim to have a privileged access to truth. Within a dialogical approach, this does not imply that truth cannot be reached. Truth is, rather, seen as the outcome of a merger of perspectives. By being open toward the perspective of the other, one may finally reach a common point of view, which surpasses the individual perspectives. The doctor acting within a dialogical style tries to get access to the story of the patient, and by communicating with it aims to enrich it. It is presupposed that the situation to which the story refers is itself ambiguous, and will be changed if a new story can be told about it. The aim is to reach a new, joint interpretation of reality.

The attitude related to this diagnostic style is engaged and personal. The doctor is involved with the patient. The corresponding interpersonal relation is one of understanding and trust. Since there is no one solution to the problem, the steps in the diagnostic process cannot be laid out by the doctor in advance. Each next move is dependent on the reactions of the patient. Doctor and patient are equal participants in the diagnostic process.

The dialogical style has its own rhetorical structure. It does not rely on objectivity (as in the rationalist style), but neither does it refer to pragmatic issues such as experience or taste (as in the relativist style). The rhetoric aims at creating mutual engagement. In a way, this style underlines that the doctor is not powerful. If the patient does not cooperate, the doctor cannot do very much. By stressing the importance of mutual engagement, however, doctor and patient are urged to communicate. Thus, the style enables the doctor to involve the patient actively in the diagnostic process.

The dialogical style is described very well by Georges Simenon in his Maigret novels. Maigret communicates with all the people involved in the crime, trying to understand their point of view. He does not deduce from clues, but tries to engage the persons he encounters in a joint search. In this quest, a mutual perspective on the events is constructed. In *Maigret et le clochard* he tries to see life through the eyes of the clochard (tramp) who is brutally attacked, by playing with the marbles found in his pocket. He spends the evening at the ship of the assailant, attempting to understand the stifling climate. Finally, he recognizes a pattern: the clochard by chance witnessed a former crime on board the ship, and although he was not interested in denouncing the crime, because he was no longer engaged in social life (for him life was just a game of marbles), he was still a potential danger to the sailor, and thus had to be suppressed. This conclusion is not brought about by a process of deduction. It is the result of engaging with both the aggressor and the victim. Interestingly, the novel does not end at this point. Although Maigret has discovered the facts, he is not able to prove them, because the sailor keeps denying the crime and the clochard, who has recovered, does not want to denounce the assailant. Maigret fails in his attempts to

convince both that they had better speak up. Because the sailor is stubborn, and the clochard is uninterested in revenge, Maigret's approach is of no use. Thus the dialogical style is dependent on the reactions of other people. Whereas Maigret usually succeeds in getting cooperation, he fails as soon as he encounters someone who, like the sailor, is totally uncommunicative, or someone who, like the clochard, is not part of ordinary bourgeois life. Both are impervious to rhetorical means which appeal to truth and understanding.

Diagnostic Styles in Gynecological Consultations

The rationalist, the relativist, and the dialogical style of diagnosis can be further illustrated by looking at concrete examples of doctor–patient interaction. In a study on doctor–patient communication several gynecological consultations were recorded (Weijts, 1993). These consultations were then transcribed. In the following we will give three examples, each exhibiting a different type of diagnostic style.

Case I

A patient consults a gynecologist for an infertility problem. The gynecologist starts by asking several questions (Are you healthy? Have you ever been hospitalized? Do you take any medicine? Is the cycle regular? Is your husband healthy? What does he do for a living?). The patient answers his questions. Then the doctor explains what will be done. First, there will be an internal examination. Then the husband's sperm will be analyzed. Next there will be a hormonal test, to check ovulation. Finally, the permeability of the uterus-membrane will be examined. During this explanation, the patient answers by either approving (saying "yes") or humming. When the explanation is completed, the internal examination takes place. Since nothing abnormal is found, the consultation ends by making an arrangement about the next steps to be taken in the procedure, as explained before.

The style involved in this case may be called rationalist, in that the process of diagnosis is ordered in clearly defined steps, which are all supposed to contribute to the discovery of the relevant facts. The doctor's attitude is marked by control of the situation. The patient is seen as a source of information. She is supposed to carry out the instructions of the doctor. The whole consultation rests on the rhetorically powerful suggestion that there is one definite cause of the problem, which will inevitably be found if the right steps are taken.

Case II

A patient comes to a gynecologist complaining about irregular menstruation with much loss of blood and abdominal pains. Three months ago she underwent curettage, but that did not help very much. The doctor proposes to regulate her periods by using oral contraceptives. The patient is not satisfied with that measure. She protests that it will not take away the cause of her complaints, which, according to her, is her uterus. Moreover, she says that she is afraid of cancer. She tells the doctor that she and her husband prefer a definite solution, and asks for a hysterectomy. The doctor warns her that a removal of the uterus will not guarantee that she will be free of all complaints in the future. Furthermore, he assures her that there is no real danger of cancer even if the uterus is not removed. He mentions several possible complications of an operation (slight incontinence, sexual problems). The patient, however, sticks to her decision. Although the doctor again mentions that the use of oral contraceptives is a more elegant solution, he does not press the matter. He asks her whether she has any more questions. This leads to a discussion about some technical details. In the end an appointment for the operation is made.

In this case, as in the former one, the doctor is less prone to drastic measures than the patient. However, the doctor does not really dissuade her from having the operation. He seems to imply that he is not in a position to do so. The style involved in this case is relativist. The doctor is aware of the different perspectives, and sees no use in pressing the matter. His solution may be more elegant, but that does not make it more valid. If the patient has a

decisive wish, he can do nothing else than to obey it, albeit reluctantly. Both doctor and patient present their arguments. They try to defend their own view as long as possible, but are prepared to give in, if necessary. In the end, it is not so hard to give up one's position, because it is seen as relative.

Case III

A patient consults a gynecologist for abdominal pains. She says she does not understand the pains, since she had her uterus removed by a hysterectomy. The doctor asks several questions (How long has this been going on? Is the pain there every day? Is it always the same place?). The patient answers, and also tells him that she has constipation. Then the doctor asks whether she is worried about something. The patient answers that she is afraid of having cancer. The doctor says that he will examine her thoroughly. He proposes to do an internal examination. The patient is rather reluctant. She doubts whether an internal examination will give enough information, and asks for a laparoscopy. The doctor says that each method has its specific advantages, and that he has to examine her first in order to be able to decide on further steps. After the examination, he proposes to consult a dietician in order to do something about the constipation. He advises against a laparoscopy, because it requires anesthesia. As he says that such drastic steps can better be postponed until later on, the patient agrees.

In this case both doctor and patient actively participate in the decision-making process. The doctor is clearly more cautious in his proposals than the patient. The patient asks for drastic measures, since she wants to get to the bottom of the problem. The doctor says that complicated examinations are not necessarily better, and that he prefers to start with simple methods. The doctor manages the situation by using the dialogical style. By giving attention to the wishes and anxieties of the patient, without giving up his own views, the doctor is able to convince the patient. The approval of the patient is secured by the assurance that the methods she proposes can always be tried later. By this rhetorical turn, the doctor can combine the patient's perspective and that of himself, and thus reach a mutual agreement.

Conclusion

In clinical interaction medical doctors apply various diagnostic styles. Doctors use different procedures in order to make clear the patient's condition. These procedures imply specific preconceptions about the nature of disease and about the doctor–patient relationship. They also imply specific rhetorical elements. This shows that doctors' actions are not idiosyncratic. They are part of a tradition. In acting, doctors rely upon a tradition, and apply the tradition to the concrete case.

Medical practice is diverse. Doctors take up various diagnostic styles. Above, we sketched three of them: the rationalist, the relativist, and the dialogical style. These different styles show that medicine is pluriform. From this perspective one can criticize approaches which presuppose that medicine implies only one specific kind of action. According to some authors, medicine is instrumental action, in which the patient is the object of medical interventions (Parsons, 1951). According to others, it is a process of negotiation between doctor and patient (Freidson, 1970). These approaches are too simple: they overlook important diversities. Authors who pay more attention to diversities in medicine tend to relate differences in approaches of medical doctors to differences in illnesses, for example acute illness versus chronic illness (Szas and Hollander, 1956). As the cases show, this distinction is still too crude, since it overlooks the fact that the same kind of illness can be the object of different interventions.

The notion of style enables us to make visible and to analyze various medical practices, each having a specific conception of disease, a spe-cific doctor–patient interaction, and a specific rhetorical structure. As with detectives, these styles have their attractions and their limitations. The challenge of medicine is to develop each of the styles separately, and combine them in such a way that diseases are treated creatively and patients are helped to live their lives in a meaningful way.

REFERENCES

Fleck, L. (1935) *Entstehung und Entwicklung einer wissenschaftlichen Tatsache* (Frankfurt am Main: Suhrkamp).

Frank, M. (1980) *Das Sagbare und das Unsagbare* (Frankfurt am Main: Suhrkamp).

Freidson, E. (1970) *Professions of Medicine* (New York: Dodd).

Gadamer, H.-G. (1960) *Wahrheit und Methode* (Tübingen: J. C. B. Mohr).

Hacking, I. (1985) Styles of reasoning. In J. Rajchman and C. West (eds.), *Postanalytic Philosophy* (New York: Columbia University Press), pp. 145–64.

Hacking, I. (1990) *The Taming of Chance* (Cambridge: Cambridge University Press).

Merleau-Ponty, M. (1945) *Phénoménologie de la perception* (Paris: Gallimard).

Merleau-Ponty, M. (1968) *Résumés de cours (Collège de France, 1952–1960)* (Paris: Gallimard).

Oderwald, A. K. and Sebus, J. H. (1991) The physician and Sherlock Holmes. *Journal of the Royal Society of Medicine* 84: 151–2.

Parsons, T. (1951) *The Social System* (New York: Free Press).

Schleiermacher, F. D. E. (1977) *Hermeneutik und Kritik* (Frankfurt am Main: Suhrkamp).

Szasz, T. S. and Hollander, M. H. (1956) A contribution to the philosophy of medicine. The basic models of the doctor–patient relationship. *Archives of Internal Medicine* 97: 585–92.

Weijts, L. B. M. (1993) Patient participation in gynaecological consultations: studying interactional patterns. PhD, University of Limburg, Maastricht.

26

"Not Clinically Indicated": Patients' Interests or Resource Allocation?

TONY HOPE, DAVID SPRIGINGS, AND ROGER CRISP

A report from the Royal College of Physicians recommended that elderly patients should have better access to cardiological services, including coronary angioplasty and cardiac surgery.[1] It also noted, however, that the facilities presently available are inadequate to provide for the patients of all ages who could benefit from these procedures.

It is clear that some elderly patients can benefit from surgery that may previously have been denied on the grounds of age alone. Patients in their 80s now constitute 3.5% of those undergoing coronary artery bypass grafting at the Mayo Clinic; 79% of 115 survivors were free of angina after a mean period of 29 months.[2] The risks of surgery are undoubtedly higher in patients of this age – in two series the hospital mortality was around 10% and the incidence of postoperative stroke was 4%.[3]

An increased use of angioplasty may limit the number of elderly patients with coronary disease who need bypass grafting for refactory angina, but there is no effective alternative to surgery for the large number of patients in their 70s and 80s with symptomatic aortic stenosis. When stenosis is the cause of severe symptoms, the prognosis without valve replacement is worse than that of many cancers, with a three

year mortality around 75%.[4] Balloon valvoplasty offers only short term palliation.[5] In published series of patients aged 80 years and over undergoing aortic valve replacement[6] the operative mortality was around 15% (compared with around 4% for patients under 70[7]). By three to five years after surgery the actuarial survival rate exceeded that of a control population.[8] This enhanced survival may reflect the fact that patients referred for surgery were highly selected, and an important limitation of these data is that the selection criteria were not explicit.

Two Different Points to Consider

For many elderly patients it will be decided that cardiac surgery is not clinically indicated. But the use of the phrase "not clinically indicated" often conceals and confounds two quite different points. The first point is that the operation is not of overall benefit to the patient – for example, the risk of death during the operation outweighs the likely benefit of the operation for the patient. The second is that it is not the right allocation of available resources to use them for this patient. Both these statements have important ethical dimensions, and they require separate analysis.

In general, where the patient's welfare is the crucial issue the patient should judge. This is a central value in a liberal society. The role of the doctor is to give as accurate and helpful information as is possible to enable the patient to come to a decision.

Even though a patient aged 80 years will usually face a higher operative mortality and a shorter expectation of life than a patient aged 40 years, it does not follow that surgery is not worthwhile for the 80-year-old. Paradoxically, the older person might be willing to take a higher risk of death during surgery than a younger person. Indeed surgery, offering, in simplified terms, either a quick death or good health, may be particularly attractive to the old.

Some people aged 80 would not consider major surgery worthwhile because their life is near to close, but others would judge quite differently. If our interest is what is of benefit to the individual patient we must take these differences into account, and in general that means allowing the patient to decide.

Carrying Out Surgery on an Old Person is the Wrong Allocation of Resources

Old people might be denied surgery on the grounds that the available resources are better spent on younger people. But what ethical principles should guide the allocation of resources? We shall briefly discuss some of the main theories of allocation that have been suggested and examine their implications for elderly people with aortic stenosis.

QALYS

Quality adjusted life years (QALYs) form the core of the most thoroughly articulated theory of allocation in health care. On this theory one year of healthy life is taken to be worth 1. A year of unhealthy life is considered to be worth less than 1: the value is lower if the quality of life of the unhealthy person is worse. A beneficial

health care activity is one that generates a positive number of QALYs, and an efficient health care activity is one for which the cost per QALY is low. QALYs are, in effect, units of welfare. A given budget will buy the maximum amount of QALYs if resources are spent on those aspects of care with the least cost per QALY. In this way welfare is maximised.

The application of QALY theory would result in old people having less chance of cardiac surgery than younger people for two main reasons: firstly, the operation is likely to have a higher mortality and morbidity for older people; secondly, older people have in general a shorter life expectancy and therefore fewer life years to gain from the operation.

The main criticisms of QALYs focus on two central points: firstly, that QALYs are unfair because they do not take into account who gains the QALYs; secondly, that "welfare" is not the only value to be put into the equation. Critics have argued that QALY theory is attractive as long as we are considering one person who is weighing up the likely outcomes with different treatments. It is eminently reasonable for an individual to choose the treatment that is likely to generate the most QALYs. But applying QALYs to the allocation of resources is quite different because it involves a choice between the welfares of different people. Thus, for example, those with mental handicap would obtain fewer resources because one year of mentally handicapped life would rate as lower in quality than one year of normal life. Similarly, people with physical handicap affecting the quality of life would have less claim on resources. This would result in those already unfortunate in having one handicap then being less entitled to further medical care.[9]

The fact that old people would lose out with QALY theory has been given as a further example of injustice. The reverse has, however, also been argued: that QALY theory does not discriminate enough against old people. This argument, which has been called "the fair innings argument," was summarised by Lockwood: "To treat the older person, letting the younger person die, would thus be inherently inequitable in terms of life lived: the younger person would get no more years than the relatively few he has already had, whereas the older person, who has already had more than the younger person, will get several years more."[10]

It follows from this that younger people will normally take preference over older people in the allocation of resources that would postpone death. Is this fair? Do we not all face the same loss, namely death? And do we not all have the same right to be saved? This raises the fundamental issue of how, ultimately, the value of life is to be determined. Harris has argued that the value of life can only sensibly be taken to be that value that those alive place on their lives.[11]

To avoid some of these difficulties with QALYs, Nord has recently suggested the "saved young life equivalent" (SAVE).[12] Instead of requiring a figure to be placed on quality of life, the SAVE approach requires a direct comparison to be made between the value of a given intervention (for example, valve replacement in an 80-year-old with severe aortic stenosis) and saving the life of a young person, restoring him or her to full health. Any particular evaluator is free, therefore, to rate a treatment for an 80-year-old as equally valuable as the equivalent treatment in a 20-year-old, or as less valuable, or as more valuable. The SAVE approach gives a way of obtaining the views of a population sample. However, it does not help individual evaluators in deciding on what basis to make their evaluations.

Needs theories

Needs theories arise from the second major criticism of QALY theory: that "welfare" is not the only value. A distinction is drawn between needs and benefits. In allocating resources, needs should be met before benefits.

This theory requires an account to be given of this central distinction. There may be clear cut cases, but there is likely to be a large area where it is unclear whether something is a need or a benefit. Furthermore, the theory is unlikely to be comprehensive. If the total resources are insufficient to meet all needs then how does one choose the needs that should take precedence? And if there are sufficient resources to meet all needs how does one choose which benefits should be funded? It is unclear whether aortic valve replacement, for example, should be classified as a need or a benefit. If replacement is a need it will in general be such for old and young alike, and similarly if it is classified as a benefit. Thus needs theories are likely to share resources equally between young and old. If aortic valve replacement were classified as a need and not simply a benefit, then needs theories, if implemented, might lead to an increased total budget for such surgery to meet the needs of old people with aortic stenosis.

"Sanctity of life" theory

This theory states that, above all, life must be saved. It is a type of needs theory in which the most important need is to save life. It suffers therefore from the same problems as all needs theories. A further difficulty is that it would apparently require us to put enormous resources towards trivial increases in length of life. Indeed, the whole idea of "saving life" is rejected by some philosophers and replaced by that of "postponing death." It does not seem, in general, valuable to postpone death by a few hours at enormous cost. In the context of valve replacement in old people, the sanctity of life theory would give high priority to a person of any age who is in imminent danger of dying. In other situations it gives no guidance.

The lottery theory

The lottery theory is a reaction to the perceived injustices of QALY theory.[13] Where QALY theory concentrates on welfare and ignores justice, the lottery theory concentrates on justice and ignores welfare. It originates from considering, for example, the situation where an older and a younger person would benefit equally from treatment but resources allow only one to be treated. Rejecting the QALY calculation, Harris suggests that since there is no rational way of choosing between the two people the way closest to being just is to choose randomly. Hence the lottery. Thus, an 80-year-old and a 40-year-old should have an equal chance of being offered cardiac surgery in equivalent circumstances. Many people believe that a lottery is no more just than any other way of choosing – perhaps less so than many other ways. But even if it is just, it does not seem to be comprehensive. It may give a method for allocating resources in a situation like that described, but it is quite unclear how it could be used to allocate resources in general.

Market forces

Market forces are part of a vision of a health care system in which individuals buy the care they can afford. With this view, if the 80-year-old or the 40-year-old can pay for the surgery then it is offered. Otherwise it is not available. This way of allocating resources faces the problems of justice in the same way as the QALY view, but immensely increased. In effect the distribution and quality of health care will be entirely on the basis of personal wealth.

Conclusion

Doctors may feel that in many cases surgery is not clinically indicated. The word "clinically" here can be dangerously misleading, for the decision being made has a major ethical component. It is as important to clarify the ethical judgments being made as it is to understand the basis for technical decisions.

NOTES

1 Royal College of Physicians Working Group, "Cardiological intervention in elderly patients," *J R Coll. Physicians Lond.* 25 (1991): 197–205.

2 Mullany, C. J., Darling, G. E., Pluth, J. R., Orszulak, T. A., Schaff, H. V., Ilstrup, D. M., et al., "Early and late results after isolated coronary artery bypass surgery in 159 patients aged 80 years and older," *Circulation* 82 (suppl. 4) (1990): 229–36.

3 Ibid; Weintraub, W. S., Craver, J. M., Cohen, C. L., Jones, E. L., and Guyton, R. A., "Influence of age on results of coronary artery surgery," *Circulation* 84 (suppl. 3) (1991): 226–35.

4 Turina, J., Hess, O., Sepulcri, F., and Krayenbuehl, H. P., "Spontaneous course of aortic valve disease," *Eur. Heart J.* 8 (1987): 471–83; O'Keefe, J. H. Jr., Vlietstra, R. E., Bailey, K. R., and Holmes, D. R. Jr., "Natural history of candidates for balloon aortic valvuloplasty," *Mayo Clin. Proc.* 62 (1987): 986–91.

5 Kuntz, R. E., Tosteson, A. N. A., Berman, A. D., Goldman, L., Gordon, P. C., Leonard, B. M., et al., "Predictors of event-free survival after balloon aortic valvuloplasty," *N. Eng. J. Med.* 325 (1991): 17–23.

6 Rich, M. W., Sandza, J. G., Kleiger, R. E., Connors, J. P., "Cardiac operations in patients over 80 years of age," *J. Thorac. Cardiovasc. Surg.* 90 (1985): 56–60; Tsai, T. P., Matloff, J. M., Gray, R. J., Chaux, A., Kass, R. M., Lee, M. E., et al., "Cardiac surgery in the octogenarian," *J. Thorac. Cardiovasc. Surg.* 91 (1986): 924–8; Edmunds, L. H. Jr., Stephenson, L. W., Edie, R. N., and Ratcliffe, M. B., "Open-heart surgery in octogenarians," *N. Engl. J. Med.* 319 (1988): 131–6; Levinson, J. R., Akins, C. W., Buckley, M. J., Newell, J. B., Palacios, I. F., Block, P. C., et al., "Octogenarians with aortic stenosis: Outcome after aortic valve replacement," *Circulation* 80 (suppl. 1) (1989): 49–56; Fiore, A. C., Naunheim, K. S., Barnes, H. B., Pennington, D. G., McBride, L. R., Kaiser, G. C., et al., "Valve replacement in the octogenarian," *Am. Thorac. Surg.* 48 (1989): 104–8; Freeman, W. K., Schaff, H. V., O'Brien, P. C., Orszulak, T. A., Naessens, J. M., Tajik, A. J., "Cardiac surgery in the octogenarian: Perioperative outcome and clinical follow-up," *J. Am. Coll. Cardiol.* 18 (1991): 29–35; Culliford, A. T., Galloway, A. C., Colvin, S. B., Grossi, E. A., Baumann, F. G., Espositi, R., et al., "Aortic valve replacement for aortic stenosis in persons aged 80 years and over," *Am. J. Cardiol.* 67 (1991): 1256–60.

7 Magovern, J. A., Pennock, J. L., Campbell, D. B., Pae, W. E., Bartholomew, M., Pierce, W. S., et al., "Aortic valve replacement and combined aortic valve replacement and coronary artery bypass grafting: Predicting high risk groups," *J. Am. Coll. Cardiol.* 9 (1987): 38–43; Craver, J. M., Weintraub, W. S., Jones, E. L., Guyton, R. A., Hatchet, C. R. Jr., "Predictors of mortality, complications, and length of stay in aortic valve replacement for aortic stenosis," *Circulation* 78 (suppl. 1) (1989): 77–90.

8 Levinson, et al., "Octogenarians with aortic stenosis"; Culliford, et al., "Aortic valve replacement for aortic stenosis in persons aged 80 years and over."

9 Harris, J., "QALYfying the value of life," *J. Med. Ethics* 13 (1987): 117–23.

10 Lockwood, M., "Quality of life and resource allocation," in J. M. Bell and S. Mendus (eds.), *Philosophy and Medical Welfare* (Cambridge: Cambridge University Press, 1988), pp. 33–5.

11 Harris, J., *The Value of Life* (London: Routledge, 1985).

12 Nord, E., "An alternative to QALYs: The saved young life equivalent (SAVE)," *BMJ* 305 (1992): 875–7.

13 Broome, J., "Good, fairness and QALYs," in J. M. Bell and S. Mendus (eds.), *Philosophy and Medical Welfare* (Cambridge: Cambridge University Press, 1988), pp. 57–73.

27

Body Language

PRISCILLA ALDERSON

The sight of very premature babies and children with serious mental and physical disabilities raises crucial questions: why is the human spirit trapped in such a puny, frail body? Is the stark contrast between spirit and body a tragic paradox or a cruel joke?

One age-old response has been to separate mind from body and to see the body as little more than an unfortunate package for the mind.

Traditionally, it was widely believed that the more we exist in our heads as purely rational intellectuals and the less we are affected by our bodies, the more fully human we are. Western philosophy and religion are riven by the mind–body split. Scientific understanding of humanity is similarly divided between medicine and psychology.

However, the essence of humanity is the spirit that fuses mind and body, that can relate and celebrate, laugh and grieve, aspire and imagine, question and create. This elusive spirit slips through the grid of scientific analysis.

Although poetry and music have a deep symbiosis with human nature, science scarcely has words or methods to address this 'soft' subject.

Care of the body and attention to patients' knowledge gained through their bodies are crucial to informed nursing practice. Yet knowledge gained and communicated through the body tends to be denigrated and mistrusted in science and philosophy and, paradoxically, even in medicine and medical ethics.

Since young children are liable to learn and speak through their feelings and body language, their knowledge tends to be devalued. We all exist in and through our bodies and, indeed, we are our bodies, although adults often try to deny or disguise this. Another effect of the mind–body split is that we have lost sight of the whole thinking, feeling person in the child. We see infants primarily as bodies and childhood as a prelude to the full blossoming of the mind.

This split creates great problems when listening to sick children if they are seen in terms of physical malfunction and rudimentary cognition. When words are the only valid currency for communication, body language is seen as counterfeit, to be mistrusted as valueless and misleading.

Yet words, too, can be misleading, confusing and misunderstood. The first barrier to overcome when taking children seriously is to rethink the mind–body split and to see the body as much more than a mere container.

Bodies can be the source of profound knowledge when children learn through their illness and disability and express themselves physically. [...]

During a study of children's consent to surgery, 120 children aged eight to 15 having elective orthopaedic surgery were interviewed.[1] Half had two or more chronic diseases or disabilities. The group included many remarkable, exceptionally mature young people.

As one mother remarked: 'He may have a small body but he has a great personality.' They had courage, compassion and good sense. The study found that 13 of the 120 believed that they were the main decider about whether to accept treatment proposed by the surgeon and 13 parents thought that their child was 'the main decider'. 'Main deciders' were aged from eight upwards.

The children were then asked who they thought should be the main decider. After surgery, 21 said that they wanted to be the main decider, 47 wanted to share making decisions with adults, and 45 wanted adults to decide for them.

Before surgery, only two children wanted their parents alone to decide, although this rose to seven when they were asked again after surgery. They seemed to have more confidence in their doctor's judgement than their parents'.

This raises questions as to whether children see their parents less as decision makers and more as mediators, interpreters, support-givers or advocates. The research was not about the final stages of life-saving treatment, although three children knew that without spinal surgery they would not have long to live.

An unpublished study of children with cancer in Bristol found that even two-year-olds understood the names of drugs and their purpose, and cooperated with treatment. Some made a fuss over washing and feeding, perhaps to compensate, but to judge them as immature because of this would be mistaken.

Most of the young people in the surgery study, although they complained at times, showed dignity and stoic courage when they faced repeated surgery. Nurses and parents commented on children who, in order to protect their parents, would not talk of their own distress.

One nurse asked a boy with cystic fibrosis whose older brother had died of the disease if he really wanted to have the heart-lung transplant he was about to undergo. He did not reply directly, but said: 'I've got to have it or my mother would be so sad.' This courage is a great strength but it is also a barrier that can make it harder to listen perceptively to children.

In the past few decades, health professionals have become more interested in listening to adult and, more recently, to child patients and sharing information and decisions with them.

There are many barriers to overcome: lack of time, skill and confidence; problems with communicating with people who speak other languages, and adults' anxiety that they may look foolish or lose control if they risk allowing children to influence decisions.[2] When children are extremely ill and possibly very distressed, the pressures increase.

Many health professionals overcome these barriers, but others find them daunting. Before trying to overcome the practical barriers, it is useful to recognise some of the psychological ones, such as anxieties and prejudices.

Is it worth listening to children? What should be done if their views seem to involve self-harm? What if the parents object? Can young children have any idea of what is meant by death? Reports from clinicians who do listen to children show how worthwhile and important their work is when they take children's minds and bodies seriously.

NOTES

1 Alderson, P., *Children's Consent to Surgery* (Buckingham: Open University Press, 1993).
2 Alderson, P., Montgomery, J., *Health Care Choices: Making Decisions with Children* (London: Institute for Public Policy Research, 1996).

28

Baby Poop

PERRI KLASS

There are a million stories in the naked city, and some of them are about baby poop. I'm sorry, I try to keep these hospital anecdotes I tell relatively uncrude, but hospitals are hospitals, and sometimes things do get a little bit graphic. But bear with me, because this particular story is fraught with meaning.

Well, there we were on the neurology consult team, a senior attending neurologist, a resident in the neurology program, a resident in the general pediatrics program who was doing a month of neurology, and two medical students, one of them me. And we got called down to the newborn nursery to do a neurological exam on a baby. And we strode in, a phalanx, our reflex hammers peeking from our pockets. We wrapped ourselves in clean hospital gowns and regrouped around the bassinet holding the baby in question, ready to bring all our different levels of expertise to bear on the problem.

I looked down at the baby. My years as a mother have trained me in certain rapid diagnostic methods. I sniffed the air over the bassinet. "This baby is poopy," I announced to the assembled doctors. "He needs to be changed."

No one acknowledged my statement, and I realized that in allowing my private life to contribute to my hospital work, I had used the

wrong vocabulary. I tried again. "This baby has apparently had a bowel movement," I said. "Let me just put a clean diaper on him."

This time I got a response. No, no, said all the doctors. They shook their heads, they motioned to me not to bother. Don't change him. We'll just do our exam, and then the nurses will take care of it.

Well, after all, I was only a lowly medical student. So I nodded, and we turned our attention to the neurological examination. We shined lights in the baby's eyes, we tapped for reflexes. We picked him up and held him in the air to assess his muscle tone. We discussed what we thought we saw. We repeated any doubtful tests. In all, we stood around that bassinet for a good forty minutes.

Now, at the risk of making this story even cruder, I have to point out that the atmosphere around that bassinet was really not very pleasant. I mean, you didn't have to be an expert parental type to detect the contents of that diaper. What I mean is, that baby smelled. I mean stank. I mean, even in the hospital, I have been in pleasanter places for forty minutes. But none of us admitted in any way that there was anything to smell except the standard aroma of disinfectant. We stood tall. We were doctors. We did not hold our noses. And finally we finished our exam and marched out; as we left the room, a nurse came hurrying over to the bassinet, carrying a paper diaper.

I have to admit, this is one of my very favorite doctor stories. I have told it several times, and it has elicited a couple of responses I hadn't counted on. So first of all, I want to tell you my interpretation of the story, the interpretation I was forming as I stood by that bassinet. And then, I want to turn the story inside out a couple of times, to suggest other meanings.

I stood by that bassinet, thinking, I cannot believe this. I wasn't so much concerned for the baby – as far as I can tell, small babies are not nearly as eager to have their diapers changed as their parents are to do the changing. But I couldn't believe this group of doctors was choosing to spend forty minutes in this poopy ambience, when thirty seconds of work with a paper diaper would have taken care of the problem.

It occurred to me that perhaps the doctors were squeamish about seeing a diaper changed. I didn't know for sure that any of them had children of their own, and I have encountered people before who imagine that the changing of a diaper is a lengthy and profoundly disgusting process. But still, I reminded myself, these men were *doctors*. They had dissected cadavers, put in their time in the operating room, coped with all the sounds and sights and smells of the hospital. They ought to be able to take it, I thought; they won't faint at the sight of baby poop.

Well, that wasn't really what it was about, I knew. What it was about was dignity. *Doctors don't change diapers.* That's all there was to it; I had offered to do a job that would have compromised my professional status, and by extension theirs, since I was on the same career path as they. I don't mean to suggest they had actually thought it through; I think it was the instinct of professional self-defense that prompted their response. Probably at home they would have changed a baby's diaper – maybe one or two of them had children at home and changed diapers all the time, I didn't know. I'm not sure it would have made any difference; the business executive who at home is fully capable of answering the phone will sometimes let it ring forever in the office if the secretary isn't there.

Part of prestige is the jobs you do; the other part is the jobs you don't do. And the strong smell of baby poop is better than a whiff of cleaner air from lower down the totem pole.

So that was the conclusion I reached as we stood in the newborn nursery. That to me was the point of the story: in my naivete as a medical student, allowing my parental responses to take over, I had made a suggestion which was incompatible with doctorly dignity. I thought it was funny because it was so indicative of the flip side of dignity, the pompous determination to preserve prestige at any cost, even if the prestige you preserve only makes your life unpleasant. I would have told the story with a punch line something like this: doctors – they'll save the baby's life, but they won't change the baby's diaper.

So I told the story, and a gentleman who is a professor of philosophy promptly informed me that if this had happened in his department, he and his colleagues would have prevented me from changing the baby too. I will leave aside the question of how it could have happened in his department; I have never studied philosophy and so have no idea what goes on behind those doors. Anyway, he told me, if there had been a baby who needed changing, and if I, the only woman in the room, had offered to do it, they would never have let me. Even if all the male philosophers had been unwilling or unable to diaper that baby, they would not have permitted me to do the dirty work. It would have looked too much like making the woman do the woman's work, he explained to me. It was too sensitive an issue; people were too self-conscious about it. My immediate response to this was that doctors were certainly *not* too self-conscious about it – I had no fear that they had stopped me for such politically advanced reasons. I suppose you could argue in fact that just the opposite was going on; as a doctor-to-be, I was "elevated" to the status of an honorary male. Or at least, I had joined the traditionally male profession, and they were not about to let me demean it with women's work; the diaper was changed by a nurse, a woman doing a woman's job.

Again, I don't mean that any of those doctors actually thought this through. I just mean that the political dynamic that was operating around that bassinet was in fact the traditional dynamic of sexual differentiation.

But when I thought further about this philosopher's comment (still resisting the temptation to imagine what the poopy baby might have been doing in the philosophy colloquium in the first place), it occurred to me that in fact my willingness to change the baby's diaper had something to do with my own attitudes toward the sexual politics of medicine. A year earlier, I'm not sure I would have offered. When I first started out in the hospital, I wouldn't have offered, simply because I never offered to do anything unless I was sure it was my place. If none of the doctors had mentioned it, I wouldn't have either; I would have been worried that perhaps my diaper-changing technique was not smooth enough to show off in front of an attending. And then, after I got over those first-time jitters, I went through a period in which I was very sensitive about sexism. I worried that if I did anything that marked me too distinctly as female, I would be respected less. I resented being mistaken for a nurse. I didn't talk much about my own child. When I wanted to leave the hospital a little bit early to meet his day-care teacher, I said I wanted to go over to the medical school library to look up some articles. When some doctor complimented me on my knowledge of the pediatric dosage schedule of a particular antibiotic, I didn't say, my kid takes that when he gets an ear infection.

But I got over most of this nonsense. By the time I met the baby in my story, I think I had honestly come to believe that both my experiences as a woman and my special skills as a parent add something to my abilities as a doctor. Being able to diaper a baby (and being willing to diaper a baby) is a skill, and a skill it is better to have than not to have. I offered to diaper that baby because I wasn't worried that I was being pressured into doing it because I was a woman; I

offered to do it because I knew I could do it and I wanted the baby to be wearing a clean diaper. And if anyone had made any cracks about female doctors, I would have despised him, and not myself. It's not a very high peak to have scaled, but I'm glad to have attained that vantage point.

Well, so much for my various kinds of arrogance: the medical student who sees through the doctors, the woman who sees through the men, the sensitive human being who sees through everyone. I told this story one more time, to someone who is not a doctor and not a professor of philosophy. She heard me through to the end, smiled but didn't laugh, and then asked, in a worried tone of voice, "Was the baby okay?"

"What do you mean?" I asked, thinking that sitting around in a poopy diaper for a while never really hurt anyone.

"You were called to do a neurological exam on a newborn baby, you said. Was the baby okay?"

What can I say? Isn't that obviously the right question to ask? Isn't that the detail I completely omitted from my story? Did it in fact occur to me as relevant, when I was doing my cute imitation of the doctors standing around the bassinet, inhaling baby poop? In fact, this particular baby was fine, or at least we couldn't find anything wrong with him, though we spent forty minutes trying. I can't remember what had originally made them suspicious that he was not neurologically intact, but whatever it was, he seemed to have gotten over it. But the fact is, I would probably still have thought I had a good story if the baby hadn't been okay. Someone else had to hear the story to point out to me that actually I and all the other doctors were peripheral characters. And when I was congratulating myself on my ability to escape the doctor's perspective, just because I offered to change the diaper, I was in fact as caught up in my own performance as any of those doctors.

29

Ethnicity and Attitudes Toward Patient Autonomy

LESLIE J. BLACKHALL, SHEILA T. MURPHY, GELYA FRANK,
VICKI MICHEL, AND STANLEY AZEN

For the past 25 years, ethical and legal analysis of medical decision making in the United States has revolved around the idea of patient autonomy. The principle of patient autonomy asserts the rights of individuals to make informed decisions about their medical care. Thus, patients should be told the truth regarding their diagnosis and prognosis, as well as the risks and benefits of proposed treatments, and should be allowed to make choices based on this information. Although this ethical ideal is imperfectly realized in actual practice, the standard of care in the USA is to tell patients the truth about even fatal illnesses,[1] to obtain their informed consent for major procedures,[2] and to involve them in decisions about withholding resuscitation.[3] The ideal of patient autonomy is so powerful that attempts have been made to extend patient control over medical decision making even to those circumstances in which the patient has lost the capacity to make decisions through advance care directives, such as the durable power of attorney for health care.[4] A federal statute, the Patient Self-determination Act, has been enacted to enhance and preserve patient autonomy. Recently, however, it has been suggested that this focus on patient autonomy has become overly narrow and that other values, such as family integrity[5] and physician responsibility,[6] have been ignored. In particular, some have argued that this preoccupation with individual rights to the exclusion of other values may reflect a cultural bias on the part of the Western medical and bioethics communities.[7] To determine the attitudes of individuals of varying ethnic backgrounds toward patient autonomy in medical decision making, we surveyed 800 Korean-American, Mexican-American, African-American, and white (European-American) subjects as part of a larger study examining the attitudes of older Americans of varying ethnicities toward health care and medical decision making.

[...]

The dependent variable – attitudes toward patient autonomy – was measured as responses to a series of questions regarding attitudes toward truth telling (diagnosis and prognosis) and toward decision making with respect to the use of life support (table 29.1).

Interviews were conducted with 200 individuals aged 65 years and older who identified themselves as belonging to one of the following four ethnic groups: African American, European American, Korean American, and Mexican American (N = 800). Care was taken to

Table 29.1   Measures of patient autonomy

Diagnosis: A physician diagnoses a person as having cancer that has spread to several parts of their body.

  (a) The physician believes that the cancer cannot be cured. Should he or she tell the patient that they have cancer? *Yes or No*

  (b) Should the physician tell the patient's family about the cancer? *Yes or No*

Prognosis: The physician believes that the patient will probably die of the cancer.

  (a) Should the physician tell the patient that he or she will probably die? *Yes or No*

  (b) Should the physician tell the patient's family that the patient will probably die of the cancer? *Yes or No*

Decision regarding life-prolonging technology: The patient becomes very ill and a decision must be made about whether to put the patient on life-prolonging machines. The machines will prolong the patient's life for a little while but will not cure the illness and may be uncomfortable. Who should make the decision about whether to put the patient on the machine?

  (a) It should be mainly the physician's decision.

  (b) It should be mainly the family's decision.

  (c) It should be mainly the patient's decision.

include an equal number of men and women within each group and to maintain a similar age distribution across all four groups. Because a simple random sample of individuals older than 65 years would have yielded a sample that was heavily skewed in terms of sex and age, a stratified quota sampling technique was used. Attempts were made to minimize selection bias by sampling from a wide range of sites.

[. . .]

Table 29.2 describes the characteristics of the survey sample, and figure 29.1 displays the effect of ethnicity on measures of attitudes toward patient autonomy. Korean Americans (47% ± 4% [SE]) were less likely than African Americans (89% ± 2%) and European Americans (87% ± 2%) to believe that a patient with metastatic cancer should be told the truth about

that diagnosis ($P < .001$). Similarly, Korean Americans (35% ± 3%) were less likely than African Americans (63% ± 3%) and European Americans (69% ± 3%) to believe that the patient should be informed of a terminal prognosis and were also less likely to believe that the patient should make the decision about the use of life-supporting technology (28% ± 3% vs 60% ± 3% and 65% ± 3%, all $P<.001$). Instead, most Korean Americans (57% ± 3%) believed that the family should make decisions about the use of life support.

Mexican Americans tended to fall between African Americans and Korean Americans, with 65% ± 3% supporting truth telling in diagnosis (statistically different from European Americans and African Americans at the $P< .001$ level). Forty-eight percent (± 3%) of Mexican Americans believed that the patient should be told the truth about the prognosis, and only 41% (± 3%) chose the patient as primary decision maker. Forty-five percent (± 3%) of Mexican Americans believed that the family should make such decisions. Although the groups differed in their opinions about whether the patient should be told the truth, 90% or more of the subjects in all ethnic groups believed that the family should be told the truth about the patient's diagnosis and prognosis. The difference was that the Korean-American and Mexican-American subjects were more likely to believe that only the family, and not the patient, should be told the truth.

To determine whether acculturation (as measured by the Marin Short Acculturation Scale) affected the attitudes of Mexican Americans toward truth telling and decision making, subjects were categorized as "high" (score ≥3) vs "low" (score <3) acculturation. The majority (79%) of the Mexican-American subjects had low Marin Short Acculturation Scale scores. Acculturated Mexican Americans (i.e., those who spoke and read more English and associated more with "Anglos") were more likely to believe that the patient should be told the truth about the diagnosis (83% vs 60%, $P = .005$) and prognosis (62% vs 44%, $P<.05$). Choice of patient as primary decision maker was not affected by acculturation (36% vs 42%, $P = .42$). Analyses could not be performed for

Table 29.2 Demographic characteristics of ethnic groups (n = 200/Group; N = 800)*

| Characteristic | Ethnic group, no. (%) | | | | P |
	African American	European American	Korean American	Mexican American	
Age, y					
64–70	57 (29)	57 (28)	57 (29)	64 (32)	
71–75	56 (28)	49 (25)	54 (27)	57 (29)	.96
76–80	49 (25)	57 (28)	53 (27)	46 (23)	
≥81	38 (19)	37 (19)	36 (18)	33 (17)	
Religion					
Protestant/ Christian	188 (94)	81 (40)	39 (19)	5 (2)	
Catholic	4 (2)	58 (29)	10 (5)	195 (98)	
Jewish	0	48 (24)	0	0	<.001
Buddhist	0	0	92 (46)	0	
Other	8 (4)	13 (7)	59 (30)	0	
Schooling, y					
1–6	23 (11)	6 (3)	53 (29)	116 (61)	
7–12	132 (66)	103 (51)	89 (49)	57 (30)	<.001
>12	45 (23)	91 (46)	39 (22)	16 (8)	
Personal annual income					
<$10,000	106 (55)	87 (45)	192 (96)	153 (84)	
$10,000–$25,000	81 (42)	80 (42)	8 (4)	25 (14)	<.001
>$25,000	5 (3)	25 (13)	0	5 (3)	
Functional status					
Katz Index	11.9 (0.4)[a]	11.4 (1.0)[b]	11.8 (0.6)[a]	11.3 (1.2)[b]	<.001
Duke Index	22.0 (10.6)[b]	23.5 (10.9)[a,b]	20.6 (8.6)[b]	27.4 (9.9)[a]	<.001
Personal experience with illness					
0 = none	22 (11)[a]	9 (5)[a]	88 (44)[b]	45 (23)[a]	<.001
≥1 = some	178 (89)	191 (95)	112 (56)	155 (77)	
Personal experience with withholding care					
0 = none	166 (83)[b,c]	89 (45)[a]	181 (91)[c]	136 (68)[b]	<.001
≥1 = some	34 (17)	111 (55)	19 (9)	64 (32)	
Access to care					
Structural	4.3 (2.1)[a]	3.6 (2.2)[a]	3.4 (1.8)[a]	6.3 (2.9)[b]	<.001
Financial	0.3 (0.3)[b]	0.1 (0.2)[a]	0.5 (0.0)[c]	0.4 (0.2)[d]	<.001

*Means with the same letter (a, b, or c) are not significantly different at the P < .001 level with use of the Scheffé multiple comparison procedure.

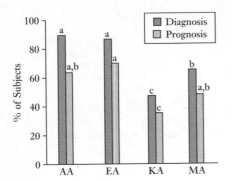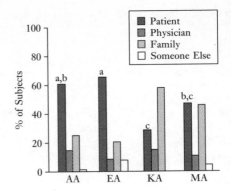

Figure 29.1 Top: The percentages of African-American (AA), European-American (EA), Korean-American (KA), and Mexican-American (MA) subjects who believe that the physician should inform the patient that they have cancer (diagnosis) and that the physician should inform the patient that they will probably die (prognosis). Bottom: The percentages of subjects who believe that the decision about whether to put the patient on a life-support machine should be made by the patient, physician, family, or someone else. Differences in percentages of subjects who believed in patient autonomy with regard to diagnosis, prognosis, and the use of a life-support machine were assessed with use of one-way analysis of variance. Pairwise comparisons across ethnic groups used Scheffé's multiple comparison procedure, with a significance level set at $P<.001$. For each measure of patient autonomy, ethnic groups that were not significantly different are indicated in the figure with the same letter (a, b, or c).

Korean Americans because 100% of this group had scores below 3 on the Korean version of the Marin Short Acculturation Scale.

To better understand the relationship between acculturation and socioeconomic status in the Mexican-American population, we analyzed the correlation between the Marin Short Acculturation Scale score, personal income, and education. Mexican-American subjects with annual incomes above $10 000 ($P<.01$) or more than 6 years of education ($P<.001$) were more likely to have a high Marin Short Acculturation Scale score. Acculturation does not appear to be a simple function of years lived in the United States. The majority (66%) of Korean Americans had lived in the country for more than 10 years. Likewise, more than 90% of the Mexican-American sample had lived in the United States at least 10 years; of those, 78% had a low Marin Short Acculturation Scale score.

Differences in attitudes toward patient autonomy among the ethnic groups are borne out in the logistic regression analyses presented in

table 29.3. Relative to European Americans, Korean Americans and Mexican Americans were less likely to favor telling the truth about diagnosis and prognosis and less likely to choose the patient as primary decision maker (ORs<1, $P<.001$). Religion and socioeconomic status were also related to our measures of patient autonomy. Because these variables were strongly associated with ethnicity, multivariate and within-group analyses were performed and are reported below. With respect to age, the oldest subjects (aged 81 years and older) were less likely to believe that the patient should be told the truth about a terminal prognosis than were the youngest subjects (ORs <1, $P<.001$). Subjects with personal experience with illness and withholding and withdrawing care were more likely to favor truth telling (ORs <1, $P<.001$). No relationships were found for sex, functional status, and access to care.

To further examine the relative contribution of each of the factors related to our measures of autonomy, we performed a stepwise logistic regression (table 29.4). Because no associations

Table 29.3 Odds ratios (95% confidence intervals) of measures of autonomy

	Tell diagnosis	Tell prognosis	Decision maker about life support
Ethnic group			
European American	1.0	1.0	1.0
African American	1.2 (0.7–2.3)	0.8 (0.5–1.1)	0.8 (0.6–1.2)
Mexican American	0.3* (0.2–0.5)	0.4* (0.3–0.6)	0.4* (0.3–0.6)
Korean American	0.1* (0.1–0.2)	0.2* (0.1–0.4)	0.2* (0.1–0.3)
Sex			
Male	1.0	1.0	1.0
Female	1.1 (0.8–1.4)	0.8 (0.6–1.1)	1.2 (0.9–1.5)
Age, y			
64–70	1.0	1.0	1.0
71–75	1.1 (0.7–1.7)	0.8 (0.6–1.2)	0.9 (0.7–1.4)
76–80	1.0 (0.7–1.6)	0.9 (0.6–1.4)	0.8 (0.6–1.2)
≥81	0.7 (0.4–1.0)	0.6* (0.4–0.9)	0.7 (0.5–1.1)
Religion			
Protestant/Christian	1.0	1.0	1.0
Catholic	0.6* (0.4–0.8)	0.7 (0.5–1.0)	0.6* (0.5–0.9)
Jewish	1.0 (0.5–2.2)	0.7 (0.4–1.3)	1.3 (0.7–2.4)
Buddhist	0.2* (0.1–0.3)	0.2* (0.1–0.4)	0.4* (0.2–0.6)
Schooling, y			
1–6	1.0	1.0	1.0
7–12	2.1* (1.4–3.0)	1.3 (0.9–1.8)	1.8 (1.2–2.5)
>12	3.3* (2.1–5.4)	2.0* (1.4–3.1)	2.5* (1.7–3.8)
Personal annual income			
<$10,000	1.0	1.0	1.0
$10,000–$25,000	4.3* (2.7–7.0)	2.4* (1.7–3.4)	2.4* (1.7–3.3)
>25,000	3.1 (1.2–8.0)	2.3 (1.1–4.8)	2.0 (1.0–4.1)
Functional status			
Katz Index	0.9 (0.8–1.1)	1.0 (0.8–1.1)	1.1 (0.9–1.3)
Duke Index	1.0 (1.0–1.0)	1.0 (1.0–1.0)	1.0 (1.0–1.0)
Experience with			
Illness	3.0* (2.1–4.3)	2.1* (1.5–3.0)	1.3 (0.9–1.9)
Withholding care	2.1* (1.3–3.0)	1.8* (1.3–2.6)	1.5 (1.0–2.1)
Access to care			
Structural	1.0 (0.9–1.0)	1.0 (0.9–1.0)	1.0 (1.0–1.0)
Financial	1.1 (1.1–1.1)	1.1 (1.0–1.1)	1.0 (0.9–1.1)

*Odds ratio significantly different from 1, $P<.001$.

were found for sex, functional status (Katz Index of Activities of Daily Living and Duke Activity Status Index), and access to care indexes in the univariate analysis (table 29.3), these variables were not included in the model. Years of schooling and income were analyzed as continuous (rather than categorical) variables.

For all three measures of attitudes toward patient autonomy, the primary factor related to attitude was ethnicity. Relative to European Americans (the reference group), Korean Americans and Mexican Americans were least likely to favor truth telling about the diagnosis and prognosis and least likely to believe that the patient should make the decision about the use of life support. After controlling for ethnic differences, the second most important factor associated with attitudes toward truth telling was years of education. Patients with more education were more likely to favor telling the truth about the diagnosis and prognosis. In contrast, years of education did not predict who would be selected to make the decision about the use of life-sustaining technology. Finally, patients with some personal experience with illness were more likely to favor truth telling with respect to diagnosis.

To further explicate the relationship between socioeconomic status, ethnicity, and attitudes, we performed within group χ^2 analyses to examine the relationship between these and our measures of patient autonomy within each ethnic group. Socioeconomic status (as measured by income and years of schooling) was not related to attitudes in the European-American and African-American groups. In the Korean-American and Mexican-American groups, however, some relationships emerged. Mexican Americans with more years of education (≥ 7 years) were more likely to believe that the patient should be told the diagnosis (79% vs 57%, $P<.05$), and those with higher annual incomes ($\geq \$10\,000$) were more likely to favor truth telling about the diagnosis (93% vs 61%, $P<.001$) and prognosis (70% vs 45%, $P<.01$). Korean Americans with higher levels of education were more likely to believe that the patient should make the decision about the use of life support (32% vs 19%, $P<.05$). Similarly, within-group analyses of age revealed that al-

though age was not related to attitudes in the European-American and African-American subjects, it was a predictor in the Korean-American and Mexican-American groups. Older Korean Americans and Mexican Americans (81 years or older) were less likely than younger subjects of the same ethnicity to favor telling the patient the diagnosis (25% vs 52%, $P<.01$, for Korean Americans; 45% vs 69%, $P<.01$, for Mexican Americans).

In the European-American and Korean-American groups, religion was related to differences in attitudes toward some of the autonomy indexes. In the European-American group, Protestants were more likely than non-Protestants to believe that the patient should be told about a terminal prognosis (81% vs 61%, $P<.01$) and were more likely to believe that the patient should be the primary decision maker (73% vs 59%, $P<.05$). Jewish subjects were less likely than non-Jewish subjects to believe in telling the truth about the prognosis (52% vs 75%, $P<.01$). In the Korean-American group, Buddhists were less likely to believe that the patient should be told the prognosis (27% vs 41%, $P<.05$). The African-American and Mexican-American groups had very little religious diversity, with 98% of the Mexican-American group being Catholic and 94% of the African-American group being Protestant; thus, further analyses of religious differences within these groups could not be conducted.

Comment

Korean-American and Mexican-American subjects were less likely than European-American and African-American subjects to believe that the patient should be told the truth about the diagnosis and prognosis of a serious illness and were less likely to believe that the patient should make decisions about the use of life support. Within the Korean-American and Mexican-American groups, older subjects and those with lower socioeconomic status tended to be opposed to truth telling and patient decision making even more strongly than their younger, wealthier, and more highly educated counterparts.

Table 29.4 Stepwise multiple logistic regression analysis of factors predictive of measures of autonomy

Step	Variable	Odds ratio (95% confidence interval)	P	Model P
		Diagnosis		
1	Ethnic group			
	European American	1.0	. . .	
	African American	1.4 (0.7–2.7)	.31	
	Mexican American	0.5 (0.2–0.9)	<.02	<.001
	Korean American	0.2 (0.1–0.3)	<.001	
2	Years of schooling	1.1 (1.0–1.1)	<.01	
3	Personal experience: illness	1.7 (1.0–2.5)	<.03	
		Prognosis		
1	Ethnic group			
	European American	1.0	. . .	
	African American	0.8 (0.5–1.3)	.39	
	Mexican American	0.6 (0.3–0.9)	<.03	<.001
	Korean American	0.3 (0.2–0.4)	<.001	
2	Years of schooling	1.0 (1.0–1.1)	<.05	
		Patient as decision maker		
1	Ethnic group			
	European American	1.0	. . .	
	African American	0.8 (0.5–1.2)	.27	<.001
	Mexican American	0.3 (0.2–0.6)	<.001	
	Korean American	0.2 (0.1–0.3)	<.001	

Our study suggests that the attitudinal differences among these ethnic groups are related to cultural rather than demographic variables, such as socioeconomic status, which tend to vary with ethnicity. In the Mexican-American group, in which the subjects had variable levels of acculturation, more acculturated subjects were more likely to share the patient autonomy model with the European-American and African-American subjects. As they begin to speak, think, and read more in English, and associate more with Anglos, they tend to take on the attitudes that are expressed by the English-speaking groups in our study. Socioeconomic status does not predict attitudes in the European-American and African-American groups. Instead, socioeconomic status may be acting as a marker for acculturation. Wealthier, more educated Mexican Americans are more

likely to speak English and be in contact with values promoted in the English-speaking sectors of American society and more likely to adopt those values with respect to medical decision making.

There are several limitations to the generalizability of our data. Subjects aged 65 years and older are more likely to be faced with serious health care decisions for themselves or their loved ones; younger subjects may hold different views. Moreover, to prevent skewing our population toward younger, female subjects, we used a quota sampling technique rather than a true random sample of the entire elderly population of these four ethnic groups. Although we attempted to minimize selection bias by sampling from a wide variety of sites, our subjects may not represent all portions of those groups. Finally, our sample was from urban southern

California; the attitudes of the elderly may differ by geographic location.

The decision-making style exhibited by most of the Mexican-American and Korean-American subjects in our study might best be described as family centered. Although the patient autonomy model does not exclude family involvement, in this family-centered model, it is the sole responsibility of the family to hear bad news about the patient's diagnosis and prognosis and to make the difficult decisions about life support. Several prior studies of the issue of telling the diagnosis of cancer with different ethnic groups have yielded similar results. In one recent report, an Italian oncologist described the approach toward decision making in Italy as one in which the patient is frequently "protected" from bad news by the family and physicians.[8] Autonomy is not viewed as empowering. Rather, it is seen as isolating and burdensome to patients who are too sick and too ignorant about their condition to be able to make meaningful choices. In a survey from Greece, only a third of those questioned believed that patients should be told the truth about a terminal illness.[9] As in our study, older subjects with less education were more likely to be opposed to truth telling. Anecdotal reports also note the tendency of Chinese and Ethiopian families to oppose truth telling on the grounds that it harms the patient by causing them to lose hope.[10] Other studies have shown that Latinos are more likely than Anglos to believe that cancer is a death sentence.[11] Finally, studies of physicians' attitudes and practice show that those in Spain, France, Japan, and Eastern Europe rarely tell patients with cancer their diagnosis or prognosis, usually informing the family instead.[12]

Thus, belief in the ideal of patient autonomy is far from universal. In this country, as recently as 1961, Oken[13] documented that 90% of physicians did not inform their patients of the diagnosis of cancer. By 1979, when this survey was repeated, this attitude had completely reversed. By 1979, 97% of physicians made it their policy to inform patients with cancer of their diagnosis.[14] Most of the literature that discusses this change views it as simple progress from an uninformed paternalism to a more enlightened and respectful attitude toward patients. Indeed,

there have been many benefits to more open discussion and increased patient involvement in medical decision making. It is probably impossible to completely deceive seriously ill patients when, despite all reassurance, they continue to deteriorate physically and to require hospitalization and medical care. Acknowledgment of the truth lets patients express their feelings and receive the emotional and spiritual comfort appropriate to the crisis they are experiencing. Allowing patients to choose from the range of treatment options available ensures that the treatment will conform to their preferences. However, the high value placed on open expression of emotion and on the rights of individuals to control their destiny is not necessarily shared by all segments of American society. For those who hold the family-centered model, a higher value may be placed on the harmonious functioning of the family than on the autonomy of its individual members. Although the patient autonomy model is founded on the idea of respect for persons, people live, get sick, and die while embedded in the context of family and culture and inevitably exist not simply as individuals but in a web of relationships. Insisting on the patient autonomy model of medical decision making when that model runs counter to the deepest values of the patient may ironically be another form of the paternalistic idea that "doctor knows best."

Many questions remain to be answered about how this family-centered model functions in actual practice. Do patients who are not told the diagnosis usually know it anyway? Is this information later communicated by verbal or nonverbal means? Is the interaction between patient and family different when the patient is the head of the household? What is the perceived harm when the medical community violates cultural conventions and insists on telling the truth to the patient? What disruptions occur in the coping mechanisms of the individual and the family? In what ways does acculturation change the beliefs of patients of various ethnicities, i.e., how are the cultures of immigrants transformed and combined with the culture of their adopted country? We plan to explore these and other issues through in-depth ethnographic interviews with 10% of the study sample.

The purpose of our study was not to convince ethicists that there should be one set of moral rules for Korean Americans and another for European Americans, and we do not expect that the information we have obtained will allow physicians to predict with certainty the attitude of any given person from a particular ethnic group. As our study demonstrates, much diversity of opinion about these issues occurs not only between ethnic groups but also within each ethnic group. Rather, we believe that it is vital to uncover the usually unspoken beliefs and assumptions that are common among patients of particular ethnicities to raise the sensitivity of physicians and others who work with these groups. Understanding that such attitudes exist will allow physicians to recognize and avoid potential difficulties in communication and to elicit and negotiate differences when they occur. In particular, we suggest that physicians ask patients if they wish to be informed about their illness and be involved in making decisions about their care or if they prefer that their family handles such matters.[15] In either case, the patient's wishes should be respected. Allowing patients to choose a family-centered decision-making style does not mean abandoning our commitment to individual autonomy or its legal expression in the doctrine of informed consent. Rather, it means broadening our view of autonomy so that respect for persons includes respect for the cultural values they bring with them to the decision-making process.

NOTES

This project was supported by grant 1 R01 HS07001 01A1 from the Agency for Health Care Policy and Research, Washington, DC. We thank Alex Capron, LLB, David Goldstein, MD, Barbara Malcolm, MA, and Elena Taylor-Muñoz, MA, for their help and support.

1 Novack, D. H., Plumer, R., Smith, R. L., Ochitill, H., Morrow, G. R., and Bennett, J. M., "Changes in physicians' attitudes toward telling the cancer patient," *JAMA* 241 (1979): 897–900; President's Commission for the Study of Ethical Problems in Medicine and Biomedical and Behavioral Research, *The Ethical and Legal Implications of Informed Consent in the Patient–Practitioner Relationship* (Washington, DC: US Government Printing Office, 1982), pp. 74–6.

2 Cobbs v. Grant, 8 C. 3d 229, 242–3 (1972); Beauchamp, T. L. and Faden, R. R., *A History and Theory of Informed Consent* (Oxford: Oxford University Press, 1986), pp. 88–98.

3 American Thoracic Society, "Withholding and withdrawing life-sustaining therapy," *Ann. Intern. Med.* 115 (1991): 478–84; Council on Ethical and Judicial Affairs, American Medical Association, "Guidelines for the appropriate use of do-not-resuscitate orders," *JAMA* 265 (1991): 1868–71.

4 Steinbrook, L. and Lo, B., "Decision-making for incompetent patients by designated proxy," *N. Engl. J. Med.* 310 (1984): 1598–1601; Schneiderman, L. J. and Arras, J. D., "Counseling patients to counsel physicians on future care in the event of patient incompetence," *Ann. Intern. Med.* 102 (1985): 693–8; Annas, G. J., "The health care proxy and the living will," *N. Engl. J. Med.* 324 (1991): 1210–13; Emanuel, L., "Does the DNR order need life-sustaining intervention? Time for comprehensive advance directives," *Am. J. Med.* 86 (1989): 87–90; Emanuel, E. and Emanuel, L., "Living wills: Past, present and future," *J. Clin. Ethics* 1 (1990): 9–18.

5 Sehgal, A., Galbraith, A., Chesney, M., Schoenfeld, P., Charles, G., and Lo, B., "How strictly do dialysis patients want their advance directives followed?" *JAMA* 277 (1992): 59–63; Nelson, J. L., "Taking families seriously," *Hastings Center Report* 22 (1992): 6–12; Orona, C. J., Koenig, B. A., Davis, A. J., "Cultural aspects of nondisclosure," *Camb. Q. Health Ethics* 3 (1994): 338–46.

6 Blackhall, L. J., "Must we always use CPR?" *N. Engl. J. Med.* 317 (1987): 1281–4; Schneiderman, L. J., Jecker, N. S., and Jonsen, A. R., "Medical futility: Its meaning and ethical implications," *Ann. Intern. Med.* 112 (1990): 949–54.

7 Hlatsky, M., Boireu, R. E., Higgenbotham, M. B., et al., "A brief self-administered questionnaire to determine functional capacity (the Duke Activity Status Index)," *Am. J. Cardiol.* 64 (1989): 651–4; Orona et al., "Cultural aspects of nondisclosure"; Levine, R. J., "Informed consent: Some challenges to the universal validity of the Western model," *Law Med. Health Care* 19 (1991): 207–13.

8 Surbone, A., "Truth telling to the patient," *JAMA* 268 (1992): 1661–2.

9 Dalla-Vorgia, P., Katsouyanni, K., Garanis, T. N., Touloumi, G., Drogari, P., and Koutselinis, A., "Attitudes of a Mediterranean

population to the truth-telling issue," *J. Med. Ethics* 18 (1992): 67–74.

10   Muller, J. H. and Desmond, B., "Ethical dilemmas in a cross-cultural context: A Chinese example," *West J. Med.* 157 (1992): 323–7; Beyene, Y., "Medical disclosure and refugees: Telling bad news to Ethiopian patients," *West J. Med.* 157 (1992): 328–32.

11   Pérez-Stable, E. J., Sabogal, F., Otero-Sabogal, R., Hiatt, R. A., and McPhee, S. J., "Misconceptions about cancer among Latinos and Anglos," *JAMA* 268 (1992): 3219–23.

12   Holland, J. C., Geary, N., Marchini, A., and Tross, S., "An international survey of physician attitudes and practice in regard to revealing the diagnosis of cancer," *Cancer Invest.* 5 (1987): 151–4; Estapé, E., Palombo, H., Hernández, J. et al., "Cancer diagnosis disclosure in a Spanish hospital," *Ann. Oncol.* 3 (1992): 451–4; Thomsen, O., Wulff, H., Martin, A., and Singer, P., "What do gastroenterologists in Europe tell cancer patients?" *Lancet* 341 (1993): 473–6.

13   Oken, D., "What to tell cancer patients," *JAMA* 175 (1961): 86–94.

14   Novack et al., "Changes in physicians' attitudes toward telling the cancer patient."

15   Freedman, B., "Offering truth: One ethical approach to the uninformed cancer patient," *Arch. Intern. Med.* 153 (1993): 572–6.

30

Power Plays

PERRI KLASS

Oh, someday we too will be attendings, and we will stride through the hospital corridors in the long white coats which are badges of status (even medical students can wear the short white ones) and smile absently at the various peons we pass, the residents and nurses and students and the occasional patient, and we will stride onto the ward and bring order out of chaos, rebuking the house staff (interns and residents) who in ignorance, overeagerness, or sloth (it hardly matters which) have done too little of the right thing or too much of the wrong. We will listen ceremoniously (or is that ceremonially?) to our patients' chests and then reassure them gently that they are in excellent hands – nodding politely to the house staff, but really meaning, of course, ourselves. And we will conduct our formal teaching sessions (attending rounds) and grill the medical students, for their own good, of course, showing them again and again how little they really know, and then when we get tired of the game, we will lecture for a while on our own research interests, and no one will dare fall asleep. (And then we will stride off the ward, making a great show of hurry and importance, and have a nice lunch, and as soon as we are gone, the resident will express himself in scato-

logical terms as regards all emendations made to house-staff management of patients and also as regards attendings who do so much research that they forget what little they ever knew about patient care and, incidentally, say a couple of scathing words to the medical student about a pretty weak showing.) Oh, someday we too will be attendings, and we will have *power*.

Medicine in a large teaching hospital is structured as a rigid hierarchy. The medical student of course is at the bottom; the term "scut-puppy" comes to mind. The hierarchy ascends in order of seniority: the intern, the junior resident, the senior resident, the fellows, the attending. The official expectation is that all doctors will teach medicine to those less experienced than themselves, and that there will also be lessons in the art of being a doctor, in what can be called bedside manner, in all sorts of intangible subjects that can be taught only by example. And one end result is that a lot gets taught and learned about how to handle power.

But wait a minute. Wasn't one group left out of that description of the hospital hierarchy? After all, doctors may flatter themselves that they are the centers of creation (How many Harvard medical students does it take to change a light bulb? One, to stand there and hold it while the world revolves around him), but surely they don't flatter themselves that hospitals exist only for their benefit. Well, no, there are the patients. The patients are outside the hierarchy, but sometimes they can also be found at its most subterranean level, below even the subbasement of the medical students. After all, the lowly medical student often knows more than the patient about the patient's prospects, about possible diagnoses, about tests in the offing, maybe painful or dangerous.

And patient care can be influenced by the issues of power which entangle the various doctors, by the little dramas of territoriality and one-upmanship which sometimes emerge from unfortunate combinations of personalities. Patients can be seen as territory, decisions as power, medical disagreements as personal challenges. An illustrative story, extreme but real:

Mr. Rachmaninoff has been finding himself a little short of breath lately. Of course, he's getting on, and in spite of what he knows about cigarette smoking being bad for your health, he hasn't been able to give up his pack-a-day habit. Otherwise he's in pretty good shape, really, lives alone, does his own shopping, takes the stairs slowly but surely, pays frequent visits to his children and grandchildren. It seems to be a close family; in fact, it's his older daughter who has dragged him to the doctor to have this shortness of breath investigated; Mr. Rachmaninoff has been inclined to write it off as old age. Anyway, as part of the doctor's investigation, a chest X-ray is done, and when the chest X-ray is read, there is a round lesion in the left upper lobe of the lung. This can mean any number of things, but one of the things it can mean is, of course, lung cancer. And in a gentleman in his late sixties with a heavy smoking history – well, it's worrisome. Mr. Rachmaninoff's doctor decides to admit him to Major University Hospital for fuller investigation of this lesion. For reasons best known to himself, Mr. Rachmaninoff shows up at 10:00 P.M., when the intern on call, who is trying to work up one emergency room admission before she gets hit with the next, is not too happy to see him. As she is rushing down to the emergency room, she runs into the Pulmonary Fellow, who is still in the hospital because it has been an

exceptionally busy day, and she remembers that in the note he wrote about Mr. Rachmaninoff, the private physician asked for a pulmonary consultation. So she stops for a minute and tells the Pulmonary Fellow about Mr. Rachmaninoff, and the Fellow, who is young and enthusiastic, says, what the hell, I'll go see the guy now, before I leave. So the intern rushes away, happy, number one, to have fulfilled the request of the private physician, and number two, to have gotten someone knowledgeable to see her patient, which will help her to be on top of the case for the next morning's rounds.

The Pulmonary Fellow leaves a long note in the chart. (The intern copies from it extensively for her own note, which she of course sticks into the chart before the other note, since hers is the admission note, and the medical student curses himself for not having been around when Mr. Rachmaninoff arrived – he was at the free late-night supper the hospital provides for people on call, and for the sake of a lousy turkey-loaf sandwich, he has missed this nice straightforward admission, and the intern will make him do some awful old emergency room gomer – hospital slang for a very debilitated, no longer mentally intact patient; stands for "Get Out of My Emergency Room" – with five volumes of past medical charts to review and multisystem disease to read up on.) The gist of the Fellow's note, which learnedly summarizes all the possibilities, obscure and more obscure, to be considered in the differential diagnosis of a lesion like Mr. Rachmaninoff's, is that the Fellow thinks the guy has lung cancer, and he wants to do a bronchoscopy to prove it – that is, stick an instrument down the patient's bronchus and take a biopsy.

The next morning, on work rounds, all hell breaks loose. The resident is furious at the intern for calling the consult. Now these Pulmonary guys are gonna come in and take over *our* patient, and they're gonna want to make all the decisions. Four or five times he tells the chastened intern, and her colleague, the other intern, I don't want you guys calling *any* consults till you check with me. Got that? *No* consults unless I say so.

As work rounds are finishing (the resident has just blown off a little steam by letting the medical student have it for taking more than ninety seconds to present the patient he worked up, the one with five volumes of old chart and the multisystem disease), the Pulmonary team turns up. With rather elaborately casual intellectual interest, the resident informs them that he is dubious about the value of bronchoscopy in Mr. Rachmaninoff's case, and he wants to go with a transtracheal needle biopsy – that is, he wants to stick a needle into the lesion from outside and take a tissue sample that way. The Pulmonary people begin talking about which test is more likely to give definite results with a lesion in this particular location, which test is more dangerous to this patient. There is a rather tense little scene as they and the resident quote journal articles back and forth. Finally the resident, who is not known for his good manners or his subtlety, says, well he's *our* patient and we make the decisions, so tough luck, guys. You don't get to bronchoscope this one.

At attending rounds, the resident tells the story to the attending, casting the Pulmonary Fellows as lawless marauders and the intern as a foolishly ineffectual guard. Now, if the resident is a notoriously bad-tempered would-be cowboy, the attending is deeply concerned with his own diagnostic brilliance, with demonstrating the breadth and depth of his knowledge, with posing questions he can himself answer at length. The attending is roused to furious scorn of the Pulmonary Fellows – why are they so sure this lesion is malignant? (He demands a list of nonmalignant possibilities from the medical student, who has unfortunately fallen asleep, and who wakes up only in time to hear the word "possibilities," spoken with the little interrogative lift which tells him that he has been asked a question. Unfortunately, he guesses the question wrong and begins to list possible types of lung cancer; he is cut off with a few sarcastic words and the attending lists the possibilities he wants himself.) He and the resident are both working themselves up into a fever of hope that they can pull the rug out from under Pulmonary by establishing that Mr. Rachmaninoff in fact has not cancer but tuberculosis (the medical student is told to give him a TB test – a little scut) or

some rare fungal infection (the medical student is told to draw blood for a series of antibody tests) or some benign slow-growing kind of tumor (the medical student is told to track down Mr. Rachmaninoff's old chest X-rays, which are apparently at a hospital not too far away, so they can be compared with this new one). Mr. Rachmaninoff doesn't know it, of course, but by the time attending rounds are over, he has a large group of doctors cheering for him with a passion no other patient on the floor can even approach. Everyone bustles around, arranging new and different kinds of X-rays, hoping to show aspects of the lesion which make malignancy unlikely, drawing blood and ordering more tests, tracking down old chest films and getting radiologists to read them. The Pulmonary people show up in Radiology just as the team is going over these films, and again express a wish to do a bronchoscopy. Absolutely not, says the resident, folding his arms. The intern whispers something apologetic when the resident isn't looking, and the Pulmonary Fellow replies with something short and pointed.

And so it goes on. Unfortunately for the resident and the attending, and even more unfortunately for Mr. Rachmaninoff, none of the benign possibilities pans out. The needle biopsy is attempted without success, and the resident has to allow a bronchoscopy to be done after all – though he makes it clear that he considers it all, including the failure of the needle biopsy, to be the intern's fault for calling in the consult. The bronchoscopy shows that Mr. Rachmaninoff has lung cancer. The attending has changed his tune and begins to insist that he saw it coming all along. He gives a learned little lecture on why lung cancer was always the most likely diagnosis in this patient, and the medical student manages to stay awake and correctly, this time, provide the four possible types of lung cancer when asked.

Mr. Rachmaninoff passes into the hands of the surgeons, who are fighting over whether he is a "surgical candidate" – that is, are his lungs, apart from the cancer, good enough to stand the surgery? And back on the home team, the attending pontificates about how much everyone has learned from this patient, about what good "bread-and-butter medicine" this was, and the resident takes the opportunity to get in a few more digs about people who call in consults and get the patients snatched away from under our noses. And the intern stares straight ahead, and the medical student begins to drift off to sleep. Someday we will be residents. Someday we will be attendings.

Mr. Rachmaninoff, in the end, probably got the same care he would have gotten without the power struggle. Oh, maybe an extra test or two, and certainly a whole lot of extra attention from doctors. He will never know the details of the controversy that raged around his lungs – but of course, from his point of view, he is caught up in a very different and much more serious drama.

31

The "Kinder Egg": Some Intrapsychic, Interpersonal, and Ethical Implications of Infertility Treatment and Gamete Donation

JOAN RAPHAEL-LEFF

"You are extra special in that you have been created with the participation of not two, but three people," writes a woman in an imaginary letter to the possible offspring of her donated eggs. "I see my involvement as that of an architect. I supplied your mother with the plans she needed, that was all. It was she who did the building, who nurtured, nourished and housed you; she who made that all important life connection, who allowed you to develop safely inside her womb, and ultimately brought you into the world. . . . All I can say is that I supplied those 'plans' with love. Love of humanity, love of life, and a compassion and empathy for all women who have been denied their right to have their own baby. . . . So just remember you are part of the whole. Not one of us can really trace our origins. *In the final analysis we are all of us related to each other.*" (Giles, 1994)

We are living through strange times when eternal facts of life have changed dramatically. Babies may now be created without sex and in the case of gamete donation by three or even four contributors, not counting the fertility team. Delayed reproduction has spawned a virtual industry with a momentum and ethos of its own. New reproductive realities are being spun of the stuff of unbridled imagination and reality is racing ahead, at times changing faster than the unconscious can keep up: fertilization outside the body is taken for granted, as is trans-plantation of long-stored deep-frozen embryos. Surrogates have been known to gestate their own grandchildren. Identical twins may be born years apart. Multiple gestations hitherto unknown to humankind (a side effect of fertility drug hyper-stimulation) have resulted in the practice of selective fetocide and genetic manipulation; pre-implantation diagnosis, sex-selection, and prenatal screening raise ethical issues about acceptable levels of congenital abnormality. Postmenopausal mothers give birth to genetically unrelated offspring and, despite recent decline in the quality of sperm, infertile men may now sire through sub-zonal insemination and even posthumous fathering is possible.

A great diversity of personal values is revealed by different reactions to this illusion of omnipotent control – around 20 percent choose not to procreate, or, if faced with infertility, do not avail themselves of reproductive technologies; some people limit their expenditure of hopes, time, and resources; others feel desperate and will go to great lengths to have a child of their own despite the odds, or settle with reservations for gamete donation.

In the light of this plurality of reactions, traditional conceptualizations of sex, gender, sexuality, and procreativity are having to be revised. Procedures such as sperm or egg donation, or surrogacy, which distinguish genetic, uterine, and social aspects of parenthood, provide us with an inkling of the corresponding intrapsychic and interpersonal complexities around the seemingly simple wish for a child. These observations are based on my own psychoanalytically oriented therapeutic work with some 150 individuals and 30 couples seen 1–5 times a week in a clinical practice specializing in emotional aspects of reproduction for over 25 years. Over a third of these had therapy over a very prolonged period of infertility, including 28 infertile women in long-term analysis, some of whom were seen through several pregnancies, while others had to come to terms with involuntary childlessness.

For some people, prolonged failure to conceive and diagnosis of "infertility" constitute fundamental threats. The inability to procreate undermines "generative identity," as I have described that aspect of gender identity which provides a sense of oneself as a potential progenitor (Raphael-Leff, 1996, 2000). When, for a variety of psychohistorical reasons, this is a pivotal part of their identity, a person may feel devastated by the idea of being unable to procreate, and/or to perpetuate their own genetic line. The intensity of these desires may apply differentially to partners in a couple, which in itself may pose difficulties.

The crisis of diagnosis and stress of fertility treatments are inadequately documented and we are not always aware of the wear-and-tear effect on a couple's sexual and emotional life of finding themselves unable to be fruitful together without external intervention. The painful gap occupied by the fantasy baby haunts their daily relationship, impelling them to actualize the child of their dreams at all costs. Loss of control, frustration, deep shame, and ferocious envy may spill over into other areas of their lives, inducing couples to restrict social contacts, avoiding childbearing couples and family or friends oblivious to their predicament. Depression, anxiety, panic attacks and agitation, magical thinking, paranoid anxieties, depersonalization, and derealization may prevail intermittently (see Raphael-Leff, 1986, 1991, 1992, 1996).

The monthly necessity for a conscious re-examination of the desire to have a child can erode a precarious relationship, particularly when the needs of partners differ. If treatment is advocated in addition to repeated reaffirmation of their respective inclination to persevere, even the most egalitarian couple experience strain and some emotional split, with inevitable gender polarization of fertility treatments.

With the medicalization of their problem, dependency, vulnerability, and infantalization inherent in any bodily care is exacerbated, retriggering intense feelings towards the powerful mediators who seem to have the power to give or withhold a baby. Reactions range from idealization of specialists and excessive gratitude for this "gift" of the yearned-for baby, to acute distress at "disappointing" the doctor's hopes and/or rage at prohibitions or negative pronouncements. Heightened emotion and the unceasing round of investigations and proposed solutions may result in some people persevering with treatment under the unstoppable momentum of enthusiastic fertility experts pursuing their own false criteria of statistical success. I have at times been consulted both by despairing women seeking termination following a long-pursued conception, and by puzzled consultants, who say indignantly: "It took me [!] three years to get this patient pregnant and do you know what she went and did? she had an abortion! Now how do you explain *that?!*." Very simply. For unknown complex reasons which may be to do with need for proof of fecundity, fear of failing, compliance with authority, or unconscious anxieties about usurping her own parents, a woman may desperately wish to conceive – but not necessarily want to have a baby. Indeed, caught up in the round of medical regimes fueled by such single-minded propulsion to circumvent obstacles and correct deficits, it is not difficult to lose sight of a baby as the ultimate goal of the intervention.

The situation is further complicated when only one of the partners is infertile. This exacerbates feelings of resentment, envy, and even suicidal despair. Gamete donation is one solution to the prospect of childlessness, but increases the discrepancy between the fertile and the infertile partner within a relationship. The baby will provide lifelong testimony of *lack* in one parent and evidence of their failure to blend their own joint genetic inputs in creating a celebratory third.

In addition to these fertile/infertile distinctions there is another fundamental reproductive asymmetry – the recipient of the donation (whether sperm, eggs, or embryo) is always the *female* partner (in a heterosexual pair). Distanced by intervention and technologically evicted from feeling at home in her own body, a woman has nonetheless to offer "hospitality" to the foreign element that holds her only hope of becoming a mother. Contradictions abound and, in the case of the ovum-donation, a recipient must open her womb to a cuckoo egg as to her own while yet acknowledging it as another's. Through her physical and psychic receptivity, she has to enable the embryo to implant, mentally transforming the gift into a baby of her own gestation, and herself into the mother. "Last week it was like falling in love," says a woman who conceived with her husband's sperm and the egg of an anonymous donor. "I felt lucky to be having such creative input in producing this baby – feels so much closer than for a father with a donor sperm . . . but suddenly, I've plummetted into a colourless pit – it's wiped out all my feelings about the baby. Just feel fraudulent, a total hypocrite, unworthy, unable to do it myself."

Clearly, the ineluctable gift of a gamete is not without its negative side for the recipient, as it highlights their asymmetry – humiliation and rage at being needy and incomplete and envy of the casual abundance of the donor coupled with worries about screening; curiosity, idealizing, or denigrating fantasies about the unknown donor, concern about the child's genetic heritage and future well-being, and with known donors, anxieties about obligations commensurate with the enormity of the offering.

Paradoxes abound. There is a strange phenomenon that happens when the donor is herself undergoing fertility treatment and agrees to share her eggs with an anonymous woman in the same program. Statistics from both large and small fertility centers show a consistently higher rate of pregnancies in recipients, possibly related to antithetical effects of ovarian stimulation (for egg production) and implantation. These facts are not made known to the women involved nor are other egg donors warned of possible risks. Ironically, despite running its own fertility program, one London hospital refused to display a private notice calling for egg donors on the grounds that "ovarian stimulation might cause cancer," a fact it neglects to convey to its own patients.

And even in relation to psychotherapy unforeseen complications may arise. A supervisee contacted me in a panic when two of her patients seemed about to collide as, unbeknownst to each other, in the same week one was being primed to receive a donated ovum and the other, by chance a nurse in the same hospital, had decided to donate her eggs to the program.

Gamete donation raises questions not only for the recipient, but for all participants – the woman's partner (if she has one), the donor and her own family, and for the child born of this procedure. Not least of these are issues of genetic origins, confidentiality, motivations for donating gametes, for childbearing, for telling or not telling their family, friends, and offspring, etc. A donor expresses surprise at the rejection of her offer of baby photos of herself and her four children at various ages:

> If it is true [as the clinic said] that couples really do only want to know those few particulars [heights, build, and coloring] then is it just that they'd rather not know?

That they want to ignore the fact that genetically it will carry an unknown set of information? ... If recipients and donors personally know each other, the connection between them will be forever present, it will be impossible not to look for resemblances, and the burden of gratitude, though certainly not demanded, could nonetheless be oppressing. The beauty of anonymous donation is that it is a benevolent act, without financial reward, and there are no future demands, obligations or expectations from either party.

But human emotions are not simple. As the same candid woman confesses after her donation:

> I understood when I signed that I would be given no information about the recipients. ... I relinquished all legal rights and claims over any offspring that may result ... when I donated my eggs, they were sexless, there was no emotional attachment to them. They were only half the equation. ... My donation did not leave me with any sense of loss, bereavement, or despair – it is something I am well used to experiencing every month. It is rare that I stop to imagine what potential child has flowed away ...
>
> Then she adds: "Though I've said that I would like to know, to be truthful I'd only like to know if it has been successful." (Giles, 1994)

These are situations without precedent: There are anthropological questions about new kinship categories (Strathern, 1992) and moral ones about a child's entitlement not to be deceived or to the right to know her or his origins. We are only beginning to find out the effects of disclosure for donor children of the circumstances of their origins. In the UK, 40 percent of the 230 families which belong to the Donor Insemination Network in London do tell their children that they were conceived by donor (DIN, 1996). In the United States this varies regionally. We are yet to discover what it might feel like for a child to know he or she has originated from an unknown "egg" or "seed" or even a known "uncle" or "auntie" for that

matter. To date there has been little feedback from children since the first baby conceived with donated eggs was born in 1984. We are yet to learn how deep unconscious implications might be different for those who originate from artificial insemination, donated egg, or embryo from those who have been adopted.

Adopted children have been vocal about their emotional experiences, and successful in establishing legal access to knowledge about their origins (in the UK since 1976, but in the USA, to date, only in Alaska and Kansas). "I think there are two reasons why genetic roots matter so much," writes a 42-year-old adoptee campaigning for gamete donation offspring to have access to records of origin:

> Firstly, our blood family connects us to the rest of the human race, on the most fundamental level. Indeed, without them, we have no absolute proof that we are human beings at all. Secondly, it is in our blood family that resides the mystery of our existence ... [where] adoption-related problems remained under the surface, including the adoptive parents' unresolved problems about their own infertility ... the damage done by adoption is so serious, and happens so early that the adoptee's problems are very deep seated. They begin in the unconscious, as a baby, and for many years that is where they remain. (Rushbrooke, 1999: 30)

Given the complexity of emotions all round, it is hardly surprising that far from assisted conception being the "happy ever after" solution, people embarking on these new journeys do so with some trepidation and a sense of loss of generative identity, ambivalence, and, in the case of recipients (inevitable and necessary) mourning for the genetically related child they will never have. A woman, faced with donor insemination, muses:

> Why am I not over the moon? ... so complicated. Can't blank my mind to the existence of another man and just focus on us and our future baby. It means blanking out REALITY. There is a *third party* in our lovemaking. I can't help but wonder who he is, what he's

like, why he's done this. My husband finds insemination painful. He almost experiences the procedure as adulterous. As for me – I know myself: I could deny the whole thing – just go into freeze mode, endure it and not crack through until I'm told I'm pregnant and only *then* react – but that's too late; this foreign life would be growing there and I would have to deal with it. Sometimes, tensing up inside it feels I'm even attacking it. . . . I'm at war with myself – feel I have to trick one part of myself to gain what the other part wants.

In the case of sperm donation, maternity demands that the woman takes into herself the raw material of a man's sperm, giving it space in her mind, her body, and possibly her marriage, as it infiltrates her ovum.

For her male partner, paternity necessitates overcoming his fear of invasion of another's seed into the ovum of his woman, finding sufficient personal authorship to inscribe the baby with a patronym of his own making despite its unknown source and his anxieties about his rival as proprietor of his partner's womb.

The unprecedented issues and bizarre nature of these innovations mean that those undergoing fertility treatment often lack psychological tools to process them. Given the rapidity of reproductive changes and difficulty in grappling with that which has neither psychic corollary nor totally positive outcome, I argue that for some, pre-conceptual and perinatal psychotherapy (rather than the statutory one-off counseling session) may be a vital necessity, providing a safe place for emotional exploration of some of the highly perplexing questions posed by these new possibilities for the individuals involved.

NOTE

A version of this paper was presented at the Tavistock Marital Studies Institute day conference on "Psychological issues for the couple surrounding donated gametes," Oct 20, 1996.

REFERENCES

DIN (Donor Insemination Network) (1996) London: personal communication.

Giles, C. (1994) On the contemplation and experience of egg donation (unpublished paper).

Raphael-Leff, J. (1986) Infertility: Diagnosis or life sentence? *Brit. J. Sex. Med.* 13: 28–30.

——(1991) *Psychological Processes of Childbearing* (London: Chapman and Hall).

——(1992) The baby-makers: An in-depth single-case study of conscious and unconscious psychological reactions to infertility and baby-making technology. *Brit. J. Psychother.* 8/3: 278–94.

——(1994) Transition to parenthood: Infertility. In *Infertility and Adoption* (Seminar Series, Post-Adoption Centre: London).

——(1996) *Pregnancy – The Inside Story* (New York: Jason Aronson).

——(1997) The casket and the key: Thoughts on gender and generativity. In J. Raphael-Leff and R. Jozef Perelberg (eds.), *Female Experience: Three Generations of British Female Psychoanalysts on their Work with Female Patients* (London, New York: Routledge).

——(2000) "Behind the shut door": A psychoanalytical approach to premature menopause. In D. Singer and M. Hunter (eds.), *Premature Menopause – A Multidisciplinary Approach* (London: Whurr Publishers).

Rushbrooke, R. (1999) Towards an open infertility industry. *J. Fertil. Couns.* 6: 29–31.

Strathern, M. (1992) *Reproducing the Future: Anthropology, Kinship and the New Reproductive Technologies* (Manchester: Manchester University Press).

32

Gynaecological Gatekeepers

NAOMI PFEFFER

An urge to pass moral judgement is evident in gynaecologists' role as gatekeepers of medical procedures relating to women's fertility. The same set of principles governed doctors' attitudes towards abortion: many gynaecologists were loath to terminate the pregnancy of a married woman, yet willing to do so if the patient was unmarried. Similarly, many doctors who frowned on abortion for social reasons sanctioned it where screening for neural tube defects indicated an abnormality in the foetus, even though most terminations on social grounds are performed at a far earlier gestational age than abortions performed for medical reasons. When asked their opinion of abortion in the early 1980s, a majority of gynaecologists supported a doctor's right to choose to prevent the birth of a child with a disability, even when the severity of the disability was unknown; a minority supported a woman's right to exercise control over her own destiny.

The long-established right of clinical freedom to do what they believe is in the best interests of their patients justifies doctors' pursuit of their own interests, even at the expense of their women patients. Yet in important respects gynaecologists were working on behalf of politicians, addressing a problem of population as if it were a medical concern. Successive governments have benefited from doctors' tenacious hold on their right both to exercise clinical freedom and to make moral judgements of their women patients, as it absolves politicians of responsibility for controversial policies. It is doctors, and not politicians, who appear to be making the difficult decisions. The process of depoliticization is at its most visible in relation to abortion. By introducing the question of a pregnant woman's mental health and her 'actual and reasonably foreseeable environment', for example, the 'special clause', in the 1967 Abortion Act gave doctors greater scope in making covert moral, as opposed to technical, decisions about women's suitability as mothers. The Act also respected doctors' right to follow the dictates of their own conscience; anyone troubled by the ethics of abortion did not have to perform it.

Judgements of the moral status of women patients are used by enthusiasts to explain why the new assisted conception technologies are necessary. These technologies include fertilization in vitro, embryo transfer and similar procedures involving the manipulation outside the body of human sperm, eggs and embryo; from here on they are referred to collectively as assisted conception technologies. Broadly speaking, assisted conception technologies substitute insemination by means of heterosexual intercourse with other methods through which fertilization may take place either within the woman's body – for example, gamete intrafallopian transfer (GIFT), where sperm are injected directly into the woman's pelvic cavity – or outside of it – for example, in vitro fertilization (IVF), where eggs removed from a woman's body are fertilized in a petrie dish, and the resulting embryos placed in the uterus through the cervix. In almost all methods, women take drugs such as gonadotrophins and clomiphene citrate in order to 'superovulate', that is, produce several eggs. Some require the woman to undergo surgery under anaesthesia.

Robert Edwards, the pioneer of the embryological aspects of the research which led to the development of the techniques culminating in the fertilization in vitro of a human egg, described his primary preoccupation as 'to study human embryology and allow women, who were seemingly condemned for ever to a life of infertility, to bear their own children fathered by their husband'.[1] And Edwards' colleague, the gynaecologist Patrick Steptoe (1913–88) persisted in the face of opposition from the medical establishment and, later, ill-health: 'What kept him going was that he was determined to help his patients.'[2] According to the modern representation of infertility, infertile women are 'desperate', 'sufferers of infertility' or 'victims of childlessness'. Thankfully, assisted conception technologies can provide them with a 'miracle baby'; only the heartless and ethically rootless would ban them. As the anthropologist Sarah Franklin has pointed out, the modern myth of infertility cites 'the emotions of the couple, their "longing" and "hope" as a way into a discussion of medical achievements, thereby providing an apparently natural and obvious link between the "hope for a medical cure" and the capability of medical science to provide one'.[3] Yet in the 1950s despair and hope were incorporated into a different infertility myth: British gynaecologists were advised that withholding treatment which had only a small chance of working was in the patient's best interests; it would discourage the development of an unhealthy, obsessive

longing for a child, and encourage women to seek and develop other sources of meaning and fulfilment in their lives.

Gynaecologists offering assisted conception technologies publicly parade their concern about the moral status of patients, although this tendency is more pronounced in doctors working within the National Health Service than in the private medical sector. A woman with a criminal conviction for running a brothel and soliciting for prostitution was refused IVF by a National Health Service gynaecologist on the grounds that she would fail the criteria of suitable motherhood set by an adoption society. Similarly, the media debated the suitability for treatment with assisted conception technology in the National Health Service of a woman who gave birth to quads: her moral status was considered ambiguous because she already had children from a first marriage, was divorced and had undergone voluntary sterilization.

Enthusiasts of assisted conception are well rehearsed in the delivery of moral messages about their patients. However, they have added to their authority by spending considerable energy and resources on psychological research to demonstrate that in married women, involuntary childlessness causes high levels of anxiety and depression, and creates marital and sexual difficulties. Enthusiasts of assisted conception technologies claim to seek to restore marital harmony and create nuclear families in circumstances hitherto deemed hopeless. Paradoxically, this moral enterprise sanctions procedures such as egg donation between sisters, and between mother and daughter, and surrogacy arrangements, which rewrite the rules of conception and birth and are effectively turning family relationships on their head.

[. . .]

Claiming to be working in the interests of suitable women patients, and conveying the impression that opponents of the new technologies are reactionary, are two of several different strategies which have effectively obscured the real interests pursued by enthusiasts of the new reproductive medicine. Another is to accuse opponents of human embryo research of being ignorant of the facts, of muddying the waters and misleading the public. Yet clarity is not evident in the propaganda produced by supporters of assisted conception. Enthusiasts insist on declaiming who they are not; they rarely reveal what they as individuals, a profession or an industry stand to gain from the technology. The public is given only negative reassurances: enthusiasts are not the crazy sort of scientists found in science fiction: human embryo research is not being exploited in order to bring into existence a race of subhuman slaves of a mad dictator, nor as a way of conceiving a monstrous chimera.

[...]

During the 1980s, the ethics of human embryo manipulation and research received unprecedented attention in the media, and in parliamentary, medical, ethical, and natural and social scientific circles. However, in retrospect, it is clear that opponents of assisted conception technologies had the cards stacked against them. One reason for their failure to influence development is that opposition to assisted conception technologies proved a weaker mobilizing force than the other concerns exercising what was a very broad church. It was pointed out earlier in this chapter that by the 1970s opposition to materialist interventions into reproduction had ceased to be a predominantly Roman Catholic movement; instead, it was made up of a motley collection of activists including radical feminists, Catholics, neo-conservatives hostile to the liberal attitudes typified by the 1960s, and people with physical and mental disabilities – groups which had little in common save this one issue, and which were all wedded to their own campaigning strategies. Furthermore, opposition to assisted conception technologies did not necessarily top their agenda: people with physical and mental disabilities, for example, were more exercised about the implications of immediate threats to resources and diminishing opportunities than about assisted conception technologies which promise to ensure that, in the future, people like them will not be born.

The most vocal opponents of the technologies were the anti-abortion lobby, who represented the human embryo as a person endowed with a soul. In effect, the embryo was subjected to a process similar to that which had redefined the foetus as a person. 'Foetal personhood', the concept of the foetus as a child capable of independent existence waiting to be born – rather than a developing bundle of tissues and cells, wholly dependent for survival on its mother's body – was first exploited in order to mobilize a public attack on abortion. The anti-abortion lobby used emotive images of a child-like foetus in order to encourage people to think of abortion as infanticide. Feminists have developed a powerful critique of the concept of foetal personhood, in particular its implications for women's civil rights. Sarah Franklin puts the argument forcefully:

> Fetal citizenship contradicts the citizenship of women; indeed, it contradicts their individuality. Endowing fetuses with full civil rights ironically confers upon them a status in relation to the patriarchal social contract *which women never had to begin with*. It is thus a double blow, extending feminine disenfranchizement from the patriarchal state, and locating within their bodies a citizen with greater rights to bodily integrity than they have.[4]

Enthusiasts of research on and manipulation of human embryos deployed a metaphysical argument in order to defeat concerted campaigns to have research on and manipulation of human embryos outlawed. The term 'pre-embryo' was developed as a way of distinguishing human embryos which had not developed a 'primitive streak' from those that had. The primitive streak, which emerges when the human embryo is fourteen days old, is the earliest manifestation of a nervous system, which in turn could be said to be the first moment at which a bundle of embryonic cells takes on human aspects. The Warnock Committee chose this stage as the cut-off point after which research on human embryos was forbidden. By conceding the possibility that once the primitive streak has developed an embryo may have human attributes, gynaecologists held on to a concept of foetal personhood which is crucial in their other work as obstetricians. In obstetrics, an image of foetal personhood has been constructed by a range of visual techniques which provide obstetricians with a 'window on the womb' through which to survey and even treat the developing foetus. It leaves the status of abortion ambiguous, but enormously extends obstetricians' authority over women during pregnancy.

NOTES

1 Robert Edwards and Patrick Steptoe, *A Matter of Life: The Sensational Story of the World's First Test-tube Baby* (London: Sphere Books, 1981), p. 91.

2 Robert Edwards, quoted in Steptoe's obituary: A. Veitch, 'A man who made thousands of babies', *Guardian*, 23 March 1988, p. 19.

3 Sarah Franklin, 'Deconstructing "desperateness": The social construction of infertility in popular representations of the new reproductive technologies', in M. McNeil, I. Varcoe, and S. Yearley (eds.), *The New Reproductive Technologies* (London: Macmillan, 1990), p. 214.

4 Sarah Franklin, 'Fetal fascinations: New dimensions to the medical-scientific construction of fetal personhood', in S. Franklin, C. Lury, and J. Stacey (eds.), *Off-Centre Feminism and Cultural Studies* (London: Harper Collins Academic, 1991), p. 201.

33

Fertility Zone

PATRICIA EAKINS

"Harley," I said when I'd crawled home through the dewy petunias, "Harley, you know that dead woman?"

"Mmmmmm," says Harley, who stuffs the covers in his mouth.

"That dead woman went and had her baby."

"Is it all right?" asks Harley, sitting right up.

"Born with everything where it should be! Dr. Conroy says it's the easiest birth ever, even if it was a Caesarian. Says he wished they were all like her – never a groan. 'Course they had her under drugs; I don't know why, if her brain was dead."

"How could the baby be all right if the mother was dead?"

"Well, her chest was going up and down, and they were feeding her through that I. V., all what the baby needed. That baby got better nourishment than she would have at home. You know what people eat – tortilla chips and beer."

"I don't like it," Harley says.

"You don't have to," I say.

But there's that motherless child, born from a brain-dead anonymous, they're going to shove in an orphanage; here's me and Harley sticking teddy-bear decals on a brand-new crib. Makes me spit. But no use arguing once Harley gets that tone to his voice.

"I'm going to fix my breakfast and turn in," I say, and I go about getting my rice puffs and raisins – you can see I eat like an elf on a mushroom. It's my glands pump me up to two-twenty-five. Harley reads the scale because I can't see past my stomach. I *look* pregnant, but I been trying for seven years.

First thing you wake, before you even tinkle, you take your temperature. And you better have remembered to shake that mercury down when you put out the light. You can't shake it down just before you jab the thermometer under your tongue, because shaking drives your heat up. You're trying to record it unaffected, at waking's first calm, before the hot presence of mind moves you to rub the hard sleep from the corners of your eyes. You're trying to find your true underlying temper, so you'll notice one day when your degrees drop. That's when your egg is falling through your tubes, falling and falling, like an astronaut, falling toward what he doesn't know. After, your temperature leaps, and then you conceive.

So Harley and I keep track of tenths of degrees, and make a graph, connecting dots. I let Harley do that part.

The night the dead woman gave birth, we were in my fertility zone, so I gulped my cereal, 'cause if I don't crawl in with Harley right off the bus, nothing's going to happen. Harley ambles off to work when he's sober – an outdoor job at Robbins's Nursery – lots of shoveling. I always say we got something in common, him spreading manure and me collecting bedpans. I've got a hoister's biceps from lifting and turning the patients, washing them, changing their bedclothes – I don't mind. Because you're helping out, as I see it, helping the needy. Not like working in the five-and-dime. There you say, "Can I help you?" But what do you have that anyone needs?

Anyway. Running home to Harley from work, I'm still painted up, my eyelashes curled, my lips bee-stung. I'm not trying to woo with my hair in rollers, lure with a hairnet over the lumps.

"Harley," I coo, and I can pout so's you'd think of a doll. "Harley," I drawl, "how you feeling, honey, can I get you something?"

"Just knead this pain in my shoulder," he says. Or his foot or his stomach. He's been home in bed all night, and I've been hefting trays and cranking beds, but I don't mind. I rub him where it hurts and hope. He talks to me, and if he's been drinking he cries a flood. Sooner or later he passes out, snores like a giant lizard stalking his dinner on the late-late show, but I let it be. I don't question. Oh, I might hint now and then. "Harley, those names you call me when you're tight . . ." And he feels so bad to hear he crowned me Miss Dual-Wheel-Stomach. He swears he loves me; just the liquor talked. I pray he don't drink around our little girl.

It's going to be a little girl, I know, just like I knew the dead woman's baby would be a girl. I could see it in the air around the mother, a soft shine like the glow of a new spring leaf.

It was just a girl-glad luster she had, though her face, it's still, without expression. Like nothing affects her, sorrow or joy, except way far in where her soul shines, that one little candle in the dark of the song, beyond caring. But who am I to say she doesn't care? Maybe she does. I'm sure she does! But her feelings aren't connected to facial expressions. Her face and all you can see is so tired, so tired from the shock and the stress of the accident, tired to dying and death.

That's how her brain died, an accident. Hit-and-run in the rain on the freeway. What was she doing jerking her thumb on that access ramp, pregnant? Trying to get somewhere good from somewhere bad? Well, aren't we all?

I hear they brung her in in thrift-shop clothes – nothing matching, all outmoded, smelling like inside abandoned cars, all wet and mousy and old – she was too young to smell so old. The rain soaking her hair down over her eyes, she may not have seen the car that would hit her. Maybe among the patter-splatting raindrops she couldn't hear the car's purr, couldn't even hear her own heart beat.

Last night her heart was beating still. They talked of disconnecting her – the baby was safe by then, you know – but they left her till the committee meets, tomorrow. Oxygen tubes jammed up her nose, the I.V. tube needled into her veins, a suction tube poked down her throat. That one's connected to a mopping machine goes *Zub! Zub! Zub!* just like a washer. Anyone would be depressed to wake up tumbled and spun to the sound of washing. Brain-washing – before you know it, you're clean of thoughts, words, and deeds, your life is bleached and plain. I wish I'd brought that woman some of those sweet peas I've been growing near the birdbath, just brought them in an old jelly glass, plunked it near her call button, case she did have some little shred of who she is left.

"Harley," I say, "you watch any good shows last night?"

"The ball game," he says, "but I slept right through."

Sometimes me and Harley, I feel we're in the two worlds, the matter and the antimatter, you read about in his comics. And I wonder where our little girl would live – in the cracks between?

I used to think, I'll quit work and take care of her, long as Harley's at the nursery. But now I think different, 'cause he's been laid off from two nurseries. And the *Nurseries* in the Yellow Pages isn't that long. For a while I thought he could sit with her nights while I was at work. But what if she choked, and he'd passed out? Now I think our little girl, Mary Ellen, she'd have to stay with Alma Parker, the widow who drives me to the Laundromat so I can flip through her photos and coo. Those little shifty-eyed gap-toothed grand-kids visit, so Mary Ellen could have slumber parties. Oh, how I like to think of them all in pajamas with feet!

In the Sears catalog's a little pink suitcase with doggies dancing I want her to have. And a little pink phone! Harley says my gears are stripped, buying so much in advance, but I want the girl to know, her mother didn't just make do at tag sales, Second Time Around. Oh, I'll take hand-me-downs, but I've knit seven pair of booties, three receiving blankets, a playsuit, a bunting, a snowsuit, and four kimono sweaters, two with matching hats, all pink, though I did knit one blue sweater set in case.

Harley laughs, but who do you think put that swing out back and damn near fell out of the tree doing it? It was Harley built that little table and chairs and painted them white, but I found the tea set. Aren't those the cutest little tiny flowered cups? When Harley's figuring out what lumber he needs for Mary Ellen's sand-box, he doesn't drink; it's only when he's watching TV and reading comics. Well, I'd drink too if I read G.I. Joe meets the insects from Mars. G.I. Joe, always escaping from trapped cars underwater, he's hardly human. And those ball-players, in helmets, pads, gloves, and masks, tiny and faraway on TV, their humanity is suspect too.

"It's time to build a dollhouse," I say as I cuddle on Harley's back. "Mary Ellen will cry for it soon."

"Mary Ellen Pig Flap," he says.

Harley, Harley. If I didn't have him, I'd be burning in a narrow bed, twitching to amble over to Bea's, drape myself around a bar stool, pretend to listen while Bea rambles on about Ed. As long as I can remember, Ed's been lying in the back near the radio tuned to the country and western station. He breathes like the dead woman, no expression even when it's all static, but Bea says the love is still in their marriage, thank God. Now Bea's is where I met Harley. Oh, I was never one of those waiting for her to open at ten A.M., never one to stretch the happy hour till closing, not even on vacation days. I only started dropping by when the bowling

lanes asked me to hang up my shoes. Said the leagues complained about my bulk shaking alleys, knocking over pins, and changing the path of balls. *Anyway*.

"Harley," I say, cute as a buttercup, "Harley, honey."

"We've got all day. I'm not going in."

He pulls the covers over his head.

"What'd you do, Harley?"

"What do you mean, what'd I do?"

"To lose it."

"Lose what?"

"Harley, don't be cute."

"I didn't do a goddamn thing. That Robbins never liked me. Well, I'm as strong as I ever was. I'm going to try for the roads next spring."

"What are we going to do till spring?"

"I'll get odd jobs."

"There might be something steady at the school —"

"Oh, cootie catchers."

I used to cut the Jell-O cubes and smear the baloney with mayo for the kids' free lunch, but Harley said I smelled like government cheese and teacher perfume.

"We can build a henhouse, you can have chickens in back."

"Neighbors too close."

"We could move."

"Moving costs."

"As much as loafing?"

"My neck is stiff. I need my sleep."

"You watch the late, late show, that golden oldies special offer one too many times?"

"Mind your mouth or I swear, I'll smack it."

"What's come over you?"

"You, waking me up to yap about a dead baby."

"Nobody —"

"I know you. I know you. I know how your pea-brain flashes signals through your fat!"

"Harley, I'm a woman with human desires, and when you're not drunk, you're human too."

"One hundred and ten percent, drunk or sober," he says. "Now quit mouthing off. Get some sleep, or you'll lose your job."

And he turns over. And that's that. I'm staring at his spine, which is stiff and still. *We're together*, I want to say. *Remember that comic "Grunts on the Moon?" We're wearing our life suits, walking on the bottom of the Sea of Fertility, marooned in a cold, dead place, beaming S.O.S., S.O.S., Mayday! Mayday! Help!* But I don't say it. I don't say a thing. I don't even tell him what I did on my break.

I started off to see Mary Ellen – that's what everyone else was doing on their break. The miracle baby, born from the dead. But something just drew me to the mother, her mouth so dumb around the suction tube, the breath rattling in her chest. I sat by her bed and I picked up her hand, her pale, freckled hand, so limp.

"Honey," I said, "I know you've had a hard life, else you wouldn't have been out on the highway so far along. You'd have waited close to home, to the little pink room with the little pink bed. Not that you're to blame.

"Now you're dead, and tomorrow you'll be deader. I'm worried no one told you right out, you gave birth to a fine girl. I know you'd like to hold her, your good red kid bawling for life. I'd like to hold her myself. To tell you the truth, I was headed that way, but then I saw the nurses huddled around her, even those starchy R.N.'s. And I had to admit she was cared for. She was set. You were the one alone.

"So here I am, a walking, talking, jumbo-sized greeting card. If you want, pretend I'm someone else. But, honey, I'm here for all my break. Yes," I said, "for now I'll stay."

And I swear she was listening, her breathing so quiet. I edged her suction tube aside and kissed her on the mouth.

Part V

Deciding What the Problem Is

Introduction

As we describe in the Introduction to this volume, bioethics has traditionally focused more on issues of treatment (deciding what should be done about the problem) rather than of diagnosis (deciding what the problem is). The readings in Part V illustrate just how deeply issues of meaning, significance, and value enter into diagnosis.

Our continuing narrative in verse, from Jenny Lewis's *When I Became an Amazon*, reaches a fork in the woods. Following her mastectomy, Lewis is "left alone to face the night" in hospital. She longs to escape, "far away from this grim country / where fear and death / gather like ancient pools / on harsh, ancient leaves."

> *The wildness calls me with primal voices*
> *But is it asking me to leave — or come home?*

What would it be to come home to the wildness? Would it be to accept death? In this poem the companion figure of the Amazon warrior-priestess is absent; there is no comforter. Lewis is left alone to decide for herself.

The next selection is also from literature: Amy Tan's novel, *The Hundred Secret Senses*. Set in the Chinese American community, the novel concerns half-Chinese Libby and her much older half-sister, Kwan. The girls' father abandoned Kwan and her mother in China in order to emigrate to the United States; now Kwan has unexpectedly rejoined the thoroughly Americanized family following her mother's death. She brings with her a baggage of myths and ghosts, albeit friendly ones, which the 7-year-old Libby finds terrifying. The family decides that Kwan must be suffering from mental illness, although the tales she tells are true enough to her, and in her native culture. Attempting to deal with her psychiatric referral as best she knows how, Kwan decides to treat the psychiatrists as ghosts: "I don't see them, don't hear them, don't speak to them. Soon they'll know they can't change me, why they must let me go." But instead the psychiatrists diagnose Kwan as catatonic, and administer electric shock therapy. Deciding what the problem is, in Kwan's case, went wrong from all sides: the psychiatrists', Libby's, and Kwan's own. The "case" hearkens back to the argument made by Jackson and Fulford in chapter 20: psychotic diagnoses are shaky unless they incorporate the values and spiritual experience of the person concerned.

The third literary selection in Part V is Anne Sexton's "The Abortion." Fairy-tale figures such as Rumpelstiltskin dominate this short poem, but from the nightmare side of fairy tales: the dark woods in which children such as Hansel and Gretel get lost, like the "somebody who should have been born." But even this grim reading of what abortion means is insufficiently draconian for Sexton. In the last stanza she refuses to allow herself the excuse of calling the aborted fetus merely "somebody," or the narrative merely one of loss:

> Yes, woman, such logic will lead
> to loss without death.
> Or say what you meant,
> you coward ... this baby that I bleed.

All three of these literary selections, then, concern naming the problem in terms that are somehow true to the patient's innermost feelings.

"Consent as Empowerment: the Roles of Postmodern and Narrative Ethics," by John McMillan and Grant Gillett, takes this concern into the process of obtaining informed consent, stressing the need for the physician to explore the patient's understanding of the problem in this context of his or her illness narrative. Rather than viewing the doctor as the one who holds information, a necessary modicum of which is to be released to the patient, who has the final power of veto, the authors argue for a different approach to informed consent: one that recognizes the power imbalance in the doctor–patient relationship. Here there are echoes of Howard Brody's argument in "My Story is Broken" (see chapter 19), but the concern in the case study presented by McMillan and Gillett is not with establishing a diagnosis so much as with ensuring that the patient is sufficiently empowered to give a meaningful consent once diagnosis is established and a treatment plan recommended.

A first-person narrative, "Life-size," by Jenefer Shute, confronts us in chapter 38 with the absolute refusal of consent to treatment by an anorexic woman and her strategies to get round the imbalance in power between herself and clinicians. Control is everything, control over her own appetite included. When presented with her supper by the hospital nurse,

Shute writes: "I concentrate on controlling this food. If I don't deal with it soon, it will exert a magnetic pull on me, commanding me to eat it, filling my consciousness until the only way I could escape would be to run shrieking into the street." Her "picture" of her "illness" is inked in with shocking clarity in the first few paragraphs: an iconography of skeletal asceticism. "One day I will be thin enough. Just the bones, no disfiguring flesh, just the pure, clear shape of me. Bones. That is what we are, after all, what we're made of, and everything else is storage, deposit, waste."

Chapter 39, "But Didn't You Have the Tests?," by Joanna Richards, compares first-person reflection on one's own narrative with typical bioethical analyses of the rights and wrongs of preventing the birth of a child with disability. If there is nothing potentially wrong with preventing the birth of a "handicapped" child, and if much good can be done by having antenatal testing, why would a woman refuse testing? Yet this is exactly what Richards did. She now writes from the perspective of a parent of a child with Down's syndrome, reflecting back on the motives for her decision. Essentially, she argues that prevention of the birth of a child with disability is not what the decision whether to seek testing felt like to her. Nor does the common reaction to her daughter's condition, "But didn't you have the tests?," feel anything but judgmental. Richards wrote this article as a course paper during her study on a master's course in healthcare ethics at the University of Reading, UK. It seemed to us a particularly perceptive and acute application of theory not so much to practice as to personal experience.

Even in jointly deciding between doctor and patient what the problem is, there is a preliminary question: does the patient have the capacity to take part in this joint decision? In "Capable People: Empowering the Patient in the Assessment of Capacity," the academic lawyer Dermot Feenan puts forward a negotiated model of mental capacity assessment which does not elevate the physician above the patient in power terms, unlike conventional models. This model takes into account recent developments in "action theory" and the work of Priscilla

Alderson (also represented in this volume), who has challenged the traditional Piagetian approach to children's cognitive capacity.

The final chapter in Part V, like the first three, comes from literature: "Kelly," from Rafael Campo's *What the Body Told*. Under the clinical language with which the poem begins, Campo seems to be suggesting, lurks a callousness almost as shocking as that of the father who has sexually abused and impregnated his 12-year-old daughter. In deciding what the problem is, we must decide to what extent clinical medicine and its distancing terminology is the problem.

READING GUIDE

Priscilla Alderson's innovative work in children's capacity has already been mentioned in Part III's Reading Guide, as has Howard Brody's analysis of power in the doctor–patient relationship. The importance of empowerment in assessing children's capacity is discussed in D. Dickenson and D. Jones, "True wishes: The philosophy and developmental psychology of children's informed consent," *Philosophy, Psychiatry, and Psychology* 2/4 (1995): 287–304. The irreducible place of meaning, significance, and values in psychiatric assessment is described in chapter 4 ("Diagnosis, values and rationality") and in chapter 5 ("Causal and meaningful interpretations of aetiological factors"), in D. Dickenson and K. W. M. Fulford, *In Two Minds: A Casebook of Psychiatric Ethics* (Oxford: Oxford University Press, 2000); and in psychotherapy in R. D. Hinshelwood, "Primitive mental processes: Psychoanalysis and the ethics of integration," *Philosophy, Psychiatry, and Psychology* 4/2 (1997): 121–44, and R. D. Hinshelwood, "Response to the commentaries," *Philosophy, Psychiatry, and Psychology* 4/2 (1997): 159–66.

The growing literature on narrative ethics in medicine, in which McMillan and Gillett locate their model of informed consent, includes Adam Zachary Newton, *Narrative Ethics* (Cambridge, MA: Harvard University Press, 1995) and the collection edited by Hilde Lindemann Nelson, *Stories and Their Limits: Narrative Approaches to Bioethics* (London: Routledge, 1997).

34

Becoming an Amazon
23rd March, 1985

JENNY LEWIS

So I am left alone to face the night
with only a glowing ceiling eye to watch me,
like Charon, awaiting his passenger.
Shiny patches on the white metal cabinets
look like maps of desert islands
when I half close my eyes.
I long to escape and find the sun,

far away from this grim country
where fear and death
gather like stagnant pools
on harsh, ancient leaves.

The wildness calls me with primal voices
but is it asking me to leave – or come home?

35

The Hundred Secret Senses

AMY TAN

One night, when my eyelids were already heavy with sleep, she started droning again in Chinese: 'Libby-ah, I must tell you something, a forbidden secret. It's too much of a burden to keep inside me any longer.'

I yawned, hoping she'd take the hint.

'I have yin eyes.'

'What eyes?'

'It's true. I have yin eyes. I can see yin people.'

'What do you mean?'

'Okay, I'll tell you. But first you must promise never to tell anyone. Never. Promise, ah?'

'Okay. Promise.'

'Yin people, they are those who have already died.'

My eyes popped open. 'What? You see dead people? . . . You mean, *ghosts*?'

'Don't tell anyone. Never. Promise, Libby-ah?'

I stopped breathing. 'Are there ghosts here now?' I whispered.

'Oh yes, many. Many, many good friends.'

I threw the covers over my head. 'Tell them to go away,' I pleaded.

'Don't be afraid. Libby-ah, come out. They're your friends too. Oh see, now they're laughing at you for being so scared.'

I began to cry. After a while, Kwan sighed and said in a disappointed voice, 'All right, don't cry anymore. They're gone.'

So that's how the business of ghosts got started. When I finally came out from under the covers, I saw Kwan sitting straight up, illuminated by the artificial glow of her American moon, staring out the window as if watching her visitors recede into the night.

The next morning, I went to my mother and did what I promised I'd never do: I told her about Kwan's yin eyes.

Now that I'm an adult, I realize it wasn't my fault that Kwan went to the mental hospital. In a way, she brought it on herself. After all, I was just a little kid then, seven years old. I was scared out of my mind. I had to tell my mother what Kwan was saying. I thought Mom would just ask her to stop. Then Daddy Bob found out about Kwan's ghosts and blew his stack. Mom suggested taking her to Old St. Mary's for a talk with the priest. But Daddy Bob said no, confession wouldn't be enough. He booked Kwan into the psychiatric ward at Mary's Help instead.

When I visited her there the following week, Kwan whispered to me: 'Libby-ah, listen, I have secret. Don't tell anyone, ah?' And then she switched to Chinese. 'When the doctors and nurses ask me questions, I treat them like American ghosts – I don't see them, don't hear them, don't speak to them. Soon they'll know they can't change me, why they must let me go.' I remember the way she looked, as immovable as a stone palace dog.

Unfortunately, her Chinese silent treatment backfired. The doctors thought Kwan had gone catatonic. Things being what they were back in the early 1960s, the doctors diagnosed Kwan's Chinese ghosts as a serious mental disorder. They gave her electro-shock treatments, once, she said, then twice, she cried, then over and over again. Even today it hurts my teeth to think about that.

The next time I saw her at the hospital, she again confided in me. 'All that electricity loosened my tongue so I could no longer stay silent as a fish. I became a country duck, crying *gwa-gwa-gwa*! – bragging about the World of Yin. Then four bad ghosts shouted, "How can you tell our secrets?" They gave me a *yin-yang tou* – forced me to tear out half my hair. That's why the nurses shaved everything off. I couldn't stop pulling, until one side of my head was bald like a melon, the other side hairy like a coconut. The ghosts branded me for having two faces: one loyal, one traitor. But I'm not a traitor! Look at me, Libby-ah. Is my face loyal? What do you see?'

What I saw paralyzed me with fear. She looked as if she'd been given a crew cut with a hand-push lawn mower. It was as bad as seeing an animal run over on the street, wondering what it once had been. Except I knew how Kwan's hair used to be. Before, it flowed past her waist. Before, my fingers swam through its satin-black waves. Before, I'd grab her mane and yank it like the reins of a mule, shouting, 'Giddyap, Kwan, say hee-haw!'

She took my hand and rubbed it across her sandpapery scalp, whispering about friends and enemies in China. On and on she went, as if the shock treatments had blown off the hinges of her jaw and she could not stop. I was terrified I'd catch her crazy talking disease.

To this day, I don't know why Kwan never blamed me for what happened. I'm sure she knew I was the one who got her in trouble.

After she came back from Mary's Help, she gave me her plastic ID bracelet as a souvenir. She talked about the Sunday-school children who came to the hospital to sing 'Silent Night,' how they screamed when an old man yelled, 'Shut up!' She reported that some patients there were possessed by ghosts, how they were not like the nice yin people she knew, and this was a real pity. Not once did she ever say, 'Libby-ah, why did you tell my secret?'

Yet the way I remember it is the way I have always felt – that I betrayed her and that's what made her insane. The shock treatments, I believed, were my fault as well. They released all her ghosts.

That was more than thirty years ago, and Kwan still mourns, 'My hair sooo bea-you-tiful, shiny-smooth like waterfall, slippery-cool like swimming eel. Now look. All that shock treatment, like got me bad home permanent, leave on cheap stuff too long. All my rich color – burnt out. All my softness – crinkle up. My hairs now just stiff wires, pierce message to my brain: No more yin-talking! They do this to me, hah, still I don't change. See? I stay strong.'

Kwan was right. When her hair grew back, it was bristly, wiry as a terrier's. And when she brushed it, whole strands would crackle and rise with angry static, popping like the filaments of light bulbs burning out. Kwan explained, 'All that electricity doctor force into my brain, now run through my body like horse go 'round racetrack.' She claims that's the reason she now can't stand within three feet of a television set without its hissing back. She doesn't use the Walkman her husband, George, gave her; she has to ground the radio by placing it against her thigh, otherwise no matter what station she tunes it to, all she hears is 'awful music, boom-pah-pah, boom-pah-pah.' She can't wear any kind of watch. She received a digital one as a bingo prize, and after she strapped it on, the numbers started mutating like the fruits on a casino slot machine. Two hours later the watch stopped. 'I gotta jackpot,' she reported. 'Eight-eight-eight-eight-eight. Lucky numbers, bad watch.'

Although Kwan is not technically trained, she can pinpoint in a second the source of a fault in a circuit, whether it's in a wall outlet or a photo strobe. She's done that with some of my equipment. Here *I* am, the commercial photographer, and *she* can barely operate a point-and-shoot. Yet she's been able to find the specific part of the camera or cable or battery pack that was defective, and later, when I ship the camera to Cal Precision in Sacramento for trouble-shooting, I'll find she was exactly right. I've also seen her temporarily activate a dead cordless phone just by pressing her fingers on the back recharger nodes. She can't explain any of this, and neither can I. All I can say is, I've seen her do these things.

The weirdest of her abilities, I think, has to do with diagnosing ailments. She can tell when she shakes hands with strangers whether they've ever suffered a broken bone, even if it healed many years before. She knows in an instant whether a person has arthritis, tendinitis, bursitis, sciatica – she's really good with all the musculoskeletal stuff – maladies that she calls 'burning bones,' 'fever arms,' 'sour joints,' 'snaky leg,' and all of which, she says, are caused by eating hot and cold things together, counting disappointments on your fingers, shaking your head too often with regret, or storing worries between your jaw and your fists. She can't cure anybody on the spot; she's no walking Grotto of Lourdes. But a lot of people say she has the healing touch. Like her customers at Spencer's, the drugstore in the Castro neighborhood where she works. Most of the people who pick up their prescriptions there are gay men – 'bachelors,' she calls them. And because she's worked there for more than twenty years, she's seen some of her longtime customers grow sick with AIDS. When they come in, she gives them quickie shoulder rubs, while offering medical advice: 'You still drink beer, eat spicy food? Together, *same* time? Wah! What I tell you? Tst! How you get well do this? Ah?' – as if they were little kids fussing to be spoiled. Some of her customers drop by every day, even though they can receive home delivery free. I know why. When she puts her hands on the place where you hurt, you feel a tingling sensation, a thousand fairies dancing up and down, and then it's like warm water rolling through your veins. You're not cured,

but you feel released from worry, becalmed, floating on a tranquil sea.

Kwan once told me, 'After they die, the yin bachelors still come visit me. They call me *Doctor* Kwan. Joking, of course.' And then she added shyly in English: 'Maybe also for respect. What you think, Libby-ah?' She always asks me that: 'What you think?'

No one in our family talks about Kwan's unusual abilities. That would call attention to what we already know, that Kwan is wacky, even by Chinese standards – even by San Francisco standards. A lot of the stuff she says and does would strain the credulity of most people who are not on antipsychotic drugs or living on cult farms.

But I no longer think my sister is crazy. Or if she is, she's fairly harmless, that is, if people don't take her seriously. She doesn't chant on the sidewalk like that guy on Market Street who screams that California is doomed to slide into the ocean like a plate of clams. And she's not into New Age profiteering; you don't have to pay her a hundred fifty an hour just to hear her reveal what's wrong with your past life. She'll tell you for free, even if you don't ask.

Most of the time, Kwan is like anyone else, standing in line, shopping for bargains, counting success in small change: 'Libby-ah,' she said during this morning's phone call, 'yesterday, I buy two-for-one shoes on sale, Emporium Capwell. Guess how much I don't pay. You guess.'

But Kwan is odd, no getting around that. Occasionally it amuses me. Sometimes it irritates me. More often I become upset, even angry – not with Kwan but with how things never turn out the way you hope. Why did I get Kwan for a sister? Why did she get me?

Every once in a while, I wonder how things might have been between Kwan and me if she'd been more normal. Then again, who's to say what's normal? Maybe in another country Kwan would be considered ordinary. Maybe in some parts of China, Hong Kong, or Taiwan she'd be revered. Maybe there's a place in the world where everyone has a sister with yin eyes.

36

The Abortion

ANNE SEXTON

Somebody who should have been born
 is gone.

Just as the earth puckered its mouth,
each bud puffing out from its knot,
I changed my shoes, and then drove south.

Up past the Blue Mountains, where
Pennsylvania humps on endlessly,
wearing, like a crayoned cat, its green hair,

its road sunken in like a grey washboard;
where, in truth, the ground cracks evilly,
a dark socket from which the coal has
 poured,

Somebody who should have been born
 is gone.

the grass as bristly and stout as chives,

and me wondering when the ground would
 break,
and me wondering how anything fragile
 survives;

up in Pennsylvania, I met a little man,
not Rumpelstiltskin, at all, at all...
he took the fullness that love began.

Returning north, even the sky grew thin
like a high window looking nowhere.
The road was as flat as a sheet of tin.

Somebody who should have been born
 is gone.

Yes, woman, such logic will lead
to loss without death. Or say what you
 meant,
you coward...this baby that I bleed.

37

Consent as Empowerment: The Roles of Postmodern and Narrative Ethics

JOHN McMILLAN AND GRANT GILLETT

Informed consent is a byword for patient-centered clinical practice, but it is time for it to be superseded in favor of a more effective understanding of medical decision-making which allows the patient to take control of that part of his or her life narrative that must be spent in medical treatment. Beauchamp and Childress (1994) have outlined the necessary conditions for informed consent, but they have not gone on to develop the idea of empowering the patient. We will outline a case in which a physician observes the requirements of informed consent: but in which the patient's role is not ideal. The assumption in this case – which involves a decision about brain surgery – is that the information is too "technical" to be shared with the patient. But we will suggest that it is, above all else, important to empower the patient instead of merely "obtaining" informed consent.

Informed Consent

Beauchamp and Childress outline seven elements of informed consent (1994: 145). First there are *threshold elements* (preconditions):

1. Competence to understand what is at issue and make a reasoned decision.

2. Voluntariness in deciding what is at issue and make a reasoned decision.

Second there are *informational elements*:

3. Disclosure of *material information* where this should be understood as that information which might make a reasonable person change their mind. This will usually involve the clinician presenting his view of the information that has been gained about the patient and then elaborating in terms of the questions asked by the patient.

4. The *clinical recommendation*: the doctor has a duty to make a recommendation and also to make it clear that that is what it is. The patient should not feel that they "have to have the operation" because the doctor says so, but, equally, the patient is entitled to know what the doctor thinks should be done.

5. The patient's *understanding of the problem* as part of the unfolding story about their illness is very important. Here there should be an attempt by the doctor to convey why the recommendation has been made and what it implies about the future and the prospects of intervention.

Third there are *consent elements*:

6. The decision in favor of a plan, usually a plan formulated by the doctor. Here the patient is often hampered by a lack of medical knowledge even though they have the right to "make the decision."
7. The authorization of the chosen plan.

The problem is not with these elements considered separately but with the presumption that there are two distinct parties, one of whom holds information and formulates plans of treatment and the other of whom may have access to some of that information and has the power of veto over any plans that might be formulated. We can best appreciate the need for a different approach if we consider a concrete case.

The Story of Stephanie

Stephanie has consulted her general practitioner because she was suffering from headaches and problems with her vision. She is 38, married and has three children. She tends to be a fairly introverted person and is not known for making a fuss about problems. Her general practitioner referred her to the neurology unit at the local hospital for assessment. After the assessment was completed Stephanie had an appointment with a neurosurgeon. Stephanie had a glioma (a tumor of the central nervous system) which the neurosurgeon was prepared and keen to operate on. The neurosurgeon knew about informed consent, so was careful to ensure that the information he provided to Stephanie was sufficient for making a decision about whether or not to have this surgery. He told her about her tumor and the aim of the operation: to attempt to remove as much of it as possible. He warned about the risk of damage to the brain during the surgery as being of the same order as a stroke, but said that this was unlikely, with a probability of about 5 percent. The neurosurgeon was careful to ensure that the information he volunteered to Stephanie was what a "reasonable patient" in that situation would have needed to know (as is the legal requirement). Stepha-

nie's neurosurgeon was also aware that it is important when asking for informed consent to present the information that a patient needs in a manner such that the patient can understand. So he was careful to explain medical terms in lay language and wrote down some of the more important medical terms on a piece of paper. The neurosurgeon even drew a picture of the lobe of the brain in which the tumor was found.

Stephanie was visibly upset by the information that the surgeon had given her, but agreed to the surgery. Although she was upset, the surgeon judged that she was in a competent state to make this decision. As she was competent and had agreed to the surgery (having asked one or two questions) the neurosurgeon was satisfied that Stephanie's consent was informed and voluntary. Thus he had no qualms about proceeding with arrangements for Stephanie's surgery.

The neurosurgeon's actions *appear* to be consistent with the requirements for informed consent, Stephanie appeared to give consent voluntarily, on an informed basis and while in a competent state. The conclusion that the neurosurgeon reached was, given the way Stephanie acted and responded in the clinic, not unreasonable. She gave no obvious signs that she was not participating in the decision-making process as fully as she might. However, even in this apparently ideal situation there are features that effectively disempower patients and may become important in clinical practice.

Empowerment and Consent

Much has been written about the power imbalance that exists in the patient–physician relationship. William May (1983) does a fine job of unpacking some of the subtleties in the patient–physician relationship within a covenant model. That model recognizes the power imbalance and its inevitability, compensating for it by building a fiduciary and care-oriented attitude on the side of the most powerful so that the weaker member of the covenant can have justified trust in the outcome. In some medical curricula, attention is paid to helping medical students come to recognize the fact that when they deal with patients they will be entering into a relationship in which they will usually hold great influence. What is less common is explicit acknowledgment of the power dynamics in the physician–patient relationship in preconditions for informed consent. As we have suggested, Stephanie's surgeon would seem to have reasonable grounds for *believing* that she has given a valid consent, but she might not have been sufficiently empowered to make a meaningful decision.

Usually the physician knows much more about the medical condition at issue, and Stephanie must trust the neurosurgeon to give her the information that she needs. But in the normal situation there is a message conveyed by the fact that he sees the information and she does not; she only hears about it from him. The implicit message is that the information belongs on the powerful side of the medical relationship and must be rationed out in a form suited to the uninitiated.

The Remedy

The change of attitude and approach required to remedy this situation are complex and need new skills of communication, understanding, and insight. There are often, though, relatively straightforward changes of practice that will greatly improve the patient's experience. In Stephanie's case, for example, the surgeon could have shown her the investigations (such as MRI scans) which delineate her problem, and explain, with their aid, what the problem is and what surgery hopes to accomplish. This achieves several things:

1. It tells the patient that the information is accessible and that they can take an intelligent interest in it.
2. It allows the patient to see the difficulties and uncertainties involved in medical diagnosis and treatment.
3. It tends to dissipate rather than increase the stress on patients, just as one feels less stressed the more one understands where one is on a trying journey.
4. It means that the patient can feel free to inquire about their tests and their medical

decision; they have, as it were, crossed the divide in terms of access to information.
5. The patients find, often to their surprise, that they can understand what is going on and claim some ownership of the decision being made.
6. Ownership and responsibility go hand in hand: therefore the patient tends to share the burden of decision-making and relieves some of it for the clinician.

We could think of it as the difference between playing a hand of cards close to one's chest and laying it down to play in a cooperative manner for the purposes of instructing a novice. If Stephanie's neurosurgeon adopted the open-handed attitude and practice in these situations, it would be possible for her to take a more active role in deciding about treatment options. Drawing Stephanie into the appreciation of tests and the planning of intervention empowers her not just to consent (in a way that is informed and voluntary) but to assume some control over this clinical and medicalized part of her autobiography.

When we look at this piece of her life story from Stephanie's perspective, the issues come into clear focus. Will she take the risks and side effects that will go along with the surgery or live out the rest of her life, albeit short, with the tumor? She has the same problem faced by many with less serious conditions such as back pain, headache, gall-bladder disease, and so on. The importance of empowerment in this process is that it enables patients to settle on the course of action that is the best option for them in the light of all their other commitments and concerns. Every medical intervention involves conflicting reasons, some recommending action and others inaction. The aim of empowerment is to enable patients to be part of the development of a management plan that leads to the outcome most congenial to their own perceptions and values.

A Narrative Approach and Empowerment

The approach to ethics most congenial to empowerment as a desired feature of the physician–patient relationship is either postmodern ethics or narrative ethics. These are closely related approaches. Postmodern ethics emphasizes the power differentials that can distort moral relationships and silence the voices of those who are traditionally disempowered by an institution and its discourses (Gillett, 1997). Within postmodern ethics the difficulty of someone like Stephanie being able to perceive or state what she found unsatisfactory about her informed consent might become evident, although the language of autonomy, beneficence, and so on would not make it visible. It is not even that Stephanie can clearly define what is wrong with her clinical care, it is just that she feels "at sea" or "out of control" in a way that she need not. Postmodern theorists address the problems of naming aspects of discourses in which certain types of people have been traditionally relegated to a powerless position, although there is no intention to marginalize them by those who hold the power; indeed the powerful players may not realize what is going on.

Narrative ethics is difficult to define (Murray, 1997), but common to most approaches that stress narrative is centering the situation on a narrative subjectivity, highlighting the ways in which events might be experienced by that person. Murray suggests that narratives put us in touch with "stories and images of good, fulfilling, meaningful lives" (1997: 54). The stories that we encounter in clinical practice, particularly when we hear the multiple voices that make up those stories, give us insight about complex moral dilemmas in a way that moral beliefs expressed in fairly clear-cut propositional terms may fail to do. Such insights are immediately relevant to the plights of the marginalized and powerless because they capture the lived experience of the person who is vulnerable, or, alternatively, the truncated narrative of the powerful, allowing us to appreciate the moral challenge that must be faced in this situation. Postmodern and narrative ethics enable us to claim "I've looked at life from both sides now" and have some hope of telling the truth.

REFERENCES

Beauchamp, T. and Childress, J. (1994) *Principles of Biomedical Ethics*, 4th edn (New York: Oxford University Press).

Gillett, G. (1997) Is there anything wrong with Hitler these days? Ethics in a postmodern world. *Medical Humanities Review* 11/2: 9–21.

May, W. (1983) *The Physician's Covenant: Images of the Healer in Medical Ethics* (Philadelphia: Westminster Press).

Murray, T. (1997) What do we mean by narrative ethics? *Medical Humanities Review* 11/2: 44–58.

38

Life-Size

JENEFER SHUTE

[...]

One day I will be thin enough. Just the bones, no disfiguring flesh, just the pure, clear shape of me. Bones. That is what we are, after all, what we're made of, and everything else is storage, deposit, waste. Strip it away, use it up, no deposit, no return.

Every morning the same ritual, the same inventory, the same naming of parts before rising, for fear of what I may have become overnight. Jolting out of sleep – what was that dream, that voice offering me strawberries and cream? – the first thing I do is feel my hipbones, piercingly concave, two naked arcs of bone around an emptiness. Next I feel the wrists, encircling each with the opposite hand, checking that they're still frail and pitiful, like the legs of little birds. There's a deep hollow on the inside of each wrist, suspending delicately striated hands, stringy with tendon and bone. On the outside of the wrist, I follow the bone all the way up to the elbow, where it joins another, winglike, in a sharp point.

Moving down to the thighs, first I feel the hollow behind the knee to check that the tendon is still clean and tight, a naked cord. Then I follow the outside of each thigh up toward the hips: no hint of a bulge, no softening anywhere.

Next I grab the inner thigh and pinch hard, feeling almost all the way around the muscle there; finally, turning on one side and then the other, I press each buttock, checking that the bones are still sticking through.

Sitting up in bed, a little more anxiously now, I grasp the collar bones, so prominent that they protrude beyond the edges of the shoulders, like a wire coathanger suspending this body, these bones. Beneath them, the rows of ribs, deeply corrugated (and the breasts, which I don't inspect). Then I press the back of my neck and as far down my spine as I can, to make sure the vertebrae are all still there, a row of perfect little buttons: as if they held this body together, as if I could unbutton it and step out any time I wanted to.

Dinner is as bad as I was afraid it would be. At precisely six o'clock, Squeaky squeaks in with a big tray, which she puts down next to the bed where I am floating again, on my back, imagining myself somewhere else altogether, cool and perfectly hard in a silk-lined gown. Firmly she says "Josie, I hope you're going to eat your salad tonight, otherwise the medical team will have to make a decision tomorrow about hyperalimentation."

I look in horror at the huge bowl of salad on the tray. *It's possible to slow yourself down by eating too much salad.* "This *is* hyperalimentation," I say: a mound of lettuce with chunks of pale tomato, shards of green pepper, hunks of purplish raw onion, and – they must be nuts if they think I'm going to eat any of this – gobs of cheese and hard-boiled egg, with a bruise-colored line where the white pulls away from the yolk. Even though I didn't ask for it, there's a big, stale-looking roll and butter, an apple, a dish of vanilla ice cream, a glass of milk, and a plastic container of some urine-colored oil labeled "Italian."

"I can't eat if you're watching me," I say, which is true.

"Okay," she says, "I'll be back in half an hour to see how you're doing."

As soon as she leaves, I draw the curtain around my bed: No one must ever see me eat, no one must ever catch me in the act – especially now that my appearance excites so much attention, with people always staring at me, willing me to weaken.

The Trobrianders eat alone, retiring to their own hearths with their portions, turning their backs on one another and eating rapidly for fear of being observed.

With the curtains drawn, my heart slows down a little and I concentrate on controlling this food: If I don't deal with it soon, it will exert a magnetic pull on me, commanding me to eat it, filling my consciousness until the only way I could escape would be to run shrieking into the street.

There is a big paper napkin on the tray, so I scrape exactly half the salad out of the bowl and into the napkin, along with half the roll. I bundle this mess up and start looking for a place to hide it: not easy in this cell. My clothes locker is locked and I don't have the key – of course not: this is going to be one of my little "rewards." (Even my shoes have been locked away, my socks.) Under my pillow would be too risky, because the napkin could leak or break, making a big lettucey mess that would be hard to explain. So the only place I can think of is the drawer of the nightstand next to the other bed, the unoccupied one, the one as flat and empty as I would like mine to be.

Once that little bundle is out of the way, I can relax a bit and start working on what's left. I separate the mound of food into piles: lettuce on one side, tomato on the other, pepper pieces neatly stacked and segregated from the rank, juicy onion. The egg and cheese I pick right off and banish to the bread plate: evil. *Cheese is the hardest food to digest, and it contaminates everything you eat it with.* Then I cut the lettuce, tomato, and pepper into tiny pieces, deciding I won't even pretend to eat the onion because lots of people don't like raw onion: It's legitimate, it's "normal." I cut the half-roll into four sections and decide I will eat only one. Of the ice cream, I will eat exactly two spoonfuls, and the apple I will save for another time. So I put it away in my nightstand drawer along with the piece of roll I picked off the lunch tray: just in case.

Now that these decisions have been made, now that the bad stuff has been removed, now that the food is separated, with white space showing on the plate, now I can start eating: one piece at a time, and at least three minutes (timed on a second hand) between mouthfuls, with the fork laid down precisely in the center of the plate after each bite.

Of course the nurse comes back before I'm done and, without even asking, swishes back the bed curtains, revealing me shamefully hunched over the tray, chewing. I freeze, unable to meet her eyes. She says, gently, "There's really no need to close the curtains, dear, when you're alone."

Sullenly I push the tray away and lie back on the pillow, staring up at the mangy acoustic tile.

"Don't stop," she says. "I'll come back in fifteen minutes or so." She leaves, but it's no good: I can't eat any more; I feel sick and upset, with the undigested salad sitting scratchily, bulkily, inside me. My stomach is beginning to swell: I feel it anxiously, palming the dip between my hipbones, sensing a new curvature, a new tightness there. Panicky, before I know what I have done, I have wolfed down three teaspoons of the now almost entirely melted ice cream.

I put the tray on the other bed and draw the bed curtains around it so I don't have to be reminded of my gluttony; climbing back onto my own bed, I draw those curtains too, wanting to be alone, to hide where no one can find me, can tempt me, can torment my will. I want to find a cave or burrow somewhere where the idea of food becomes an abstraction, and this body, ever clearer and purer, evaporates finally into the dark, leaving only consciousness behind.

When the nurse comes back, I ask her to take me to the bathroom (another of these laws under which I now live: I can't leave the ward unaccompanied). This is partly a diversionary tactic, but partly also because I'm desperate to wash my hands and face: My skin feels oily and slimy, as if the fat in the food is oozing out through my pores. She helps me tie on my hospital-issue robe, with a faded blue design that makes my skin look even more cyanotic than it is. I'm cold but she won't let me put on any more clothes. So we walk slowly to the bathroom and she stands near the door while I go into a cubicle, where I'm not allowed to close the door in case I make myself vomit (which I've never been able to do – though not for want of trying). I can't pee under these conditions, so I give up and comb my hair instead (it's still coming out, in dry hanks), tying it back tightly with an elastic band. Then I scrub my face and hands once, and again, then again, until the nurse says sharply "That's enough now" and we trudge back to the cell.

She bustles about, making a big deal of flinging back the curtains on both beds, plumping up pillows, straightening the limp covers. Then, tilting her head to one side, she contemplates the tray and says, "Well, Josie, you did a good job on your dinner."

Relieved, I climb back on the bed and pick up a *Vogue* that's been lying around – I got away with it! again! – when she says "I'm going to have to take a look around, if you don't mind. It's one of the rules."

If I don't mind! What choice do I have, powerless as a child, forced to lie and scheme simply to exercise the elementary – the alimentary – right to determine what does and doesn't go into my body?

She looked quickly under both beds and behind the curtains, checks the lock on the clothes locker, runs her hand between the end of the mattress and the metal railing at the foot of both beds, and then, of course, opens the nightstand drawer on the far side.

"What's this?" she says, though she knows.

"I was saving it for later," I say. "I couldn't eat it all now, so I was going to have some more later, before bed."

She says nothing but just stands there, shaking her head, holding the imperfectly closed bundle of salad and bread, already soggy in spots. Then she dumps it on the tray and says, "Anything you don't eat, just leave on the tray." She seems about to pick up the tray and go, but then, as an afterthought, comes over to the side of my bed, opens the screeching drawer – is there no place that's mine? – and finds the apple and the piece of roll I took from lunch. "This is hoarding," she says. "You can have anything you want to eat at any time – just ask, but don't hoard."

Angry and humiliated and bereft, I don't answer. I put the *Vogue* over my face so I won't have to see her, wondering what I must look like, lying here flat in a faded robe, my fragile limbs sticking out like a grasshopper's, my skin a dry grayish white, netted with veins, my fingertips and nails blueberry-hued, the crook of each arm a purplish mess dotted with bloody pinpricks, and on top of this all, superimposed over my face, the vivid face of the *Vogue* cover, each eyelash alert, each tooth a dazzling, clunky tile like a Chiclet, the skin a sealed and poreless stretch of pink, and the ripe, shiny lips curved into a radiant smirk.

39

But Didn't You Have the Tests?

JOANNA RICHARDS

Three years ago, at the age of 40, I gave birth to my second daughter, Saskia. I had refused pre-natal testing, basing my decision more on the feeling that I would not wish to terminate the pregnancy whatever the findings, than on any very detailed consideration of the various implications and options. And had Saskia been a "normal" baby, I would probably have given little further thought to that decision. In the event, however, the fact that our little girl has Down's Syndrome, further complicated by brain damage following heart surgery, means that we live with the ongoing consequences, trying to balance meeting her very complex needs with maintaining an ordinary family life. Generally, my interest, concern, and effort are concentrated on the here and now, with increasing thought and planning for the future; the past has considerably less relevance. Nevertheless, there is a sense in which I feel it is important for me to look back and revisit the decision I made prior to her birth in order to clarify how I now view my own position within the wider context of the debate on the prevention of disability.

If we take as our starting point Harris's (1993) definition of disability as a physical or mental condition which we have a strong ra-

tional preference not to be in, a condition which is in some sense a "harmed condition," literally "disabling," then surely it is only right that we should try to prevent it wherever possible. And, indeed, there seems to be nothing very controversial nor ethically problematic about many interventions which are aimed, directly or indirectly, at preventing the onset of disabling conditions (for example, road safety and accident-prevention campaigns).

However, when we switch our attention to congenital, lifelong forms of disability, referred to as that "great evil" by Wynn and Wynn (1979), the question suddenly takes on a greater complexity. Why is this? What exactly is it about the prevention of disabling conditions at the outset of life which raises complex ethical issues? For, in the same way that none of us would wish to become disabled ourselves, so, surely, none of us would wish to give birth to a child with a disability.

In addressing these questions, Harris (1993) and Parfit (1976) adopt quite similar lines of argument. Harris asks the question whether there is anything morally wrong in the desire to have a "fine baby girl or boy," and to hope that one's baby will not be born disabled. Turning the question around, what would we think of someone who actually wished that their child would be born with a disability?

Accepting this as a starting point, we can then move on to ask what is our view of someone (like myself) who, while hoping for a "normal" healthy baby, decides not to take all the necessary steps to ensure this outcome, even though the option of doing so is freely available to them? On the face of it, such a stance may well seem "utterly incomprehensible" (Purdy, 1995).

Parfit (1976) gives the example of a woman planning to stop taking the contraceptive pill because she wants to have a child. The doctor warns her that, because of a temporary medical condition, any child she conceives now will have a disability. But if she waits three months, the condition will resolve itself and a child conceived after that time will be unaffected. Would we not all agree that she should wait the three months before becoming pregnant?

And we can think of other similar hypothetical situations, where, for example, the advice might be to adopt a certain diet, or to take a course of tablets for a period of time before becoming pregnant, in order to prevent disability in the fetus. Again, would we not agree that the woman should follow the regime advised to her?

Harris (1993) includes an example from IVF treatment to illustrate the point further, asking whether a doctor would be right to choose embryos randomly for implantation if he knew that some embryos had defects and some did not. Given that knowledge, would it be morally defensible to implant embryos with disabilities?

The answers to these questions might seem very obvious, but the responses are, in fact, dependent on our accepting not only that disability is an undesirable state, but also that the course of action on offer to ensure that a baby is not born with a disability is a morally acceptable one. And it is this last point that is at the heart of the current controversy concerning the prevention of congenital disability. For, while the examples outlined above are clearly of relevance to the debate, they do not accurately reflect the circumstances of the majority of prospective mothers in the UK. The actual course of action which medical science currently has to offer consists of prenatal diagnosis of a disabling condition in the fetus, followed by termination of the pregnancy.

This interpretation of the term "prevention" certainly feels very different in essence from the kind of prevention which seemed quite unproblematic in the context of acquired disability or pre-conception counseling. Applying a model of prevention well known within the field of healthcare, the latter are examples of primary prevention, where the target groups consist of well persons, and the aim is to prevent the onset of problems. By contrast, the kind of intervention which involves screening for a detectable disorder is an example of secondary prevention, where the aim is to treat promptly to prevent the condition worsening.

Considerable confusion and distress can be caused if misleading or incomplete information is given to prospective parents about antenatal screening. "Prevention" to a lay person is generally understood in the sense of primary prevention. Some women do not fully understand that prenatal tests will not, as some doctors may ambiguously suggest, "prevent" the baby being affected (Birke et al., 1990). The prevention of congenital disability, in the form it currently takes, is an example of secondary prevention: prenatal diagnosis of a disability already evident in the fetus followed by termination of the pregnancy. Termination classed as a form of treatment may sound wrong, but that is exactly what the term "therapeutic abortion" means.

The ethics of prenatal diagnosis has stimulated a great deal of debate, a debate which, inevitably, has close links with the ongoing abortion debate. At either end of the spectrum of opinion, the two issues overlap completely: at one extreme are those who believe that abortion should be available on demand in any circumstances, while at the other are those who believe that every fetus has an absolute right to life and who effectively judge any termination of pregnancy to be indistinguishable from murder. In the middle ground, views on abortion are anything but fixed, decisions being influenced much more by the context within which they take place than by any single factor (Rothman, 1988).

The number of terminations of pregnancy carried out following prenatal diagnosis actually constitutes only a very small proportion of the total number of abortions performed, a fact that has prompted some people to question whether it is really an area worthy of any concern or interest; if up to 200,000 terminations of pregnancy are performed each year in the UK, largely for social reasons, why should anyone worry if a few more are being added to the statistics, particularly if the justification for doing them seems so sound to most people?

Yet there is a crucial sense in which this small minority of abortion cases do raise especially complex and specific ethical problems. What is particularly significant is that the entire context in which termination of pregnancy takes place shifts when the reason is because a fetal abnormality has been detected. In the vast majority of abortion decisions, the woman chooses to have an abortion because she does not wish to be pregnant at that particular time; it is not a question of any characteristic of the particular fetus which she has conceived, but rather the fact that she does not want any baby at all.

In the context of prenatal diagnosis, by contrast, the pregnancy is in all likelihood a welcome occurrence, and the baby wanted, maybe even longed for. The only reason for deciding to have the pregnancy terminated is specifically to avoid giving birth to that particular fetus, because he or she would be born with a congenital defect, would become a person with a disability.

So it is the particular condition of the fetus and the future for the child that are seen as central to the decision whether or not to continue the pregnancy. And the legal position in the UK is that if there is "substantial risk" that the child will be "seriously handicapped," the law permits termination of pregnancy at any time up to birth.

But just how serious does the fetal condition have to be before abortion is justified on these grounds? Is it the particular characteristics, or the probable extent, of the future child's anticipated disability that is the deciding factor? In my case, supposing I had opted to go down the prenatal diagnosis route, is it really acceptable that I might have decided not to abort on grounds of Down's Syndrome alone, but that I could subsequently have reversed that decision had my child's major heart defect been detected on ultrasound scan?

It may well be that terminating the pregnancy is seen to be in the best interests of the fetus, with the aim of preventing future pain and suffering;

many, including Harris (1991), defend this view. It may be that the anticipated quality of life for the future child is judged to be unacceptably low. Although many of us might feel instinctively that this is a valid and humane consideration, certainly in extreme cases, the subjective nature of quality of life judgments makes it very difficult to come up with any firm criteria. Someone who has profound intellectual and multiple disabilities, such as my daughter has, is functioning at a level which doubtless seems unacceptably low to many people. Yet those of us who are close to Saskia take a very different view, knowing subjectively that she has a good quality of life. It is a life with very obvious limitations, but that does not mean that it is a life with no value. Were it possible to elicit Saskia's own view, I find it hard to believe that she would opt for no life rather than the life she has. For that would have been the only alternative.

We are told that one of the leading aims of the new reproductive technologies is to provide people with more information and, consequently, with greater choice. But, in reality, how open are these choices? Is there not a real danger that refusing antenatal screening for fetal defects, or refusing to terminate a pregnancy where the fetus is known to be affected, may be judged less and less acceptable as valid choices in our society?

What is undoubtedly true is that the existence of a disabling condition in the fetus is already widely accepted by the majority of the population as justifying termination of pregnancy, even among those who say they are against abortion in other contexts. How can this be? Are we to suppose, for example, that the "responsibility objection" (Boonin-Vail, 1997) to abortion no longer applies if the fetus is found to have a disabling condition? Certainly, the prevailing view would seem to suggest exactly that, to the extent that the interpretation of "responsibility" switches from meaning a responsibility towards the fetus which is contravened by abortion, to a very different sense of "responsibility" which actually demands termination of the pregnancy.

After Saskia was born, several people asked me: "But didn't you have the tests?" Somehow, the implicit judgment within that question did not fully strike me at the time. Looking back, however, I am acutely aware of just how value-laden a question it is, translating only too easily into: "You should have had the tests and terminated the pregnancy. I judge that you were wrong to have given birth to this baby."

Writing this chapter has helped me to look afresh at a very significant decision which I made without great deliberation, and whose true import has only really become apparent in the light of its consequences. The crucial question which remains for me to answer is whether, with the benefit of hindsight, and having spent time considering some of the key ethical issues surrounding prenatal diagnosis, I would make the same decision again. My response is unequivocal: I would still refuse to have the tests.

REFERENCES

Birke, L., Hemmelweit, S., and Vines, G. (1990) *Tomorrow's Child: Reproductive Technologies in the 90s* (London: Virago Press).

Boonin-Vail, D. (1997) A defense of "A defense of abortion": On the responsibility objection to Thomson's argument. *Ethics* 107: 286–313.

Harris, J. (1991) Ethical aspects of prenatal diagnosis. In J. O'Drife and D. Donnai (eds.), *Antenatal Diagnosis of Fetal Abnormalities* (London: Springer-Verlag).

Harris, J. (1993) Is gene therapy a form of eugenics? *Bioethics* 7/2, 3: 178–85.

Parfit, D. (1976) Rights, interests and possible people. In S. Gorovitz et al. (eds.), *Moral Problems in Medicine* (New Jersey: Prentice-Hall).

Purdy, L. (1995) Loving future people. In J. Callahan (ed.), *Reproduction, Ethics and the Law* (Indianapolis: Indiana University Press).

Rothman, B. (1988) *The Tentative Pregnancy: Prenatal Diagnosis and the Future of Motherhood* (London: Pandora Press).

Wynn, M. and Wynn, A. (1979) *Prevention of Handicap and the Health of Women* (London: Routledge and Kegan Paul).

40

Capable People: Empowering the Patient in the Assessment of Capacity

DERMOT FEENAN

Introduction

Medical writing on assessment of a patient's mental capacity, or competency, to make decisions about treatment tends to uncritically adopt an approach in which the doctor controls the timing and method of assessment. Such an approach has three main implications. First, it precludes or inhibits the patient's power regarding his or her mental status. Secondly, it affects his or her decision-making capacity in respect of health care generally. Thirdly, it reinforces the unequal, but alterable, power relationship between doctor and patient.

[. . .]

A fresh approach is required. The concept of empowerment is attractive. It represents an effective means by which to complement the benefit to patients afforded through the principle of self-determination and associated facets of the various meanings of autonomy. [. . .]

Patient Empowerment

Generally, the term and practice of empowerment exists across a range of fields, principally mental health advocacy,[1] and within distinct organisations, particularly nursing[2] and social work.[3] However, its usages within these fields and organisations reveals a term whose purposes and applications are invariably problematic and sometimes contradictory.[4] Servian, for instance, proposes that empowerment occurs where individuals are able to follow their own interests, to feel fulfilment or to meet their own material needs.[5] This appears to be insufficient. Such a definition might equally connote liberty or freedom – quite different concepts to empowerment. Moreover, controversy surrounds the issue of who would empower. Some nursing literature, for example, uncritically assumes that nurses can empower the patient.[6] This claim is advanced despite substantial sociological literature on the different roles of nurse and patient, and in particular, the professional and institutional constraints experienced by nurses in their relationship with their patients. Such a claim by nurses also assumes that empowerment is appropriately effected by health care providers. Many patients, consumers or clients within the health care sector challenge the idea of professional control over the process of empowerment.

Empowerment: Theoretical Starting Points

The term 'empowerment' is adopted in this [chapter] as a response to the unequal power relations in society generally, with particular reference in the present context to the disequilibrium of power between medicine (understood as medical knowledge and professional practice) and health care patients, clients or consumers. It draws from wider sociological attempts to understand professional occupations in terms of their power relations in society[7] and in terms of authority to construct modes of medical knowledge.[8] This theoretical approach would be open to seeing individuals as having some ability to apply power rather than to see individuals in health care encounters, as Lukes[9] and Foucault[10] might suggest, as necessarily victims of other people's power.[5]

Empowerment and Capacity

My focus on capacity is an attempt to isolate one of the events in doctor–patient relations where power issues are at stake. In this context empowerment starts from acknowledging power relations, honouring a patient's actual and/or potential power in decision-making, and respects a patient's exercise of greater control over the process of assessment. Control here does not mean domination. Rather, it conveys effective involvement and authority in communication and decision-making. Control is not necessarily equivalent to an autonomous decision to consent to or refuse medical treatment. It is embedded in a process rather than an isolated event. It may serve as a vehicle by which an autonomous decision on a proposed treatment or series of treatments is achieved. It can be viewed, to paraphrase from the psychological literature on self-control:

> as a process through which an individual becomes the principal agent in guiding, directing, and regulating those features of his [sic] own behavior that might eventually lead to desired positive consequences.[11]

Roberts et al. treat powerlessness in the health care encounter as an absence of control. In their study of the effects on a small sample of patients of negotiated and non-negotiated nurse–patient interactions, they found that subjects in the negotiated group expressed greater perceptions of control over decisions occurring within the interaction than did subjects engaged in a non-negotiated approach. The feeling of control was a function of the interactive approach with the caregiver, and not based on subject personality alone. While the study did not show that the perception of empowerment affected agreement with treatment, the authors suggest that studies may show that nurses could, by increasing patients' responsibility for and involvement in their treatment, be instrumental in improving patient compliance and satisfaction.[12] Empowerment would seek to address the complexity of psychological factors implicated in decision-making which arise from, and could be remedied through, the dynamics of power. For instance, learned helplessness theory casts light on the inhibition of human action through historical explanation of lack of control and negative consequences following attempts to gain control.[13] As Servian points out, this may be relevant to empowerment when: '[c]arers and users in many cases may feel stigmatised by historically unresponsive and uncontrollable services'.[5]

This may affect patients' requests for support and their decision-making ability generally. An empowerment approach would seek to respond to the patient's sense of powerlessness by addressing these psychological (as well as structural) inhibitors. Conventional doctrine on self-determination and patient autonomy tends not to do so, though in fairness it should be added that modern conceptions of self-determination and respect for autonomy in medical ethics generally did not attempt to do more than secure limited, though laudable, objectives for patient decision-making.[14]

Empowerment and Action Theory

This awareness of the complexity of decision-making reflects recent developments in action

theory. While different meanings are attached
to action theory, a common denominator reveals
an aim to analyse human action broadly, in
response to the historically narrow approaches
of philosophers, jurists and psychologists, particularly behaviourists.[15,16,17] It incorporates
examination of volition, intention, goals, means,
potential consciousness and responsibility;[18]
informed, though not necessarily jointly, by
sociological, psychological[19] and philosophical[20]
perspectives. In addition to its sensibility to
complexity, it is relevant to the present discussion because some of its proponents explicitly
acknowledge the importance of addressing the
issue of power in decision-making both at an
individual level[21] and in terms of social action.[22]

Empowerment also goes beyond the atomistic
individualism of self-determination and patient
autonomy by recognising the need for individuals to have access to resources, including affective support, needed to effect their own control.[23]
Internally, the patient experiencing disrupted
capacity may need to adjust and find a new, or
re-establish a familiar, centre from which to make
clear, autonomous choices. Externally, the patient may need to control influences on capacity.
For instance, Alderson observes in the context of
children – a group traditionally assumed to be
incompetent – that some facing surgery used
patient-controlled analgesia pumps or practised
their own hypnotherapy, which 'literally put the
child in charge'.[24] Old people, disillusioned with
conventional medicine and health care, have
achieved improvements in self-care decision-
making through empowering initiatives such as
peer health counselling, advocacy and support
groups for Alzheimer's sufferers.[25]

Crucially, however, the aim of empowerment
is mediated by the need to respect each patient's
well-being and long-term autonomy. At least
from the perspective of allegiance to professional
codes and avoidance of liability, the doctor who
intends to respect a patient's power in the lead up
to and process of ultimate assessment of capacity
regarding treatment would need to be satisfied
that the patient is mentally capable of doing so.
Empowerment, therefore, acts on and fosters
autonomy while also respecting patients' greater
control over the process of assessment.

[. . .]

Group and Social Empowerment

Much of the literature on empowerment emphasises empowerment at a number of social levels
of interaction and action. Athena McLean, while
noting the operation of empowerment at an individual level, also identifies three further levels:
(a) group – involving self-help and mutual aid;
(b) organisational – effecting change in the social
community; and, (c) consumer – securing
greater funding and promoting advocacy.[26]
Action at all these levels may help to effect patient empowerment in respect of capacity assessments. Consumer action, through, for example,
representative groups such as the National Association for Mental Health (MIND), can help in
altering the power relations between medical
professionals and patients by influencing legislation (as was the case with the Mental Health Act
1983 in England and Wales) and by promoting
the confidence of, and resources for, patients and
users of mental health services.

Group meetings may be a particularly useful
method for empowerment in institutional settings, such as residential homes, where lack of
extra-institutional stimulation, traditional ageist
attitudes, and a relative absence of independent
support from consumer organisations impedes
the actualisation of individual and collective
power. Ward and Mullender advance self-
directed group-work as a powerful facilitation
of empowerment.[27] They note that with
the focus on the individual the weight is too
strongly distributed in favour of individual
uniqueness and private troubles. They state
that a number of distinctive benefits follow
from self-directed group-work. Personal
troubles can be translated into common concerns. Group solidarity engenders strength and
dissolves previous apathy. A range of voices
offer, and foster, alternative explanations,
options for change and improvement. Self-
directed group-work can also lend itself to an
anti-oppressive style of working from which participants have an experiential base to challenge
oppressive practice. Rappaport, writing about
mental health, suggests that individually
oriented interventions may actually impede their
allegedly empowering mission in so far as their
limited expectations reduce the self-esteem of

individuals and increase their feelings of worth-lessness and despair.[28] He calls for a wider view of empowerment that is sensitive to the various contexts in which a person is found over time.

Group empowerment may be particularly important among social or cultural groups who experience their power with an emphasis on the collective rather than on the individual. Professional or institutional practices which effectively remove such peoples from their social network can disempower them, with resulting harmful effects on functioning and, in particular, on decision-making capacity. In the context of children's capacity, Alderson challenges the traditional Piagetian approach to cognitive development whose unconscious influence permeates much discussion about competency. She states:

> Competence is more than a skill, it is a way of relating and can be understood more clearly when each child's inner qualities are seen within a network of relationships and cultural influences.[24]

Alderson states that some of the one hundred and twenty 8–15-year-old hospital patients in her survey on capacity wanted to be the main decider, some wanted to share in decision-making, while others wanted their parents and doctors to make decisions for them.

Patient empowerment may be informed by methods of long-term enhancement of capacity. McLaughlin refers to the Jean Vanier-inspired L'Arche residences in which people with learning difficulties share their lives with others, with (mutual) advances in capacity.[29] McLaughlin notes that it often takes years for people with learning difficulties to overcome the accumulated toll of institutionalisation and over protection but that when it happens, they begin to engage once more in trial and error learning and make substantial gains in functioning ability and competence.

[. . .]

However, espousal of an apparently catch-all concept of empowerment which fails to account for disparities according to class, race, gender and education will privilege some patients over others, thus reinforcing social inequities. More-over, that assessment of capacity may be biased or impaired by culturally determined ideas of illness or intelligence and by communication difficulties between participants with different ethnic or cultural backgrounds[30] suggests the need for context-sensitive empowering strategies. For instance, group encounters among similarly affected individuals can raise consciousness about, and action in response to, such specific power issues in medicine.

Conclusion

Traditional medical writing on patients' capacity to make decisions reinforces the unequal power relation between doctors and patients. This is most clearly shown by medical control over the general process of assessment, particularly timing and location. When commentators discuss capacity within a context of normative principles, the main principles, namely self-determination, patient autonomy and well-being, do not address power at all, or, if they do, do so insufficiently.

Patients' interests in having greater control over the process of capacity assessment are substantial and pressing. A determination of incapacity can not only carry a social stigma and injury to self-esteem,[31] but may also leave an individual feeling angry and resentful,[32] particularly where he or she feels denied the opportunity to take responsibility and control in the process of assessment.

While amendment to principles of self-determination and patient autonomy and concepts such as self-help and enablement may go some way towards alleviating the problems surrounding self-actualisation, only the theory and practice of empowerment challenges and offers solutions to the power and control of the medical professional over decision-making. This is illustrated in the context of assessment of capacity by advocating that patients exercise greater control and responsibility over the timing, location and use of resources (material, emotional and social). Such power can be facilitated at a number of levels: individual, group, organisational and consumer. Some writers believe that empowerment must be taken and cannot be granted. Realistically, however, the success of any theory and practice of empowerment in medicine requires acceptance from medical professionals as much as patients, not least because courts tend to rely on medical opinion in adjudications about capacity.

REFERENCES

1 Rose, R. M. and Black, B. L. (1985) *Advocacy and Empowerment: Mental Health Care in the Community* (Boston: Routledge Kegan Paul).

2 Colman, R. (1993) Patient power. *Nursing Times* 89/47: 50.

3 Braye, S. and Preston-Shoot, M. (1995) *Empowering Practice in Social Care* (Buckingham: Open University Press).

4 Jack, E. (ed.) (1995) *Empowerment in Community Care* (London: Chapman Hall).

5 Servian, R. (1996) *Theorising Empowerment: Individual Power and Community Care* (Bristol: The Policy Press).

6 Conway, J., Williams, M., and Taylor, N. (1994) Quality, philosophy and Riehl's model of nursing. *British Journal of Nursing* 3: 1139–42.

7 Johnson, T. J. (1972) *Professions and Power* (London: Macmillan).

8 Friedson, E. (1970) *Profession of Medicine: A Study of the Sociology of Applied Knowledge* (Chicago: University of Chicago Press).

9 Lukes, S. (1974) *Power: A Radical View* (Basingstoke: Macmillan).

10 Foucault, M. (1980) *Power/Knowledge: Selected Interviews and other Writings 1972–1977*, ed. C. Gordon (Brighton: Harvester Press).

11 Goldfried, M. R. and Merbaum, M. (eds.) (1973) *Behavior Change Through Self-Control* (New York: Holt).

12 Roberts, S. J., Krouse, H. J., and Michaud, P. (1995) Negotiated and non-negotiated nurse–patient interactions. *Clinical Nursing Research* 4/1: 67–78.

13 Seligman, M. E. P. (1975) *Helplessness* (San Francisco: W. H. Freeman).

14 Hill, T. E., Jr. (1991) *Autonomy and Self-respect* (Cambridge: Cambridge University Press).

15 Eckensberger, L. H. and Meacham, J. A. (1984) The essentials of action theory: A framework for discussion. *Human Development* 27: 166–83.

16 Brand, M. and Walton, D. (1975) *Action Theory: Proceedings of the Winnipeg Conference on Human Action, Winnipeg, Manitoba, 1975* (Dordrecht/Boston: D. Reidel).

17 Linden, M. (1994) Therapeutic standards in psychopharmacology and medical decision-making. *Pharmacopsychiatry* 27 (supp): 41–5.

18 Aune, B. (1977) *Reason and Action* (Dordrecht: D. Reidel Publishing).

19 Harris, A. E. (1984) Action theory, language and the unconscious. *Human Development* 27: 196–204.

20 Care, N. S. and Landesman, C. (eds.) (1968) *Readings in the Theory of Action* (Bloomington: Indiana University Press).

21 Goldman, A. I. (1970) *A Theory of Human Action* (Princeton: Princeton University Press), p. 225.

22 Ewart, C. K. (1991) Social action theory for a public health psychology. *American Psychologist* 46: 931–46.

23 McWilliam, C. L., Brown, J. B., Carmichael, J. L., and Lehman, J. M. (1994) A new perspective on threatened autonomy in elderly persons: The disempowering process. *Social Science and Medicine* 38/2: 327–38.

24 Alderson, P. (1992) 'In the genes or in the stars?' Children's competence to consent. *Journal of Medical Ethics* 18: 119–24; p. 122.

25 Ivers, V. (1995) Practical projects for empowering people in health and social welfare. In Jack (1995), at note 4, above.

26 McLean, A. (1995) Empowerment and the psychiatric consumer/ex-patient movement in the United States: Contradictions, crisis and change. *Social Science and Medicine* 40/8: 1053–71.

27 Ward, D. and Mullender, A. (1991–2) Empowerment and oppression: An indissoluble pairing for contemporary social work. *Critical Social Policy* 11: 21–30.

28 Rappaport, J. (1987) Terms of empowerment/exemplars of prevention: Toward a theory for community psychology. *American Journal of Community Psychology* 15/2: 121, as cited in McLean (1995), at note 26, above.

29 McLaughlin, P. (1979) *Guardianship of the Person* (Toronto: Roeher).

30 Appelbaum, P. S. and Grisso, T. (1988) Assessing patients' capacities to consent to treatment. *New England Journal of Medicine* 319: 1635–71.

31 Ho, V. (1995). Marginal capacity: The dilemmas faced in assessment and declaration. *Canadian Medical Association Journal* 152/2: 259–63.

32 Pearce, J. (1994). Consent to treatment during childhood: The assessment of competence and the avoidance of conflict. *British Journal of Psychiatry* 165: 713–16.

41

Kelly

RAFAEL CAMPO

The patient is a twelve-year-old white female.
She's gravida zero, no STD's.
She'd never even had a pelvic. One
Month nausea and vomiting. No change
In bowel habits. No fever, chills, malaise.
Her school performance has been worsening.
She states that things at home are fine.
On physical exam, she cried but was
Cooperative. Her abdomen was soft,
With normal bowel sounds and question of
A suprapubic mass, which was non-tender.
Her pelvic was remarkable for scars
At six o'clock, no hymen visible,
Some uterine enlargement. Pregnancy
Tests positive times two. She says it was
Her dad. He's sitting in the waiting room.

Part VI

Negotiating a Treatment Plan

Introduction

Negotiating a treatment plan depends on "understanding the enemy," as Jenny Lewis reminds us at the beginning of this section. The nursing sister in Lewis's eponymous poem offers advice consonant with the themes of this volume: that disease management cannot proceed in a vacuum, without exploration of the patient's underpinning emotions, values, and experiences of loss. Lewis is urged to "let it all out": "my son, banished by family tradition / to prep school...the friend I'd like to be with / who is already father to another family." It might be queried, however, whether "letting it all out" and then being given "a pill – the first of many" – really represents genuine negotiation and interaction between the health professional and the patient.

Lewis's first-person account in verse is followed by what might at first appear to be an incongruously "clinical" article; but Veronica Thomas's chapter, "Patient-controlled analgesia," epitomizes the sort of issues about patient-centered, negotiated care, which, as Lewis's experience reminds us, is all too difficult to achieve in actual practice. Patient-controlled analgesia (PCA), through a syringe pump with a timing device, appears to allow the patient's own pain threshold, tolerance, and preferences greater sway in the difficult management of pain in sickle cell disease (SCD), the most common genetic disorder in the world. Loss of control is a major feature in sickle cell disease, where acute episodes are often unpredictable, and patients value the control that PCA allows them. Nevertheless, it is important to take account of some patients' adverse opinions: some, for example, feel that PCA "legitimizes the nurses' need to avoid us." Nor should it be assumed that all patients want to take an active part in their own pain management.

In sickle cell disease it is not only the clinical condition itself which is so intractable, but also the additional difficulties that arise from patients' and clinicians' expectations and attitudes. As Thomas writes, "The management of pain in this group of patients is problematic, with both patients' expectations about pain relief and staff's attitudes concerning the provision of that relief contributing to the inadequacy of the situation." In particular, there may be conflict between the "sick role" that patients are expected to assume and the more assertive attitude too often required to obtain adequate pain relief. A vicious spiral may develop in which patients inadvertently exaggerate the extent of pain in order to be listened to, confirming some clinicians' view that analgesia is not really clinically indicated. "It is understandable if SCD patients feel that they have to exaggerate their emotional reactions to pain, since the inadequate recognition and treatment of pain by healthcare professionals is influenced by a set of entrenched attitudes that warrants drastic action." Here the negotiation process has broken down, largely because healthcare professionals have not examined their attitudes toward SCD patients and toward their supposed risk of narcotic or analgesic dependency. Yet very few sickle cell patients are actually opiate-addicted. Thomas reminds us that the attitudes of some healthcare professionals might be swayed by the ethnic origin of SCD patients in the Afro-Caribbean, Asian, and Mediterranean communities. This may well be true, although, on the other hand, the hospice movement has long had to struggle with preconceived notions about supposed opiate dependence in dying people of all ethnic backgrounds (Dickenson et al., 2000; Gebhart et al., 1993).

We return to a first-person account in chapter 44, with the narrative by the feminist literary critic Sandra Gilbert of the death of her husband after a routine operation. As with many negligence actions, Gilbert and her children finally felt driven to bring a malpractice suit against the hospital in order to obtain any response to their request for further information. Her account reminds us of another sort of breakdown in negotiations to that detailed by Thomas, and of bereaved families' sense that some clinicians hide their unwillingness to be open behind terminology such as "adverse events." A particularly telling image from Gilbert's account is of waiting in the hospital lobby to see her husband after his operation, "when the elevator door slides open and the surgeon comes towards me, flanked by his resident and a strange woman carrying a packet labelled 'Bereavement Services'." No doubt the hospital thought it was demonstrating concern for patient-centered care by setting up this "Bereavement Services" unit, but it is hard to conceive of any more inadvertently callous way to inform the family of the patient's death.

Patient-centered research, rather than patient-centered care, is the focus of the next chapter: "Decisions, Decisions: How Do Parents View the Choice they Made About a Randomized Clinical Trial?" The authors, Claire Snowdon, Jo Garcia, and Diana Elbourne, discuss the difficult situation in which parents of critically ill neonates must decide not so much what is the best treatment option for their baby as whether they will leave that decision to randomization, in the hope that participation in a randomized clinical trial of an experimental treatment will be the overall best choice for their child. The study which they document concerns provision of oxygen to newborns with breathing difficulties; thus the ethical problems concerning consent were compounded by what had often been a long and exhausting labor for the mother, often ending in a Caesarean section. All the babies concerned were already on a ventilator, the conventional treatment, but were failing to make progress; against that reality, the experimental treatment (ECMO, Extra-Corporeal Membrane Oxygenation) was more invasive, although it might well have represented a last chance.

For most parents, the experimental treatment was the treatment of choice, to the extent that they sometimes felt that they would have been wronged by being placed in the non-treatment arm of the trial. "It was often inferred that simply by offering the trial the doctor must feel that it offered a better chance than the apparently failing conventional treatment. Almost all of the parents said that at the time they had felt that their baby would die without ECMO. The strength of feeling expressed on this subject was striking. It was presented in many of the interviews as something upon which the parents pinned their hopes, 'a lifeline,' and 'a ray of hope in a bleak situation'." Thus in giving consent many parents felt that they were actually giving consent to ECMO, not to being placed in a situation where there was an equal chance that the baby would or would not be given ECMO. Furthermore, "typically, parents described how once they agreed to the trial, they had to wait to find out whether or not their baby would be 'accepted' or 'rejected.' All babies who had got as far as randomization were in fact accepted on to the trial. Allocation to continue with the ventilator treatment was, however, presented or seen as being turned down for the trial." Given the assumption of equipoise in randomized clinical trials, and the difficulty of presenting what is often insufficient evidence from similar trials, how can researchers meaningfully negotiate with parents in such situations?

Issues about ethical issues in research on children are further explored in chapter 46, by Virginia Morrow and Martin Richards of the Centre for Family Research at the University of Cambridge. The dominant model of children in research calls attention to their vulnerability, but Morrow and Richards argue that this set of values is based on particular epistemological assumptions which blind us to children as subjects rather than objects, "as social actors in their own right." In particular, research has tended to focus on "problem children and children's problems"; "thus we have no baselines with which to compare the experiences of the vulnerable with the unexceptional." Ruling out clinical trials on children because they are seen as particularly vulnerable may protect them from harm and exploitation, but it also leaves them vulnerable in another sense: to inadequate medical knowledge about, for example, how pharmaceutical dosages for children differ from those for adults. Yet we must be sensitive to disparities in power and status between children and adults. Morrow and Richards borrow Allison James's model of the "social child" (James, 1995) to argue that children should be conceptualized as research subjects comparable with adults, but that research methods of communication should be tailored to children's particular skills, using drawings and stories, for example. Thus participatory research can be pursued, but in a way which "empowers" children.

In chapter 47 Priscilla Alderson and Chris Goodey continue the story of Philip and Lucy, this time exploring the kinds of information and choices offered to children and parents. Negotiating a "treatment" plan – assuming that emotional and behavioral disturbance can be encompassed under this model, which of course was questioned by Alderson and Goodey earlier – means deciding in the first instance whether the problems of disturbed young people are seen as medical, educational, or legal. In fact, young people like Philip and Lucy have little room for negotiation about which service treats them or about the wide differences between local services. The two young people represent very different ways of dealing with this disparity of power: whereas Philip expressed his consent or refusal of cooperation openly, supported by a father who attributed the problems to untrained staff rather than his son, Lucy's parents were unhappy with her special school but did not feel they could do anything to reinforce her wish to attend mainstream school. Lack of information and consultation is more widespread in education than in medicine, Alderson and Goodey assert, as is absence of specific "treatment" plans and aims. Yet decisions about children's education are presented by educational psychologists and child psychiatrists as quasi-medical "expert" decisions. On both sides there is a reluctance to confront the epistemological and value bases of decisions made in the name of the child's welfare.

Moving from power imbalances in treatment negotiation with children to those with adults, Paul Cain argues in chapter 48 that "partnership is not enough." Despite the popularity of the partnership model in conceptualizing professional–client relations, we need to think about whether the values embodied in that model are desirable for and accepted by all parties. Partnership conveys collaboration and equality, "doing with" rather than "doing to." "So the equality at issue is a moral equality," whatever the actual differences of status, knowledge, and investment between professional and client, and the model is implicitly rights-based. Cain explores alternative and overlapping models of the professional–client relationship, embodying different values: an authority relation (which is not the same as an authoritarian one), laying more stress on the virtues of the professional; a paternalistic power relationship, in which the patient's will is overridden for his or her "own good;" and a therapeutic relationship, which focuses on healing. All except the pure power relationship are compatible with partnership, but it is important to be sensitive to which model the different parties to the "partner" relationship really have in mind.

How patients actually experience nursing care, whether in a "partner" relationship or other model, is explored through ethnographic data by Stève Ersser in chapter 49, "Experiencing Care." Ersser focuses on four ways in which patients evaluate care: in terms of the nurse as a person, as an information provider, as a partner promoting patients' involvement in their own care, and as a physical and psychological therapeutic presence. Ersser's study echoes Cain's concern that a simplistic partner model may not adequately cover all these representations, and Thomas's reminder that not all patients want to be fully autonomous. As Ersser says, "enhancing patient control for therapeutic ends needs to be communicated and negotiated by the nurse. This practice must be adjusted according to the patient's prevailing needs and wishes, with control being relinquished and restored to the patient as appropriate."

In chapter 50 Thomas H. Murray and Stuart J. Youngner concentrate on negotiation not with actual patients, but with future organ donors and their families. While admitting the good intentions of American Medical Association (AMA) recommendations on mandated choice and presumed consent, the authors criticize the AMA's failure to consider the particularly sensitive value issues surrounding the deaths of desirable organ donors, who are likely to be young, healthy victims of sudden and catastrophic trauma. In particular, the AMA proposals are grounded in a notion of patient autonomy, which has little to say about what to do with a dead body. The "patient" is dead, and the "patient's" relatives must reconceive their own lives and redefine their relationship with their dying or dead daughter or son – but an ethics grounded in autonomy can offer little assistance in designing morally sensitive policies for organ donation. In the wake of the recent Alder Hey and Bristol scandals in the UK, revealing the extent to which bereaved families were shut out of the process as children's organs were "harvested" for research, Murray and Youngner's article has a wider, continuing import.

In chapter 51, "Rationing, Justice, and Ageism," the British academic lawyer John Keown considers the largely unconsidered values which underpin age discrimination in healthcare allocation. In many cases where treatment is withheld from elderly patients on the grounds of their age, there are no efficiency grounds for doing so. Clot-busting drugs, for example, actually save more lives proportionally in patients over the age of 70 than in younger patients; yet one study revealed that 40 percent of coronary care units refuse these drugs to older patients. On grounds of medical prognosis, it is wrong to assume that the elderly will not benefit from receiving treatment; but other, non-medical judgments also come into play, such as the assumption that the elderly have less to offer society because they will not live as long. (If apparently objective QALY measures are used, for example, the elderly will lose out, since they have fewer expected life-years remaining.) Using the vehicle of an imaginary courtroom confrontation between an elderly patient deprived of clot-busting drugs and counsel for the hospital, Keown produces an extensive cross-examination of the arguments for and against use of age as a device for rationing healthcare resources.

The effect of age on do-not-resuscitate (DNR) decisions is examined by Paul Cain in chapter 52, providing a specific analysis to bolster Keown's generic arguments. Many practitioners believe that age is a rightful reason for withholding cardio-pulmonary resuscitation (CPR). Cain argues that there is no clinical or moral reason to withhold CPR from older patients. Considering the argument put forward by John Harris that older people have had a "good innings" (Harris, 1985), Cain concludes that even within its own utilitarian framework, the argument fails to consider all possible utilities which might be served by offering older people treatment on an equal basis with younger people. Although younger people may contribute to more national wealth through employment, a society which patently sets no store by the lives of its older citizens will arguably produce lower overall welfare. Cain reviews studies which demonstrate that doctors also give more DNR orders to patients with AIDS or lung cancer than to those with cirrhosis, varices, or congestive heart failure, despite the fact that reviews of the literature show that all these conditions have similar prognoses. Once again, judgments about values are entering in where supposedly only clinical data play a part, and discrimination is replacing just allocation. The same, Cain argues, is true of failure to treat the elderly on the basis of age alone. If withholding resuscitation is to be justified, it is most likely to be on the basis of the patient's own wishes, but here care is called for in discussing a difficult and emotive topic.

We have primarily concentrated in Part VI on value understandings held by healthcare professionals, but negotiation over treatment plans is just as much informed by the understandings and value preferences of patients. In a study also cited by Paul Cain, presented here in chapter 53, Gwen M. Sayers, Irene Schofield, and Michael Aziz explore elderly patients' preferences regarding CPR. Existing studies had shown that widening participation of the elderly in making such decisions is desirable because "most [older people] desire CPR, most are not disturbed by the consultation, and many want to make their own decisions." Clinicians often tend to assume the opposite of all these findings, and so it is not surprising that there is poor correlation between clinicians' recommendations and patients' preferences. Sayers, Schofield, and Aziz examine the reasons behind patients' CPR preferences in an attempt to educate other physicians and bridge this gap. They find that patients who choose not to be resuscitated typically have quite explicit reasons, which they will offer unasked, such as "no, I'm old and tired of life." Patients who wanted resuscitation were less forthcoming and less definite in their reasons. Two patients out of nineteen had radically misunderstood the explanation, both giving consent because they believed that they were taking part in beneficial research. Four patients wanted CPR without understanding that the risks of the procedure were inconsistent with their other beliefs and risk preferences. Two patients had no recollection of the interview at all, and the majority of others failed to remember crucial information. This level of recall and understanding is depressingly consistent with that documented for other patients, and is not unique to the elderly (see e.g. Robinson and Merar, 1983). But it still raises profound difficulties for physicians committed to patient participation in making such important decisions as those involving cardiopulmonary resuscitation.

A similar approach to a different clinical issue, endoscopy without sedation, can be found in chapter 54, by Sam A. Solomon, Vijay K. Kajla, and Arup K. Banerjee. Since sedation increases the risk of complications following gastroscopy in elderly patients, it is important to ascertain these patients' own preferences and tolerance for undergoing the procedure without sedation, rather than simply assuming that sedation is required in the patient's best interests. In fact a similar percentage of sedated and unsedated patients described the procedure as mildly unpleasant, and the majority of unsedated patients did not want to be sedated for future examinations when the risks of complications were explained.

Patient preferences for non-conventional treatment in breast cancer are the focus of chapter 55, taken from the book *Fighting Spirit: The Stories of Women in the Bristol Breast Cancer Survey*. In September 1990 a paper was published in *The Lancet*, comparing treatment results for 334 women with breast cancer who had attended the Bristol Cancer Help Centre for complementary therapies, in addition to receiving conventional treatment, as against 461 women in a control group who received orthodox treatment alone. The report found that "the cancer was nearly three times as likely to threaten survival by spreading to other parts of the body in women attending the Bristol centre." Although it was later successfully challenged as methodologically flawed, this report received tremendous publicity and did great harm to the "fighting spirit" of women who had attended the Bristol center. The excerpts reproduced here illustrate the diversity of response to the report and its sequel: one from a doctor, Myles Harris, two from women who had attended the center – Vicki Harris and Heather Goodare.

The patient's voice is also expressed in the final chapter in this section, but in this case it is the voice of a user of mental health services, selected from an anthology of personal experiences of mental distress edited by Jim Read and Jill Reynolds for the Open University. "What We Want from Crisis Services," by Peter Campbell, begins from one minimum requirement, that care should increase the security of the person cared for. "People want more control, particularly more of their own control over crisis situations. Given that many of us are unlikely to be contemplating a future where we never have another mental health crisis, the fact that we gain confidence that further crises will not destroy us is of the greatest significance. Existing services, no matter how insensitive, do often offer that reassurance. From then onwards, the desire to increase our own control in our loss of control becomes central." Campbell ends by noting that his first crisis admission was not medical to him, but moral: "a moral event, a moral failure." His final sentence emphasizes the themes of this volume: "the crucial questions about mental health crisis services are to do not with locations and technologies but with understandings."

REFERENCES

Dickenson, D., Johnson, M., and Katz, J. T. S. (eds.) (2000) *Death, Dying and Bereavement* (London: Sage, 2nd edn).

Gebhart, G. F., Hammond, D. L., and Jensen, T. S. (eds.) (1993) *Proceedings of the 7th World Congress on Pain: Progress in Pain Research and Management* (Seattle: IASP Publications), vol. 2.

Harris, J. (1985) *The Value of Life* (London: Routledge).

James, A. (1995) Methodology of competence for a competent methodology? Paper presented at Children and Social Competence Conference, Guildford, Surrey, July.

Robinson, G. and Merar, A. (1983) Informed consent: recall by patients tested postoperatively. In S. Goroviz et al. (eds.), *Moral Problems in Medicine* (Englewood Cliffs, NJ: Prentice-Hall, 2nd edn).

READING GUIDE

A fuller account by Sandra Gilbert is available in her book *Wrongful Death* (New York: W. W. Norton and Co., 1996).

Some of the ethical difficulties arising from randomized clinical trials are presented in Michael Parker and Donna Dickenson, *The Cambridge Medical Ethics Workbook* (Cambridge: Cambridge University Press, 2001), ch. 4, "Medical research." The particular issues arising in relation to research on neonates and children are considered by the report of a working party on which one of the editors (DD) sat: British Medical Association, *Children's Consent to Medical Treatment*, ch. 7, "Sensitive or Controversial Procedures" (London: BMA, 2000). A collection of articles on these issues may be found in M. A. Grodin and L. H. Glantz (eds.), *Children as Research Subjects: Science: Ethics and Law* (Oxford and New York: Oxford University Press, 1994).

42

Understanding the Enemy
25th March, 1985

JENNY LEWIS

I struggle to the surface, burst into daylight,
as Sister asks – "Are you awake?" She sits
on my bed, then starts holding both my hands
and looking so serious, I know the enemy
can no longer be avoided. She says quietly –
"You should prepare for the worst."

Then "Cancer often follows loss. Have you
     lost
someone close to you recently? Or is there
something you feel you need but you can't have?"

I tell her about my son, banished by family tradition
to prep school; and about the friend I'd like to be
     with
who is already father to another family. I tell her
about the rage and frustration locked deep inside
     me –
a Pandora's Box waiting for someone to lift the lid.

Sister recommends I let it all out.
Then she gives me a pill – the first of many –
and leaves me to my thoughts.

43

Patient-controlled Analgesia: Advantages, Disadvantages, and Ethical Issues in the Management of Pain in Sickle Cell Disease

VERONICA THOMAS

The management of pain in sickle cell disease (SCD) is fraught with problems, and patient-controlled analgesia (PCA) is widely seen as a solution. In this chapter I describe how 10 patients with sickle cell disease perceived the benefits but also the disadvantages of PCA. The study highlights the extent to which patients' and professionals' perceptions of PCA may be at variance. I will start with a brief introduction to sickle cell disease and the use of PCA to control the painful crises which are its most common and disabling effect.

Sickle Cell Disease

Sickle cell disease is a term used to describe a group of blood disorders where an abnormal hemoglobin is inherited. There are several different genotypes. As a consequence of this abnormal hemoglobin, the subjects' red blood cells have a tendency to become distorted. The deformed cells then create blockages in the small blood vessels preventing the normal flow of blood, thus depriving the area of oxygen. Oxygen deprivation causes tissue damage associated with acute and extremely severe pain in the affected parts of the body, most commonly the arms, legs, joints, and back. Painful "crises," as they are called, are the most common manifestation of the condition and account for over 90 percent of hospital admissions (Brozovic et al., 1987). Other complications include severe abdominal pain and rapid enlargement of the spleen or liver, serious infections, delayed growth, priapism (spontaneous and prolonged and painful erections), painful hip or shoulder joints, and strokes.

SCD is thought to be the most common genetic disorder in the world and recent evaluation of data based on population modeling reveals that there are 9,000 sufferers in London alone. This figure is expected to increase to 12,500 by the year 2011 (Streetly et al., 1997). The disease primarily affects those of African origin as well as Asians, Mediterraneans, and people from the Middle East. The incidence of silent healthy carriers (i.e. people who carry the genes but do not have the disorder) as it occurs within the ethnic groupings are as follows:

- Black Caribbean: up to 1 in 10
- West Africans: up to 1 in 4–5 (Nigeria and Ghana)
- Asians: up to 1 in 20–30

The Nature of Sickle Cell Pain

Pain arising from serious injury or postoperatively is often considered less severe than sickle cell crisis pain. However, some appreciation of the nature and severity of painful episodes may be gained from African tribal names (Konotey-Ahulu, 1991), as shown in table 43.1. The average SCD patient will experience one or two severe crises per year and because of the severity of the pain, opioid analgesics are the mainstay of management of painful crises. Crises may be precipitated by such factors as infection, dehydration, exposure to extremes in temperature, physical exertion, and psychosocial stress; but in many cases the trigger mechanism is unknown.

On admission to hospital the treatment consists of three essential components: analgesia, hydration, and the identification and treatment of underlying infections (Midence and Elander, 1994). Most hospitals use either subcutaneous or intramuscular morphine, diamorphine, or pethidine for pain relief. However, PCA is being gradually introduced in many of the hospitals in London (this will be discussed below).

Problems of Pain Management

The management of pain in this group of patients is problematic, with both patients' ex-pectations about pain relief and staffs' attitudes concerning the provision of that relief contributing to the inadequacy of the situation (Weisman and Schecter, 1992). Ingrisano (1986) suggests that when patients with SCD enter the hospital in a painful crisis they are required to assume a sick role, whilst simultaneously obtaining adequate analgesia. The first is a dependent/passive role and the latter necessarily involves assertive behavior and an active role. Consequently, the pain behavior elicited frequently appears to be disproportionate to the disease process (Ingrisano, 1986; Waters, 1992) in the patient's attempt to convince the staff that the pain is real. It is understandable if SCD patients feel that they have to exaggerate their emotional reactions to pain, since the inadequate recognition and treatment of pain by healthcare professionals (Gil et al., 1989) is influenced by a set of entrenched attitudes that warrant drastic action.

Many doctors and nurses who have limited experience of managing SCD may become excessively concerned about narcotic use, and frustrated when attempting to manage painful crises (Weisman and Schecter, 1992; Waters, 1992). On the other hand, some healthcare professionals who see only a few patients with SCD may misinterpret a patient's pain behavior as "faking" or "drug-seeking." Evidence that nurses misinterpret pain behavior as "faking" or "drug-seeking" comes from a study by Alleyne and Thomas (1994). In this study, not only did the majority of patients sense that nurses doubted the authenticity of their pain status, they also stated that the nurses deliberately prolonged their suffering by extending the time taken to "check" and prepare the analgesic medication.

Healthcare professionals' fears about opiate dependence is largely based on a misconception, and yet it is a major obstacle to effective pain

Table 43.1 Meanings of African tribal names

Name	Tribal or ethnic language	English translation/meaning
Hemkom	Adangme tribe	Body-biting
Nuiduduii	Ewe tribe	Body-chewing
Chwechweechwei	GA tribe	Relentless and repetitive gnawng pain in bones and joints

control in SCD. In the USA Vichinsky et al. (1982) reported that out of 600 sickle cell patients there was no incidence of drug addiction or dependency; Brozovic et al. (1986) found 13 addicted and 7 drug-dependent cases among 101 sickle cell patients. Such conflicting evidence regarding drug-dependency and drug-addiction only serves to problematize the situation even more. Nevertheless, even the few drug-addicted or drug-dependent patients are entitled to treatment when they are in pain (Midence and Elander, 1994).

PCA in the management of sickle cell pain

Patient controlled analgesia (PCA) is delivered through a syringe pump controlled with a timing device. The patient activates the system by pressing a button. This causes a small dose of analgesic to be delivered directly into the blood. Simultaneously, the timing device is activated, insuring that another dose is not delivered until the first dose has had time to exert its full effect. This interval is usually between 10–15 minutes and is preprogramed before the therapy commences.

Clinicians in the USA have found PCA to be a successful analgesic method for controlling pain in children and adolescent SCD sufferers (Schechter et al., 1988). In the UK, its use among the SCD population has been introduced more slowly, but recently most of the London hospitals have begun to recognize its value in the management of painful crises. In the sense that the occurrence of the acute painful event is unpredictable, patients with SCD frequently experience feelings of helplessness and lack of control in their daily lives. This in turn can lead to depression, which exacerbates the pain (Thomas et al., 1998). It has been demonstrated within the context of acute surgical pain that increasing the patients' sense of control is beneficial in bringing about a decrease in the pain experience (Thomas et al., 1995). Therefore, methods such as PCA that increase personal control are very important. However, as I have argued elsewhere (Thomas and Rose, 1993; Thomas et al., 1995), control in the form of PCA should not be thrust upon individuals without determining their personal preference

and the appropriateness of its use in particular circumstances.

The Study

It was in order to determine patients' perceptions of the advantages and disadvantages of PCA in sickle cell disease that I carried out my recent study. I interviewed 10 patients in depth (7 females and 3 males) recruited from three large teaching hospitals in London. Patients were interviewed individually and were asked to give their views of the benefits and the drawbacks of PCA in the daily management of their pain.

The perceived benefits

All the patients highlighted the high degree of independence and the immediacy of treatment that is afforded with PCA. This is reflected in the following statement from one patient: "I like the fact that it is in my control and I don't have to ask the nurses for my pain killer." In addition to removing the dependence on hospital staff, the patients also recognized that PCA removed or reduced the potential for conflict or "the hassle factor" between patients and staff: "It's great not to be constantly asked 'are you sure you are due?' or to be told 'you have to wait'." The majority of patients stated that they felt more in control of their pain when compared to the conventional nurse administered injection method. They also liked the sense of privacy that is achieved with PCA's use.

The perceived disadvantages of PCA

Although PCA has been found to be associated with efficient pain control among other pain populations (Thomas et al., 1995), this benefit was not identified by these SCD patients. On the contrary, there was a general feeling that PCA was not always effective in controlling the pain, and this was identified as a disadvantage. The majority of patients were not able to provide an explanation for this inefficiency, but four patients suggested that it might be due to the small bolus dose (the dose of analgesics delivered on each demand). It appears that since the bolus dose is much smaller than they are used to getting with injections, there is a perception that this small PCA dose is "not getting on top of the pain." One patient stated: "I have to push the button a lot before I finally feel like the pain is easing." This may reflect the fact that the protocols for PCA prescriptions are usually based on post-operative pain-management strategies. The prescription may therefore not be sufficient for the severity of sickle pain, since sickle cell patients having had opioids all their life have a greater tolerance and require larger doses of opioid.

Another disadvantage identified is the fact that it increases the patients' isolation. This is graphically expressed by one patient who said: "PCA legitimizes the nurses' need to avoid us. I know that with injections, we get a lot of hassle but at least it means that they have to see us on a regular basis." In exploring this issue further, it appeared that no assessment of pain, respiration, and other vital signs are undertaken, and, therefore, opportunities for meaningful contact with nurses are rare. This point is highlighted by another patient, who stated that, "pain relief medication is the only care that we receive when we are in hospital; now that we have PCA we are totally self-sufficient."

Some patients didn't like the bulkiness of the PCA equipment because it increased their sense of invalidity, as they are unable to move around as freely as they would like. This was seen as a particular problem, since the ability to walk about the hospital and visit friends on other wards is important. For some, it is the only means of getting social support. Walking about is also an important "distraction technique," used to take the mind off the pain. Finally, a few patients felt that they just didn't like the idea of being dependent on a "machine."

Ethical Implications

It is clear that sickle cell patients value the degree of personal control and sense of privacy that is achieved with PCA. This is important because loss of control is a major feature of sickle cell disease and empowering the sickle patient with respect to his/her pain reduces helplessness. However, this has to be set against the disadvantages identified.

The first of these was lack of effectiveness. Although this sounds like a purely technical problem, it could be related to an important aspect of autonomy, i.e. the provision of information. The patients in my study had been informed of the advantages of PCA but not its disadvantages. As McCaffrey and Beebe (1989) put it, where pain control is concerned the patient is autonomous when he or she "can decide the duration and intensity of pain he is to tolerate, he is informed of all possible methods or can choose which method he wishes to try, and can choose to live with or without pain." According to Whedon and Ferrell (1991), patients' autonomy is threatened when they are in a climate of advanced healthcare technology and poor levels of information. This was precisely the situation of the patients in my study group. Hence they were disempowered rather than empowered; and hence more, rather than less, vulnerable to their pain.

A second aspect of empowerment is whether patients are actually given a choice at all in selecting PCA. As I have argued elsewhere (Thomas and Rose, 1993; Thomas et al., 1995), there is a widespread tendency to presuppose that all patients want to become active participants in their pain management. But the efficient use of PCA requires careful patient selection that takes account of the patient's wish to be an active participant. This seems especially pertinent when caring for a disempowered group such as SCD adult patients, who, due to repeated hospitalizations for pain management, may have learnt to be dependent on the hospital system and staff. To thrust PCA onto SCD patients without any negotiation or any degree of choice is to force them to become independent – this is a breach of patients' rights. There are occasions when patients do not want autonomy and will look to the physician to decide.

A third concern raised by my study was the failure to monitor side effects. Patient-controlled devices deliver opioid analgesics that are known to cause sedation and respiratory depression. Thus, in my view, PCA is only safe if patients are monitored very frequently in order to detect side effects early and to prevent morbidity. However, it is clear from the discussion of the patients' views above, and from my own observation of the clinical setting, that SCD patients using PCA do not have their vital signs monitored, nor do they have regular pain assessments. Without such assessments, nurses cannot know whether PCA is causing any unpleasant side effects such as nausea or pruritis and do not, therefore, instigate corrective treatment. They are also not in a position to allay patients' fears and offer reassurance. Nurses, however, may not consider these omissions to be violations of patients' rights and ethics, since research has shown that they perceive pain relief to be the only care that is required by SCD patients (Alleyne and Thomas, 1994; Waters and Thomas, 1995). PCA, as a technological sinecure, is thus seen as abrogating them of all their wider responsibility of care. Yet, as my study showed, it is the side effects as much as pain relief itself that are important to the patients concerned.

If there was a gap between nurse and patient in their perceptions of the importance of side effects, there was an even more serious gap in the perceptions of pain relief itself. PCA was perceived by the patients in my study to be inefficient in controlling pain. As noted earlier, this was probably due to the fact that the prescriptions were inadequate for their pain requirements. However, since PCA is viewed by nursing and medical staff as a "wonder machine that controls all pain," complaints of pain from SCD patients can be taken as confirmation that their pain is not genuine, and that sickle cell patients use opioids for "other reasons." Although none of the patients in my study experienced this directly, many did feel alienated and angry at the lack of effectiveness of their treatment, and the apparent indifference or at least lack of understanding of staff. The degree of isolation and alienation experienced by SCD patients when using PCA is particularly worrying in the light of recent research evidence which has identified high levels of anxiety and depression in patients with SCD (Thomas et al., 1998). The desperate need to avoid the sense of alienation is reflected in a comment made by the patient who considered the "hassle" of confrontation with disbelieving nurses to be better than being condemned to the isolation associated with PCA.

Alienation also limits opportunities for communication. According to Somerville (1993), it is easy to detach ourselves from those with whom we cannot communicate or those whose status or position with which we do not identify. With respect to sickle cell pain management, we must also add color and culture to this list, and these disparities adversely affect the communication process. In disidentifying with people, we are guilty of an injustice by also depersonalizing them (Somerville, 1993) and sometimes we deliberately avoid communication with others in order to take advantage of this reaction. Sickle cell patients who took part in a different study (using a cognitive-behavioral approach to manage sickle cell pain, Thomas et al., 1998), and others with whom I have a therapeutic relationship, have told me that they are not treated as individuals by healthcare professionals, but, rather, like "animals" and without respect. If a person cannot identify with someone, then it becomes difficult to be empathetic. Certainly the majority of patients in Waters and Thomas's study (1995) estimated nurses' sympathy for their pain to be very low indeed. Furthermore, patients found that nurses rarely offered comfort measures or verbal support as means of providing relief.

Conclusion

I have argued that the patient participation which is achieved by PCA is generally regarded as valuable, with many psychological benefits. In the context of SCD, the autonomy achieved with PCA is therefore valuable for the management of pain, since one of the psychosocial consequences of the illness is a sense of helplessness. PCA is also advantageous because it removes confrontation between patient and staff.

However, it may also increase isolation and remove the opportunities for meaningful communication with SCD patients who already feel deprived because of huge deficits in the care they receive. It is especially important to be aware of these dangers with this form of treatment, since individuality is essential to the concept of patient participation, which is the very basis of PCA.

REFERENCES

Alleyne, J. and Thomas, V. J. (1994) The management of sickle cell crisis pain as experienced by patients and their carers. *Journal of Advanced Nursing* 19: 725–32.

Brozovic, M., Davies, S. C., and Brownell, A. I. (1987) Acute admissions of patients with sickle cell disease who live in Britain. *British Medical Journal* 294: 1206–8.

Ingrisano, C. (1986) Planning patient care for the adolescent. In A. L. Hurtig (ed.), *Sickle Cell Disease: Psychological & Psychosocial Issues* (Illinois: University of Illinois Press), pp. 84–149.

Konotey-Ahulu, F. I. D. (1991) *The Sickle Cell Disease Patient* (London: Macmillan Education Ltd).

Midence, K. and Elander, J. (1994) *Sickle Cell Disease: A Psychosocial Approach* (Oxford: Radcliffe Medical Press).

McCaffrey, M. and Beebe, A. (1989) *Pain: Clinical Manual for Nursing Practice* (Illinois: C. V. Mosby).

Schechter, N. L., Berrin, F. B., and Katz, S. M. (1988) The use of patient-controlled analgesia in adolescents with sickle cell pain crisis. *Journal of Pain and Symptom Management* 3: 1–5.

Somerville, M. A. (1993) Death of pain. In G. F. Gebhart, D. L. Hammond, and T. S. Jensen (eds.), *Proceedings of the 7th World Congress on Pain: Progress in Pain, Research & Management* (Seattle, WA: IASP Publications), vol. 2, pp. 41–58.

Streetly, A., Maxwell, K., and Mejia, A. (1997) Sickle cell disorders in Greater London: A needs assessment of screening and care services. The Fair Shares for London Report.

Thomas, V. J. and Rose, F. D. (1993) Patient-controlled analgesia: A new method for old. *Journal of Advanced Nursing* 18: 1719–26.

Thomas, V. J., Heath, M., Rose, F. D., and Flory, P. (1995) Psychological characteristics and the effectiveness of patient-controlled analgesia. *British Journal of Anaesthesia* 74: 271–6.

Thomas, V. N., Wilson-Barnett, J., and Goodhart, F. (1998) The role of cognitive-behavioural therapy in the management of pain in sickle cell disease. *Journal of Advanced Nursing* 27: 1002–9.

Vichinsky, E. P., Johnson, R., and Lubin, B. H. (1982) Multidisciplinary approach to pain management in sickle cell disease. *The American Journal of Pediatric Hematology/Oncology* 4: 328–33.

Waters, J. (1992) The nurse role in the management of sickle cell crisis pain. BSc undergraduate dissertation. King's College, London University.

Waters, J. and Thomas, V. J. (1995) Pain from sickle cell crisis. *Nursing Times* 91/16: 29–31.

Weisman, S. J. and Schechter, N. L. (1992) Acute pain: Mechanisms and management. In A. H. Hord, B. Ginsberg, and L. M. Preble (eds.), *Sickle Cell Anaemia Pain Management* (Missouri: Mosby Year Book, Inc.).

Whedon, M. and Ferrell, B. R. (1991) Professional and ethical considerations in the use of high-tech pain management. *Oncology Nursing Forum* 18: 1135–43.

44

Grief is Carved in Stone

SANDRA GILBERT

Elliot and I had been married a little more than 33 years and he was barely 60 when he went into surgery at the University of California, Davis, Medical Center on that ill-starred February 11. He had already survived two other problematic procedures at the same hospital, the first a bone biopsy that turned out to be unnecessary, the second an attempt at prostatectomy discontinued by the surgeon when the anaesthetists botched their effort at intubation. Despite these disturbing episodes, he had no reason to suppose his life was at risk when he ceremoniously waved goodbye to me as he was wheeled towards the operating room. Yes, he had prostate cancer, but it hadn't metastasised; otherwise, he was a robust man with no history of health problems.

When we saw him next, just 15 hours later, there was a sheet tucked up to his chin, his body was beginning to chill – to turn to granite – and it seemed to me that his mouth was curved into a rueful, slightly embarrassed smile. And for five and a half years I have carried that rueful granite smile around the world, part of the stone of my sorrow.

To be sure – and the very phrase "to be sure" is one I learned to use from Elliot – I've done what I could to speak for my husband, and

specifically to tell the story of the wrong and mystery of his death. In the hope of elucidating that mystery (since we knew we could never right the wrong) my children and I brought a lawsuit against the hospital where he died. And although admitting no wrong, the institution settled almost immediately after the surgeon in charge was deposed. With the further hope of helping readers understand the terrible gravity of the phrase "medical malpractice," I wrote *Wrongful Death*, about the two years during which my children and I struggled to overcome not only our grief but also the stony silence with which hospital officials responded to every request for information about my husband's last hours.

How did we manage to learn anything at all about what happened? And how and why did "what" happen? These are questions I try to answer, while also examining the complex legal, social, and medical questions surrounding what doctors sometimes call "adverse events" like the one that killed my husband.

My memories of certain episodes are ineradicable – obdurate scenarios that repeat themselves again and again. Eight hours after we have been told that Elliot's surgery went well, my daughters and I are waiting in the hospital lobby, hoping that we will finally be able to visit him in the intensive care unit, when the elevator door slides open and the surgeon comes towards me, flanked by his resident and a strange woman carrying a packet labelled "Bereavement Services".

"We've had a problem, a big problem," the doctor says. "Dad's had a heart attack" – then confesses, minutes later, that my husband is dead in the recovery room, just hours post-op.

The next day, sitting in a daze at my kitchen table, I read an official obituary issued by the university public relations office, saying that Elliot died of "heart failure", not a heart attack. Two weeks later, shaky and grim, my daughters and I steel ourselves to study an official death certificate, in which yet another hospital spokesman has declared that my husband died of "liver failure". And that night I write to the medical center, asking for my husband's records.

Ten days later, a bulky parcel arrives and we Xerox the stacks of notes it contains, puzzling over phrases that will later come to have dire meanings ("17:30. BP: 114/70. Pulse: 126. Observations/Treatments. Feeling 'Awful.' Look Pale.") then send the materials to a close friend who is a pathologist at the National Institutes of Health in Bethesda, Maryland. Within a month I overhear my longtime collaborator, Susan Gubar, discussing the "case" on the telephone with my friend the pathologist. "Hemato-what?" she asks, pen in hand. "Hemato-crit?"

"A hematocrit is a simple blood test that can reveal internal bleeding...Bleeding was the problem with Elliot." She scribbles in a notebook.

A few minutes later, I am weeping and cursing as she tells me what my friend in Bethesda learned from the records but no one at the hospital has ever revealed: my husband was given 12 units of blood before he died – a transfusion of more than half the blood in his body.

What went wrong to cause such massive bleeding that the accurate diagnosis of cause of death was neither "heart failure" nor "liver failure" but instead "acute posthemorrhagic anemia"? And how could experienced recovery room workers have failed to detect the bleeding? To this day, no representative of the medical

center has answered these questions. After *Wrongful Death* was published in 1995 and a story about the book appeared in the *Sacramento Bee* newspaper, an inquiry into the case was opened by the California State Medical Board, the agency responsible for medical accreditation throughout the state. An investigator for the board has already interviewed some of the nurses, doctors, and interns who were in the surgery suite when my husband died. But it is getting harder to locate witnesses, while those who can be found are forgetful – or recalcitrant.

If my grief is so stony, my memories so ineradicable, why should I still want an explanation? What possible difference could a full description of the "adverse event" itself make at this point? From legal, medical, psychological, and sociological studies of malpractice and its repercussions – and perhaps, more dramatically, from the many readers of *Wrongful Death* who wrote to share their own tormenting experiences with the mystification that often surrounds medical calamities like the one that befell us – I know that accountability is both morally and emotionally crucial. A British commentator has summarised this point concisely. Noting that accountability "has proved to be [of most importance] to victims" of medical negligence and their survivors, he observes that "from the victim's point of view [this] means simply that something is done to ensure that those responsible...are required to give [an explanation] and that steps are taken to try to avoid a similar accident happening again."

Still, neither explanation nor rectification – nor, for that matter, retribution – will raise the dead or shatter stony grief. A University of Florida sociologist who has written on the meaning of the death penalty said recently that although many victims' families demanded the "closure" supposedly offered by executions, there could never really be any such resolution. "I don't even know what the term 'closure' means," he said. "Someone kills your child – there is no closure."

Someone, somehow, killed my husband. And indeed, there is no closure.

Yet that there is no closure gives special urgency to the quest for knowledge, for justice, and even for change, change not just in medical procedures but also in social attitudes towards those victims of malpractice who find it necessary to take legal action – neither out of greed nor out of gullibility (towards ambulance-chasing lawyers) but out of a passion for accountability.

And I have learned, too, in these five and a half years that even if there is no closure there is a *modus vivendi* called "survival," a way of living through and with grief that seemed absolutely impossible to me for months, even years, after February 11, 1991.

To be sure, my husband and I are irrevocably imprisoned in the events of that date carved in the stone that marks his grave: he is trapped in the granite of his death, and everywhere I go the stone self of my sorrow shadows some part of me, like the "monumental statue set / In ever-lasting watch and moveless woe" that Elizabeth Barrett Browning depicts in her powerful sonnet on "Grief".

But in these years I've learned the secret that I suppose must be known to all who have deeply mourned. One can live in the presence of that stone companion as one might live in any other circumstance, not always gesturing toward it yet not ignoring it either. Most of the time it has the impervious facticity of a massif – but now and then it takes on the terrifying beauty of a muse.

45

Decisions, Decisions: How Do Parents View the Decision They Made About a Randomized Clinical Trial?

CLAIRE SNOWDON, JO GARCIA, AND DIANA ELBOURNE

Introduction

Randomized controlled trials (RCTs) are carried out where there is uncertainty over the best approach to treatment. Typically, they involve comparison of an experimental approach and standard care, placebo, or non-treatment. Participants are randomly allocated to a group for treatment, follow-up, and analysis. The use of randomization is based primarily upon the need to avoid biasing the results of the study. None of the parties involved has any control over allocation.

When patients are offered RCT participation, they face a potentially complicated and difficult decision. There are factors to be considered that fall outside the usual framework of care, and they are asked to suppress their expectations and to view treatment in a new light. In short, the ground-rules of care have changed. In ordinary circumstances, a clinician would recommend treatment options, which the patient could accept or reject. Trials are carried out precisely because the best treatment option is not clear and so, where a treatment is part of a trial, none of the options can be recommended

as the most efficacious or the least risky. With this background of uncertainty, prospective participants have to decide not only if the treatment groups are acceptable but also if they will leave the choice of treatment to chance.

We explored some of these issues in a study with parents of critically ill newborn babies. This chapter describes the various ways in which the parents viewed their decision to consent to a trial in stressful circumstances.

The Research Trial

The research trial that these parents were involved in concerned the best way to give oxygen to newborn babies with breathing difficulties. It compared conventional management on a ventilator with oxygenation of the babies' blood through a temporary artificial lung (an external circuit known as ECMO[1]). When babies were allocated to receive this new treatment, it usually involved transfer to one of five UK centers, sometimes by air-ambulance. The babies were all at high risk of death and were already placed on a ventilator when the trial was offered. In total, the trial involved 185 babies, born between January 1993 and November 1995 in more than 80 centers; 101 babies survived to one year, and 84 died.

Methods

The study involved only parents of surviving babies. Some interviews took place as the trial was ongoing. When the trial results were published, they were communicated to the parents involved in the trial, except for those who had indicated that they did not wish to see the findings, and those whose health professionals had requested that the results should not be sent. Further interviews with parents of surviving babies who had received the results were carried out.

The interviews followed a chronological structure in which parents were asked to describe the events and were asked for their opinions. They were tape-recorded and transcribed.[2]

The circumstances of consent

Research trials requiring decisions in the face of life-threatening illnesses are inevitably difficult. In trials involving newborn babies the decision is further complicated, not only by the need for a proxy decision from fearful parents, but also by physical and emotional exhaustion which can be felt after a possibly complicated delivery.

Some of the women involved in this study had undergone Caesarean sections (often as emergencies and with general anesthetics). Many women had used pain-relieving drugs during labor or post-operatively. Some babies deteriorated rapidly in a dramatic period where ventilator pressures were continually increased; others underwent a slow and persistent decline. Decisions about whether or not to become involved in the trial could not be delayed and could take place during the night. Two women were woken after taking sleeping drugs. Some fathers who had left the hospital were recalled to discuss the trial. In most cases, quite speedy decisions were required, as the health of the baby was so severely compromised.

An important feature of the trial was that babies were already receiving conventional ventilator treatment at the time the trial was proposed to their parents. By then they could be seen to have deteriorated and a baptism was sometimes offered. Parents commonly said that they were told or felt that nothing more could be done for their baby, so that for them the new experimental treatment, ECMO, represented a last chance for survival.

What we found

In our interviews with the parents, we asked them to look back on their decision. In this [chapter], we focus on their feelings about the treatments being randomized, i.e. about having to agree to the baby being given either a new or a conventional treatment essentially on the basis of a toss of a coin.

Attitudes to the Two Treatments

There was a small number of parents who reported that they had not been keen for their baby to have ECMO, which could seem invasive and frightening. Beverley[3] was set against it and was sure her daughter would die if transferred for this treatment. She was entered into the trial when Beverley's husband consented. Angela's fears revolved around the thought that it was an experimental treatment which conjured up very negative images for her. Once her son deteriorated further, she saw it as his last chance. Jim preferred to continue with conventional treatment, feeling concern over the invasive nature of ECMO. His wife, however, wanted their son to have the new treatment and he was prepared to accept this if allocated.

A further small group of parents spoke of being neutral, feeling either unsure about which treatment would be the best or taking on board the background of medical uncertainty to the trial. These parents often referred to fate or philosophically used the phrase "what will be will be."

It is important to note that the experimental treatment was undoubtedly the treatment of choice for the majority of parents. Some based this on technical aspects such as feeling that it would be easier than the ventilator for their baby. As ventilator pressures are increased, the likelihood of a pneumothorax, or air leak, also increased. This was sometimes characterized as "the lungs bursting" and could be very worrying. The new treatment was often seen as a way to avoid this. It was often inferred that simply by offering the trial the doctor must feel that it offered a better chance than the apparently failing conventional treatment. Almost all of the parents said that at the time they had felt that their baby would die without ECMO. The strength of feeling expressed on this subject was striking. It was presented in many of the interviews as something upon which the parents pinned their hopes, "a lifeline," and "a ray of hope in a bleak situation." Adam and Ellen, for example, were very clear about this:

Adam: I'm sure that anybody that . . . puts their child through to the trial . . . is wanting their child to go on ECMO 'cos otherwise if they didn't put them through to the trial they know that they're gonna be getting whatever other treatment there was. So by putting them through to the trial, you're really saying you want them to have ECMO.

Ellen: Yeah. Well we were.

ECMO as an Experimental Treatment

Although ECMO was a relatively new concept, and the long- and short-term effects were unclear, parents expressed very few concerns about its use. Certain aspects of the treatment could be worrying in themselves – the incision in the neck for cannulae, transportation, and heparinization – but very few parents said that the risks involved played a part in their decision-making. Mary was the only parent to say that the trial was important, as ECMO could in fact be shown to be hazardous. Fatima and Andrea stated their concerns about any unknown side effects:

Andrea: [W]hat if say in 20 or 30 years time something happens? . . . I don't mean that he just gets up and dies one day, but that he contracts some form of, I don't know, any-

thing, and then it is directly linked back to the fact that he did have ECMO. It's just sort of fears like that, but they're only fleeting, they are very very fleeting. I think it's when he's at his worst of an illness –

CS: How does that connect to the fact that it was research?

Andrea: Because you just don't know do you? OK, it's all very well that the States know[4] . . . but, I mean, do they really know? They must have had to start off trialing it somewhere and I mean, God, if they were babies who went on it then, then I mean they're not going to be full adults . . . so maybe nothing's popped up in the States yet. Or, maybe it has and they just don't want to let on, but it's just anything, like a new form of cancer or blood cancer or something like that, because he has had such invasive surgery on him at 23 hours old.

Some parents said that they had been told that there was a chance of cerebral palsy associated with ECMO. Paula said that this was not related to a detrimental effect of the treatment itself, but to the fact that more babies survived. Similarly, Neil argued that brain damage could be a result of complications at delivery and not ECMO.

In contrast, Tina was pleased that she wasn't aware of such a possibility at the time. With hindsight she felt that her son would have died without ECMO but at that time of considering the trial, she would have refused and continued with conventional treatment if she had felt there were associated risks. Andrea and another parent, Pascal, mentioned the irony of a baby's life being saved but the possibility of the brain being damaged by the formation of a blood clot. Andrea was the only parent to say that she would not have wanted efforts to be made to treat her son in such circumstances. The thought of a "brain-damaged baby" meant she almost backed out at the last moment:

They gave us a lot of pamphlets to read, and the only thing that sticks in my mind is that his blood could thin and go into his brain, and that was my sticking point, 'cos I thought, OK. So we're lucky enough to get him on this trial, and we're lucky enough that a bed's [available], then I sit in fear and trembling throughout his treatment on ECMO that his blood doesn't then run into his brain.

It might have been expected that more parents would have worried about participation in treatment in the context of research, effectively an experiment. In fact there seemed to be a redefinition of the situation in two ways. ECMO was either seen as an established, non-experimental, treatment or as an important new development. In the latter case it was precisely the newness, a feeling that it must be an improvement on existing care, which made ECMO so desirable.

An important factor which clearly affected parents' views of ECMO was the information that it was available in a number of countries, including America. Three small trials had been carried out in America, but the unconventional designs meant that the resulting data were not easy to interpret. Clinicians were faced with a difficult situation, as disclosure of this information could lead parents to feel that ECMO was a proven and effective treatment; withholding this information, however, meant that they were less well informed. To the parents who were told about the use of ECMO elsewhere, the trial often seemed simply a formality and the desirability of the treatment was increased. With this information Robert saw ECMO as established: "To my eyes it's not new. It's a success in the States. I just think they're being – I can understand, why go on someone's else country record? But, no, I didn't feel it was new."

Sandra presented ECMO as something that was informally known to be effective but which had not yet been officially proven. She said that although "the ECMO trial obviously hadn't been proven as working," ECMO offered the better chance of survival:

The reason they put Sam in the trial was because they didn't think the ventilator treatment . . . would work. They said that he would only have a 5 percent chance of living if he stayed, but if he went up to [the ECMO center] his chances of survival were more.

Technological developments can be exciting, and simply by being a new treatment ECMO was sometimes perceived as superior to what one parent referred to as "the old way." Several parents described ECMO as a miracle, and Graham referred to it as "this whizzo new cure." For parents such as Paula, the fact that it offered another means of treating their baby was sufficient to make the context of experimentation simply irrelevant:

We understood that it was an experimental thing . . . but I don't think it played any part in the way I made my mind up about whether he could be considered for ECMO. It was just incidental at the time. . . . We just saw it as an alternative treatment.

Attitudes to Randomization

The experience of deciding about trial participation is very much shaped by what is known or believed about the nature of the trial, what randomization is, and why it was being used. The beliefs parents expressed are described in detail elsewhere (Snowdon et al., 1997). In brief, most knew there was some doubt about access to ECMO but not necessarily why that was so and that the choice of treatment was left to chance. It was often seen as a decision based on clinical or practical grounds. Whilst most were aware that a computer was involved, others said that a doctor or the trial staff had said which treatment the baby would have. Although the word "randomization" appeared to be familiar to all of the interviewed parents, parents of a number of babies presented the treatment decision as non-random. Some said that at the time they felt they were simply offered and accepted ECMO with no suggestion of doubt over access. Randomization was said to be used for three types of reason: scientific, e.g. to find appropriate babies for the new treatment and to avoid bias in the trial; ethical, to remove responsibility from the doctors or the parents; and clinical, a means to decide between babies competing nationwide for a limited number of ECMO beds.

Parents were thus making two quite different decisions, depending on what they felt they were being asked to consider: a choice between two treatments or forgoing a choice of treatments.

Choosing Between Two Treatments

A widespread terminological difficulty which was evident in the interviews was the way in which the concept of the trial, commonly referred to as "the ECMO trial," and the ECMO treatment itself were used interchangeably. Both could be referred to simply as "ECMO" and some parents, in describing the treatment, referred to it as "the trial." Where the distinction between the two was not clear, parents asked to agree to the ECMO trial (which included the possibility of allocation to continue with the ventilator treatment) could feel that they were simply being asked to agree to the ECMO treatment. It is not surprising that some parents described how they went through a process of considering the two treatments and making their own choice.

Marie, whose partner had not been present at the time of delivery and decision-making, felt weighed down by the huge responsibility she felt was placed on her shoulders. She said she herself, rather than a doctor, had had to decide which treatment her son would have and worried that he might die if she chose the less effective treatment. A number of fathers felt ill-equipped to make a decision. Ian felt this was due to their own lack of medical knowledge and described their decision as "the worst thing we have ever had to do." Nick said that asking parents to make the decision was "passing the buck." Simon felt that they were inappropriately left to make a decision about treatment that doctors were not prepared to make themselves:

> To leave it to parents to make the decision . . . with their limited knowledge of medicine . . . it's not on really. I mean OK if they are going to do this there should be video evidence and stuff like that available to help them to make that decision. . . . What I'm really saying is you kind of put your faith

in the medical situation to help to the best of their ability but I don't think it is really helping to ask somebody else to make the decision for them. . . . If a consultant or a doctor cannot make a decision which is best it is very hard for ordinary folk on the street to be able to do it.

Typically, parents described how once they agreed to the trial, they had to wait to find out whether or not their baby would be "accepted" or "rejected." All babies who had got as far as randomization were in fact accepted on to the trial. Allocation to continue with the ventilator treatment was, however, presented, or seen as being, turned down for the trial.

The finality of the allocation was not always clear. Liz and Carl said they would have paid to have ECMO if their daughter had not been allocated to it. Frank said that had he known that the new treatment might have been better for his son he would have fought for him to have it. Adam and Russell, whose children were both allocated to receive the new treatment, both understood the basis of randomization but did not readily believe that it was used in their cases. As Adam's son was already at a hospital where ECMO was carried out, there would be no transfer and treatment could start at any time of day or night. It seemed simply illogical that he would not be treated: "I thought it wasn't going to be a 50:50 chance. It was gonna be 100 percent chance. . . . I thought because we were there that if we decided we were going to go for the trial, that meant we were going to have ECMO." In contrast, Gary was very aware of the inability to gain access to ECMO if his baby was not allocated to it and he saw the system as very unfair:

> They came back and said she had been randomized in and there's a bed available. Even if she had been randomized out that bed would still have been available, wouldn't it! I couldn't come to terms with that at all. Now by all means fill the beds up and if the babies come along that can't get into the beds then that is fine, but this randomization of having a bed and a team and not being able to get into the bed . . . well I just couldn't come

to terms with that, which is why I would question the ... system of randomization.

Whether or not parents agree to randomization does not seem to be part of these accounts of decision-making. Rather, it is a separate event in which the parents' own decision may be acceded or blocked.

Forgoing a Choice of Treatments

Randomization could complicate the decision-making process, confusing parents about their role. This may lie in part in the presentation of the parents being asked to make a decision and the presentation of a computer or "the trial" also making a decision. Alastair was not the only one to find this layering of "decisions" confusing:

> I remember it being very very difficult to grasp the idea that we had to make this decision first of all whether or not he should be considered ... for this trial and having made that decision, he might not get it anyway. You know it was very very difficult at that time to understand what you were actually deciding because even having thought you had made a decision, it wasn't clear cut, it still had to be decided randomly.

Ellen talked of her frustration at only being able to take the decision she had made so far: "It's a strange situation to be in because you're making decisions and you're not making decisions. Yeah, you're deciding to go forward to the trial but that means not having a decision. You're deciding to give up a decision in a way." In contrast, Lorna and Neil felt that the use of randomization removed from them any responsibility for a negative outcome and greatly eased their situation. They both described it as "the easy way out."

As consent to the trial was the only possible route to the new treatment, agreement to the trial does not necessarily indicate acceptance of randomization. Parents could consent to randomization, but hate the idea. Ultimately, they had to agree to randomization or lose the only chance of gaining access to ECMO. Where the inability to transfer from one treatment to another was appreciated, it seemed particularly harsh. That such an important and irreversible decision was left to a computer amazed some parents. Angela felt the lack of human feeling in the decision made it hard to accept. There were many negative comments about randomization, but statements that they had considered rejecting the trial were rare. Instead, there was often a sense of parents simply having no choice.

The Experience of Decision-making

The decision to join the trial was presented in very different ways in the interviews. It could be an obvious and clear choice, or agonizing and burdensome. In the former instance it was seen as either no choice – that is, there was nothing else that parents could do – or the choice was so obvious that there was no decision to be made; the alternative was to continue with a treatment viewed as ineffective. Parents often said they had nothing to lose by agreeing to the trial.

Even where parents were sure that they wanted their baby to have ECMO, it was not always easy to agree to the trial. The risk of transportation to another, possibly distant, hospital was worrying. The emotional costs of separation from the baby, especially for mothers who were in a different hospital for several days after surgery, should not be underestimated. This was the case for Sandra and Nigel who felt that ECMO offered their son a better chance of survival. Despite this view, their decision was complicated tremendously by the thought that he might die with neither parent present. They described a very stressful time as they smoked heavily and held on to each other in a private room, unable to decide what to do.

Although parents were given some information about the two treatments and the trial, it was often seen as insufficient to help them decide what to do. It was the absence of precisely the information that the trial aimed to collect, for instance whether or not a baby would be more likely to survive with the new treatment, that made decision-making difficult for parents. Tina felt the information given was insubstantial in the light of the seriousness of their situation:

> Right from the minute I'd said yes, I almost wanted to change my mind, right from that second because...it's just so difficult. I mean it's not a criticism of the doctors at all because they can't give you more information than they have but...you have to decide...almost whether he's going to live or die on the basis of 2 sheets of paper and that is hard for anybody.

A few parents had to make the decision completely on their own. Babies born in smaller hospitals were usually transferred to a hospital with appropriate facilities. In two cases mothers were not moved at the same time and their partners had to make a decision about the trial themselves. Marie decided about the trial on her own, as her husband could not be with her and Lesley was under such pressure of time that she had to decide before her husband could return to the hospital. Beverley felt unable to decide and left it to her partner.

In the absence of information, parents often said that they had asked doctors what they would do in their position. Some were given answers, others were not. As noted earlier, parents sometimes concluded that the doctor must approve of the new treatment to have suggested the trial at all. Russell pointed out in a questionnaire that parents had been asked to complete 4 months after the birth that he felt a need for professional assistance in decision-making:

> The first time ECMO was mentioned by a doctor I felt the subject was presented without sufficient information. The consultant was not on duty and I was desperate for guidance. When he came in he was able to give me more background on ECMO and although I really wanted someone to tell me what was the best likely treatment for Henry I can understand that this would be impossible in the circumstances....

> I think that it is right that a parent should be given some help in making a decision.

Discussion

The results of our study highlight a distinction between the position of those developing and implementing RCTS and those considering participation. This distinction may be crudely characterized as represented by the two worlds of public and private responsibility, which are inevitably brought together in the informed consent encounter. While there is clearly important central ground, that is, the aim to provide the best and most appropriate care for the patients concerned, the two broad perspectives can differ on the means by which this may be achieved.

In the public or medico-scientific world, randomization is largely considered to be a fair means of distributing the unevaluated risks and benefits of different treatments. This was, however, simply irrelevant to most parents, who were asked to consider randomization and treatment in a very personal and private context. Where the new treatment was not viewed as risky, then randomization made little sense other than as a form of rationing. It was hard for parents to see it as a form of risk-limitation when their baby appeared to be dying when treated with standard care. They often had clear preferences and needs which were simply not met by randomization. A comment made by Robert was echoed by several parents and is indicative of the frustration felt:

> Why are they playing around with babies' lives?...Who gives them the right to sit there with say ten babies and think well this one here will...suit the trial, you know. Why not all ten of them? Why isn't it available everywhere so everybody has a fair chance?

The primary reason for carrying out a trial is to establish whether a new approach is more beneficial or more risky than standard care. The justification for the trial is that there is a state of equipoise, that is, it is not clear which treatment is best. This idea was not taken up by many parents in the study. The majority did not talk of the lack of evidence to indicate which treatment would be the better for their baby. Instead, many had quite clear ideas about the treatment they wanted their baby to have. Without the benefit of information or guidance from the scientific and medical worlds, parents fell back on their own feelings about what would be best.

Given that the study did not include parents who turned down the trial, it is not surprising to find that there were few who objected to the idea of ECMO. It was not, however, predictable that there would be so few concerns about this treatment. It was generally not viewed as an experimental approach with possible risks but as a proven, beneficial treatment. Some parents concluded that in offering the possibility of ECMO as an alternative treatment, the doctor must feel that it confers some additional benefit. Similarly it was suggested that the trial was carried out exactly because it was hoped that the new treatment would be more efficacious. The most important factor which led parents to favor ECMO was that the babies had declined to a critical state and so faith in the type of treatment they were already receiving was undermined. The scientific and ethical concept of equipoise had little relevance as parents sought to work out what would provide the best chance for their baby.

Of course, the situation was not as clear cut as this brief report suggests. There were parents who approved the use of randomization and clinicians who, according to the parental accounts, openly stated that they felt the new treatment would be the best treatment for the baby. In the parents' accounts of professional responses to the situation, there was evidence that some clinicians also found this situation extremely difficult. Not surprisingly, the boundaries between public and private responsibility can be hazy for clinicians too. They are required to make a radical change in their practice and can be faced with parents sometimes explicitly asking for information and guidance, a situation where every move or gesture can be taken as an implied recommendation.

Conclusions

The message from this study is that a public perspective cannot be simply grafted on to the private. Even though parents were forced by circumstances into a public world of clinical trials which are aimed at developing strategies of care, their primary concern remained their private world, their personal need to try to establish the best care for their own baby. This is wholly appropriate behavior for parents but it is far from clear whether these public and private perspectives are reconcilable.

Postscript

Since this report was first written, we have engaged in further research in this area. Our current study involves a larger number of parents and health professionals associated with various trials. We are finding a wider range of views, which probably relates to the circumstances of some of the trials that we are examining. There is also, however, much common ground between the views of parents involved in the ECMO trial and those of parents in our present study. This is in spite of the fact that in the current research the trials the parents were offered did not involve such dramatic and hi-tech treatments as ECMO, and that the circumstances of consent are more varied. This is in keeping with other research in the area which has recently been reported (Mason and Allmark, 2000). What is common to all of the situations we have looked at is the fear that parents have that their baby may not survive. Communication in this setting is inevitably fraught with difficulties for both parents and professionals. The challenge facing professionals is to improve the quality of consent in this area whilst maintaining a humane approach to parents who may well be distressed by the information they are given.

NOTES

1 Extra Corporeal Membrane Oxygenation (for further details, see UK Collaborative Trial Group, 1996).
2 For details of the recruitment process, study structure, and analysis of the interviews, see Snowdon et al., 1997; Snowdon et al., 1998; Snowdon et al., 1999.
3 All names are pseudonyms.
4 Trials previously carried out in the USA had supported the use of neonatal ECMO, and parents were often told this by their doctor.

REFERENCES

Mason, S. A. and Allmark, P. J. (2000) Obtaining informed consent to neonatal controlled trials: Interviews with parents and clinicians in the Euricon study. *Lancet* 356: 2045–51.

Snowdon, C., Garcia, J., and Elbourne, D. R. (1997) Making sense of randomization: Responses of parents of critically ill babies to random allocation of treatment in a clinical trial. *Social Science and Medicine* 45/9: 1337–55.

Snowdon, C., Garcia, J., and Elbourne, D. R. (1998) Reactions of participants to the results of a randomized controlled trial: Exploratory study. *BMJ* 317/7150: 21–6.

Snowdon, C., Garcia, J., and Elbourne, D. R. (1999) Zelen randomization: Attitudes of parents participating in a neonatal clinical trial. *Controlled Clinical Trials* 20: 149–71.

UK Collaborative Trial Group (1996) UK collaborative randomized trial of neonatal extracorporeal membrane oxygenation. *Lancet* 348: 75–82.

46

The Ethics of Social Research With Children: An Overview

VIRGINIA MORROW and MARTIN RICHARDS

Introduction

Our original paper provided a detailed overview of ethical issues related to social research with children. It set the discussion in the context of current debates about researching children in the UK, and explored the extent to which children should be regarded as similar to, or different from, adults in social research. It focused on how children are positioned as vulnerable, incompetent, and relatively powerless in society in general, and how this conceptualisation of children needs to be taken into account in social research. The paper concluded with some practical and methodological suggestions.

Essentially, the dilemma that was explored is that in everyday social life, we (as adults, parents, or researchers) tend not to be respectful of children's views and opinions, and the challenge is to develop research strategies which are fair and respectful to the subjects of our research. The key to such strategies is a balanced view of the relevant differences between children and adults. It is this that was the focus of section 3 of the paper, which is reproduced here in full.

Children: Different or the Same? Vulnerability, Powerlessness and Incompetence

Arguments about ethics of social research with children can effectively be reduced to the question of the extent to which children are regarded as similar or different to adults, and these discussions in turn can be reduced to two related descriptive perceptions that adults hold of children, that is, children as vulnerable and children as incompetent. These conceptualisations are reinforced by notions of childhood as a period of powerlessness and irresponsibility.

Vulnerable children

There are some thorough discussions of the ethical dilemmas raised by medical and psychological research with children, in particular Nicholson (1986), and papers in two US volumes: Grodin and Glantz (1994) and Stanley and Sieber (1992). However, such discussions are dominated by a particular conceptualisation of children as vulnerable and consequently in need of protection from exploitative researchers, and as the *objects* rather than subjects of research. In other words, the methodological starting points for such discussions, and the epistemological assumptions about what children are, are based on a specific formulation of the category 'child', which we need to move away from if we are to attempt a *social* analysis of children's experiences, and in doing so are to see children as social actors in their own right.

A second, and related, consideration is that (not least for funding and social policy reasons) research with children in the UK has tended to be dominated by concerns about groups of children who are vulnerable in some way: 'problem children and children's problems' (Qvortrup, 1987). Again a specific conceptualisation of children appears to dominate, as weak, passive, and open to abuse. Research has tended to focus on children already damaged by their experiences and this inevitably raises ethical questions, which are not always adequately addressed. Rightly, these children are seen as in need of protection from further harm by exploitative researchers, or thoughtless researchers who may cause distress by asking children to describe upsetting or damaging experiences. But the consequence of this is that we know something about certain problematic groups of children and young people, and very little at all about 'ordinary' or 'normal' children and young people, and thus we have no baselines with which to compare the experiences of the vulnerable with the unexceptional.

Lansdown (1994) suggests that children are vulnerable in two respects: they are inherently vulnerable because of their physical weakness, and their lack of knowledge and experience, which renders them dependent upon the adults around them. Secondly, they are structurally vulnerable, 'because of their total lack of political and economic power and their lack of civil rights' (1994: 35) which derives from historical attitudes and presumptions about the nature of childhood. She emphasises that 'there is a tendency to rely too heavily on a presumption of children's biological and psychological vulnerability in developing our law, policy and practice, and insufficient focus on the extent to which their lack of civil status creates that vulnerability' (ibid). As she points out, we simply 'do not have a culture of listening to children'

(ibid: 38; see also Flekkoy, 1991). The consequence of this presents a dilemma for social researchers: in the UK, we simply are not used to talking to children to try to ascertain their views, opinions and so on. There are so few attempts to understand children's lives 'in their own terms', and taking children's own words at face value, and as the primary source of knowledge about their experiences, effectively goes against a tradition in sociology in which children's voices have rarely been heard and their opinions rarely sought (cf. Mauthner (1995) on women, and Butler and Williamson, 1994). The challenge for social research is to find ways of eliciting children's opinions and experiences, to develop appropriate methods, and corresponding strategies to deal with ethical dilemmas that may arise.

A further important point to note is that an overly protective stance towards children may have the effect of reducing children's potential to participate in research. As Grodin and Glantz suggest, research with children

> presents a powerful tension between two sometimes conflicting social goals: protecting individual children from harm and exploitation, while at the same time increasing our body of knowledge about children in order to develop beneficial medical, psychological, and social interventions (1994: vi).

The consequence of such an over-protective stance may well be that there are various aspects of children's lives that we simply know nothing about.

Finally, children's perceived vulnerability means that a further fundamental difference is that the obligations, duties and responsibilities that researchers have towards their subjects are qualitatively different when working with children and relate to adult responsibilities towards children in general. Thus, if a child discloses that he or she is at risk of harm, then the assumption is that the researcher has a duty to pass this information on to a professional who can protect the child/other children at risk (see NCB Guidelines). Researchers need to recognise their moral obligations as adults to protect children at risk even when this may mean losing access to, or the trust of, the children concerned if they do intervene.

On the other hand, children expect adults to behave in certain ways and by not intervening in certain situations, adult researchers may lose credibility (Boyden and Ennew, 1996). Depending on the context, nature of the disclosure, age of the child, relationship of child to researcher, perhaps the most helpful solution in such situations is for the researcher to discuss with the child what strategy they would like to pursue (e.g. Butler and Williamson, 1994); similarly, researchers who come across adults who may be at risk in some way are presumably also likely to find some strategy for supporting a vulnerable adult. However, there must always be a danger of the research drawing attention to problematic situations which the child did not perceive as a problem in the first place.

Incompetent children?

The second key perceived (and related) difference between children and adults in research is children's assumed lack of competence: competence to make decisions about whether to participate in research, and competence to provide valid sociological data. US researchers Fine and Sandstrom, for example, in a discussion of participant observation with children, seem to perceive children as profoundly different to adults when they suggest that 'Discovering what children "really" know may be *almost* as difficult as learning what our pet kitten really knows; we can't trust or quite understand the sounds they make' (1988: 47). (Of course, the same is true with adults, but to lump children and animals together makes it sound as if it is not worth trying.)

Mainstream developmental psychology often perceives children to be less competent than adults, and developmental psychologists sometimes impose methods and interpretation on data collected from children which may be quite out of line with what the children meant – rarely do they return to their research subjects to confirm (though see Gilligan et al., 1990). Conceptualising children as less competent in this way is unhelpful, and it is important to see it critically, because it has provided teachers and

parents (and sociologists) with powerful normative models for what children are (or should be) like. It reflects a cultural reluctance to take children's ideas seriously, which in itself is not surprising, given that – at the macro-social level at any rate – adults tend to trivialise and devalue children's acts as a matter of course. As Waksler suggests, 'Adults routinely set themselves up as the understanders, interpreters and translators of children's behaviour' (1991: 62). Rather, Waksler suggests, we would be better advised to see children's competencies as 'different' rather than lesser. Recent research on children as witnesses suggests that children can give reliable testimonies (Spencer and Flin, 1990; Fielding and Conroy, 1992), provided they are not asked leading questions, and so on. Recently too philosophers have begun to criticise theories of developmental psychology for allowing no real place for philosophical thinking among young children (see Matthews, 1994; Pritchard, 1985). Sociologists too can and should take children seriously as social actors in their own right, as sources of valid sociological data.

Powerless children?

Ultimately the biggest ethical challenge for researchers working with children (and implicit in much of the preceding discussion) are the disparities in power and status between adults and children. Mayall notes that 'discussions about data collection with, and from and for children tend to focus on the following perceived problems: children can't tell truth from fiction; children make things up to please the interviewer; children do not have enough experience or knowledge to comment on their experience, or indeed to report it usefully; children's accounts are themselves socially constructed, and what they say in conversation or tell you if you ask them is what they have been told by adults' (1994: 11). She notes that all of these drawbacks, of course, apply equally when collecting data from adults. For Mayall, the differential power relationship between children and adults in the research process lies at the level of interpretation of data, rather than at the point of data collection; she suggests that whatever the data collection method,

However much one may involve children in considering data, the presentation of it is likely to require analysis and interpretations, at least for some purposes, which do demand different knowledge than that generally available to children, in order to explicate children's social status and structural positioning (ibid: 11).

Similarly, Qvortrup notes that real difficulties arise in interpreting the results of sociological data in child research: 'the question of objectivity is . . . more acute than in any other social science field, because children . . . have to leave the interpretation of their own lives to another age group, whose interests are potentially at odds with those of themselves. This is a sociology of knowledge problem, which so far is almost unexplored' (1994: 6; see also Alanen, 1992, 1994).

Recently Allison James (1995) has suggested that the ways of 'seeing children' that researchers hold have a profound impact upon the way in which we study children. Here too, of course, the power to choose which standpoint or way of seeing lies with the researcher. The methods we use, the research populations and subjects we study, and crucially the interpretation of the data collected, are all influenced by the view of children we take, and there are obvious ethical implications to this. James usefully identifies four overlapping ways of 'seeing' children, each of which combine notions of social competence with those of status to give rise to four 'ideal types' of 'the child' (1995: 4): the developing child, the tribal child, and adult child, and the social child. The developing child perspective undervalues children's competencies and when children's voices are elicited their words may not be taken seriously or even trusted. Methods here range from experimentation to observation, and the power of the researcher lies in the interpretation of data collected. The tribal child view sees children as inhabiting an autonomous world, separate from adults, in which children are competent actors, existing in a conceptually different world from that of adults, with its own rules and agendas. The method is participant observation. The ethical implications of the 'tribal child' view are that because children are 'other', inhabiting a separate world, they are essentially 'unknowable' in some way. Adult researchers are surely being misleading if they try to engage with this other world by attempting to suspend their adult status, because they cannot become children again. Attempts to do so can be as misleading and confusing for the children being studied as being deceived in experiments.

The 'adult child' view sees children as 'competent participants in a shared, but adult centred world' (ibid: 11); attention is focused on 'children's perspectives on and comprehension of an adult world in which they are required to participate' (ibid: 12). The method here is usually to assume that children are essentially the same as adults and the same tools of research can be used, from qualitative interviews to questionnaire surveys, but the ethical problem with this approach is that the differences between adult researchers and child subjects in terms of social status are not always adequately addressed. Asking children about things they have not experienced only makes it easier for adults to conclude that they are not only ignorant but incapable of understanding (Alderson, personal communication).

James's fourth model, the 'social child', offers a solution. This model envisages 'children as research subjects comparable with adults, but understands children to possess different competencies, a conceptual modification which . . . permits researchers to engage more effectively with the diversity of childhood' (1995: 14). James suggests that this has implications for the methods used in studying children: children have different abilities, and are encouraged to be skilled in different mediums of communication (drawings, stories, written work, and so on) but are nonetheless competent and confident in them, so as researchers, we need to draw on these:

Having been taught these skills, they use them daily and, unlike most adults, are accomplished practitioners. It behoves us then to make use of these different abilities rather than asking children to participate unpractised in interviews or unasked submit them to our observational and surveilling gaze. Talking with children about the meanings they themselves attribute to their paintings or asking them to write a story... allows children to engage more productively with our research questions using the talents which they, as children, possess (ibid: 15).

This needs to be qualified, because children's willingness to join in participatory research techniques may vary from age to age, drawings may be appropriate at younger ages while older children may be willing to talk freely (Alderson, personal communication). However, ethical guidelines call on researchers to avoid undue intrusion, and using methods which are non-invasive, non-confrontational and participatory, and which encourage children to interpret their own data, might be one step towards diminishing the ethical problems of imbalanced power relationships between researcher and researched at the point of data collection and interpretation.

NOTE

We gratefully acknowledge funding from the Joseph Rowntree Foundation. This paper is produced as part of a wider project, *Children's Accounts of Family and Kinship*. The authors would also like to thank Priscilla Alderson, Helen Roberts, Alan Prout, Marjorie Smith, Judith Ennew, Nina Hallowell, Ros Pickford, Frances Price, Jackie Scott, Chris Williams, and Tom Hall for their comments. An earlier version of the paper was presented at the Norwegian Centre for Child Research in Trondheim, and the first author would like to thank members of the Centre for their helpful discussion.

REFERENCES

Alanen, L. (1992) *Modern Childhood? Exploring the 'Child Question' in Sociology*, Research report no. 50 (Institute for Educational Research, University of Jyvaskyla, Finland).

Alanen, L. (1994) Gender and generation: Feminism and the 'child question'. In J. Qvortrup, M. Bardy, G. Sgritta, and H. Wintersberger (eds.), *Childhood Matters. Social Theory, Practice and Politics* (Aldershot: Avebury, and Vienna: European Centre).

Boyden, J. and Ennew, J. (1996) *Children in Focus: A Training Manual on Research with Children* (Stockholm: Radda Barnen).

Butler, I. and Williamson, H. (1994) *Children Speak. Children, Trauma and Social Work* (London: NSPCC/Longman).

Fielding, N. G. and Conroy, S. (1992) Interviewing child victims: Police and social work investigations of child sexual abuse. *Sociology* 26/1: 103–24.

Fine, G. A. and Sandstrom, K. L. (1988) *Knowing Children. Participant Observation with Minors*, Qualitative research methods series no. 15 (Newbury Park: Sage).

Flekkoy, M. G. (1991) *A Voice for Children. Speaking Out as Their Ombudsman* (London: Jessica Kingsley).

Gilligan, C., Lyons, N. P., and Hanmer, T. J. (1990) *Making Connections: The Relational Worlds of Adolescent Girls at Emma Willard School* (Cambridge, MA: Harvard University Press).

Grodin, M. A. and Glantz, L. H. (eds.) (1994) *Children as Research Subjects: Science, Ethics, and Law* (Oxford and New York: OUP).

James, A. (1995) Methodologies of competence for a competent methodology? Paper prepared for Children and Social Competence Conference, Guildford, Surrey, July.

Lansdown, G. (1994) Children's rights. In B. Mayall (ed.), *Children's Childhoods. Observed and Experienced* (London: Falmer Press).

Matthews, G. B. (1994) *The Philosophy of Childhood* (Cambridge, MA: Harvard University Press).

Mauthner, N. (1995) Postnatal depression: The significance of social contacts between mothers. *Women's Studies International Forum* 18/3: 311–23.

Mayall, B. (ed.) (1994) *Children's Childhoods: Observed and Experienced* (London: Falmer Press).

National Children's Bureau (1993) *Guidelines for Research* (London: NCB).

Nicholson, R. H. (ed.) (1986) *Medical Research with Children: Ethics, Law and Practice* (Oxford: OUP).

Pritchard, M. S. (1985) *Philosophical Adventures with Children* (Lanham, MD: University Press of America).

Qvortrup, J. (1987) Introduction. *International Journal of Sociology*, special issue, 'The sociology of childhood', 17/3: 3–37.

Qvortrup, J. (1994) Recent developments in research and thinking on childhood. Paper to ISA Conference Children and Families: Research and Policy, London.

Spencer, J. R. and Flin, R. (1990) *The Evidence of Children. The Law and the Psychology* (London: Blackstone Press).

Stanley, B. and Sieber, J. E. (1992) (eds.) *Social Research on Children and Adolescents: Ethical Issues* (London: Sage).

Waksler, F. C. (1991) *Studying the Social Worlds of Children: Sociological Readings* (London: Falmer).

47

Consent, Refusal, and Emotional Disturbance: Philip and Lucy

PRISCILLA ALDERSON AND CHRIS GOODEY

This chapter continues the experiences of Philip and Lucy (for background details, see chapter 17) and reviews the kinds of information and choice offered to children and parents. We have questioned whether emotional and behavioral disturbance (EBD) is an illness, and if it is not, how relevant is the treatment model which is commonly assumed?

The first decision about treating disturbed young people is to judge whether their problem is seen as medical and requiring clinical psychology or psychiatry treatment, as a special educational need, as a need for care and control by social services, or as delinquency to be dealt with by legal and penal systems. The same condition can be treated very differently by the four systems, and referral depends arbitrarily on the referring professional and the current pressures on each service,[1] not on the nature or severity of the problem. Severely affected students remain in mainstream schools without help, whilst less severely affected ones enter special schools or secure units.[2]

Each service also approaches consent very differently. Health professionals tend to take making a clear treatment plan and requesting parents' and often children's consent seriously;[3]

many educationalists disregard even parents' consent and, by law, parents must comply with their child's referral to special school, suggesting that the state assumes that parents are unwilling to do so and must be compelled. Young people have little choice, either about which service treats them, or about the wide differences between local services, as Philip's schooling in East City and Lucy's in West County show.

Opting In and Out

The special school Philip went to at the age of 7 was due to close and, like the other five pupils, Philip began to attend a mainstream school part time with unobtrusive support. His father said:

> He was concentrating on what he was doing, he was helping everybody else in the class, he was actually instructing the other children in the class what to do with their work, and they said that's good. He was beginning to cope with stress. If they were having a barney, Philip would sit there nice and calmly. Then he also can control his

temper. So if he was really angry he wouldn't take it out on other people. He wouldn't shout and scream or make a riot, he'd go for a little walk out of the classroom. Two minutes later he comes back in, sits down nice and calm, just as if it hadn't happened. But they did say, if people had a go at him it increased his anger.

[At a play scheme, Philip became bored and angry] and he felt picked on. He'd go off for a little walk, he liked to have his own space, calm down then he'd come back. They didn't know this so they'd go hounding him, shout and bawl at him, telling him off, things like that, giving him real bad grief, and it winds him up more. And he'd swear back at them and lose his temper, really bad, and then they'd have a go at me: "Philip's been abusive." But Philip's not like that. [I said to the staff] "You're not trained at all, you don't know what you're doing."

Philip's father thinks that his worst time was before Philip was excluded from infant school, where they were

shouting and bawling at him, screaming at him, which at the time it would make him worse. As soon as they were out of distance he would feel all right again. Nobody knew what was going on in his head . . . there was no one helping him – it was just, oh blame all of it on Philip. It would spark him off, he would just rant and rave and scream, shout, which used to make me mad; I used to think there should be someone here to help us.

The best time was when Philip started at the local secondary school without needing support. Here, the "treatment plan" was an ordinary academic and social education. Philip and his father were told what school he would go to, rather than consulted, but they were content with the service. Philip expressed his consent and refusal emphatically, by opting in or out of the classroom or play scheme. Teachers who respected him could work with him well, staff who did not respect him failed, raising questions about how far it is

possible to help pupils with EBD without their cooperation. Philip's father attributed disturbance to untrained staff rather than to Philip.

Accepting "Expert" Advice

Lucy's parents disregarded Lucy's wish to attend mainstream school, though knowing "she's set her heart on it." They were unhappy about her special school but insisted that they had no choice.

Mother: We were told it was the *only* school she could go to. . . . The LEA say she can't go to [local] school because she'll get picked on. . . . The teachers too, the doctor said they'll be cruel to her, the other girls just won't understand . . . so this is the only school that will deal with her needs.

Yet they knew that the school was not helping Lucy, and a few months later they removed her. After months at home, she began to go to a girls' EBD school. Her parents were annoyed that this option was not offered three years earlier. Her new SEN statement involved a strange mixture of clinical and social assessments. The doctor wrote: "In order to equip Lucy for a degree of adult independence I feel residential school should be at least considered, but on medical grounds there is no doubt Lucy does not merit residential education. When her social skills are examined I believe it becomes apparent that her severe need can best be addressed in a residential setting."

Interviewer: The doctor doesn't explain quite why.
Mother: She can't . . . [When the parents pressed for Lucy to go to a boarding school] she said to me that she's not allowed to put in writing what she really thinks.
Interviewer: What does she think?
Mother: She thinks Lucy should be off at boarding school for life skills because being at home, I and my husband haven't got enough to offer her . . . they can teach her a lot more than I can.

EBD Schools, Negotiation, Informed Consent, and Refusal

An essential stage of consent is to be informed about the nature and purpose of treatment, its risks and benefits, short- and long-term effects, and alternatives.[4] Yet this depends on staff having the essential information to provide to potential consent-givers. Modern evidence-based medicine's efforts to obtain such information through rigorous research is not matched in education. Schools have broader, vaguer, longer-term aims than specific medical treatments have.

Doctors and psychologists seldom knew what the special school they recommended, or the high (secondary modern) schools they advised against, were like. They worked on assessments but not in the schools. Yet when presented as a quasi-medical expert decision, however ill-informed it was, referral to "special" school tended to be accepted by West County parents as the best and often the only option for their child. It is questionable whether doctors should contribute to statements of special *educational* need unless children have an illness that affects their education.[5]

NOTES

1 NHS Health Advisory Service for Disturbed Adolescents, *Bridges Over Troubled Waters* (London: HMS, 1986).

2 Kelly, B., *Children Inside: Rhetoric and Practice Inside a Locked Institution for Children* (London: Routledge, 1992).

3 Alderson, P. and Montgomery, J., *Healthcare Choices: Making Decisions with Children* (London: IPPR, 1996).

4 World Medical Association, *Declaration of Helsinki* (Fernay-Voltaire: WMA, 1964/1989).

5 Goodey, C. and Alderson, P., "Doctors, Ethics and Special Education," *Journal of Medical Ethics* (1998).

48

"Partnership" is Not Enough: Professional–Client Relations Revisited

PAUL CAIN

Health professionals work with their clients and patients with diverse aims, in widely varying contexts, and under differing sets of constraints. The kinds of relationship involved vary enormously. Also, any one relationship may have several modes, for example requesting and responding to requests, the giving and receiving of advice, the exercise of benevolent pressure, and so on. It is, therefore, unlikely that any one way of denoting these relationships will do, and so the richer the language we have, the better.

It follows from this that although it is enjoying wide currency, the concept of a partnership may well be too limited in scope. What it highlights may be a characteristic of many professional–client relationships, and the values it embodies may be desirable for all; other conceptions are needed, however, if we are to do justice to the rich variety of practice. In this context, "doing justice" may be elusive, precisely because of the wide-ranging realities. The more modest aim of this chapter is to explore the concept of partnership and some alternative conceptions, to illustrate how these provide a conceptual framework, albeit limited, for thinking about practice.

The Concept of Partnership

To be a partner is, necessarily, to be involved with one or more other person in some joint enterprise. Partnership, therefore, implies working together, collaboration. So although the healthcare professional may be doing things *for* a client, and *to* a client, the overriding conception is that of doing things *with* a client.

As currently used, "partnership" conveys also some notion of equality. For example, Jones, as reported by Laurent (1991: 22), associates partnership with the idea of having "an equal say." More fundamentally, Strehlow (1983: 46) says that "partnership implies an egalitarian way of working, which gives full credit to clients' freedom of choice." This "egalitarian way of working" is held to involve other values: for example, nurses studied by Quilligan (1992: 7) found that a partnership approach demanded "honesty, humility and the ability to trust and to be self-aware"; Wilson-Barnett (1989: 12) picks out "trust, equality and negotiation."

At this fundamental level, therefore, a partnership conception is grounded in the basic moral principle of respect for persons: the values, perceptions, and judgments of clients are to be accorded due respect. (It could be argued that this is, in any case, logically implied by the notion of collaboration: "doing with," in contrast to "doing to," implies taking account of another person's point of view, their capacity for responsible agency, and their potential to contribute to the joint enterprise. In this sense, collaboration implies respect.)

So the equality at issue is a moral equality. It is worth emphasizing this, in view of the various inequalities (differences) that may characterize the relationship, for example a difference of status (professional–client), a difference of knowledge (it is reasonable to suppose that, qua professional, the healthcare worker has relevant expert knowledge), and a difference of investment (the health status of the client will have greater personal significance for the client than for the professional, however much the latter may care). The relationship may, also, be characterized by differing degrees of power: the client, for example, can choose not to comply, the professional may be able to impose a view of what is best.

In some extreme cases of difference – for example where a client is unconscious, or severely mentally disabled, or senile – the element of collaborative working highlighted by partnership may be impossible: "doing with" may have to give way to forms of "doing for" and "doing to." So this conception, as a description of the relationships involved, may in such cases be inapt. Needless to say, this gives added importance to the moral equality that has been highlighted.

Inequalities as such, however, don't invalidate the use of "partnership," since our use of the term allows for difference. We speak, for example, of "senior" and "junior" partners in a firm; and of a couple we may say that one is the "dominant" partner. Nevertheless, the inequalities I have referred to, in addition to the variety of relationships already noted, do suggest there is scope, and a need, for complementary conceptions, picking out potentially different aspects of the relationship, and embodying different values. An authority relation is one such conception.

An Authority Relation

In reviewing inequalities between professional and client, I claimed that "it is reasonable to suppose that, qua professional, the healthcare worker has relevant expert knowledge." For there to be an authority relation, it is necessary that the client should believe that the professional has such knowledge, and should comply voluntarily with what is perceived to be the professional's knowledgeable view. This belief and this voluntary compliance are sufficient for what I am describing as an authority relation. It follows that such a relationship can exist where the person perceived as an authority is not in any sense "in" authority, or in any sense authorized to occupy a particular role.

This account has a number of implications. First, it is not logically necessary that the professional should in fact be an authority (though this is, obviously, desirable): the client's perception is what counts. Secondly, although advice, guidance, or direction may often be a feature of an authority relation, these are not logically necessary: willing compliance with what is *taken to be* the professional's view is sufficient. Thirdly, to the extent that it involves force, authoritarianism is, logically, not a feature of this relationship, since force precludes willing consent.

It could be argued that authority, as defined, is typically a feature of professional–client relations, not least in healthcare where clients may have, perforce, to trust and comply with the judgment of those on whose expert care they must rely. As such, it calls for the exercise of particular virtues, for if clients are in a position of having to entrust their well-being to nurses, doctors, etc., then the latter must be *trustworthy*, and this, surely, presupposes at least diligence, in developing expert knowledge, and honesty, in acknowledging, to the client, areas of ignorance and uncertainty. These virtues are perhaps particularly relevant if clients are predisposed to ascribe authority to those who are authorized to speak and who are "in" authority.

A claim to authority is a claim to know; but some claims to know are suspect – for example, a claim to know what would be for the best for a client, if this claim is made in ignorance of a client's own values and lifestyle. Authority has its proper sphere. For this reason, it may be inappropriate for healthcare workers to offer guidance or advice, and it may be inappropriate for clients to comply, however willingly, since this may represent an abdication of personal responsibility.

What emerges from this analysis is that authority and partnership are not incompatible, since inequality in knowledge is consonant with moral equality, and willing compliance does not preclude collaboration. This is significant, in view of the practical importance of authority and the moral importance of partnership. Is there, nevertheless, an incompatibility if compliance is not voluntary? This is the next question to be considered, in reflecting on conceptions involving power and paternalism.

Power and Paternalism

To be perceived as an authority and to engender willing compliance is, clearly, to exercise power: there is power in authority. However, a "power relationship" I define as one where compliance is imposed on a person, i.e., where a person's will is overridden.

Evidently, such imposition can and does occur in healthcare settings. Here are some examples: a young mother cooperates reluctantly with a health visitor, knowing that legal sanctions may be applied to protect her child judged to be at risk from unsafe parenting; a frail, elderly man, judged to be a danger to himself and others, agrees to give up cooking and accept help that is organized, through fear of being put in a home; an elderly lady is benignly bullied out of bed, to prevent her getting bedsores; a mentally ill patient agrees to take his medication, under the threat of being sectioned; a woman, manic through the stress and anguish of bereavement, is found wandering the streets, and is (forcibly) taken to hospital.

Where a person's will is overridden for what is perceived to be their own good, then the exercise of power is paternalistic. The benign bullying just referred to would be a case in point. However, paternalism may take the form of lying to a person, or withholding the truth, in what is judged to be their best interests; in which case, if unwilling compliance is not involved, it will not be, strictly, a "power relationship" as defined: what is overridden may not be a person's will, but their rights – in this case, perhaps, a right to know.

Since both power and paternalism involve acting on, rather than working collaboratively with, a person, and to that extent involve a lack of respect, they fall outside the concept of partnership. There is a potential arrogance in paternalism, in the assumption to know best what is in the best interests of another person, which is at odds with partnership. Nevertheless, paternalistic actions, by definition benevolent and altruistic, may be an attempt to honor an obligation of trust to care for another person; so values fundamental to healthcare are highlighted in this relationship.

Such values are, however, not exclusive to paternalism; and whether a paternalistic relationship is a justifiable alternative to partnership depends on how much moral weight is placed on respect (respect for rights, respect for expressed wishes, respect for autonomy, etc.). If a distinction is made between what a person says he or she wants, and what he or she would want *on reflection*, a case can be made for paternalism. In the examples noted above, the old lady who is "benignly bullied" to get out of bed would not choose to have bedsores; the bereaved manic woman who, let's say, vigorously resists hospitalization, accepts, on recovering, that this was what she would have wanted. In neither case can we talk of partnership, but in each case, arguably, the action was justified.

If there is justification, this arises in part from the healthcare worker's commitment to a therapeutic task. Since this is central to many professional–client relationships in healthcare, the notion of a therapeutic relationship demands some comment.

A Therapeutic Relationship

A relationship can correctly be termed "therapeutic" in terms both of its aim (to bring about healing) and its outcome. It follows that if the focus is on its aim, a professional–client relationship in healthcare may *not* be "therapeutic," since the aim may be, for example, health maintenance (as in chronic care) or the teaching of skills (as with antenatal classes); and that, if the focus is on outcomes, *any* relationship may correctly be said to be "therapeutic," whatever its point and purpose, always provided there is some initial health deficit which is made good.

Any relationship, therefore, described as a "partnership" could also be correctly described as "therapeutic," in view of its outcome, although it would be a mistake to assume that this description can apply to all: in a particular relationship, it may be, simply, that certain skills or knowledge are acquired. Equally, not all partnerships are "therapeutic" in terms of aims: the "joint enterprise" may not involve therapy.

It may be suggested, however, that, from the outcome perspective a partnership relationship stands a good chance of being therapeutic, in view of the values it embodies – for a commitment to moral equality and respect involves valuing the client as a person.

Conclusion

The discussion has highlighted different ways of thinking of relations between healthcare professionals and their clients. A relationship may be thought of as either a partnership, or as involving authority, power, or paternalism, or as therapeutic. (Without a doubt, there are also other conceptions that have not been discussed here.) With one exception, these ways of relating are not mutually exclusive – what has emerged is the familiar point that the one relationship can be viewed under different descriptions: what from one perspective can be seen as a partnership, from another can be seen as an authority relationship, and from yet another as a therapeutic relationship. (I have argued that an exception to this is that partnership cannot accommodate paternalism.) In practice, these conceptions demand the exercise of particular virtues: these include respect, diligence, honesty, and altruistic concern.

What has not been explored is the significance of particular personal qualities that give tone to these different ways of relating to clients. Healthcare workers can be, for example, brusque or gentle, empathetic or distant, attentive or distracted. Here is yet another perspective from which to view professional–client relations.

What has been illustrated is the claim that although partnership is of fundamental moral importance, it is "not enough" to accommodate the rich variety of possible and ethically justifiable relationships.

REFERENCES

Laurent, C. (1991) Perfect partners. *Nursing Times* 87/45: 22.

Quilligan, S. (1992) Educational preparation and support for nurse–patient partnership. *Nursing Times* 8/16: 7.

Strehlow, M. S. (1983) *Education for Health* (London: Harper and Row).

Wilson-Barnett, J. (1989) Limited autonomy and partnership: professional relationships in health care. *Journal of Medical Ethics* 15: 12–16.

49

Experiencing Care

STEVE ERSSER

Ethnographic data may provide a useful source of patient-centered information on patient health and illness and their reactions to health services which are not self-evident (Ersser, 1996). Data excerpts are presented here. They are drawn from a study of nursing as a therapeutic activity, in which patients' experiences of receiving nursing care and nurses' experience of providing care have been documented systematically (Ersser, 1997). In outline, data was collected using patient-held diaries, followed up by qualitative in-depth interviews to allow for elaboration and collaboration of patients' diary entries and subject to qualitative analysis.

For the purposes of this volume four themes are selected from this study of nursing practice which have moral implications for those providing health care (see box 49.1). Each is introduced in turn, supporting data excerpts are selected from the appropriate diary or interview transcript. An explanation is given of the extract and the ethical issues or moral dimension arising from each extract is touched on briefly.

Observations and Issues

Theme 1

Patients' accounts of receiving nursing indicate that we perhaps take for granted the significance to patients of the nurse's expressive behavior for patients. Quality nursing is in part a function of what the nurse brings to the situation as an individual person, with all their strengths and weaknesses. For example, the nurse's facial expression is judged by the patient in excerpt 1. Whilst seemingly trivial, the nurse communicates to the patient that they are not valued; the patient, in consequence, does not feel valued and instead feels quite ill at ease. Another example is seen in excerpts 2, 3, and 4; these highlight the importance to patients of the genuineness and ordinariness of the nurses' actions. Others have also identified this issue (e.g.: Taylor, 1994). Aside from the fact that the psychological literature highlights the importance of genuineness in all helping and therapeutic relationships (Ersser, 1997), this raises the ethical issue of the extent to which health professionals should and can

> **Box 49.1** Selected themes from a study of patients' experiences of nursing care in hospital (Ersser, 1997)
>
> 1. *Judging the 'Nurse as a Person'*   Patients judge the way the nurse presents him or herself to the patient (*the Presentation of the Nurse*) when evaluating nursing care; this includes aspects concerned with appraising the nurse as a person and his/ her moral character.
>
> 2. *Sentiments and acts: the case of awareness of the patient's need for consistent information*   Nurses believe they benefit patients by giving them information through patient teaching, by helping them adjust to their situation and develop greater independence. However, patients highlight that such practices may be inconsistently delivered with the result that patients can receive conflicting information. As such, the patient can judge the nursing received negatively and at worst this can create distress and dependence through a failure to inform patients effectively.
>
> 3. *Patients' involvement in care – when is it desirable?*   Nurses convey that they are often keen to take opportunities to involve patients both in health care decisions and the nursing care itself because they believe it to be valuable therapeutically, however, patients indicate that they may not always be willing or able to do so.
>
> 4. *The 'Presence of the Nurse' – a valuable and limited resource*   A significant feature of the patients' experience of nursing (their *Presentation*) is the extent to which nurses convey their physical and psychological presence to patients. Such behaviour is said by patients to help them in ways, such as coping and communicating their needs. However, nurses may have significant difficulties at times responding to this level of need, occasionally due to their lack of awareness and skill, but more often due to the demands of their workload, an issue of inadequate resources.

reconcile this expectation with their true feelings about their work (e.g. disgust at seeing a severe wound). Sociologists have described this type of behavior as 'sentimental work' and 'emotional labour' (e.g.: Strauss et al., 1982; Hochschild, 1983). It raises the question of what the ethics and politics are of such work.

Excerpt 1   *Neither a smile, nor a word, nor a look*

SE: You referred Nina to the nurse Sally. You said 'neither a smile, nor a word, nor even a look' – [interrupted]

N: Oh yes I remember she used to come and do things and neither look at me, nor smile, nor speak. And that's not nice for a patient you know. It makes you feel as if you're of no consequence, you know what I mean?

SE: It does not make you feel as if you're of value?

N: Yes, that's it, that's quite right.

SE: Is that what you mean?

N: Yes I do.

SE: Did you mean that a nurse's smile or how she looks at you is an important quality?

N: Oh I think so, very important. Oh it makes me happy when they smile, look pleasant, you know. This nurse didn't have a smile on her face – it made me feel that she didn't want to do anything for me.

SE: Did that affect you more deeply in any way?

N: No, not physically, but it did bother me. [...]

N: I must say she has improved since then, she's much more pleasant. Maybe she was

feeling off that time when she was like
that and not feeling well or something.

SE: When she's like that does it have any
bearing on your health at all?

N: No – only just that it makes me feel
uncomfortable.

Laura's account of managing with a new tracheostomy illustrates the effect of the nurse's look on patient satisfaction. Both aspects of presentation operate here, facial expression (personal qualities) conveying the nurse's availability (presence).

Nurses' accounts The nurse's appearance is seen primarily as an outward reflection of the nurse's emotional state by patients. Nurses seem to place greater emphasis on the implications and possible attempts to control their emotions, such as being 'down', 'disappointed', 'frustrated' and 'being sullen'.

Excerpt 2 *A kind genuine smile*

E: My point is that as a patient one perhaps
tends to be perhaps oversensitive to what
seems unkind treatment, whereas a kind,
genuine smile from anyone does wonders
for the patient.

Excerpt 3 *Having an ordinary-friendly way:
doing something personal*

L: Hospital can be a very lonely place – you
know. I think if you sort of find one or two
nurses who are friendly in a kind of ordinary friendly way – You know what I mean,
not just a nurse being friendly but, but –
just another person being friendly to you –
know. I think that sort of makes me feel
less isolated.

Excerpt 4 *Giving you loving care like your own
people*

The following reveals the patient's satisfaction with the nurse who is caring (sensitive and responsive to the patient) and uses the metaphor of the family to describe his relationship with the nurses.

[Following on from talking about the nurse providing comfort.]

R: They will give you the loving care like your
own people, as if it were your wife, or it was

your own mother, they couldn't be finer.
They talk to you when they see you, they
look across at you and if you look uncomfortable, whether it's nurses who have been
detailed to you or not, it's done.

Theme 2

As discussed above, when patients make judgements about nursing they employ criteria concerned with the nurse's expressive-personal actions (the nurse's *Presentation*), but they are also interested in the specific technical activities nurses engage in (the *Specific actions of the nurse*). These two elements are judged as inextricably linked in a complex way when patients evaluate nursing care. Nurses place significant emphasis on a particular specific action, the importance of giving patients information in a structured way. Many nurses recognize that lack of information is a common complaint of patients in hospital and that effective patient teaching can help patients to cope with their situation (aside from their right to receive such information). However, despite these good intentions and practices the data provides evidence of the breakdown of this information in cases (where health professionals believe they are benefiting patients by giving information), because of the inconsistency of the information. As a result, patients can be left distressed and dependent (e.g. see excerpts 5, 6, 7, and 8).

Excerpt 5 *Nurses who know what they are doing*

L: I mean, when you get a nurse come in and
she's too frightened to clean it, it doesn't
make you feel sort of confident about
it...I could've done with people who
understood and could just help me to feel
happier about it.

Excerpt 6 *The nurse who knows what they are
doing*

L: You want someone who knows what they
are doing – I mean obviously it's nice to
have someone who's very professional and
who's friendly as well; but I mean you are
in hospital because you're ill, not for a good
social life with nurses. You want to feel
confident in them.

This excerpt is illustrative of the ways in which the various presentational actions of the nurse may interact in a complex way to influence the patient.

The nurse's personality or character Patients also describe the 'character' of the nurse. The disposition of the nurse may be described by patients in emotional terms, such as 'happy' or 'cheerful' or 'quieter nurse'. The value of nurse being themselves is also expressed. Patients refer to the 'different types of people who are nurses' such as the nurse who is 'quiet' or 'miserable'. While these are likely to be transient features they may be construed as typifying the nurse's personal characteristics. The nurse's personality may be seen by nurses to help indirectly to develop the patient's confidence in the nurse and as a basis for the nurse and patient to relate in a more personalised way.

Excerpt 7   *Nurse with a sense of humour*
L: 10.30 pm. Finally had my tracheostomy cleaned. The nurse said she'd only ever cleaned one years ago! Wouldn't it be nice to have someone who knew what they were doing!...She had a good sense of humour and treated me like a normal person so it didn't matter so much that she wasn't used to doing them.
    [Responding to a request to tell me more about this incident.]
L: I mean, if somebody can keep their sense of humour and deal with it, then she's obviously, not sort of fazed by it all, or frightened to death, looking at you sort of horrified....You look to other people to get confidence in it.

Excerpt 8   *Lack of clear guidance: getting conflicting advice*
L: Asked nurse to clean my tracheostomy. I don't think she'd cleaned one before. She was asking me questions about how it was done. It's taken several days to get guidance on how it should be treated. People constantly have different ideas about care and a lot of the nurses are nervous about helping me with it because they are not used to them. This has caused me a

lot of distress it's unnerving to be told different things and it doesn't help me to adjust mentally to the trachy.

Helping the patient This category has no discernible properties. The codes include the nurse helping the patient through meeting physical care needs, such as assisting with bathing and movement.

These specific examples are of a patient with motor neurone disease who had suffered a respiratory arrest; this was followed by the insertion of a tracheostomy tube. This person, Laura was fiercely independent and wished to manage her tracheostomy herself so as to be able to leave hospital as soon as possible. The data from the nurses indicated that they believed they were helping Laura by giving her information about how to manage the care of her tracheostomy tube. However, the patient's accounts reveal that despite the nurses' good sentiments they are unaware that they are giving conflicting advice about the care of the tube and the problems this is causing. This highlights the fact that despite the nurses' intentions they may not be aware that the inconsistency of their actions may leave patients worse off.

Theme 3

Nurses endeavor to empower patients and promote their ability to care for themselves by encouraging them to get involved in making decisions about their own care and taking greater responsibility for aspects of their care. However, the patient data indicate that at times nurses can be over-zealous, by trying to give patients control when they do not want it and feel it to be inappropriate. Excerpt 9 highlights the student nurse's own cynicism about patient involvement, working on a neurosurgical ward. She conveys how the patient she is looking after misconstrues her encouragement for him to go to the bathroom himself to wash, rather than have a washbowl brought along, as the nurse 'being bossy'. The therapeutic objective of the nurse appears not to have been clearly communicated to the patient. It highlights the issue that enhancing patient control for therapeutic ends needs to be communicated and negotiated by the nurse. This practice must be adjusted according to the patient's prevailing needs and wishes, with control being relinquished and restored to the patient as appropriate.

Excerpt 9   *Involvement and choice in nursing*

Nurses' accounts reveal an attitude which highlights the value of patients being more involved in their care, but patients made little mention of this. Giving the patient choice and opportunity for involvement is seen to be a way of communicating respect for the patient's autonomy and individuality. The data indicates the significance of a difference in the patient's interpretation of the nurse's motives. For example, [one nurse] highlights how 'giving a patient choice and involvement' is a part of the 'ward approach' and helps patients to feel valued ('they don't feel just another patient that's a number or a condition'). This is seen to reduce the patient's dependence and encourage them to ask questions. However, there are indications that not all nurses are convinced of the value of this approach and patients can misconstrue the nurse's intentions in getting them to become more involved in their care. This is seen in the data from the senior student nurse Sarah who describes 'the patient perceiving me as bossy' when inviting him to get his own washing arrangements organised. She says: 'I think he thought "oh sod her I'm not doing it anyway" .... They don't like this wishy washy "What do you feel you might be able to do Mr so and so?".'

Although patients do not refer overtly to their involvement in their care, they do describe how their independence and self-confidence may be enhanced through nursing.

Theme 4

The presence of the nurse is significant to patients. To create the conditions of presence requires awareness and skill on the part of the nurse and the opportunity afforded by the organisation to respond to the patient in this way. The resource of time is needed to create the conditions whereby nurses can be sufficiently responsive to patients, physically giving them time and being available for them emotionally when they need to talk or just to have someone 'be there' during their suffering.

Excerpts 10 and 11 illustrate the importance of the nurse's presence and its absence to one patient mentioned above. The significance of the nurse's presence for this patient is seen in the apparently trivial instance of her being left on the commode, but one in which there was an important but subtle therapeutic need. The context is that Laura has recently undergone a respiratory arrest. She was unable to walk, being wheelchair-bound from motor neurone disease. The patient was fearful and lacking confidence in being left alone for prolonged periods. The nurse's presence was particularly important here.

Excerpt 10   *Not being there*

L: I mean sometimes I'm just sort of on the loo and my chest's a bit rough. I know somebody might not come for a while, you know, it takes a lot of confidence to sit there, particularly bearing in mind that I, I did have a, I did stop breathing. I did have a bout in ITU and it was bound to have some effect on me. You know, I need to build up my confidence – you know that does take – ermm, quite an effort on my part, just to, you know relax and realise that nothing is going to happen.

The aspects of the property 'presence of the nurse' are now illustrated and examined. In order to present the data in a comparative way for each informant group, and given the different emphasis given to different properties a set of combined subheadings are used as noted in table 49.1.

Giving the patients time or not (patients)   A salient feature of nurses' and patients' accounts of the nurse's presence is seen in terms of the temporal or time quality of nurse–patient interaction. Emphasis is given to the nurse being available for the patient. This is not confined to the nurse simply 'being with' the patient, an aspect described later. Informants refer to nurses 'having' or more actively 'making', 'giving' and 'allowing' time to be available to respond to the patient's needs or wants, as well as the converse. They also describe the benefit gained by the patient through the nurse being available for them.

Table 49.1 Headings used to present the aspects of the property 'presence of the nurse' for nurse and patient data

Heading used	Aspect of nurse (N) and patient (P) data
1) Giving the patient time or not	Giving the patient time or not (P)
2) Being available or not	Being available or not (N)
3) Nurse as a person: aspects of the presence of the nurse (Overlapping areas of properties)	Sensitivity/insensitivity shown to the patient (P) Trying to determine the patient's viewpoint
4) Being caring	Nurse being caring (P) Caring (N)
5) Being with a patient or not (N)	Being with the patient or not (N)
6) Giving support (N)	Giving support (N)

There are two aspects to the patient accounts:

(1) giving the patient time;
(2) nurses being busy and rushed.

Excerpt 11   *Giving the patient time*
The following patient account illustrates how by the patient being given time the nurse may help them to cope with their situation.

Making time to talk to you
[*SE*: Laura was talking about being lonely at times in hospital.]

L: Obviously at times, I've felt quite depressed and I don't particularly like being in hospital. I tend to suffer quite a lot of anxiety just through being stuck in hospital and feeling, you know, a funny sort of claustrophobia and panicky at times. So I think obviously at times when I've lacked confidence that's made it feel worse. I mean, it has been very much kind of, because I'm not ill, my sort of coping with it, you know, my mental state. It's things like when they've got time to talk to you and sort things out, that'll obviously alleviate some of the stress of being in hospital.

By making herself available for the patient the nurse is seen to help alleviate some of the patient's distress. This is reinforced by Laura's diary account on nurses stopping to talk to her. For example, describing a nursing auxiliary:

'She stopped to chat for five minutes in her own time – after the morning; it was a pleasant change for someone to have time for me.'

This illustration, which is one of many on this theme, raises the issue of the limitations on the nurses' resources of time, because of the growing expectations of nurses. These reflect growing demands imposed by the need to deliver managed care, embrace technological change and to respond to pressure to accommodate the devolution of aspects of what were previously activities within the traditional medical role, in responding to the political drive to reduce junior doctors' hours (NHSME, 1991).

REFERENCES

Ersser, S. J. (1997) *Nursing as a Therapeutic Activity: An Ethnography* (Aldershot: Avebury).

Ersser, S. (1996) Ethnography and the development of patient-centred nursing. In K. W. M. Fulford, S. Ersser, and T. Hope (eds.) (1996) *Essential Practice in Patient-Centred Care* (Oxford: Blackwell Science).

Hochschild, A. R. (1983) *The Managed Heart: The Commercialization of Human Feeling* (Berkeley, CA: University of California Press).

NHS Management Executive (1991) *Junior Doctors: The New Deal* (NHSME).

Strauss, A., Fagerhaugh, S., Suezek, B., and Wiener, C. (1982) Sentimental work in technological hospitals. *Sociology of Health and Illness* 4/3: 254–78.

Taylor, B. J. (1994) *Being Human: Ordinariness in Nursing* (Melbourne: Churchill Livingstone).

50

Organ Salvage Policies: A Need for Better Data and More Insightful Ethics

THOMAS H. MURRAY AND STUART J. YOUNGNER

Salvaging organs from the bodies of the newly dead is a project of great medical urgency and cultural significance. The Council on Ethical and Judicial Affairs of the American Medical Association (AMA) has recently completed two reports on possible changes in public policy intended to increase the supply of transplantable organs. One of these reports deals with policies known as mandated choice and presumed consent.[1] The other report is on financial incentives.[2]

The two AMA reports share the same good intention. There are more people in desperate need of transplantable organs than there are organs available. Lives could be extended if more organs could be obtained. In the Council's judgment, two of the policies discussed – mandated choice and a form of financial incentive known as a future contract – hold sufficient promise that model legislation should be drafted for the former and a pilot program initiated to test the latter.

The two reports likewise share similar weaknesses, all of them related to the failure to place the problem of organ recovery in its full scientific, cultural, ethical, and historical context.

Aside from opinion polls with their obvious limitations, there are too few pertinent empirical data. We have based organ-recovery policy too often on little more than enthusiastic hunches.

A deeper difficulty with the Council reports is their thin understanding of the moral, psychological, and cultural significance of the deaths that lead to potential organ donors. Desirable organ donors are relatively young, healthy people who suffer sudden and catastrophic trauma. Their deaths are unexpected. The people closest to the newly dead person confront the urgent task of reconceiving their own lives, as they redefine their relationship with their dying or dead daughter, son, or spouse. Both Council proposals are grounded in an ethic of autonomy, which has diminished relevance to the question of what to do with a dead body – by any reasonable standard, no longer an autonomous person. This emphasis on an atomistic, individualistic conception of autonomy as the dominant moral justification for salvaging organs may hinder more than help the effort to design effective and morally sensitive policies.

There is evidence that health care professionals frequently failed to inform families that organ donation was possible. A policy requiring such requests was widely and rapidly adopted, yet seems to have had no positive impact on the number of donations obtained. Presumed consent would eliminate the need to ask survivors and therefore remove health care professionals' reluctance and family opposition as impediments to organ salvage. The AMA Council wisely, in our view, rejects this option, which is morally dubious, confronts sticky problems of implementation (if it permits opting out), and has not proven to increase the supply of organs in any event. A recent study from Europe finds "no obvious correlation between high postmortem organ removal rates and the existence of presumed consent laws."[3]

Like presumed consent, mandated choice strives to eliminate most or all of the impediments created by reluctant health care professionals and resistant families. Physicians would not be seeking anyone's permission to take organs; they would merely need to ascertain which choice – to donate or not to donate – the newly dead person had made. Families are simply excluded from any role in the decision. Future contracts would operate similarly to change physicians' roles from requesting permission to obtaining information and to eliminate any family role in the decision. Future contracts may also impose new legal liabilities on physicians. Cohen, the principal proponent of such contracts, argues that the person's heirs would have a financial interest in seeing that organs were recovered. Hospitals would be "required to take as much care with [the newly dead body] as with his wallet and watch." If negligent, they could be sued. As for physicians, "Should some doctors still feel inclined to ask the relatives of the deceased for permission, and acquiesce in a negative response, they will receive a sharp blow to their wallet when they are successfully sued by another relative who is the named beneficiary under the organ sales contract; such requests for permission will quickly become extinct."[4] Presumably physicians and other health care professionals could be sued for failing to identify someone as a candidate for organ salvage or for negligence in instituting

organ-sparing procedures or recovering organs. The economic view of human motivation, to which Cohen and presumably the AMA Council subscribe, treats the decision to donate one's organs as an unpleasant task and takes the prospect of a small addition to one's estate as a sufficient incentive for people to donate their organs. It likewise appears to presume that the best way to get health care professionals to cooperate in organ salvage is to threaten them with lawsuits.

An Adequate Ethic for Organ Donation

The AMA Council defends both mandated choice and future contracts as expressions of individual autonomy, like the Uniform Anatomical Gift Act, which favors the individual's choice. The Council sees family involvement as problematic at best. We suspect that this is an instance in which our laws have overreached our morality. Even in the presence of signed donor cards, families are nonetheless asked for permission.[5] Although there are certainly pragmatic reasons, physicians also may be reluctant to shut families out of the donation process because they recognize that autonomy has limited usefulness in such circumstances and that families have a legitimate moral interest in what happens to the body of their newly dead relative. Treating a person how they want to be treated is a persuasive argument for doing just that while they are alive; it loses much of its persuasive force after death.

Deciding what to do with a dead body is a matter that profoundly concerns the intimate survivors. Suppose that a person had discussed organ donation with his or her family and that they had all agreed that his or her organs would be donated at death. Then suppose the person dies unexpectedly and suddenly, and the family in its grief wants most of all to be with their beloved relative as that individual comes to complete biological rest, unobstructed by the paraphernalia of organ preservation. It is unlikely that either the now-dead person or the family could have predicted such a response. Yet such things can happen.[6] It seems reasonable to suppose that even the putative donor might have preferred to have his or her donation request overridden if it posed too great a burden on his or her family. In such a case, we would have honored a hollow notion of autonomy, while achieving exactly the opposite of what the donor and the family genuinely desired.

Mandated Choice and Future Contracts

Although it may be beset by implementation difficulties, we support a trial of mandated choice. Getting all adults to express their choices will be difficult. Ensuring that the record of their choice is immediately available when needed is equally daunting given our discouraging experience with donor cards.[7] The unhappy experience with the rush to adopt required request policies urges a cautious approach in a handful of jurisdictions rather than a rapid national scramble. Even in cases in which the prospective donor has indicated a desire to donate, we would not exclude the family. Rather, we would inform them of the individual's choice and our desire to honor that choice. However, when the family firmly opposes donation, we should give the family's refusal significant weight.

Future contracts, on the other hand, are a bad idea. They are premised on defective accounts of family relationships, of the newly dead human body, and of the nature of gifts.[8] They embody naive views about the ethical and social context of donation decisions.[9] They threaten to transform the meaning of organ salvage from gift to financial transaction, and they may well result in a decrease, rather than an increase, in the supply of organs.

Organ salvaging for transplant is not the first historical example of the clash between the rational ethos of medical progress and concerns about respect for dead bodies. The British historian Ruth Richardson has chronicled how for centuries British society (America's experience is similar) struggled to meet the need for fresh dead bodies to teach anatomy to surgeons. Initially, Britain reserved dissection as an add-itional punishment for executed criminals. When the demand exceeded supply, grave robbing flourished. Society's tolerance for this practice ended when Burke and Hare were convicted of killing people and selling their corpses to anatomists. Parliament considered various schemes including presumed consent, financial incentives, and importing cadavers from abroad but eventually passed the Anatomy Act of 1832, which allowed the dissection of people who died in the poorhouse without family to provide for burial expenses. Richardson notes, "What had for generations been a feared and hated punishment for murder became one for poverty."[10]

Today, voluntary donation provides an adequate supply of cadavers for dissection, but Richardson argues that the Anatomy Act may have set voluntary donation back for a century. She emphasizes that the problem was solved by appealing to the best side of human nature: voluntary gifts for the benefit of others. The appeal for organ transplantation should be easier not harder to make, but some patience may be necessary.

We must create public policies for organ salvage that are effective and sustainable and that reflect our deepest and best values. First, we need to enrich the discussion of the ethics of organ salvage. Autonomy is not the all-purpose answer to every question, certainly not about what ought to happen to the bodies of newly dead individuals and the role of their families. Second, we should encourage research that illuminates the meaning of events attending sudden and unexpected deaths and the settings in which requests to families for organ donation are made. This research should attend carefully to differences among cultures. Third, we need to create a just and efficient health care system that people trust is fair to rich and poor alike.

NOTES

1 Council on Ethical and Judicial Affairs, American Medical Association, "Strategies for cadaveric organ procurement: Mandated choice and presumed consent," *JAMA* 272 (1994): 809–12.
2 Council on Ethical and Judicial Affairs, American Medical Association, *Financial Incentives for Organ Procurement: Ethical Aspects of Future*

Contracts for Cadaveric Donors (Chicago, IL: American Medical Association, 1994).

3 Land, W. and Cohen, B., "Postmortem and living donation in Europe: Transplant laws and activities," *Transplant Proc.* 24 (1992): 2156–67, p. 2167.

4 Cohen, L. R., "Increasing the supply of transplant organs: The virtues of a futures market," *George Washington Univ. Law Rev.* 58 (1989): 1–51, p. 34.

5 Overcast, T. D., Evans, R. W., Bowen, L. E., Hoe, M. M., and Livak, C. L., "Problems in the identification of potential organ donors," *JAMA* 251 (1984): 1559–62.

6 Kunin, R. A., "Voluntary organ donation: Autonomy . . . tragedy," *JAMA* 270 (1993): 1930.

7 Overcast et al., "Problems in the identification of potential organ donors."

8 Murray, T. H., "Organ vendors, families, and the gift of life." Presented at the Park Ridge Center, Chicago, May 1, 1993.

9 Fox, R. C. and Swazey, J. P., *Spare Parts* (New York: Oxford University Press, 1992).

10 Richardson, R., *Death, Dissection and the Destitute* (London: Penguin Books, 1989), p. xv.

51

Rationing, Justice, and Ageism

JOHN KEOWN

This chapter comprises three sections. The first section provides working definitions of "rationing," "justice," and "ageism." The second section sets out evidence indicating the reality of age discrimination in healthcare. The final section addresses the question: is the denial of treatment to a person simply on account of his or her age unjust?

Definitions: "Rationing," "Justice," and "Ageism"

In every society, rationing of healthcare is both a reality and a necessity. For one thing, funding is limited: healthcare is not the only demand on the public purse; it must compete with other public expenditures such as education and defense. For another, though funding of healthcare is limited, the demand for healthcare is not. The development of expensive new drugs, such as AZT, and new technologies, such as IVF, inevitably produce a corresponding demand for them. And there is the growing number of elderly patients, whose treatment accounts for a substantial proportion of the health budget. In 1994 in the UK, those over the age of 65 made up 16 percent of the population but accounted for 40 percent of hospital and community health spending.[1]

Resource constraints and increasing demands therefore require that hard decisions be made at a number of levels. For the sake of simplicity, we can reduce these to three. We have, first, to decide how much to devote to healthcare: how much should we allocate to health and how much to, say, defense? Secondly, we must, within the health budget, set priorities within different forms of healthcare: should we have more preventive medicine or more organ transplants? Thirdly, when we have decided to allocate a certain amount for a certain treatment, and the demand for that treatment exceeds supply, we have to decide how that treatment ought to be rationed.

These are large questions requiring thoughtful, detailed, and close consideration by ethicists, economists, healthcare professionals, lawyers, theologians, laypeople, and their political representatives. My modest proposal in this chapter is to touch on the third question, the question how, once resources have been allocated as a result of the first and second decisions, we ought to ration them between potential recipients. More specifically, I shall concern myself with the question whether, in deciding whom to treat, it is just to deny treatment to the elderly solely on account of their age.

Justice requires not only that people be given what they deserve but that people be treated fairly, that like cases be treated alike. It would obviously be unjust if we denied treatment to a person on the ground of his or her color, since a person's color is an irrelevant consideration. We would rightly regard such a decision as racist. Equally, it would be unjust to deny treatment to a person because of his or her sex, an equally irrelevant consideration. We would rightly brand such a decision sexist. But can it be just to deny a person treatment on the ground of his or her advanced age? Is age a relevant consideration or would such a decision be "ageist," yet another case of unjust discrimination on the basis of a morally irrelevant characteristic? This is not merely a hypothetical question, for, as the evidence we are now to consider indicates, age discrimination in healthcare is a reality.

Evidence of Age Discrimination in the Provision of Healthcare

Over recent years, evidence has steadily amassed to show that elderly patients have been denied equal treatment purely on the basis of age. John Grimley Evans, Professor of Geriatric Medicine at the University of Oxford, wrote in 1993:

> There has long been evidence that older patients have poorer access to medical and surgical care. An American study showed that doctors spent less time on average in consultation with older patients than with younger ones, despite the fact that older patients usually have more complex problems.[2]

In April 1994, he commented that surveys showed that elderly patients had to wait longer before seeing a specialist and were offered less effective treatments for heart disease and cancer. He said that, since elderly people with cancer were expected not to do well, it was easy to overlook the fact that they were doing less well because they were getting second-rate treatment. There was, he explained, a misap-

prehension that elderly patients will not benefit from aggressive treatment or will suffer worse side-effects.[3]

The potential benefits of treatment, even at an advanced age, were royally illustrated when Queen Elizabeth the Queen Mother underwent, at the grand old age of 95, hip replacement surgery. She emerged from hospital in such a good state that she was not only able to smile and wave at the crowd in her inimitable manner, but felt able to wear a pair of black court shoes with 3-inch heels. But although Her Royal Highness is a shining example of the capacity of even the very old to benefit from treatment, not all elderly patients are treated like royalty.

In April 1994, the media exposed the case of Johnny Gray.[4] Mr Gray was a 73-year-old former saxophonist with chronic arthritis, whose physiotherapy was discontinued. Mr Gray said that when he rang the hospital he was told that he could not be treated because he was over the age of 65. Although his health authority denied age discrimination, his case produced a political storm and a stream of similar cases were exposed. *The Sunday Times* reported that pensioners across the country were coming up against arbitrary age restrictions barring their access to treatment.[5]

The stories prompted the then Health Secretary, Virginia Bottomley, to issue a press release. She stated: "The NHS provides services for everybody, on the basis of their clinical need and regardless of their ability to pay. There are no exceptions to that rule, whatever the age of the patient." That principle was the first and most important of the patients' rights as set out in the government's "Patients' Charter" and it was, she added, "the duty of all health authorities to ensure that people of all ages had access to acute care and that specialist care was available for those who suffered from chronic conditions due to the ageing process." The case of Johnny Gray did not, she explained, reflect any change of policy. Remedial action had been taken in that case, which she attributed to "local misunderstandings."[6]

The evidence suggests, however, that, despite government pronouncements, age discrimination continues to be a reality for a significant number of patients. In May 1994, a month after the Health Secretary's press release, the Royal College of Physicians published a report which stated that the elderly were regularly denied life-saving surgery and medical treatment because of their age. It quoted a study which revealed that 20 percent of coronary care units refused to treat patients above a certain age – usually 75 or 70 but sometimes as low as 65. Moreover, 40 percent refused to give clot-busting drugs to older people, prompting one of the researchers to com-ment: "There is absolutely no justification for withholding this therapy from elderly patients because studies show that it will save 80 lives in every 1,000 patients treated over the age of 70 compared with about 25 per 1,000 in younger patients."[7] In other words, not only was it effect-ive in older people; it was actually more effective. Although the situation had been improving, there were still some units imposing age bars.

The Royal College report also noted that the elderly were discriminated against in relation to kidney dialysis and organ transplantation. It concluded that age discrimination permeated society and would become worse as the propor-tion of elderly people grew and increasingly competed for healthcare resources, and it called for equal access to health services on the basis of medical need, not age.

Similarly, in September 1994 the Medical Research Council (MRC), the government's funding body for research, published a report stating that:

> There is a widespread tendency amongst healthcare professionals . . . to use age as a criterion for exclusion from certain types of health care. . . . There is a view, unsubstanti-ated by research, which is pervasive amongst health and social service professionals and the population at large, including older people themselves, that elderly people bene-fit less from medical and surgical interven-tions than do younger age ones. This may in turn contribute to an attitude that older people are less deserving than younger people because they may be viewed in some respects as having less to offer society.[8]

As an example of explicit inequality, it cited the inclusion rules for screening programs. The guidelines, issued by the Health Secretary's own department, exclude women over the age of 65 from regular invitation to breast screening. Nor are they recommended for regular follow-up for cervical screening. The MRC report observed that the limit persisted despite evi-dence establishing the benefits of screening up to the age of 74.[9] Similarly, Age Concern, the major pressure group for the elderly in the UK, published a report arguing that as many as 2,000 women's lives could be saved each year if women over 65 were invited for screening.[10]

It seems clear that age discrimination in healthcare exists (though its extent requires much more research). But is it unjust? Not all discrimination is unjust. There are often good reasons for discriminating between people. In admitting students, for example, universities discriminate in favor of those with the highest academic grades and against those with lower grades. Is denying healthcare because of ad-vanced age just or unjust discrimination?

A convenient vehicle for addressing this question is to imagine how a court – a court of *justice* – would decide it. Let us imagine a hypo-thetical case before an imaginary court. Our focus will be on general principles of justice rather than particular rules of law.

Unjust?

Imagine a woman of 66, Alice, who has suffered a heart attack. She is admitted by her local hospital, the General, but the casualty doctor, Dr Young, tells her that, as it is not hospital policy to admit those over 65 to the coronary care unit (CCU) or to give them clot-busting drugs, she is simply to be placed on a general ward, even though there is indeed a bed avail-able in the CCU. Alice is eventually sent home, but her condition deteriorates. The medical evi-dence is that her condition would not have deteriorated had she been admitted to the unit and received the clot-busting drug.

Alice challenges the hospital's policy in the courts, claiming it is ageist and unjust. The hos-pital defends its policy, claiming that its funds are limited and must be rationed somehow, and that in imposing an age limit of 65 it is only following the practice of other hospitals.

You are the judge. Whether you would strike down the hospital's age discrimination policy as unjust might well turn on what arguments counsel for the hospital could advance in its defense.

Counsel for the hospital, Miss Cash, raises five arguments. She argues, first, that rationing decisions have to be made and are so complex that you are not competent to pronounce on their justice. The decisions ought to be left to the hospital, particularly if the hospital is simply following the practice of some other hospitals. Miss Cash cites two cases in which the courts refused to strike down decisions not to fund treatment. The first involved a 37-year-old woman seeking IVF who was denied treatment because of an age limit of 35 on the provision of such treatment,[11] the second a 10-year-old girl with leukaemia seeking chemotherapy and a bone-marrow transplant.[12]

Counsel for Alice, Mr Noble, counters Miss Cash's argument. He argues that, while you might understandably be *hesitant* to interfere, you are nevertheless capable of identifying and remedying obvious instances of injustice. Indeed, English judges have long held that they can intervene where a hospital's decision is so unreasonable that no reasonable hospital could have made it. Furthermore, he adds, the courts in the two cases cited by Miss Cash held that they had the jurisdiction to intervene, although they did not exercise it because the decisions in those cases, based on the relative lack of benefit of the respective treatments, were in fact reasonable. In the former case, although the judge held that it was not unreasonable to deny IVF to women over 35 on the ground that it is generally less effective in such women, "a clinical decision on a case-by-case basis is clearly desirable and, in cases of critical illness, a necessary approach."

There can be little doubt, continues Mr Noble, that if, for example, the General hospital barred from treatment all Afro-Caribbeans, you would strike its policy down as racist, even if it were following the practice of other hospitals. Or, if it excluded all women, that you would strike it down as sexist. If, then, it excludes all those over 65 from the coronary care unit, why would you not strike it down as ageist, not least when age discrimination is contrary to stated government policy?

Miss Cash might argue, secondly, that the claims of the elderly to healthcare are less strong than those of younger patients on the ground that the elderly have already received a fair share of the benefits of the healthcare system. However, Mr Noble might reply that it is simply not true that all those over a certain age have so benefited: some lead healthy lives and make little use of healthcare until old age. Consequently, a blanket age ban is unjustifiable.

Miss Cash might argue, thirdly, that the elderly are in a poorer state of health than the young and are therefore less capable of benefiting from healthcare. But Mr Noble might reply that some elderly people are in a perfectly fit condition to undergo even serious procedures and that some younger people are not. The elderly comprise a diverse group, he stresses, and many are quite capable of benefiting. He cites the MRC report we noted earlier, which states:

It is on average true that unselected groups of older patients do less well after hazardous medical or surgical procedures than their younger counterparts, because physiological impairment increases with age, and the ability to adapt to challenges or changes within the environment is reduced.... However, at no age – "young" or "old", and it must be recognised that such a distinction in this context is arbitrary – will such impairments affect all individuals equally. It is important to acknowledge that, like younger individuals but perhaps to a greater degree, older people are a heterogeneous group and should be considered as such.[13]

It adds:

Using age rather than physiological status to determine the care given to an individual appears not to be based on solid foundations. It is partly the result of ignorance in many areas of medical care of the physiological variables of relevance to the prediction of

outcome. Less active treatment for the elderly may arise out of low social worth of the
old in society.[14]

And, Mr Noble adds, in Alice's case, there
would certainly appear to be no evidence that
she would have benefited any the less from
admission to the CCU and from the clot-
busting drug than a person under 65.

Miss Cash might argue, fourthly, that even
though the old may be in as fit a state to undergo a procedure, they will benefit from it less,
because of their shorter life expectancy. But Mr
Noble might reply that it is not true that all
elderly people have a shorter life expectancy
than the young. Alice at 66 might well, for
example, have a significantly longer life expectancy than a newborn baby with AIDS.

Fifthly, Miss Cash might argue that the
young have greater social obligations to fulfill
than the elderly. Not necessarily, Mr Noble
might reply: some elderly people have more
obligations than some younger people.

Undaunted, Miss Cash calls an expert witness, indeed a star witness. She calls Dan Callahan, President of the Hastings Center, New
York, and one of the world's leading ethicists.
Holding a copy of his book *Setting Limits*[15] in
his right hand, he defends the thesis he advances in that book which seeks to justify the
denial of treatment to the elderly. The argument runs that we acknowledge the idea of a
"tolerable death," that is, a death that is not
premature, a death that takes place after what
Callahan calls a "natural life span." A "natural
life span" is completed when the projects and
commitments which constitute a person's life
are largely completed, which usually happens
by a person's late 70s or early 80s. When a
person has completed a natural life span, Callahan argues, medical care should not be used to
prevent death but only to palliate suffering.
This is, it seems, because the proper purpose
of medicine is not to extend life beyond its
natural span. Moreover, the denial of life-
extending treatments to the elderly beyond a
natural life span does not harm them, because
the proper purpose of old age is not relentlessly
to stay alive but, for example, to prepare for
death.

Not to be outdone, Mr Noble calls an expert
witness of his own, Professor Boyle of the University of Toronto, who contradicts Callahan's
thesis.[16] Professor Boyle testifies that, while it
may be true that some elderly do not want life-
extending treatment and wish to prepare for
death, this is not true of all the elderly, many
of whom have different evaluations of their lives
and want treatment. He adds that even if there
were such things as proper purposes of medicine and of ageing, this still would not show it
was just to refuse life-extending treatment to
those elderly people who want it. Boyle concludes that there is a strong presumption that
the use of age to ration healthcare is unjust.
There are, he adds, fairer criteria, such as assessing the benefit of treating one person rather
than another.

Professor Boyle ends with a warning about
the negative impact that ageist rationing would
have on the elderly, and social attitudes to them.
He quotes one physician who has written:

> Only if routine medical care were withheld
> would the savings be substantial. The non-
> economic costs of a national policy to restrict
> routine care for the elderly would be high.
> To achieve acceptance of such intuitively
> distasteful measures would require a societal
> reeducation (brainwashing) effort that would
> exacerbate tensions between the generations
> and further devalue the status of the eld-
> erly.[17]

Having heard the arguments of counsel for
the General hospital and counsel for Alice, and
the two expert witnesses, you must now retire
and consider whether the hospital's policy
which denied her admission to the CCU is
ageist and unjust. What will your judgment be?

NOTES

1   Department of Health press release, 1994, p. 182.
2   "Dangers of Ageism," *Care of the Elderly* (June
    1993): 217, citing Keeler, E. H., Solomon, D. H.,
    Beck, J. C. et al., "Effect of patient age on dur-
    ation of medical encounters with patients." *Med-
    ical Care* 20 (1982): 1101–8.

3   *The Times*, April 15, 1994. See also I. S. Fentiman et al., "Cancer in the elderly: Why so badly treated?" *Lancet* (April 28, 1990): 1020–2.

4   *The Times*, April 15, 1994.

5   *The Sunday Times*, April 17, 1994.

6   DH press release 94/182.

7   Royal College of Physicians, *Ensuring Equity and Quality of Care for Elderly People* (1994), quoted in the *Daily Telegraph*, May 11, 1994.

8   Medical Research Council (MRC), *The Health of the UK's Elderly People* (London: MRC, 1994), p. 37.

9   Ibid, p. 38.

10 Age Concern, *Not at My Age: Why the Present Breast Screening System is Failing Women Aged 65 or Over* (London: Age Concern, 1996).

11 *R v. Sheffield Health Authority, ex parte Seale* (1995) 25 BMLR 1.

12 *R v. Cambridge Health Authority, ex parte B* [1995] 6 Med LR 250.

13 MRC, *The Health of the UK's Elderly People*, pp. 39–40.

14 Ibid, p. 40.

15 *Setting Limits* (New York: Simon and Schuster, 1987).

16 "Should age make a difference in health care entitlement?" in Luke Gormally (ed.), *The Dependent Elderly* (Cambridge: Cambridge University Press, 1992).

17 Ibid, p. 157.

52

Cardiopulmonary Resuscitation

PAUL CAIN

Since its inception as a life-saving procedure in 1960, cardiopulmonary resuscitation, or CPR as it has come to be termed, has been a focus of professional and ethical concern. One of the key questions that it has raised is what would be morally acceptable grounds for decisions not to resuscitate a patient? This is the issue I wish to explore. Initially, some illustration of how this particular question has emerged out of (sometimes harrowing) experience may be useful in setting a context for the discussion.

As early as 1966, a survey by the RCN Ward and Departmental Section, promoted in part by nurses' dilemmas over who should be resuscitated, elicited comments of relief that "something is being done about the problem." A report of the survey (*Nursing Times*, 1966) referred to "nurses' concern about their responsibility in resuscitating patients suffering from cardiac arrest." The report noted that "their concern is not only in defining their responsibility, it is for the patients and their relatives and for the young and inexperienced student or pupil nurses who may have to make a life and death decision without the necessary experience or guidance to influence that decision."

In 1977, a research study (Gaskell) involving 103 nurses in three hospitals found that a ma-jority of the nurses (88 percent) sometimes had to decide for themselves whether or not to initiate resuscitation: for the most part, instructions were lacking: 54 nurses were only "occasionally" told in advance who they should or should not resuscitate.

The dilemmas that resuscitation decisions may raise, particularly for young and inexperienced nurses, is highlighted by Canham and Gunga (1985), who write:

> Doctors and experienced nurses are rarely present when a patient's life comes to an unexpected end. They escape the torment of deciding whether to confer a peaceful demise or the dramatic mobilisation of hospital forces upon a lifeless body. The person at that bedside may be only 19 and no one will be there to tell her with absolute authority what action she should take.

Two particular cases presented by Dolan (1988) illustrate vividly the anguish that resuscitation attempts may provoke. In a hospital where there was a policy of resuscitating everyone regardless, a nurse was haunted by the memory of having to attempt resuscitation on a patient with infectious hepatitis and AIDS.

She said: "It was terrible. With every compression, blood flowed from his mouth, so giving him oxygen was nearly impossible.... Wasn't our futile attempt to save his life unfair to him and to us?" Another nurse spoke of doing CPR on a patient riddled with bone cancer: "I could feel the crunch of broken bone on each compression. What was I doing?"

In the above cases, the nurses followed policy against their better judgment. However, where a nurse exercises his or her own judgment, in order to safeguard what, in their view, are the best interests of a patient, this may be professionally risky. The *Nursing Times* (1983) carried a report of a nurse who chose to let an elderly man die rather than call an emergency resuscitation team. She was dismissed on grounds of gross misconduct. At the industrial tribunal considering her appeal against unfair dismissal, a hospital registrar said she had no right to decide whether or not a patient should be resuscitated. The nurse had told the tribunal, "I thought I would let him die peacefully. In my mind he was already dead."

These references highlight why it is that the practice of cardiopulmonary resuscitation has provoked professional and ethical concern. In particular, they highlight the particular question that concerns us here: on what grounds would it be justifiable to withhold resuscitation?

In the discussion that follows, I consider four possible grounds: the patient's age; the patient's condition; the patient's quality of life; and the patient's wishes. There is, however, a view that should be considered first – that is, the view that *no reason* is good enough to justify decisions not to resuscitate.

No Reason is Good Enough to Justify "Do Not Resuscitate" Orders

The two distressing cases cited above (Dolan, 1988) support the view that there must be some circumstances in which resuscitation should not be attempted. However, a particular understanding of the sanctity of life principle implies that resuscitation should *never* be withheld. J.

David Bleich (1989), a Jewish rabbi, expresses this clearly:

> Not only is life in general of infinite and inestimable value, but every moment of life is of inestimable value as well. The quality of life which is preserved is thus never a factor to be taken into consideration. Neither is the length of the patient's life expectancy a controlling factor.

Consistent with this, he claims that the physician's duty is to work for "not simply ... the restoration of health, but ... the restoration of even a single moment of life." The implication of this is that if we are to hold open the possibility that in some circumstances withholding resuscitation might be morally justifiable, we have either to abandon the sanctity of life principle or to dissent from the particular understanding placed upon it by Bleich.

I would argue for the latter option in the following way. A distinction can be drawn between life as an organic metabolic process and human life. From this perspective, life in the first sense has instrumental value as a necessary means to the possibility of human life. Distinctively human life has intrinsic value because of its particular potentialities and capacities, for example, the potential and capacity to form relationships, to exercise choice, to be happy. Hence respect for life, as entailed by the sanctity of life principle, implies, overridingly, valuing the potentialities and capacities that constitute the value of personal life. Where these are absent, or are seriously eroded, for example by chronic illness, withholding resuscitation might, therefore, not conflict with a sense of the value of life and respect for life; and further, if a patient expressed a clear wish not to be resuscitated, to administer CPR would be a violation of the duty of respect.

On this view, the principle of respect for life and a conviction of the value of life do not necessarily imply resuscitation at all costs; indeed, they may require, in particular circumstances, that resuscitation is not attempted. Just what these circumstances may be can be explored by returning to the question: on what grounds would it be justifiable to withhold resuscitation?

The Patient's Age

Research, for example Stewart and Rai (1985), has shown that many healthcare practitioners believe that age should be a factor in resuscitation decisions; it has also shown, for example Candy (1991), that in the practice of healthcare age may well be a factor. However, although at least three arguments might be advanced in support of such belief and practice, none is persuasive.

It might be argued, first, that the age of the patient may make a good outcome of resuscitation attempts unlikely; however, in a review of research on this question, Bayer at al. (1985) concluded that "most studies have failed to confirm that age has an independent influence on the prognosis for survival after resuscitation" (see also Murphy et al., 1989; McIntyre, 1993).

It might be argued, secondly, that old people, generally speaking, would not want to be resuscitated. Again, such a claim is not supported by research, which confirms, unsurprisingly, the fact that people differ and that whereas some old people might wish to be resuscitated, others would not (see, for example, Fusgen and Summar, 1978; Gunasekera et al., 1986; Sayers et al., 1997).

A third argument in favor of age as a reason might be a version of the "good innings" argument, according to which old people have had their "innings," there are limited resources, and, therefore, it is only fair that these should go to younger people who have their life ahead of them. This argument might find support in a utilitarian perspective. From this point of view, the overriding concern is to maximize welfare, and it could be argued that younger people have greater social utility than older people (they are more likely to be in employment, or to be bringing up children) and that, therefore, welfare would be maximized if an age-based rule were applied to decisions about resuscitation. A counter-argument, though, could claim that social utility is not just a matter of making an economic contribution or bringing up children; it could plausibly claim that old people make an invaluable contribution to society, for example as grandparents; and that a society which made

every effort to value old people would be happier (have more welfare) than one which systematically denied them access to particular benefits. Since one benefit is provided by the availability of resuscitation, this should, therefore, not be denied to them on the basis of age.

The difficulty here is in weighing up and quantifying the consequences for welfare of having an age-based standard, and then comparing these with the consequences of having some other standard which does not discriminate against people on the basis of age. And, as has been seen, another difficulty is that what values should go into the calculation is controversial.

The utilitarian perspective does at least rescue the age-based standard from a charge of arbitrariness: it gives it a rationale. But it does not rescue it from the charge of being unfair, since fairness is not simply a matter of applying the same rules (whatever these may be) equally to all; it is also a matter of what the rules are, and whether they discriminate on morally acceptable grounds between individuals and groups.

The three arguments in favor of age as a reason for withholding resuscitation thus fail to be persuasive. Can a more plausible reason be found?

The Patient's Condition

For some patients, the likelihood of recovery after resuscitation is minimal, and a number of research studies have demonstrated that failure to recover is correlated to their condition (see, for example, Bedell and Delbanco, 1984; Murphy et al., 1989). Reviewing these studies, Blackhall (1987) concluded that "survival after CPR is related to the underlying illness that leads to the arrest, and ... patients with certain conditions very rarely survive." Experience thus confirms what, a priori, appears likely to be the case, that the patient's condition may provide a good reason for "do not resuscitate" decisions. Given the invasiveness of CPR, the threat to dignity, and the risk of part survival in a deeply damaged, possibly vegetative, state, let alone the potential cost involved, it is hard to justify an attempt at resuscitation where it appears to be futile.

There are, however, two points to be made. First, it is the prognosis to which the condition gives rise that is the relevant point. This should be emphasized in view of research (Wachter et al., 1989) which found that physicians tended to give "do not resuscitate" orders much more frequently to patients with AIDS or lung cancer than to those with cirrhosis and varices or congestive heart failure with coronary artery disease in spite of the fact that reviews of the literature indicate that all these diseases have similar prognoses. The possibility of subjective bias in relation to disease categories must, therefore, be held in check by reference to the prognosis. Secondly, the claim that patients with certain conditions very rarely survive implies that some patients with those conditions do survive; hence we have to ask, are condition and prognosis necessarily *sufficient* grounds for a decision not to resuscitate? Is there not moral space for the claim that, even where there is much risk and a poor prognosis, a patient's wishes should, at the very least, be taken into account?

Quality of Life

I claimed above that "respect for life...implies...valuing the potentialities and capacities that constitute the value of personal life," and that, "where these are absent, or are seriously eroded," withholding resuscitation might not conflict with respect for life. It follows from this that a severely curtailed quality of life, whether in terms of the patient's current state or in terms of his or her predicted state following resuscitation, could provide grounds for withholding resuscitation. This conclusion may follow, also, from two of the principles that many would hold to be of fundamental importance in healthcare: beneficence and non-maleficence. If quality of life were very poor indeed, to take active steps to prolong that life might well violate these principles.

There is, however, a worry about this, which can be put in the form of a question: which of the many factors that contribute to a person's quality of life is morally relevant to a decision to withhold resuscitation? Farber et al. (1985) have shown that resuscitation decisions may be influenced by whether the patient lacks support systems (e.g. he or she is a "street person," or is mentally retarded or institutionalized); and yet such factors are not, surely, sufficient to sanction a negative view of the patient's quality of life, even if, which is not obviously the case, they were morally relevant. The worry of being on a slippery slope here underlies the reservation that some writers have expressed about quality of life judgments. Kass (1980), for example, writes that:

> Such a move...invites considerations of "social worthiness" or other alien matters to contaminate medical decisions, with not only individual lives, but our very reverence for life, in jeopardy. The consideration in medicine of quality of life, it is correctly said, was the fundamental error of the Nazi physicians.

What is to be made of this worry about allowing quality of life judgments to count in resuscitation decisions? The worry is, clearly, well founded: the scope for subjective and morally questionable judgments is evident. And even where factors less controversial than social worth are in view, such as level of pain, capacity for enjoyment, or ability to relate to others, even here there is scope for disagreement about what weight these should be accorded in particular cases: what level of incapacity is acceptable? how much pain? what degree of inability to relate?

The dangers of a slippery slope are, surely, minimized if account is taken of the patient's own valuation of his or her life, where this is available (it may of course be hard or impossible to have access to this, if, for example, the patient is senile, comatose, or profoundly mentally retarded). A person's life may lack many of the features that, it would generally be agreed, are objectively important and desirable, but may still be *experienced* as valuable.

To affirm this, i.e. to bring into prominence the patient's own valuation of their quality of life, is to bring into focus a further possible reason for withholding resuscitation, namely the wishes of the patient.

The Wishes of the Patient

Often, and perhaps typically, patients' wishes in relation to CPR are not sought (see, for example, Bedell and Delbanco, 1984; Evans and Brody, 1985; Candy, 1991); and it is not hard to find plausible reasons to account for this apparently widespread failure to consult.

Apart from particular difficulties of communication arising from the state of the patient (for example, where the patient is anxious or depressed) or the status of the patient (for example, where the patient is a young child, or mentally impaired), there are difficulties intrinsic to what is to be communicated. Nolan (1987) draws attention to the fact that resuscitation and its withholding can have "multiple and sometimes conflicting meanings for patients, families and clinicians;" she notes the risk that attempts at resuscitation can carry, risk "of the most fearful aspects of impending death: pain, isolation, violence and loss of control," the balancing of the certainty of death if resuscitation is not attempted against the risk of a process of dying that is "lonely, mechanical and dehumanised" (Kubler-Ross, 1969).

Practitioners may reasonably fear, therefore, that the process of seeking the patient's wishes about resuscitation would be distressing. That such fears may be justified is borne out by research. For example, Schade and Muslin (1989), in discussing seven cases where the issue was broached with patients, found that discussion for some provoked "psychological discomfort and disarray," "anguish," and depression and fright; and Sayers et al. (1997) found that some patients with whom the issue was broached were "emotionally unable to deal with it" and experienced "psychological pain."

Nevertheless, what the patient wishes must, surely, be held to constitute a good reason for a decision not to resuscitate, in view of the principle of respect for autonomy: as I claimed above, "if a patient expressed a clear wish not to be resuscitated, to administer CPR would be a violation of the duty of respect." This being so, identifying what the patient wishes is a moral imperative, as is providing accurate information, and ascertaining whether the patient's con-

sent (or dissent) is informed. The possibility of misunderstanding, and so of patients making non-autonomous choices, is highlighted by Sayers et al. (1997), who report that one patient opted for CPR because he thought this would be helping medical science: he would be " 'allowing his heart to be taken out and fastened up this way or that. I may as well have it. Somebody's got to learn. Somebody's got to try them out'."

Thus the fact that discussions about resuscitation may be upsetting does not entail that such discussion should not take place: it *may* imply that in particular cases discussion should not be taken very far; it *might* justify in particular cases a decision not to engage in discussing the issue at all; but, given the importance of autonomy as a value, all that is implied *as a general rule* is that the way in which such discussions are initiated and carried through is all-important. (Schade and Muslin (1989), who, as has been noted, highlighted the potential distress such discussions may cause, propose a "careful and cautious delivery of information, guided by patient feedback.")

What this implies is the importance of a relationship between practitioner and patient in which judgments about what the patient can cope with – and understand – can accurately be made, and of good communication between medical and nursing staff, so that knowledge of the patient as a person can be shared, and damaging errors of judgment avoided. Also implied is the importance of context – a point which has been well made by Nolan (1984):

> Given some capacities for autonomous action, whatever can be made comprehensible and refusable by patients can be treated as subject to their consent – or refusal. This may require doctors and others to avoid haste and pressure, to counteract the intimidation of unfamiliar, technically bewildering and socially alien medical environments. Without such care in imparting information and proposing treatment, the consent patients give to their treatment will lack the autonomous character which would show that they have not been treated paternally but rather as persons.

Conclusion

The question that has been in focus is on what grounds it would be justifiable to withhold resuscitation. Four possible grounds were considered: the patient's age, condition, quality of life, and wishes. I argued that the first of these, the age of the patient, does not provide good grounds. The other three, I argued, are, each in their way, problematic: judgments based on the patient's condition that resuscitation would be futile are vulnerable to the charge that particular patients with the condition in question may survive even though most would not; quality of life judgments risk unacceptable bias and subjectivity; seeking the patient's wishes risks emotional harm and misunderstanding. As I have shown, however, all three may provide a good reason for withholding resuscitation. In particular, in view of the principle of respect for autonomy, the importance of the patient's wishes has been underlined.

Thus where, for whatever reason, the patient's perspective is not available, decisions based on judgments relating to quality of life or the patient's condition may be morally defensible. Where the patient's perspective *is* available, the problematic nature of these factors as grounds can be mitigated, removed even, if the patient's own perspective is given weight: bias and subjectivity in relation to quality of life judgments can be countered by the patient's own valuation of his or her life; and judgments based on the patient's condition can be made morally more secure if the patient's viewpoint is sought.

REFERENCES

Bayer, A. J., Ang, B. C., and Pathy, M. S. J. (1985) Cardiac arrests in a geriatric unit. *Age and Ageing* 14: 271–6.

Bedell, S. E. and Delbanco, T. L. (1984) Choices about cardiopulmonary resuscitation in hospital: When do physicians talk with patients? *New England Journal of Medicine* 310/17: 1089–93.

Blackhall, L. J. (1987) Must we always use CPR? *New England Journal of Medicine* 317/20: 1281–5.

Candy, C. E. (1991) "Not for resuscitation"; The student nurses' viewpoint. *Journal of Advanced Nursing* 16: 138–46.

Canham, J. and Gunga, D. (1985) A matter of life or death. *Nursing Times* 81/46: 52.

Dolan, M. B. (1988) Coding abuses hurt nurses, too. *Nursing* 18/2: 47.

Evans, A. L. and Brody, B. A. (1985) The do-not-resuscitate order in teaching hospitals. *Journal of the American Medical Association* 253/15: 2236–9.

Farber, N. J., Weiner, J. L., and Boyer, E. J. (1985) Cardiopulmonary resuscitation. Values and decisions – a comparison of health care professions. *Medical Care* 23/12: 1391–8.

Fusgen, I. and Summar, J. D. (1978) How much sense is there in an attempt to resuscitate an aged person? *Gerontology* 24/1: 37–45.

Gaskell, M. (1977) An investigation into the problems of deciding which hospital patients are/are not to be resuscitated. Unpublished MSc dissertation. University of Manchester, UK.

Gunasekera, N. P. R., Tiller, D. J., and Clements, L. T.-J. (1986) Elderly patients' views on cardiopulmonary resuscitation. *Age and Ageing* 15: 364–8.

Kass, L. R. (1980) Ethical dilemmas in the care of the ill: What is the good of the patient? *Journal of the American Medical Association* 244/17: 1946–9.

Kubler-Ross, E. (1969) *On Death and Dying* (New York: Macmillan).

McIntyre, K. M. (1993) Failure of "predictors" of cardiopulmonary resuscitation outcomes to predict cardiopulmonary resuscitation outcomes. *Archives of Internal Medicine* 153: 1293–6.

Murphy, D. J., Murray, A. M., and Robinson, B. E. (1989) Outcomes of cardiopulmonary resuscitation in the elderly. *Annals of Internal Medicine* 111: 199–205.

Nolan, K. (1987) In death's shadow: the meanings of withholding resuscitation. *Hastings Center Report*, Oct/Nov: 9–14.

Nursing Times (1966) Resuscitation – The nurse's responsibility. No. 62 (Nov 11): 1497.

Sayers, G. M., Schofield, I., and Aziz, M. (1997) An analysis of CPR decision-making by elderly patients. *Journal of Medical Ethics* 23: 207–12.

Schade, S. G. and Muslin, H. (1989) Do not resuscitate decisions: discussions with patients. *Journal of Medical Ethics* 15/4: 186–90.

Stewart, K. and Rai, G. (1985) A matter of life and death. *Nursing Times* 85/35: 27–9.

Wachter, R. M., Luce, J. M., Herst, N., and Lo, B. (1989) Decisions about resuscitation: Inequities among patients with different diseases but similar prognoses. *Annals of Internal Medicine* 111: 525–32.

53

An Analysis of CPR Decision-making by Elderly Patients

GWEN M. SAYERS, IRENE SCHOFIELD, AND MICHAEL AZIZ

Introduction

In recent guidelines on withholding cardiopulmonary resuscitation (CPR), Doyal and Wilsher draw attention to the potential clash between respect for individual autonomy and a tradition of clinical discretion which continues to deprive patients of any knowledge of their CPR status.[1]

They propose that informed consent must be obtained in the case of patients where CPR is withheld on grounds other than futility, and in cases where the clinicians do not know the true wishes of the patients.

Generally when patients are admitted to hospital they are understood to be for resuscitation as part of a duty of care unless otherwise explicitly stated. In young patients, withholding resuscitation is largely based on the chances of successful outcome being negligible, that is to say of CPR being considered futile. In America such patients are required to provide informed consent to their do not resuscitate (DNR) orders, but in this country it has been stated that consent is neither morally nor legally required under such circumstances.[2]

In geriatric medicine it is relatively uncommon for non-resuscitation decisions to be made on the basis of futility. Most are based on a variety of considerations such as frailty, disability, extreme old age and multiple pathology, all of which may reduce the likelihood of successful outcome but would not necessarily predict failure with certainty.[3]

This allows discretionary space for clinicians to decide, on the basis of their own values and principles, that resuscitation is not in the patient's interest. Such decisions may be based on the perceived poor quality of life before resuscitation, or the expected poor quality of life after resuscitation.

Further, both for this group of patients and for those for whom resuscitation may be considered a reasonable option, no clinician can be said to know a patient's true wishes without consultation with the individual concerned.

There has been a burgeoning number of studies which have supported the participation of elderly patients in CPR decision-making. Such studies have been questionnaire-based and have sought to assess patients' attitudes regarding their resuscitation preferences. These studies have shown that most patients want to be consulted regarding CPR decision-making, most desire CPR,[4] most are not disturbed by the consultation,[5] and many want to make their own decisions.

However, none of the studies has indicated whether the patients' preferences had been used in any way in the recorded CPR status although there is clear evidence of poor concordance when comparing the patients' preferences with those of the clinicians.[6] In an American study which considered hypothetical outcomes, 25 percent of elderly patients questioned said they would not opt for CPR even if there were 100 percent chance of survival.[7]

Although the guidelines[8] have stressed the need to obtain consent for DNR where futility is not the issue (assuming the patient can then indicate a preference for resuscitation, which would be respected) it seems that a simpler approach would be rather to ask the patient whether he/she wants resuscitation. The same would apply to those patients whose true wishes are not known which, from the evidence derived from the above studies, would be a fair proportion of elderly patients.

When treating acutely ill elderly patients, we have found that there are few who, at the time of admission, are well enough to be consulted or be able to decide. Less than 50 percent of the patients admitted were able to participate in decision-making in the only British study which determined the views of acutely ill patients.[9] However, following the acute phase of illness most elderly patients spend a further 7–14 days in hospital prior to discharge. Some elderly patients spend months in hospital. These patients by necessity still require a CPR status.

On our service we have been approaching such competent patients, whose discharge was not imminent, to gauge their resuscitation wishes. It was made clear to these patients that such decisions had been formerly made by the doctors and if they so wished we would still decide. However, if they wanted to choose their own CPR status, we would implement their choice. On this basis we changed a number of the resuscitation orders held by such patients.

We found that none of the patients was upset by the consultation. Most made their own decision, and those choosing not to be resuscitated usually elaborated their answers unasked, with reasons such as, "No, I'm old and tired of life", or "No, definitely not. I have nothing to live

for." The patients who wanted resuscitation were less specific, simply replying in affirmative terms.

We therefore chose to examine the reasons patients may have for their resuscitation preference and to see whether decision-making correlates with measurable anxiety or depression ratings using the Hospital Anxiety and Depression scale (HAD).[10]

Since CPR decision-making implies informed consent, we decided to measure the degree to which the patients were informed, whether their reasoning was consistent with their beliefs and whether their decision was based on such reasoning. We were interested in whether the choice was stable or whether a change had occurred one week after decision-making.

Methods

Patients with a mental test score of >8 on an Abbreviated Mental Test[11] were eligible for the study. However, we excluded patients whom we considered overtly anxious or depressed, or whom we thought might be upset at participating in such decision-making. The patients were interviewed during the rehabilitation phase of their illness when medically stable, usually within 2–7 days after admission to hospital.

They were initially approached by the registrar responsible for their care (MA) in order to obtain their preference regarding CPR. It was explained that "occasionally patients have a cardiac arrest. This means that the heart stops beating and, as no blood is pumped around the body, death occurs. In hospitals we usually try to start the heart up again by using various techniques", and described were cardiac massage, bag mask ventilation, drug therapy and defibrillation. "In about one out of ten cases of cardiac arrest we manage to start the heart up again. The procedure itself may have complications such as broken ribs and sometimes brain damage. I would like to ask you whether you would like us to try and start the heart up again if you had a cardiac arrest?"

The patients were reassured that this was not expected in their case but that their opinion

Table 53.1   Analysis of CPR decision-making by elderly patients

Patient	Age	AMT score	HAD score		Patient decision	Unsolicited reasons given by patients at first interview	Stability of choice	Recall score
			Anxiety	Depression				
LN	78	9	9	12	FR	I think I would, I've got everything to live for	–	–
LB	94	10	13	14	FR	Of course I want to live	–	–
AH	83	10	–	–	FR	Oh yes	–	–
HRM	85	10	7	6	FR	I think so	–	–
LH	80	10	7	12	FR	I suppose so	–	–
BD	83	9	–	–	NFR	Finish me off. I've had my life. I've got little to live for	–	–
RH	84	8	–	–	FR	I would, I've got all my friends and neighbours	NFR	4
PH	85	10	6	10	FR	Yes but it's up to you	FR	2
PP	92	10	11	10	Unsure	If I would cause aggravation I would call it a day	Unsure	3
NF	73	10	2	2	FR	Oh yes	FR	2
FM	81	10	7	6	FR	No not really but it's worth a try	NFR	2
ME	85	10	–	–	FR	Life is important, age does not matter	FR	1
EW	93	10	7	7	ER	I suppose so. I don't want to die yet	FR	4
EP	81	9	4	5	FR	Yes but I'm not too sure	FR	4
RM	80	9	11	5	FR	I don't want to die	FR	0
FC	86	10	8	4	FR	Oh yes there is life	FR	4
AS	80	10	14	13	NFR	I've got a strong heart. I feel so tired I don't want to go on	NFR	3
JW	75	10	10	4	FR	I think so, where there is life there is hope	FR	6
KC	80	10	5	2	FR	Life is sweet	FR	0

was important in letting us know what they wanted done for them and that we would abide by it.

The HAD testing was done two or three days later.

One week after the initial interview the patients were approached by one of us (IS) who obtained informed consent in order to discuss with them the reasons for their CPR decision and their recall of the information provided by MA. These interviews were taped. The patients were asked whether they remembered discussing CPR with the doctor, what was said, what they decided, the reasons for their decision and whether they still stood by their decision.

Results

Nineteen patients entered the study, 14 females and 5 males. Ages ranged from 73 to 94. Mean age 83. (See table 53.1.)

Our CPR decisions, based on the likelihood of a successful outcome, favoured CPR in 18 of the patients. In one case (LH) we would have chosen not to resuscitate the patient because of underlying heart disease and her bed-bound state, but not because of a predictably futile outcome.

Eighteen patients were able to make their own decision and one patient was unsure. Three of the patients' decisions differed from ours. Unsolicited comments were made by all of the patients at the time of the initial interview, and these are recorded in the table. No patient appeared distressed at the initial interview.

The HAD questionnaire was administered to 15 of the patients and the results are tabulated. A score of seven or less indicates non-cases, scores of 8–10 indicate doubtful cases and scores of 11 or more indicate definite cases. Using this scale, two patients present as definite cases of depression, two as anxious and two had high scores for both anxiety and depression. One of these patients chose not to be resuscitated at first interview.

Six patients refused the second interview but nevertheless five made revealing comments reflecting disturbance:

LN said "I'm up to here with everything. I have no more to say. I said it all to Dr Aziz. I spent two hours with him."

AH found the question about CPR disturbing and did not want to talk any further about it. She said the subject upset her and she could not sleep that night. She wanted to block the matter out of her mind.

LB volunteered that "he (MA) was funny. Not a proper doctor. What was he talking about?" She said she had a pacemaker so her heart would not stop. "I should not be here. I've lived too long. I've been lost since my husband died."

HRM said "I don't want to answer any questions. It played on my mind and it makes me feel sick to think about it. I wish I hadn't said yes."

LH remembered talking to the doctor, but not about heart massage and refused to be further interviewed.

BD said he could remember discussion with the doctor but not the topic. When prompted he said "When you're dead that's it."

Thirteen patients were interviewed in depth regarding their recall of the information given and the reasons for their decision-making. Two patients had changed their minds from wanting CPR to not wanting it. One patient was still unsure and thought the doctor should decide. Twelve patients thought they should decide.

On testing for content recall using eight categories of content: 9/13 patients remembered

that the heart stopped and could be restarted; 10/13 patients remembered about heart massage; 5/13 remembered an electric shock was used; 2/13 recalled that the procedure could be complicated by brain damage; 1/13 recalled artificial breathing. No patient recalled the use of drugs or the chances of success.

Of the 12 patients who were able to decide, 8 were debatably not providing fully informed consent. In brief:

Two patients appeared not to have understood the explanation:

PH said his reasons for wanting CPR were that he thought he would be helping with an experiment involving research on the heart and "Why not? It helps you, and you are helping me." When asked whether he thought CPR would help him he answered "Yes and no."

NF thought he was helping medical science by having a donor card and "allowing his heart to be taken out and fastened up this way or that. I may as well have it. Somebody's got to learn. Somebody's got to try them out."

Four patients wanted CPR without appreciating that the risks of the procedure were not consistent with their beliefs:

ME, when asked about her conversation with MA, said "He didn't tell me anything about it but asked what I thought. And I said life's happy yet and I would like to be resuscitated. The only thing is if I were to go really into a coma I'd like to be left."

EP, when asked for her reasons, said "You've got to make up your mind if it's really going to be helpful or not". When asked if the doctor had given any indication of how helpful it could be, she said "No, he was very careful not to do that so that he wouldn't put me in a spot. I decided beforehand that if anything was available to me and I needed it I'd use it."

FC said "I would want to be brought back. Where there's life there's hope even if someone is in a coma. I thought it was a funny question to ask. It frightened me a bit. If you can save a life, I don't care how much it costs but I wouldn't like to be a cabbage."

EW said "I've seen it on television. He asked if my heart stopped beating would I want it restarted and I said 'yes, wouldn't you?'" The interviewer asked if she remembered any risks to the procedure. The patient said, "Are there risks to it then? No I can't remember. I knew what he meant about he restarted it and I said yes but I didn't know anything about it being dangerous you know."

Two patients had no recall of the first interview:

KC had no recollection of cardiac massage ever having been mentioned. On being reminded she said that she thought it was all hypothetical and that God decides. However, she would expect to be helped and still chose resuscitation.

RM could not remember heart massage ever being mentioned to her. When reminded of the procedure and asked if she would still want it, she said "Yes, if it happens. I know I'm not young, but if my heart stopped something would have to be done because I have a family, two brothers I like to be with as much as I can."

Two patients changed their mind at the second interview, one of whom was upset:

RH became tearful when approached for the second interview because she could not read the consent form, never having learned to read or write. She did agree to further discussion at which time she said she wouldn't want to be brought back if she died, but would want a proper burial to be with her husband.

FM said "I first thought yes, if it's going to help after I died. But if you are already gone what's the good of fetching you back. That's what I've been thinking. When you are old what's the good of fetching you back. It would be better in a younger person."

Two patients could be said to have given consistent and informed consent:

AS said "I don't want anyone jumping and bumping on my chest bringing me back from the dead. I live alone. When my time has come I want to go. At my age and with the pain, there's no need to come back. The decision is final. I've read a lot about it."

JW said "The doctor told me about brain damage and I think that where there's life there's hope. The brain damage is a minimal risk and with a lot of people, they would rather have an old person who is with them even in an institution or hospital where they could visit. They've still got that time with them. I think

some may think they are better off dead, but most people would want it."

Discussion

Most British studies, although asking patients for their resuscitation preference, do not specify whether this preference was used in decision-making or whether the patients were necessarily aware that they were deciding on their own outcome.

One study, in which 92 percent of the patients wanted CPR, attributed this to the fact that the patients were not considering their circumstances to be hypothetical.[12] Yet this study, after broadly informing the patients about CPR, without indicating the chances of success, obtained the data by asking four questions dealing with general issues pertaining to CPR and a fifth question asking "Would you wish CPR if you had a cardiac arrest?" These patients, in keeping with the other studies, were happy to discuss their views. The authors do not indicate whether they acted on the patients' wishes.

In our study all except one patient indicated their CPR preference and none seemed upset at the time of questioning. However, one week later six patients appeared to have been distressed by the decision-making, two patients in an unequivocal fashion. Four patients had no recollection of the discussion regarding CPR although two continued to express a wish for active intervention.

Difficulties With Recollection

In a paper by Schade and Muslin,[13] in which resuscitation was thought to be a hopeless option, six patients who were asked to consent to NFR orders became disturbed. In three of the patients there were difficulties with recollection or processing of the information given. Some of our patients' responses were similar in this respect, suggesting psychological harm.

An explanation for the distress invoked by asking patients to determine their own resuscitation status, which is not apparent in the questionnaire-based studies, might be the immediacy of the possibility of cardiac arrest for this patient group. In the large group studies the patients were being canvassed regarding their views, and the inclusion of their CPR preference amongst a wide variety of issues relating to CPR may not have been perceived by them to have much bearing on what would ultimately happen to them in the event of a cardiac arrest.

In asking patients to make CPR decisions we are subscribing to the principle of autonomy. Even if there is only a marginal chance of success, it may be argued that it is only the patient who ought to decide whether to accept or reject this chance.

Failure to involve competent patients in end-of-life decisions has been described as generally, but perhaps not always, a form of crass paternalism.[14] Paternalism is regarded as being wrong because it interferes with the right of individuals to control aspects of their lives in accordance with their own values.

The exercising of autonomy requires both intellectual and emotional competence as well as the opportunity for action. We would deprive a person of the opportunity for action by choosing for him, as one would do by non-consultation in CPR decision-making.

However, if an individual makes a choice, without understanding the implications of that choice, or because of emotional factors which impair judgment, that person may not be functioning with the degree of autonomy we would normally expect to be present in a competent adult.

Hospers[15] points out that we can accept the truth of a moral principle, but that instances reflecting the exercise of that moral principle are empirical and hence need to be individually evaluated and can only be evaluated in terms of the agent concerned.

Hence:

1. Allowing patients to exercise autonomy in CPR decision-making is right.
2. This act is a case of the exercising of autonomy in CPR decision-making.
3. Therefore this act is right.

Premise three depends on the truth of premise two and the nature of the act will differ for different agents. As it is a false assumption to believe that all individuals are equally autonomous in their behaviour, the rightness or wrongness of the act depends on the particular case rather than the broad moral principle.

Our results tend to show that individuals manifest differing degrees of competence, both intellectual and emotional, in that some of our patients were intellectually unable to grasp the situation and others emotionally unable to deal with it. As competence and autonomy are inter-related the autonomy of decision-making in such cases becomes suspect.

Fitten and Waite[16] showed the decision-making capacity of elderly hospitalised patients to be impaired when compared with a matched non-hospitalised group. Their study cast strong doubts about such patients' capacity to give truly informed consent, particularly where complex or risky treatments, such as resuscitation, were involved. They also showed that neither physicians' evaluations nor results of a mental state examination could identify the seriously decisionally impaired patients. Attention is drawn to these marginally competent patients, so that their limited autonomy can be respected and appropriate protection instituted where necessary. They accept, however, that we have no prospective means of identifying such patients.

It is a pity that elderly patients have served as the focus of this debate. This is because they are in a number of senses a vulnerable patient population. They are often chronically ill and suffer from a significant degree of unrecognised depression. Although our measures of cognitive function exclude obvious dementing disease, they do not reflect subtle memory and judgment failure and the poor educational opportunities experienced by some people born at the beginning of [the last] century.

On the other hand this is the population in whom it appears some people would not wish for CPR whatever the outcome, and in whom CPR has poorer prospects of success, particularly when viewed against a background of general debility and multiple pathology.

Loewy points out that forcing patients to make a choice in a situation in which they would prefer not to choose is not an exercise in autonomy, rather another type of paternalism.[17]

On the basis of respecting the wishes of those patients who would not want to be involved in such decision-making, perhaps some form of invitation might be provided to those entering the hospital. This would explain the existence of a resuscitation policy, and offer them the opportunity to discuss it with their doctor if they want to be instrumental in determining their own resuscitation status.

Although an obvious limitation to this study is the small number of patients entered, we believe these patients to be representative of apparently cognitively intact elderly individuals who might be thought capable of participating in their own decision-making regarding CPR.

Our results prove contrary, both in highlighting the faulty reasoning employed by some patients, and in demonstrating psychological pain which has been said to be the only justification for paternalism in these circumstances. We suggest further work directed at identifying those patients who want to be involved in determining their own CPR status, and how best to inform them, before approaching mentally alert patients (as Mead and Turnbull have proposed) in order to identify in advance those who would not desire CPR in the event of a cardiac arrest.[18]

NOTES

1 Doyal, L., Wilsher, D., "Withholding cardiopulmonary resuscitation: Proposals for formal guidelines," *British Medical Journal* 306 (1993): 1593–6.
2 Ibid.
3 McIntyre, K. M., "Failure of 'predictors' of cardiopulmonary resuscitation outcomes to predict cardiopulmonary resuscitation outcomes," *Archives of Internal Medicine* 153 (1993): 1293–6.
4 Mead, G. E., Turnbull, C. J., "Cardiopulmonary resuscitation in the elderly: Patients' and relatives' views," *Journal of Medical Ethics* 21 (1995): 39–44; Bruce-Jones, P., Roberts, H., Bowker, L., and Cooney, V., "Resuscitating the elderly: What do the patients want?" *Journal of Medical Ethics* 22 (1996): 154–9; Liddle, J., Gilleard, C., and Neil, A., "The views of elderly patients and their relatives on cardiopulmonary resuscitation," *Journal of the Royal College of Physicians of London* 28 (1994): 228–9; Potter, J. M., Stewart, D., and Duncan, G., "Living wills: Would sick people change their minds?" *Postgraduate Medical Journal* 70 (1994): 818–20.
5 Hill, M. E., MacQuillan, G., Forsyth, M., and Heath, D. A., "Cardiopulmonary resuscitation: Who makes the decision?" *British Medical Journal* 308 (1994): 1677; Bruce-Jones et al., "Resuscitating the elderly."
6 Hill et al., "Cardiopulmonary resuscitation"; Morgan, R., King, D., Prajapati, C., and Rowe, J., "Views of elderly patients and their relatives on cardiopulmonary resuscitation," *British Medical Journal* 308 (1994): 1677–8; Bruce-Jones et al., "Resuscitating the elderly"; Liddle et al., "The views of elderly patients and their relatives on cardiopulmonary resuscitation"; Potter et al., "Living wills."
7 Murphy, K. J., Burrows, D., Santilli, S., Kemp, A. W., Tenner, S., and Kreling, B., "The influence of the probability of survival on patients' preferences regarding cardiopulmonary resuscitation," *New England Journal of Medicine* 330 (1983): 545–9.
8 Doyal and Wilsher, "Withholding cardiopulmonary resuscitation."
9 Potter et al., "Living wills."
10 Zigmond, A. S. and Snaith, R. P., "The Hospital Anxiety and Depression Scale," *Acta Psychiatrica* 86 (1983): 1–10.
11 Hodkinson, H. M., "Evolution of a mental test score for assessment of mental impairment in the elderly," *Age and Ageing* 1 (1972): 233–8.
12 Potter et al., "Living wills."
13 Schade, S. G. and Muslin, H., "Do not resuscitate decisions: Discussions with patients," *Journal of Medical Ethics* 15 (1989): 186–90.
14 Loewy, E. H., "Involving patients in do not resuscitate decisions: An old issue raising its ugly head," *Journal of Medical Ethics* 17 (1991): 156–60.
15 Hospers, J., *Human Conduct. An Introduction to the Problems of Ethics* (London: Rupert Hart-Davis, 1963).
16 Fitten, L. J. and Waite, M. S., "Impact of medical hospitalization on treatment decision-making capacity in the elderly," *Archives of Internal Medicine* 150 (1990): 1717–21.
17 Loewy, "Involving patients in do not resuscitate decisions."
18 Mead and Turnbull, "Cardiopulmonary resuscitation in the elderly."

54

Can the Elderly Tolerate Endoscopy Without Sedation?

SAM A. SOLOMON, VIJAY K. KAJLA, AND ARUP K. BANERJEE

Oesophago-gastro-duodenoscopy (OGD) is an established and useful investigation for upper gastrointestinal disorders. In experienced hands it is a safe procedure, with a mortality rate of about 0.01%.[1] The majority of deaths are due to cardiorespiratory complications related to sedation rather than to perforation or haemorrhage.[2] Patients with ischaemic heart disease, stroke, gastrointestinal bleeding and anaemia are considered to be at risk, as are the elderly. They should be given little or no sedation and carefully monitored during the procedure.[3] The overall feasibility and acceptance of OGD in the elderly without sedation need to be evaluated further as it could potentially increase the number of patients examined as day cases.

Patients and Method

Sixty-two patients (42 women), mean age 79 years (range 72–97), undergoing diagnostic OGD were included in the study which was approved by Bolton Health Authority local ethics committee. Informed written consent was obtained from all patients. Details of age, sex, medical history, clinical diagnosis, indication for OGD, endoscopic findings and results

of full blood count, urea and electrolytes were recorded. Pre-existing ischaemic heart disease, obstructive airways disease and anaemia (Hb < 10 g/dl) were present in 21 (34%), 7 (11%) and 16 (26%) subjects, respectively. Endoscopy was performed by the consultant author using an Olympus GIF.XQ 20 flexible gastroscope in a dedicated endoscopy suite with full support staff and resuscitation facilities. All patients had their pharynx sprayed with lignocaine prior to OGD. The examination was undertaken in the left lateral position. At baseline, during, at extubation and five minutes after OGD, blood pressure, oxygen saturation and cardiac rhythm were recorded as previously described.[4]

The patients were randomised into two groups to receive either:

- sedation with intravenous midazolam (mean dose 2 mg), given as a slow injection over two minutes to produce drowsiness or slurred speech (group A); or
- no sedation prior to OGD (group B).

The two randomised groups were similar in age, sex distribution, risk factors and vital signs at baseline (table 54.1).

On recovery from the procedure, and prior to transfer from the recovery ward, responses to the following questions were recorded:

- What degree of discomfort did you experience while swallowing the instrument?
- What degree of discomfort did you experience during the examination?

Choices for response to both these questions were: tolerable; mildly unpleasant; very unpleasant.

- If given the choice in the future, would you prefer to be sedated or not?

Any volunteered comments on this question were recorded.

Data on oxygen saturation and haemodynamic changes from two patients in group A who were sedated and subsequently given supplementary oxygen were excluded from analysis. However, their responses to the questionnaire were included in the analysis.

Statistical analysis

Differences in continuous variables between the two groups were compared by Student's t-test, and categorical variables by χ^2 test where appropriate.

Results

Sedation did not ameliorate the discomfort suffered by patients during intubation; 78% and 80% in groups A and B respectively found intubation mildly unpleasant (table 54.2), and almost the same percentage of patients in both groups described the procedure as tolerable (16% vs 13%). No significant differences were noted in the percentage of patients in the two groups who found the examination mildly unpleasant (63% vs 57%). Surprisingly, although the majority of patients in group B described the intubation and examination as unpleasant, when given the choice of having sedation for future OGD almost three-quarters did not want to be sedated. Eighteen patients in this group gave the

following reasons for their choices: five found the procedure bearable and not a problem; 10 wanted to be aware of the procedure and avoid the inconvenience of a recovery period; and three had not known about the effects of sedation. Five patients in group B who had had OGD under sedation in the past expressed a preference for sedation for any future OGD as they did not recall the procedure being as unpleasant as it was on this occasion. The main reason given by the group A patients for future preference for sedation was apprehension by 10 (48%). Eleven (52%) gave no reason, probably because of partial or total amnesia of the procedure, and five wanted no sedation in future because of curiosity. Six group A patients did not record a preference.

Oxygen saturation

There were no significant differences in oxygen saturation during OGD between the groups, although there was a slight transient fall in oxygen saturation in group A after sedation and during OGD, which returned to baseline after extubation (table 54.3).

Blood pressure, heart rate and arrhythmias

Heart rate increased transiently in both groups during OGD, more so in group B, but the differences between the groups were not significant (table 54.3). One patient in group B with a history of chronic obstructive airways disease developed transient self-terminating supraventricular tachycardia of 180 beats/min lasting for 30 seconds during antral biopsy; no treatment was required. No other serious arrhythmias were noted.

Discussion

In experienced hands, OGD without sedation is acceptable in elderly patients with or without co-existing anaemia and cardiorespiratory disorders. The examination was successful in nearly all subjects and sedation did not seem to influence tolerability. A similar study in unselected patients, mean age 57 years (range 15–85), showed that OGD without sedation was feasible without complications, although the patients'

Table 54.1 Comparison of randomised groups; values are means (±sd) unless otherwise stated.

	Group A (sedated, $n = 32$)	Group B (unsedated, $n = 30$)
Age (years)	79 (range 72–89)	79 (72–97)
Male/female	10/22	10/20
Blood pressure (mmHg)	148 (±25)/74 (±18)	146 (±30)/77 (±17)
Pulse (bpm)	88 (±16)	89 (±15)
Haemoglobin (g/dl)	12.2 (±2.5)	11.6 (±2.7)
Blood urea (mmol/l)	8.1 (± 3.6)	8.1 (±3.4)
Oxygen saturation (%)	93 (±2)	93 (±3)
Midazolam (mg)	2 (range 1.0–2.5)	
Medical history		
IHD/heart failure	9 (28%)	12 (40%)
COPD/asthma	3 (9%)	4 (13%)
Stroke/Parkinson's disease	1 (3%)	1 (3%)
Anaemia (Hb < 10 g/dl)	7 (22%)	9 (30%)

IHD = ischaemic heart disease
COPD = chronic obstructive pulmonary disease

Table 54.2 Tolerance to oesophago-gastro-duodenoscopy; responses to questionnaire.

	Group A (sedated, $n = 32$)	Group B (unsedated, $n = 30$)
Intubation		
Tolerable	5 (16%)	4 (13%)
Mildly unpleasant	25 (78%)	24 (80%)
Very unpleasant	1	2
Unrecorded/don't know	1	0
Examination		
Tolerable	10 (31%)	12 (40%)
Mildly unpleasant	20 (63%)	17 (57%)
Very unpleasant	1	1
Unrecorded/don't know	1	0
Future choice		
Sedation	21 (66%)	5 (17%)
No sedation	5 (16%)	22 (73%)
Unrecorded/don't know	6 (19%)	3 (10%)

assessments of the procedure were not recorded.[5] The elderly tolerate oesophageal intubation without sedation better than younger patients during trans-oesophageal echocardiography.[6] With adequate counselling and explanation, the anxiety and apprehension generated prior to the procedure could be alleviated. OGD without sedation is less likely to cause severe oxygen desaturation which is believed to precipitate cardiac ischaemia and arrhythmia.[7]

Conclusion

Some elderly patients may not wish to be sedated during OGD and should be given the choice of undergoing the procedure without sedation. Those who are at particular risk of cardiorespiratory complications could be examined safely without sedation. Full counselling and frank explanation of the procedure are,

Table 54.3   Changes in oxygen saturation, heart rate and blood pressure; values are means ($\pm$ sd).

	Group A (sedated, $n = 30$)*	Group B (unsedated, $n = 30$)
Oxygen saturation (%)		
Baseline	93.0 ($\pm$2.4)	93.0 ($\pm$3.0)
After sedation	92.8 ($\pm$3.0)	
During gastroscopy	92.3 ($\pm$3.5)	92.5 ($\pm$3.2)
After extubation	94.0 ($\pm$2.5)	93.9 ($\pm$2.6)
Blood pressure (mmHg)		
Baseline	148 ($\pm$25)/74 ($\pm$18)	146 ($\pm$30)/77 ($\pm$17)
After sedation	156 ($\pm$27)/86 ($\pm$21)	
During gastroscopy	155 ($\pm$30)/79 ($\pm$26)	158 ($\pm$34)/86 ($\pm$19)
After extubation	144 ($\pm$28)/79 ($\pm$26)	153 ($\pm$26)/81 ($\pm$13)
Heart rate (bpm)		
Baseline	88 ($\pm$16)	89 ($\pm$15)
After sedation	90 ($\pm$14)	
During gastroscopy	93 ($\pm$16)	98 ($\pm$25)
After extubation	84 ($\pm$20)	86 ($\pm$17)

*Excludes two patients given supplemental oxygen.

however, even more important if the procedure is undertaken without any sedation.

NOTES

Technical assistance from the nursing and theatre staff of the endoscopy suite at Bolton General Hospital is gratefully acknowledged.

1   Silvis, S. E., Nebel, O., Rogers, G., Sugawa, C., and Mandelstan, P., "Endoscopic complications: Results of the 1974 American Society for Gastrointestinal Endoscopy Survey," *JAMA* 235 (1976): 928–30.

2   Ibid; Daneshmend, T. K., Logan, R. F. A., and Bell, G. D., "Sedation for upper gastrointestinal endoscopy: The results of a national survey," *Gut* 32 (1991): 112–15.

3   Bell, G. D., McCloy, R. F., Charlton, J. E., and Campbell, D. et al., "Recommendations for standards of sedation and patient monitoring during gastrointestinal endoscopy," *Gut* 32 (1991): 823–7; Solomon, S. A., Isaac, T., and Banerjee, A. K., "Oxygen desaturation during endoscopy in the elderly," *J R Coll. Physicians Lond.* 27 (1993): 16–18.

4   Solomon et al., "Oxygen desaturation during endoscopy in the elderly."

5   Pecora, A. A., Chiesa, J. C., Alloy, A. M., Santoro, J., and Lazarus, B., "The effect of upper gastrointestinal endoscopy on arterial oxygen tension in smokers and non-smokers with and without premedication," *Gastrointest. Endosc.* 30 (1984): 84–8.

6   De Belder, M. A., Leech, G., and Camm, J. A., "Transoesophageal echocardiography in unsedated outpatients: Technique and patient tolerance," *J. Am. Soc. Echo.* 2 (1985): 375–9.

7   Liberman, D. A., Wuerker, D. K., and Katon, R. M., "Cardiopulmonary risk of oesophago-gastro-duodenoscopy: Role of endoscopic diameter and systematic sedation," *Gastroenterology* 88 (1985): 468–72; Rostykus, P. S., McDonald, G. B., and Albert, R. K., "Upper intestinal endoscopy induces hypoxaemia in patients with obstructive pulmonary disease," *Gastroenterology* 78 (1980): 488–91; Fleischer, D., "Monitoring the patient receiving conscious sedation for gastrointestinal endoscopy: Issues and guidance," *Gastrointest. Endosc.* 35 (1987): 262–6; Bell, G. D., Brown, N. S., Morden, A., Coady, T., and Logan, R. S., "Prevention of hypoxaemia during upper gastrointestinal endoscopy by means of oxygen via nasal cannulae," *Lancet* i (1987): 1022–4.

55

Fighting Spirit: the Stories of Women in the Bristol Breast Cancer Survey

MYLES HARRIS, VICKI HARRIS, AND HEATHER GOODARE

When the Kind Cure May Kill
Dr Myles Harris

The astonishing news that counselling, holistic medicine and spiritual support might make cancer worse seems scarcely credible. But it may be so.

In a report published in the *Lancet* two groups of women suffering from breast cancer were compared. One group received the normal treatment – radiotherapy, surgery and drugs. The other received the standard treatment plus being offered attendance at the Bristol Cancer Help Centre. The centre, opened by the Prince of Wales seven years ago, offers patients counselling, spiritual and emotional support and treatments with diet, touch and holistic remedies. The disease-free survival of these women was, the report concludes, 'significantly poorer' than those women who got the no-frills therapy.

While the youth of patients attending the centre may have been a factor, 'It is certainly possible,' concludes the report, 'that the BCHC attenders may, in some subtle way, have worse diseases than our controlled series [*sic*], the possibility that some aspect of the centre's regimen may be responsible for their decreased survival must be faced.'

Statistics are slippery things. I have on my desk a paper that shows Vitamin C to be marvellously beneficial in the treatment of cancer, and one, equally authoritatively, demonstrating that it is about as useful as a glass of cold water at the bottom of a swimming pool.

But not all statistics are wrong. The Bristol study was conducted by reputable people of good faith. It appears to be sound. It also shows a healthy respect for the truth by the centre that it offered to take part. If we are to assume what was found was true, it is important to speculate why.

Alternative medicine is, next to Islam, the fastest growing religion – albeit a secular one – in Britain. Counselling, a large element of alternative medicine, is a form of confessional capitalism, an idea that illness is caused by consumerism and can only be cured by a form of secular love from strangers called 'caring'.

There are counselling chapters in almost all towns. In London it supports an expensive PR organisation and no tragedy is ever enacted on

TV without the reporter genuflecting to the need for the victims to be counselled. But if it becomes evident that such popularist support groups, however well-intentioned, can do harm, then we need to know quickly.

If the Bristol Cancer Help Centre adheres to the principles of the easy democracy of self-help and alternative medicine it will emphasise the informal. There will be none of the usual signs of a hospital; the clanking of trolleys, the mysterious, dimly frightening noises of crashing metal, the sweet sour medical smells or bowel-loosening signs to places like 'Main Operating Theatre'.

In alternative centres there will be no sisters in blue with clipboards, nor spotty medical students nor doctors waving terrifying looking X-rays. Instead the unit will be as much like home as possible.

The staff at such centres tend to be inflexibly informal, smiling people who insist on the use of Christian names. Elitist authority symbols such as 'Doctor', 'Nurse' or 'Father', they will tell you, only serve to distance the patient.

How on earth could such inoffensive methods affect the progress of a tumour? One alarming possibility is that the centre quite inadvertently attracts people with a greater liability to die from cancer than normal. How could that be?

The answer may lie in the work of Professor Hans Eysenck and Grossarth-Maticek at the Institute of Psychiatry in London. They have controversially described personalities that are 'overly cooperative, weak, unassertive, over-patient, defensive, harmony seeking and compliant' as particularly prone to cancer.

Studies of such people over 20 years suggest that they have a much higher incidence of cancer than aggressive or well-balanced personality types.

It is not unreasonable to speculate that this is where a flaw in the alternative treatment of cancer might lie. For holistic and 'support' therapies, far from being radical alternatives to conventional treatment, are the essence of consumerist compliance. Instead of such therapies teaching the patient to get up and fight – Eysenck's categories of personality suggest that aggressive hostile people and well-adjusted people are many times less likely to get cancer – alternative medicine's emphasis on 'non-confrontational techniques' may teach the cancer victim to lie down and whisper comfortable phrases about 'caring' or being 'in touch with himself'.

Such instructions may well send his natural killer cells, designed to destroy cancer, to sleep. Thus the poor prognosis.

This is unlikely to happen in a normal hospital. They are not meant to be frightening, but they inadvertently show you just enough of 'the instruments' to make you aware of danger.

The figures from this study show that the fear-inspiring conventional hospital may have over the centuries evolved at least part of the correct mixture of order, rank and discipline to offer at least some hope of a cure. People are reassured by uniforms, stimulated by struggles and needled by fear. In the midst of such struggles they often discover who really among their relatives and friends loves them. In such lessons lie the roots of personality change.

Another alternative exists, but for it to happen it would mean the 'carers' having to lie down with the psychological school of Professor Eysenck, a man whose wildly controversial work on race and intelligence and demolition of the idea that you can measure any effect from conventional psychotherapy (such therapy must, I believe, include a good deal of counselling and alternative medicine) rank him almost as the Beast of the Apocalypse in Left-wing eyes.

Eysenck of course is no beast, but a scientist before his time. His worse sin in caring eyes is his advocacy of behaviour therapy – a highly modified form of conditioning which involves learning to recognise and alter disabling personality traits. It has been used, successfully, to lower the risk of cancer in vulnerable groups, and improve prognosis in patients with cancer. Breast cancer patients on chemotherapy showed an increase in survival (over an average of 11.28 months) of 2.8 months. On behaviour therapy the increase was 3.64 months. Together the two treatments reinforced each other, resulting in a mean survival time of 22.4 months.

The holistic movement, if it has ignored such studies, cannot afford to do so any longer.

Having had the courage to submit their work to ruthless scientific scrutiny they must now, like any other medical discipline, be willing to throw untested, well-meaning assumptions overboard in favour of facts. Eysenck may be their man.

[...]

A Cancer in Medical Statistics
Vicki Harris

As I was one of the women involved in the Bristol Cancer Help Centre mentioned by Dr Myles Harris, I would like to put the other side of the story.

I attended Bristol in April 1987 at the age of 37 having undergone a mastectomy and radiotherapy treatment for breast cancer. The centre puts the patient back in control, something that the negative attitudes of doctors and nurses cannot do. (I even comforted a crying nurse who became upset when hearing of my poor prognosis.)

Bristol does not have magic cures, nor does it promise to extend life span, but it does give one the opportunity to reassess the situation, release any old emotions and help the patient face prospective death as positively as possible.

Emotions obviously run high, but if the media knew what damage is done to patients by surveys and statistics that don't give the full story then I am sure reporting would be handled with more care.

Over the past three years, through connections with Bristol, I have met many people with cancer, some of whom have died, but they died by their rules, being able (thanks to the teachings of Bristol) to go with no guilt and the ability to look loved ones in the eye to say goodbye. How can this be so badly criticised?

Coda
Heather Goodare

'It is when I am weak that I am strong' – 2 Corinthians 12:10

So can the self affect the course of cancer? Logically, if psychological factors can contrib-

ute to the onset of cancer, they can also play a part in recovery. A recent study looked at 33 individuals who have lived for an extended period despite a 'terminal' medical prognosis.[1] The author, Warren Berland, tackles the question of how far retrospective self-reports are accurate: the same question arises with this book. Looking back at my own contribution, I acknowledge freely that I have been selective in my self-report (it would otherwise have been far too long). But I have tried to be honest, and where possible I have checked it against notes made contemporaneously.

Berland also asks 'How can we know whether patients' self-reports have any relation to factors that actually influence healing and survival?' To what extent do patients distort their narratives? I don't think it matters very much if there is distortion: this will inevitably occur. People will select or 'distort' for two main reasons: to preserve privacy or avoid offence, and to attribute meaning to their own experience. (In what way can the opinion of the consultant who sees the patient for a few minutes in each year of follow-up be more 'true' than the patient's own self-report?) I do find it very interesting, though, that Berland's key findings were that 'support of family and friends, and changes in attitude, were the most significant attributions regarding recovery – surpassing even the role of medical treatment, both conventional and alternative.'

We also need to ask to what extent adverse events can affect survival after the onset of illness.[2] The stories here seem to point to a connection in some cases. Sigyn's long struggle to have her disease acknowledged, let alone treated, must have been a serious setback emotionally, as well as saddling her with the huge physical handicap of a very late diagnosis. Those who knew her would not have characterised her as bitter (quite the opposite), but she must have borne much inward stress.

It is important too to try to assess the emotional damage done by the *Lancet* report itself to the women who willingly participated in the study. Among this small sample, Joanna seems to have been the one who was the most deeply affected, perhaps because she had taken the whole Bristol programme so very seriously, especially in her own work as a counsellor.

'I believe the *Lancet* report was a major blow to her', writes her husband, implying that this may have accelerated the disease process.

There may have been others who lost faith in what they were doing; who, while not believing the report, felt perhaps there could not have been smoke without fire. The Centre itself seemed to waver, and made modifications to its programme: the impact on the staff was severe. There was also an impact not just on women who had taken part in the survey, but on other patients who had visited Bristol, especially women with breast cancer. In one case, while the woman herself remained emotionally robust, her teenage daughter became distraught, thinking her mother must be about to die. This girl needed professional counselling before she could regain mental health.[3]

As to whether or not people who go to Bristol are 'different' in some way from the general population of cancer patients, we still have no clear evidence one way or the other. Sir Walter Bodmer, the then director of research at the ICRF, reckoned that a 'useful observation to emerge from the study' was that 'patients are attracted to complementary medicine when they feel their outlook is unpromising'.[4] We surely did not need such a report to tell us anything so obvious. Indeed, some people only seek the help of the Centre on the recurrence of their cancer, or when all else has failed and orthodox doctors have declared 'There is nothing more we can do.'

However, 'disasters can lead to opportunities',[5] and the Bristol study is no exception. The work of the Bristol Survey Support Group has shown that the subjects of research must be respected as more than mere statistics. Indeed, a rich vein of material lies unexploited unless such subjects are truly listened to, and researchers would do well to make better use of them as a resource for designing research that is both more relevant to patients' needs and avoids obvious and preventable pitfalls.[6]

Further than this, we might with profit engage the conscious cooperation of patients right from the start in any research that has a psychosocial component. The major complaints of the women in this survey were not just that the statistics were poor, but that the methods

used were inappropriate and that the promised quality of life study was never undertaken. The study of holistic medicine demands holistic research methods. New ways must be found of marrying qualitative and quantitative approaches: both have something to contribute.

Finally, what this book clearly illustrates is that the naïve research subject is a myth. The 'father' of client-centred therapy, Carl Rogers, went further, saying:

> *Suppose we enlisted every 'subject' as an 'investigator'!* Instead of the wise researcher measuring changes in his subjects, suppose he enlisted them all as coresearchers. There is now ample evidence that the so-called naïve subject is a figment of the imagination. The moment a person becomes the object of psychological investigation he starts developing his own fantasies as to the purpose of the study. Then, depending on his temperament and his feeling for the researcher, he sets out either to help develop the finding he thinks is wanted, or to defeat the purpose of the study. Why not bypass all this by making him a member of the research team?[7]

If this had been done in the case of the Bristol study, perhaps some worthwhile findings might have emerged. The anonymous 'controls' whose data were simply culled from cancer registries without their knowledge or consent might also have had something useful to say on the matter.

The women in this survey were distressed at the way in which they were used as pawns[8] in what they saw as a stage battle between orthodox and so-called 'alternative' practitioners. They saw the Bristol Centre not as 'alternative' but as complementary to mainstream medicine, which indeed it has always been. In nearly every case the women went to Bristol to find something not readily available to them locally in National Health Service settings. However, in the past few years the value of complementary approaches in the care of cancer patients has been recognised,[9] and many hospices and cancer centres now offer a range of gentle therapies. This is surely as it should be: as Rachel remarked in our film *Cancer Positive*, 'We should all be working together.'

NOTES

1 Berland, W., 'Can the self affect the course of cancer? Unexpected cancer recovery: Why patients believe they survive', *Advances* 11/4 (1995): 5–19.

2 Ramirez, A. J. et al., 'Stress and relapse of breast cancer', *British Medical Journal* 298 (1989): 291–3.

3 The story was told by Lynda McGilvray in *The Cancer War Story*, BBC 2, May 23, 1995.

4 Bodmer, W., 'Bristol Cancer Help Centre' (letter). *Lancet* 336 (Nov. 10, 1990): 1188.

5 Goodare, H. and Smith, R., 'The rights of patients in research', *British Medical Journal* 310 (1995): 1277–8.

6 Bradburn, J., Maher, J., Adewuyi-Dalton, R., Grunfeld, E., Lancaster, T., and Mant, D., 'Developing clinical trial protocols: The use of patient focus groups'. *Psycho-oncology* 4/2 (1995): 107–12.

7 Rogers, C. R., *Encounter Groups*, 1973 edn (Harmondsworth: Penguin), p. 167 (first published 1970).

8 Bourke, I. and Goodare, H., 'Bristol Cancer Help Centre' (letter). *Lancet* 338 (Nov. 30, 1991): 1401.

9 Expert Advisory Group on Cancer to the Chief Medical Officers of England and Wales, *A Policy Framework for Commissioning Cancer Services* ('The Calman Report') (Department of Health, 1995), para 4.2.17.

56

What We Want from Crisis Services

PETER CAMPBELL

This [chapter] outlines some of the things some or perhaps many mental health service users/survivors want from crisis services. It is influenced by my own experience of receiving mental health services over the last twenty-eight years (sixteen admissions onto acute wards) and by my involvement in the user/survivor movement in the last ten years. It is also particularly informed by the following facts: I am a man; I am white; my crises would usually be described by most experts in terms of psychotic episodes.

I am not able to address precise definitions of mental health crisis here, but the reality that a proportion of those who are deemed to be having a mental health crisis resist such an attribution must be openly acknowledged. Numerous recipients of crisis services are not just unwilling recipients but are compelled recipients. Such disagreements have traditionally been explained through the lack of insight within the distressed persons, their inability to know what is really going on and what is in their best interests. While this approach has been very convenient in justifying control of unco-operative people, it is not the most encouraging starting-point for responses sensitive to individual wants and needs. A more sophisticated ap-

preciation of insight and a willingness to address the range of reasons why people may deny they are in a mental health crisis would be most helpful. It is certainly possible that these denials are not so much because people do not think they are in difficulty as because they object to their problems being characterised as mental illness ones or dislike the interventions being offered.

Although the manifestations of mental health crises have a wide range and may be strongly contrasted, the basic wants and needs of people in crises of this kind are probably very similar. I have regularly asked groups of survivors, groups of mental health workers and mixed groups to do an exercise imagining themselves in a mental health crisis and then drawing up lists of wants and not wants. Overall the lists are always very much the same, although people who have been through services usually have a sharper idea of what they do not want. The fact that people in crisis may have difficulty communicating or talk of worlds, concepts and perceptions with which mental health workers have limited natural sympathy should not lead to assumptions that their wants and needs are extraordinary or esoteric or that there is inevitably a gulf between what people say they want and what they really need.

On the other hand, individual wants and needs do conflict and compete. How can you reconcile someone's desire for space with someone else's desire for a feeling of physical limitation and safety in the same location and with extreme limitations on the number and flexibility of staff? It is hard to see how the traditional acute ward, wherever located, can possibly provide a sensitive response to crisis within its contradictory imperatives for supervision and privacy, containment and renewal, peace and quiet and restimulation. The widespread demand for alternative approaches and different destinations is rooted in personal experience of the barren, ordered chaos of the acute ward. When mental health service users talk about their crises, several strong themes tend to emerge and these have a vital relevance to crisis provision.

People want more control, particularly more of their own control over crisis situations. Given that many of us are unlikely to be contemplating a future where we never have another mental health crisis, the fact that we gain confidence that further crises will not destroy us is of the greatest significance. Existing services, no matter how insensitive, do often offer that reassurance. From then onwards, the desire to increase our own control in our loss of control becomes central. Recently there have been encouraging signs of a move away from approaches seeing people with a mental illness diagnosis as uncomprehending victims of outbreaks of inscrutable illnesses, towards responses asserting our essential competence and capacity to moderate our crises. Examples of this (coming perhaps from rather different perspectives) are: *Inside Out – A Guide to Self-management of Manic Depression* (Manic Depression Fellowship, 1995) and work on intervention in the preliminary (prodromal) phases of psychotic episodes (Bradshaw and Everitt, 1995).

People want to gain understanding of and from their crises. We want to learn from our crises things that are relevant to the rest of our lives. We want to integrate these experiences into the weave of all our other experience and not to carry them around with us as some separate and unsightly garment. In this regard I feel crisis services, indeed mental health services as a whole, remain clearly deficient. I remember the frequent use of the phrase 'Och, it's not the real you' to limit and circumvent aspects of my concerns when going through crisis in acute wards. Sadly, I am convinced that for many mental health workers it remains true that they do not think the content of our crises, particularly those they define as psychotic, are real, relevant or of anything but negative value. It is ironic that while increasing numbers of people in the user/survivor movement are seeking new meanings in their most vivid personal experiences, so many mental health workers continue to look the other way.

People want to be treated with respect and dignity. Clearly there are many levels to this demand. For myself, the lack of respect I now perceive is related to concerns expressed in the previous paragraph. For others the denial of respect may be far more blatant. In particular, I often wonder how different my journey through the crisis services would have been if instead of being a six-foot-four-inch white, Protestant Scotsman, I had been a six-foot-four-inch Black Rastafarian man.

No one would deny the very real difficulties of always providing a sensitive response to people in crisis. Nevertheless we should also not overlook the fact that crisis responses are still occurring that are quite obviously going to increase the trauma of those experiencing them. How is it still possible for someone in crisis picked up under section 136 of the Mental Health Act 1983 to be kept in solitary confinement for a period of hours in a police station cell while awaiting assessment?

How can anyone with a caring imagination possibly think such destinations are places of safety? It is also important that the quality of crisis care being given to people who go through Accident and Emergency Departments continues to be scrutinised. Evidence of the mistreatment of people who self-harm (including the sort of misunderstanding of people who self-harm without suicidal intent that can involve endless waiting at the bottom of the queue and being stitched up without an anaesthetic) suggests that the scope for re-education is very large.

People, particularly people involved in the user/survivor movement, want twenty-four-hour non-medical crisis services. This remains a key issue for the future of crisis services in the United Kingdom. For, although in the last ten years the demand for twenty-four-hour services has gradually gained acceptance, the demand for non-medical provision has stayed very much at the margins. This may be partly due to the refusal of psychiatrists to consider approaches challenging their reliance on medication. (It is interesting how the medical establishment's clarion cry of 'Antipsychiatry' so quickly paralyses the faculty of rational consideration.) But it is also due to a failure to define more carefully what people mean by non-medical services. Does this mean absolutely no use of medication? Does it mean not using medication as the standard first resort? Does it mean having medical and complementary approaches? Does it mean having staff teams that are not led by psychiatrists? Does it mean an open employment of the expertise of local users/survivors?

At the moment, debate on these questions does not seem to be very open and it is not easy to discover what progress has been made in different localities. Although there is evidence from other countries that it is possible to support people through crises without using neuroleptics (Mosher and Burti, 1994; Podvoll, 1990), our NHS system seems reluctant to innovate. As it stands, using the expertise of survivors and not using medication appear to be the most likely elements to be dropped from new crisis services.

I conclude on a personal note. My first crisis admission was not a medical event. For me, it was a moral event, a moral failure. All my subsequent admissions have contained shadows of that first failure. None of the important implications have been medical ones. In my view, the crucial questions about mental health crisis services are to do not with locations and technology but with understandings.

REFERENCES

Bradshaw, T. and Everitt, J. (1995) Early intervention to prevent psychotic relapse. *Mental Health Nursing* 15/6: 22–5.

Manic Depression Fellowship (1995) *Inside Out. A Guide to Self-Management of Manic Depression* (Manic Depression Fellowship).

Mosher, L. and Burti, L. (1994) *Community Mental Health – A Practical Guide* (London: Norton).

Podvoll, E. M. (1990) *Seduction of Madness – A Revolutionary Approach to Recovery at Home* (London: Century).

Part VII

Continuing Contact: Getting Well

Introduction

Jenny Lewis's story of her recovery from breast cancer continues in chapter 57 with "Wounded in Action." In this poem, describing the moment when she first sees the results of her mastectomy, Lewis appropriates a masculine discourse: she is the wounded soldier. Whereas men's war wounds can be referred to, indeed rewarded with medals and praise, a mastectomy was traditionally something best kept quiet about. By setting her story in the context of epic and martial valor, Lewis claims the right to confront her loss in a public discourse. That discourse, however, turns wryly comic with the final stanza.

As in Part V (see chapter 36), first-person poetic narrative is represented here, in chapter 58, by an account by Anne Sexton, "Flee On Your Donkey." Whereas Lewis valorizes her surgery into a kind of victory, Sexton's poem is about defeat, as she construes her readmission to the mental hospital where she has previously spent six years. "Six years of such small preoccupations! / Six years of shuttling in and out of this place!... It was a long trip with little days in it / and no new places." Once Sexton had apotheosized the clinicians: Howard Brody's warning about "the healer's power" is mirrored in her lines: "But you, my doctor, my enthusiast, / were better than Christ; / you promised me another world / to tell me who / I was." But that is an impossible burden for any human being to bear, and now Sexton sees through her old naivete: "I have come back / but disorder is not what it was / I have lost the trick of it! / The innocence of it!" Turning to Rimbaud's lines, "Anne, Anne, flee on your donkey," she rallies herself to make herself well: "Ride out / any old way you please!"

Another first-person selection, "Quickening," by Oliver Sacks, describes the moment when Sacks, who has severely injured his leg in a fall, first confronts the result of his "recovery." Like Lewis, Sacks must come to terms with a radically altered body, so changed as to be almost no body at all. While his leg is in its cast, he is racked by dreams in which the leg itself rots away, or turns to air, or becomes one with the cast. The procedure of removing the cast begins horrifically, but is quickly over. What remains is Sacks's disquiet with his leg, his sense that "though it was 'there' – it was not really there." Sacks is eventually able to recover both the sensation in his leg and the sensation that this *is* his leg, but the process is intermittent: "Power was returning, but it was still labile, unstable, not yet securely fixed in my nervous system or mind. I was beginning to remember, but the memory came and went."

The exploration of Philip and Lucy's stories, begun by Priscilla Alderson and Chris Goodey in Part III, continues in chapter 60 with an assessment of the role that education can play in ameliorating or worsening emotional and behavioral disturbance. "Meanings of 'getting well' are complicated by the difficulties, already discussed, of defining and assessing mental health and normal behavior, and of agreeing how expert doctors, parents, teachers, and young people themselves are at doing so." Like Sacks and Lewis's psychological accounts of physical loss, and, even more clearly, Sexton's account of her psychotic illness, Alderson and Goodey's chapter relates to mental health broadly construed. This emphasis, a consistent thread throughout the volume, is in line with our view that ethical issues in mental health are neglected and under-conceptualized (Dickenson and Fulford, 2000). Alderson and Goodey remind us that in relation to emotional and behavioral disorder, the conventional sickness model of falling ill and getting well can be misleading. We might say that this is more generally true of physical and mental "illness."

Two further poems follow these prose sections: William Shakespeare's "That Time of Year Thou Mayst In Me Behold" and W. B. Yeats's "When You Are Old." Seeking the meaning of ageing well, both bring us naturally to Daniel Callahan's canonical chapter on ageing, a selection from his controversial book *Setting Limits*. A focus on narrative such as we have espoused in this volume should alert us to the individuality of how each person's narrative ends. Not everyone will or should want to go on forever like Gulliver's Struldbrugs: differences in how we conceive of ageing should be allowed to flourish. The relevance of this argument to Part VII, "Getting Well," lies in the meaning of "getting well" as one grows older. Does it always mean the preservation of life at all costs? "Just what is good for us as we age? What should we hope for? What is the human meaning of old age?" This component of Callahan's argument seems harmless enough; what has caused the controversy are the implications when we extend the argument from individual difference to collective social policy. We suggested in the Introduction to this volume that there are dangers in absolutism. Here, though, Callahan argues that we need to move beyond relativism not only for reasons of resource allocation, but also in order to give the aged themselves a "thick" notion of what is good in ageing, a model to follow where there is now a void.

The notion that "getting well" is consistent with accepting physical limitations drives the next selection, Rainer Maria Rilke's poem "Going Blind." From his initial pity for the blind woman's condition, when her half-smile pains him, the poet moves to an admiration for the hope with which she approaches the obstacles that bar her stride: "as if she on the farther side / Might not be walking any more, but flying."

A short first-person account in chapter 65 by Margaret Allott, who developed breast cancer in her thirties, raises another issue to do with getting well: the decision whether or not to have reconstructive surgery. Once the trauma around the chances of survival ceased, with a good prognosis announced, and once Allott had adjusted to her mastectomy, did she want to go through further trauma, further reminder of her disease? "After all, I was alive and healthy; the physical effects of the operation made no difference to those who knew me, they liked me or not, just as before." However, the opinion of others, even supportive others, is not all-determining. "The first conclusion I came to is that a decision to have any sort of optional surgery must be made for oneself, not for how it looks or seems to others but how it feels to you. Following this, I was forced to reappraise my own sense of body image." This long process of evaluation took place during a period when Allott was heavily involved in producing an Open University course on "Death and Dying," confronting her daily with other people's narratives about loss and death. Her account stresses that every day of using the prosthesis reminded her of her own loss; reconstruction allowed her to return, "physically, at least," to the time before she had cancer.

What does getting well mean in the context of child sexual abuse? Is it ever possible to return to a lost state of innocence? – as in a way reconstruction allowed Margaret Allott to do.

Gill de la Cour, who is both a counselor working with clients who have experienced sexual abuse as children and a survivor herself, raises such issues in chapter 66, "Survivor or Expert? Some Thoughts on Being Both." De la Cour cautions against regressing to "splitting," a psychological defense mechanism from an early stage of child development and an inadvertent cause of further, emotional abuse by professionals dealing with abuse survivors. But survivors, too, may fall into the same trap, mythologizing the counselor into a psychologically perfect being. We are reminded of Sexton's initial, naive belief that her psychiatrist was greater than Christ, in that he could tell her who she really was.

The final chapter in this section is again literary: Robert Hass's brief allegory, "A Story About the Body." Is it about lost sweetness? – symbolized by the dead bees. Or perhaps the young man's inability to see beyond the superficial indication of womanliness? We leave it to you to judge.

READING GUIDE

The importance of individual values and meanings in determining what counts as recovery is highlighted by psychiatry: see, for example, Moore, A., Hope, T., and Fulford, K. W. M., on mania in "Mild Mania and Well-Being," *Philosophy, Psychiatry, and Psychology* 1/3 (1994): 165–78; and Hinshelwood, R. D., on difference between psychotherapy and brainwashing in his *Therapy or Coercion? Does Psychoanalysis Differ from Brainwashing?* (London: Karnac Books Ltd, 1997). The central place of empowerment as a goal of psychotherapy is described by Holmes, J. and Lindley, R. in *The Values of Psychotherapy* (Oxford: Oxford University Press, 1989).

A moving collection of their individual routes to recovery by accounts by survivors of child abuse is Malone, C., Farthing, L., and Marce, L. (eds.), *The Memory Bird* (London: Virago, 1996). The collection of first-person accounts by breast cancer survivors in the Bristol Cancer Centre collective's collection, *Fighting Spirit* (London: Scarlet Press, 1996), is also highly recommended.

REFERENCES

Dickenson, D. and Fulford, K. W. M. (2000) *In Two Minds: Case Studies in Psychiatric Ethics* (Oxford: Oxford University Press).

57

Wounded in Action
30th March, 1985

JENNY LEWIS

*When you're gone, Matron helps me remove
the bandage, then holds me in kind, starched
arms as I register my loss in the hard stare
of the bathroom mirror – a wounded soldier
who can no longer be kissed better.*

*All afternoon I play Mozart loudly
on my headphones, trying to staunch
the rising tides of panic and hoist myself
to a higher plane from which it might
be easier to jump – when the time comes.*

*At last I hear the comforting rattle
of the tea trolley and think to myself –
"Thank God, here comes the cavalry!"*

58

Flee On Your Donkey

ANNE SEXTON

Ma faim, Anne, Anne,
Fuis sur ton âne . . . Rimbaud

Because there was no other place
to flee to,
I came back to the scene of the disordered
    senses,
came back last night at midnight,
arriving in the thick June night
without luggage or defenses,
giving up my car keys and my cash,
keeping only a pack of Salem cigarettes
the way a child holds on to a toy.
I signed myself in where a stranger
puts the inked–in X's –
for this is a mental hospital,
not a child's game.

Today an interne knocks my knees,
testing for reflexes.
Once I would have winked and begged for dope.
Today I am terribly patient.
Today crows play black–jack
on the stethoscope.

Everyone has left me
except my muse,
that good nurse.

She stays in my hand,
a mild white mouse.

The curtains, lazy and delicate,
billow and flutter and drop
like the Victorian skirts
of my two maiden aunts
who kept an antique shop.

Hornets have been sent.
They cluster like floral arrangements on the
    screen.
Hornets, dragging their thin stingers,
hover outside, all knowing,
hissing: *the hornet knows.*
I heard it as a child
but what was it that he meant?
The hornet knows!
What happened to Jack and Doc and Reggy?

Who remembers what lurks in the heart of man?
What did The Green Hornet mean, *he knows?*
Or have I got it wrong?
Is it The Shadow who had seen
me from my bedside radio?

Now it's *Dinn, Dinn, Dinn!*
while the ladies in the next room argue

and pick their teeth.
Upstairs a girl curls like a snail;
in another room someone tries to eat a shoe;
meanwhile an adolescent pads up and down
the hall in his white tennis socks.
A new doctor makes rounds
advertising tranquilizers, insulin, or shock
to the uninitiated.

Six years of such small preoccupations!
Six years of shuttling in and out of this place!
O my hunger! My hunger!
I could have gone around the world twice
or had new children – all boys.
It was a long trip with little days in it
and no new places.

In here,
it's the same old crowd,
the same ruined scene.
The alcoholic arrives with his golf clubs.
The suicide arrives with extra pills sewn
into the lining of her dress.
The permanent guests have done nothing new.
Their faces are still small
like babies with jaundice.

Meanwhile,
they carried out my mother,
wrapped like somebody's doll, in sheets,
bandaged her jaw and stuffed up her holes.
My father, too. He went out on the rotten blood
he used up on other women in the Middle West.
He went out, a cured old alcoholic
on crooked feet and useless hands.
He went out calling for his father
who died all by himself long ago –
that fat banker who got locked up,
his genes suspended like dollars,
wrapped up in his secret,
tied up securely in a straitjacket.

But you, my doctor, my enthusiast,
were better than Christ;
you promised me another world
to tell me who
I was.

I spent most of my time,
a stranger,

damned and in trance – that little hut,
that naked blue-veined place,
my eyes shut on the confusing office,
eyes circling into my childhood,
eyes newly cut.
Years of hints
strung out – a serialized case history –
thirty-three years of the same dull incest
that sustained us both.
You, my bachelor analyst,
who sat on Marlborough Street,
sharing your office with your mother
and giving up cigarettes each New Year,
were the new God,
the manager of the Gideon Bible.

I was your third-grader
with a blue star on my forehead.
In trance I could be any age,
voice, gesture – all turned backward
like a drugstore clock.
Awake, I memorized dreams.
Dreams came into the ring
like third string fighters,
each one a bad bet
who might win
because there was no other.

I stared at them,
concentrating on the abyss
the way one looks down into a rock quarry,
uncountable miles down,
my hands swinging down like hooks
to pull dreams up out of their cage.
O my hunger! My hunger!

Once,
outside your office,
I collapsed in the old-fashioned swoon
between the illegally parked cars.
I threw myself down,
pretending dead for eight hours.
I thought I had died
into a snowstorm.
Above my head
chains cracked along like teeth
digging their way through the snowy street.
I lay there
like an overcoat
that someone had thrown away.

You carried me back in,
awkwardly, tenderly,
with the help of the red-haired secretary
who was built like a lifeguard.
My shoes,
I remember,
were lost in the snowbank
as if I planned never to walk again.

That was the winter
that my mother died,
half mad on morphine,
blown up, at last,
like a pregnant pig.
I was her dreamy evil eye.
In fact,
I carried a knife in my pocketbook –
my husband's good L. L. Bean hunting
    knife.
I wasn't sure if I should slash a tire
or scrape the guts out of some dream.

You taught me
to believe in dreams;
thus I was the dredger.
I held them like an old woman with arthritic
    fingers,
carefully straining the water out –
sweet dark playthings,
and above all, mysterious
until they grew mournful and weak.
O my hunger! My hunger!
I was the one
who opened the warm eyelid
like a surgeon
and brought forth young girls
to grunt like fish.

I told you,
I said –
but I was lying –
that the knife was for my mother . . .
and then I delivered her.

The curtains flutter out
and slump against the bars.
They are my two thin ladies
named Blanche and Rose.
The grounds outside
are pruned like an estate at Newport.

Far off, in the field,
something yellow grows.

Was it last month or last year
that the ambulance ran like a hearse
with its siren blowing on suicide –
Dinn, dinn, dinn! –
a noon whistle that kept insisting on life
all the way through the traffic lights?

I have come back
but disorder is not what it was.
I have lost the trick of it!
The innocence of it!
That fellow-patient in his stovepipe hat
with his fiery joke, his manic smile –
even he seems blurred, small and pale.
I have come back,
recommitted,
fastened to the wall like a bathroom plunger,
held like a prisoner
who was so poor
he fell in love with jail.

I stand at this old window
complaining of the soup,
examining the grounds,
allowing myself the wasted life.
Soon I will raise my face for a white flag,
and when God enters the fort,
I won't spit or gag on his finger.
I will eat it like a white flower.
Is this the old trick, the wasting away,
the skull that waits for its dose
of electric power?

This is madness
but a kind of hunger.
What good are my questions
in this hierarchy of death
where the earth and the stones go
Dinn! Dinn! Dinn!
It is hardly a feast.
It is my stomach that makes me suffer.

Turn, my hungers!
For once make a deliberate decision.
There are brains that rot here
like black bananas.
Hearts have grown as flat as dinner plates.

Anne, Anne,
flee on your donkey,
flee this sad hotel,
ride out on some hairy beast,
gallop backward pressing
your buttocks to his withers,
sit to his clumsy gait somehow.

Ride out
any old way you please!
In this place everyone talks to his own mouth.
That's what it means to be crazy.

Those I loved best died of it —
the fool's disease.

59

Quickening

OLIVER SACKS

On Monday morning, the fourteenth day after surgery, I was due to go down to the Casting Room, to have the wound inspected and the stitches removed. In these two weeks, indeed since the night of the accident, I had not actually been able to see the leg – it had always been covered and encased in a cast. There was something about the cast – its smooth featurelessness, its sepulchral whiteness, and its shape, which was like a vague and obscene parody of a leg – which invested it with horror: and indeed, as such, it played a great role in my dreams.

The night before I was due to be taken down, and uncasted, these dreams rose to a frightful climax: I dreamed, woke briefly, fell into the same dreams – hundreds of times I must have dreamt of the cast as empty, or solid all through, or filled with a disgusting verminous mass of rotting bones, bugs and pus. When the dim grey dawn of Monday finally came, I felt shuddery and weak, too sick to have breakfast, to say anything, or think. I lay like a corpse in my bed, waiting to be carried out.

The very term 'casting room' had a grim and frightful resonance. Even the word 'cast' took on disquieting other meanings. I found unbidden images rising in my mind – of the Casting Room as a place where they cast and cast away; where new limbs and bodies were cast by the Caster, and old and useless ones were cast away. Such fancies kept bursting into my mind, and I could not dismiss them, absurd though they were.

It was a relief, but also a terror, when the orderlies finally came for me and heaved me on to a stretcher and out of the room. Out of my room! For the first time in fifteen days. I caught a brief glimpse of the sky as we waited to go down. The sky! I had forgotten it, forgotten the outside world, as I lay in my small windowless cell, in solitary confinement, excited, obsessed, my mind a pressure-cooker of thoughts. The rumbling of the stretcher-trolley seemed monstrously loud, and kept suggesting to me the roll of tumbrils, the sense of being taken to my death – or something worse than death: to the realisation of an abominable nightmare, where all my fantasies of the uncanny, the unalive, the unreal, would turn out true.

The Casting Room was small, white, featureless, somewhere between a surgery and a workshop, with shears and other implements hanging on the wall – the strange, frightening tools of the Caster's Art. The orderlies shifted me on to a raised block in the centre – something between a catafalque and a butcher's block, I felt – and went out, shutting the door behind them. I was suddenly alone in this uncanny silent room.

And then I realised that I was not alone. The Caster, in a white gown, was standing in a corner. I had somehow failed to notice him when I was wheeled in. Or, perhaps, he had come in without my noticing. For, in a curious way, he did not seem to move, but to materialise suddenly in different parts of the room. He was here, he was there, but I never caught him in transit. He had a strangely immobile, carven face, with features of a medieval drawing. It might have been the face of Dürer, or of a mask or gargoyle imagined by Dürer.

I summoned up a social manner and said, 'Hello, Mr Enoch. Funny weather we're having.'

He made no response – not a movement, not a flicker.

I made some further desultory comments, and then tailed off as he made no reply but continued to stand motionless in the corner with his arms folded and his eyes fixed on mine. I found myself increasingly unnerved – it crossed my mind that he might be mad.

And then, suddenly, without any intermediate movement, he was no longer in his corner, but by the wall where the shears and other tools hung. And now, in a flash, he had the shears in his hands. They looked monstrously large to me – and he looked vast too. I felt that with a single cut he could shear off my leg, or slice me in two.

A single bound and he was on me, shears wide open, for the first cut. I wanted to yell 'Help! someone, anyone, come in! I am being attacked by a madman with a pair of shears.' My reason told me that this was all fancy, that Mr Enoch might be a little odd and taciturn, but was assuredly a skilled and responsible craftsman. So I controlled myself, and smiled, and said not a word.

And then I heard a reassuring sound – a gentle crunching, as the cast was snipped open. There had not been any terrible attack! Mr Enoch was quietly doing his business. He slit open the cast from top to bottom, and then gently pulled it open, exposing the leg. The cast itself he tossed lightly in a corner. This as-tounded me, for I had imagined it was enormously heavy, forty or fifty pounds at the least. Friends, at my request, had lifted the two legs, and said 'Blimey! That one in plaster weighs a ton – at least forty pounds heavier than the other one.' From the way Mr Enoch held it up and flicked it in a corner, it evidently weighed almost nothing at all, and the dead weight of the leg, that extra forty pounds, must have been due entirely to its total lack of muscular tone – that normal postural tone which one finds even in the deepest relaxation or sleep.

Mr Enoch stepped back, or, rather, suddenly disappeared, and reappeared as suddenly in his original corner, with a faint enigmatic smile on his lips.

And now Sister and the Surgical Registrar came bustling in, smiling and chatting as if nothing had happened – nothing *had* happened.

Sister said she was going to remove the stitches, but the Registrar interposed: 'Don't you want to *look* at your leg? After all, you haven't seen it for more than two weeks!'

Did I? Most assuredly, and passionately and eagerly; and yet I feared, shrinking, not knowing what I would see; and admixed with both feelings was a curious lack of feeling – a sort of indifference, real or defensive – so that I hardly cared what I would see.

With the Registrar's help, I raised myself on one arm, and took a long, long look at the leg.

Yes, it was there! Indisputably there! The cast was neither empty nor solid, as I had feared, nor did it contain a mass of earth, or dung, or rotting chicken bones. It contained – a leg, of approximately normal dimensions, though greatly wasted in comparison with its fellow, and with a long, clean scar about a foot long. A leg – and yet, not a leg: there was something all wrong. I was profoundly reassured, and at the same time disquieted, shocked, to the depths. For though it was 'there' – it was not really there.

It was indeed 'there' in a sort of formal, factual sense: visually there, but not livingly, substantially, or 'really' there. It wasn't a real leg, not a real thing at all, but a mere semblance which lay there before me. I was struck by the beautiful, almost translucent, delicacy of the limb; and I was struck by its absolute, almost appalling, unreality. It was exquisite, lifeless, like a fine wax model from an anatomy museum.

Gingerly I put out my hand to touch it – and touch was as uncanny and equivocal as sight. It not only looked like wax, but it felt like wax – finely-moulded, inorganic and ghostly. I could not feel the feeling fingers with the leg, so I squeezed the leg, pinched it, pulled out a hair. I could have stuck a knife into it for all the feeling it had. There was absolutely no sensation whatever – I might have been squeezing and kneading lifeless dough. It was clear that I had a leg which looked anatomically perfect, and which had been expertly repaired, and healed without complication, but it looked and felt uncannily alien – a lifeless replica attached to my body.

'Well,' said the Registrar. 'You're looking hard enough. What do you think of it? We did a nice job, eh?'

'Yes, yes,' I replied, bemusedly trying to gather my thoughts. 'You did a very nice job, beautiful, really beautiful. I do thank and congratulate you. But –.'

'Well, what's the "but"?' he asked with a smile.

'It looks fine – it *is* fine, surgically speaking.'

'What do you mean – "surgically speaking"?'

'Well, it doesn't *feel* right. It feels – sort of funny, not right, not mine. Difficult to put into words.'

'Don't worry, old chap,' the Registrar said. 'It's done beautifully, old fellow. You'll be right as rain. Sister will take the stitches out now.'

Sister advanced, with her gleaming instrument tray, saying, 'It shouldn't hurt too much, Dr Sacks. You'll probably just feel a tweaking sensation. If it does hurt we can put in some local.'

'You go ahead,' I answered. 'I'll let you know if it hurts.'

But, to my surprise, she didn't seem to be going ahead, but fiddling around, with her scissors and forceps – fiddling in the strangest, most unintelligible way. I watched her, perplexed, for a time and then closed my eyes. When I opened them, she had stopped her unconscionable fiddling, which, I supposed, must have been some sort of 'warm-up' or preparatory activity: I presumed she was now ready to take out the stitches.

'You going to start now?' I enquired.

She looked at me in astonishment. 'Start!' she exclaimed. 'Why, I just finished! I took out all the stitches. I must say, you were very good. You lay quiet as a lamb. You must be very stoical. Did it hurt much?'

'No,' I answered. 'It didn't hurt at all. And I wasn't being brave. I didn't feel you at all. I had no sensation whatever when you pulled the stitches out.' I omitted to say, because I thought it would sound too strange, that I had entirely failed to realise that she *was* taking them out, indeed that I had failed to make any sense of her activity whatever, or to see it as having any sense or relation to me, so that I had mistaken all her motions as meaningless 'fiddling'. But I was taken aback, confounded, by the business. It brought home to me once more how estranged the leg was, how 'alien', how 'exiled' from myself. To think that I could have seen Sister making all the characteristic motions of snipping and pulling out stitches, but only able to imagine she was 'warming up' in readiness for the 'real thing'! Her activity had seemed meaningless and unreal, presumably, because the leg felt meaningless and unreal. And because the leg felt senseless, in all senses of senseless, absolutely senseless and unrelated to me, so had her motions which had been related to it. As the leg was merely a semblance, so her motions, her taking-out stitches, seemed merely a semblance. Both had been reduced to meaningless semblance.

Finding my horrible fears and phantasms unfounded, finding the leg at least formally intact and there, finding finally an infinite reassurance when Mr Enoch lifted the heel off the block, and the knee locked firmly, precisely, in place, and that the horror of kneelessness, dislocation, disarticulation, was gone – I suddenly felt an infinite relief: a relief so sweet and intense, so permeating my whole being, that I was bathed in bliss. With this sudden sweet and profound reassurance, the sudden and profound change of mood, the leg was utterly transformed, transfigured. It still looked profoundly strange and unreal. It still looked profoundly unalive. But where it had previously brought to mind a corpse, it now made me think of a foetus, not yet born. The flesh seemed somehow translucent and innocent, like flesh not yet given the breath of life.

Theoretical as yet, the flesh was there, healed anatomically, but not yet quickened into action. It lay there patient, radiant, not yet real, but almost ready to be born. The sense of dreadful, irretrievable loss was transformed into a sense of mysterious 'abeyance'. It lay there, in a strange suspension, or limbo, a mysterious landscape between death and birth...

> ...between two worlds, one dead
> The other powerless to be born
>
> (Arnold)

Flesh which was still as unliving as marble but, like the marble flesh of Galatea, might come to life. And even the new plaster partook of this feeling: I had hated the old one, feeling it putrid, obscene, but I immediately took a liking to the new one which Mr Enoch was now carefully applying, laying layer upon layer round my new pink leg. This cast I thought elegant, shapely, even smart. More important, I thought of it as a sort of good chrysalis, which would sheathe the leg and let it develop completely, until it was ready to hatch, to be reborn.

As I was wheeled back from the Casting Room, and up in the lift, we paused by the broad windows, which were open now to the air. The sky had been dark and charged before; but now the storm had broken, and it was heavenly calm and clear. I felt the very elements themselves had had their crisis at precisely the same time as I had had mine. All was resolved now, the heavens clear and blue. A lovely breeze came through the great windows, and I felt intoxicated as the sun and wind played on my skin. It was my first sense of the outside world in more than two weeks, two weeks in which I had mouldered, in despair, in my cell. And there was music, a new radio, when I returned to my room – wonderful Purcell, *Dido and Aeneas* – and this too, like the wind and the sun and the light, came like a heavenly refreshment to my senses. I felt bathed in the music, penetrated by it, healed and quickened through and through: divine music, spirit, message and messenger of life!

Relieved of all my anxieties and tensions, sure and confident that the leg would come back, and

that I would recover and walk again – though when, and how, God only knew – I suddenly fell into a deep blissful sleep: sleeping in trust, cradled in God's arms. A deep, deep, and in itself healing, sleep – my first proper rest since the day of the accident – my first sleep uninterrupted by hideous nightmares and phantoms. The sleep of innocence, of forgiveness, of faith and hope renewed.

When I awoke I had an odd impulse to flex my left leg, and in that self-same moment immediately did so! Here was a movement previous impossible, one which involved active contraction of the whole quad – a movement hitherto impossible and unthinkable. And yet, in a trice, I had thought it, and done it. There was no cogitation, no preparation, no deliberation, whatever; there was no 'trying'; I had the impulse, flash-like – and flash-like I acted. The idea, the impulse, the action, were all one – I could not say which came first, they all came together. I suddenly 'recollected' how to move the leg, and in the instant of recollection I actually did it. I suddenly knew what to do – and, in that instant, I did it. The knowing-what-to-do had no theoretical quality whatever – it was entirely practical, immediate – and compelling. And it came to me without the slightest premeditation or warning, without any calculation or contrivance on my part. Suddenly and spontaneously – out of the blue.

Excited, I rang my bell and called for the Nurse.

'Look!' I exclaimed. 'I did it, I can do it!'

But when I tried to show her, nothing happened at all. The knowledge, the impulse, had departed as it came, suddenly, mysteriously. Mortified, and puzzled, I returned to my book – and then about half an hour later, and again in mid-word, unbidden, unconsidered, I had the same impulse again. The impulse, the idea, the remembrance, flashed back – and I moved my leg (if 'moved' is not too deliberate a word for the utterly *un*deliberated, spontaneous movement which 'occurred'). But a few seconds later it was impossible again. And so it was throughout the rest of the day. The power of moving, the idea of moving, the impulse to move, would suddenly come to me – and as suddenly go – as a word, or a face, or a name, or a tune, can be at the tip of one's tongue, or in the immediate ambit of one's vision or hearing, and then, as suddenly, disappear. Power was returning, but it was still labile, unstable, not yet securely fixed in my nervous system or mind. I was beginning to remember, but the memory came and went.

60

Emotional and Behavioral Disturbance: Philip and Lucy

PRISCILLA ALDERSON AND CHRIS GOODEY

This chapter continues the experiences of Philip and Lucy (for background details see chapters 17 and 47) and examines the part education can play in reducing, increasing, or recovering from emotional and behavioral disturbance (EBD). Meanings of "getting well" are complicated by the difficulties, already discussed, of defining and assessing mental health and normal behavior, and of agreeing how expert doctors, parents, teachers, and young people themselves are at doing so. Apparently disturbed young people challenge conventional ideas about the sick role and functionalist faith in a well-ordered, benign society. Should they be blamed or pitied when they do not fit adults' expectations? Should they be regulated, punished, counseled, or calmed by drugs such as ritalin? Or should the context to which they are reacting, or the inappropriate roles assigned to them, be seen as the main problems?

Policies are influenced by historical and religious beliefs about "can or will,"[1] about whether disturbed young people *cannot* help behaving badly (they are sick and to be pitied) or could *will* themselves to behave better (they are naughty and must be corrected or punished). Staff in EBD schools veer erratically from one assumption to the other, pitying one minute and punitive the next. At a broader level, just as prisons emphasize reform in one decade and punishment in another, claiming to reflect public opinion, it is likely that attitudes in and toward EBD schools follow similar patterns. Currently, with soaring school exclusion rates, the stress is on punishment and away from a more caring, "sickness" model of "they cannot help it." So "getting well" can be harder, when disturbed young people feel that they are punished rather than being encouraged and helped toward better behavior.

The great increases in disturbance as measured by school exclusions or prescribed ritalin[2] have to be understood in the context of great increases in poverty, deprivation, and physical restriction for children in the UK;[3] and increasingly intolerant regimentation in school.[4] Most EBD "treatments" are controversial.[5] We are cautious about generalizing from our research project. However, Philip who originally appeared to be much more disturbed, and Lucy who had much longer and more severe "treatment" illustrate the experiences of many other young people in their respective East City mainstream schools and West County special schools.

Philip in East City

After a short time in a special school which was closing, at the age of 7 Philip returned to mainstream school with support, and is now at secondary school, full time and with no extra support. The interviewer asked Philip about his SATs (standard attainment tests) and Philip showed his SATs work, saying in a pleased tone, "English I got 3, science I got 4, maths I got 3." At the age of 12, he takes the 25-minute walk to school, likes exploring the city using his travel card, and no longer needs to attend hospital for the bowel problem. He likes writing and making up games. "He'd rather be the team leader telling everybody what to do, organizing, that's what he's good at, putting rules down. He doesn't like it if somebody disagrees with his rules," said his father. Philip's father was helped by a parents' group at the special school where "we learned about our rights." They visited their MP and by talking together felt less isolated.

Philip thinks the secondary school teaching is rather boring and strict, and says aggressively, "Just get on with your work. Just put down what's on the board and GET ON WITH YOUR WORK!" He enjoys lunch time breaks most, talking with his friends. His father said:

> He now has no problems like what he'd been through. He's settled in, he's just like any normal kid, without anything wrong with him and any problems.... With Philip, I talk to him like an adult now, I mean I always have. To me, he's just another adult but with a younger brain. Because they are *people*.... Even though his brother's eight, he's still a person. Now if you treat them like an idiot, they'll look at *you* like an idiot.

When talking about the family budget or planning weekends or attending a funeral, "they understood and we all talked about it like adults."

Lucy in West County

Although Lucy attended an EBD school, it was not at all clear that she was disturbed. Lucy was interviewed again at home when she was 15, and the researcher spent days observing both of her EBD schools. After 10 years in special schools was she "getting well"? Her parents said they found her easier to live with, but were unsure how much this was due to her growing up. The head teacher of her second school was asked about the "treatment program" in terms of the aims of the school. He spoke about the therapy of art and sports sessions, free from pressures of much academic work. Girls do not do GCSEs in case they fail, he said, and he stressed social skills:

Head teacher: However young they are, when they leave school, to prepare each girl socially in their relationships with their parents and their peers, with adults... to find their way round work experience.
Interviewer: Find their way round?
Head teacher: Find their way round the locality and the town. There's a lot of that in the 24-hour [boarding] education, access to leisure facilities, to prepare them educationally to find their way around.... The concentrated [boarding] social program is to drive towards independence, concerned with their ability to relate towards one another outside the normal classroom, drawing out situations which normal young people, teenagers, experience, of trying to get to manage their behavior, manage their emotions in a less formal way than in the classroom.

Day girls who do not improve are recommended to have more of the same by becoming boarders. Like Lucy's mother, the head teacher speaks in contradictions, since boarders actually have much less, not more, opportunities to travel around the town and surrounds, use local facilities, relate to their parents, and have "normal" experiences outside formal school. "Life skills" courses in the 16–19 age group train the girls in skills they would have learnt already if they had not been boarders or lived such a restricted life on the advice of teachers and doctors. The head teacher added: "We're kind to them, we look after them, we like them and in a way this cushions their behavior. We're trying to fill in all the gaps, repair all the damage. However, we must make sure they don't become over-protected; [at times] we stand back and give her that push." The staff veer between pushing and cushioning and, as the words suggest, treating the girls rather as objects.

The school uses a behavior modification system (BMS). Everyone is assessed each week on a 5-star system, with rewards for 5- and 4-star girls, "normal privileges allowed" for 3-star girls, and punishments for 2- and 1-star girls. The head teacher said:

> We try to create as stress free an environment as possible [in contrast to] the conflict and abuse and rejection . . . at home. . . . [The BMS] gives added structure and security for the girls. . . . They're very accepting. . . . The girls are happy here. . . . There are clear unambiguous guidelines and they're all told what is acceptable behavior, and the youngster needs to know "Cross that line and the consequences will be so and so." . . . We're constantly monitoring and evaluating and changing the system.

BMS is meant to be a tool for change, used for a set period rather than indefinitely, and aimed not at perfection but at an achievable standard, with careful assessment before and afterwards. If the target cannot be reached, it is supposed to be lowered. If the intended change does not occur, the BMS is assessed as too ambitious or as ineffective. Rewards have greater effect than punishments.[6] However, this school uses the BMS permanently to manage-control rather than to modify-change behavior, in that, for example, the proportion of girls at each star level remains fairly constant. The ideal of clear guidelines conflicts with the claim that the system is constantly changed. Teachers were observed to vary unpredictably and arbitrarily in giving rewards and punishments.

Girls find the system confusing and oppressive. "Someone tells a teacher you've done something and you get a cross and when you try to say you didn't do it you get another cross, so it's not worth trying." "A cross cancels out a tick but I don't think a tick cancels out a cross."

Lucy: When the teachers shout at you, the girls get so angry they shout back and the teachers don't like it. And if you say something and the teacher shouts and you say, "Don't shout," she takes it the wrong way and says, "Right, you get a cross!" And everyone thinks it's so stupid, 'cos every time you do something you get a cross for it. We don't like it. . . . For the little ones, yes, but the grown ups, no, 'cos I think we should behave ourselves. We should learn without needing this.

The complications in the system can increase its power, and the girls' anxieties about being marked down appeared to make them feel cautious and unconfident, rather than secure as the head teacher believed. When asked about permitted activities, the girls' typical reply was, "I don't know, you have to ask." Lucy was frequently in trouble and on the lower star levels.

Ambiguities in the remit and aims of these schools do not help the pupils to be informed or prepared for their "treatment." It is harder for them to have clear goals or to take personal decisions, in even the smallest things, when they are constantly reprimanded for any sign of independence, walking across a room to fetch a pencil, helping another pupil, speaking without permission. Self-control, suppression of feeling and impulse are stressed, rather than positive responses. The girls are constantly reminded of their own weaknesses and failings, and are also warned against "being too friendly" with one another. "My key worker says I mustn't trust anyone here. I mustn't tell them too much; it only leads to rows and people telling on you," was a typical comment. Continual uncertainty and doubt undermine the self-esteem and confidence that are part of mental health.[7]

Recovering From Emotional and Behavioral Difficulty

Special schools are assumed to be the best places for disturbed pupils because, after expert selection, they can benefit from specially trained staff, using special techniques and resources, following a specially tailored curriculum in a school where the whole remit is to cater for their special needs. The schools are seen as havens from the rigors of competitive exams and sports and the full national curriculum, as refuges from the risks of failure, stress, bullying, and poor self-esteem presented by "normal" school. In this model, the pupils are seen as sick and the schools as places of expert treatment, care, and healing.

Our evidence challenges all these assumptions. We found arbitrary selection of students, meagre resources, and no obvious extra teaching skills or techniques beyond those that skilled mainstream teachers use. Few lessons were either interesting or challenging, boredom and frustration increased disruptive behavior, which was pathologized as totally irrational.

In contrast, Philip illustrates the common finding that when people feel respected, trusted, and treated reasonably as an ordinary person in an ordinary setting, they feel better able to behave "normally," reliably, and maturely and to benefit from the diverse opportunities of a busy, ordinary school. When people are not divided by exaggerated labels – good stable staff/bad disturbed pupils – then it is easier for disturbed students to become part of the wide range of "normal" people who have good and bad times. When schools can support everyone, staff and students, during their times of stress and distress, all students learn to respond positively to difficulties, their own and other people's. Some children and teenagers have severe mental illness which needs psychiatric treatment, but Philip and Lucy belong to a great EBD majority whose problems are increased when they are treated as if they are ill and abnormal.

The sickness model or metaphor of falling ill and getting well needs to be applied with caution to the thousands of students every year who are described as EBD. It privatizes EBD, isolating it as a problem in each individual. A more efficient and economical approach would attend to the difficult social and political contexts of their lives, to ways of preventing disturbance, and helping ordinary schools to support disturbed students. The medical model of consent, if applied to schools, could help students to become more informed and involved in decisions about their schooling. This is as long as the importance of the informed and voluntary nature of valid consent is understood by all concerned, and the consent form is not simply used to transfer power to the professional and responsibility for any adverse later events to the client.[8] More families are being asked to sign "contracts" before the school will accept a student. Educationalists appear to be using a spurious model of consent to enforce their control and to increase discrepancies of power and knowledge between teachers and students, which denies the voluntary nature of education – people cannot be forced to learn. Schools urgently need to develop positive rather than pathologizing ways of helping disturbed students.

NOTES

We are grateful to everyone who helped with the research study "Which kind of school is best for me?" and to the Gatsby Trust for sponsorship.

1   Goodey, C. F., "From natural disability to the moral man: Calvinism and the history of psychology," *History of the Human Sciences* 14/3 (2001).

2   Levy, F., "Attention deficit hyperactivity disorder," *British Medical Journal* 315 (1997): 894–5.

3   Lansdown, G. and Newell, P., *UK Agenda for Children* (London: Children's Rights Office, 1994); Wilkinson, R., *Unfair Shares* (Barkingside: Barnardo's, 1994).

4   Jeffs, T., "Children's educational rights in a new ERA?" in B. Franklin (ed.), *The Handbook of Children's Rights* (London: Routledge, 2001, pp. 25–39).

5   Christensen, C. and Fazal, R., *Disability and the Dilemmas of Education and Justice* (Buckingham: Open University Press, 1996); Hornby, G., Atkinson, M., and Howard, J., *Controversial Issues in Special Education* (London: David Fulton, 1997).

6   Ayers, H., Clarke, D., and Murray, A., *Perspectives on Behaviour: A Practical Guide to Effective Interventions for Teachers* (London: David Fulton, 1995).

7   Seligman, M., *Helplessness: On Depression, Development and Death* (San Francisco: Freeman, 1975).

8   Dickenson, D., *Moral Luck in Medical Ethics and Practical Politics* (Aldershot: Avebury, 1991).

61

Sonnet LXXIII

WILLIAM SHAKESPEARE

That time of year thou mayst in me behold
When yellow leaves, or none, or few, do hang
Upon those boughs which shake against the
  cold,
Bare ruin'd choirs, where late the sweet birds
  sang.
In me thou see'st the twilight of such day
As after sunset fadeth in the west;
Which by and by black night doth take away,
Death's second self, that seals up all in rest.
In me thou see'st the glowing of such fire,
That on the ashes of his youth doth lie,
As the death-bed whereon it must expire
Consum'd with that which it was nourish'd by.
This thou perceiv'st, which makes thy love
  more strong,
To love that well which thou must leave ere
  long.

62

When You Are Old

W. B. YEATS

When you are old and gray and full of sleep,
And nodding by the fire, take down this book,
And slowly read, and dream of the soft look
Your eyes had once, and of their shadows deep;

How many loved your moments of glad grace,
And loved your beauty with love false or true,

But one man loved the pilgrim soul in you,
And loved the sorrows of your changing face;

And bending down beside the glowing bars,
Murmur, a little sadly, how Love fled
And paced upon the mountains overhead
And hid his face amid a crowd of stars.

63

Setting Limits: Medical Goals in an Aging Society

DANIEL CALLAHAN

Individualism, and the classical political liberalism of the eighteenth and nineteenth centuries upon which it is based, rests upon the right of individuals to seek that which in their private judgment will bring them happiness. The only limit upon that right is that they may not do harm to others in seeking their personal self-fulfillment. [...] The search for the good of human life, for its purposes and ends and meaning (if any), is left to the individual. The search for the good is not, and must not become, a collective enterprise to be pursued by the community as a whole, much less by the state.

An equivalent thin theory of aging and health care would say something more or less like the following. Individual people will look upon aging in different ways, express different tolerances for the burdens of old age, seek different goals and lifestyles in old age, and differ about how long they want to live and about the medical conditions under which they are willing to die. It is perfectly fitting in a pluralistic society – one dedicated to individual liberty and opposed to a coerced notion of a good life – that such differences should exist and be allowed to flourish. Medicine should serve that diversity, which does not in any case admit of a single right answer about what people ought to want.

Save for evidence that satisfying the desires of some, or many, for a longer and healthy life would do harm to others (surely a difficult fact to establish), medicine should give people what they want. And what do they want? Simply life and good health, themselves perfectly traditional goals even if variously interpreted.

That is a powerful philosophy for the provision of health care, all the more because it makes the values in medicine consistent with the kinds of freedom available in other parts of the society. Yet it also assumes we can afford to leave some basic questions publicly unanswered and unasked. Just what is good for us as we age? What should we hope for? What is the human meaning of old age? The mounting problem of providing health care for the elderly in the setting of an ever-expanding scientific frontier, limited resources, and the inexorable demography of an aging society shows the limitations of a thin theory. Medicine cannot give every person what he or she may desire. Lacking a direction, goals cannot be set. Lacking a deep purpose, coherence cannot be found. Rational priorities can then not be set, or sensible principles of allocation devised. Even within the terms of conventional individualism, there is good reason to believe that satisfying all the desires of the elderly for health care and life extension can do harm to the health needs of other groups and to social needs other than health, such as education, housing, and public transportation. Unlike those of younger age groups, the needs of the elderly for continuing good health are of their very nature open-ended: in old age, the conquest of one disease only guarantees death from some other disease, one which, if conquered, will give way to some further lethal condition. As our present experience demonstrates, the logic of a medical progress set to conquer all disease – in combination with a growing proportion of elderly people – guarantees an ever-rising budget and ever more ways of spending more money. In the absence of unlimited resources, therefore, some degree of harm to other groups must be an inevitable outcome even in the face of efforts to deny the existence of a problem or to imagine a utopian solution.

There is another thin theory which is no less harmful, one that has nothing to do with resources. The price we pay for our individualism in an aging society is that our culture provides neither the elderly nor anyone else with a clear picture of what they should be able to hope for from society in their old age or of the way they might make social sense of their illnesses and eventual death. Given the great importance of meaning for the aged – meaning in their lives and about their place and value in society – there is a harm in the implicit relativism of the diversity itself. There is at present no meaning for the aged unless they can supply it for themselves. Where there should be a public conception of the nature of a good life for the elderly in their weakness and not just in their strength – including the significance of the decline of the body – there is mainly a void. It may be, in fact, that our present, supposedly neutral thin theory actually coerces the elderly by social pressure, particularly in the direction of a forced acceptance of youthful vigor as the ideal of old age. When one sort of aging and death is deemed as good in principle as another, all are increasingly deprived of significance. That some form of rationing of expensive high-technology medicine may be necessary provides still another reason to look for a greater social consensus

than a thin theory would countenance. A capricious method of allocation, or one unjustly based on wealth alone, would clearly do harm to many. Even a system that tried to act more fairly (but still had to set some limits) would do harm to the self-worth of the aged unless based on some solidly accepted, dignity-enhancing consensus. Individualism should, in sum, give way to a community-based and affirmed notion of the value of the aged in society and, with that, an acceptance of limits to health care for the aged and medical research of benefit to them. That requires a thick, not a thin, theory of the good.

Medicine is perhaps the last and purest bastion of Enlightenment dreams, tying together reason, science, and the dream of unlimited human possibilities. There is nothing, it is held, that in principle cannot be done and, given suitable caution, little that ought not to be done. Nature, including the body, is seen as infinitely manipulable and plastic to human contrivance. When that conception of medicine is set in the social context of an individualism which is, in principle, opposed to a public consensus about any ultimate human good, it is a potent engine of endless, never-satisfied progress. Yet such a consensus about the human good at least of medicine and aging is exactly what the management of an aging society and of health care for the aged requires. Both the welfare of the elderly for their own sake and the need to allocate resources in some rational and moral way demand that medicine have a clear direction and purpose.

[...]

As it confronts aging, medicine should have as its specific goals averting premature death, understood as death before the fulfillment of a natural life span, and the relief of suffering. It should pursue those goals in order that the elderly can finish out their years with a conviction that their lives have meaning and significance, with as little suffering as possible, with as much vigor as possible in contributing to the welfare of the young and the community of which they are a part. By vigor I do not exclusively mean active, physical vigor. Beyond some point of physical decline and with the approach of death, there may be little of that left. I take it also to be vigor of a no less valuable kind, to present to the young a model of what it means to decline gracefully, to relinquish roles and visibility, and to reflect on the way death closes out a life. Even that latter kind of vigor, which may be manifest only as a struggle for some kind of tranquillity, may well require the ministrations of medicine. Medicine cannot bring happiness, but it can help provide the physical substrate of a tolerable aging and death. Those in the process of aging, or already aged, should ask of medicine not a longer life, but help in maintaining a life that can complete its work as close to the time of death as possible. More needs to be said, however, about the relief of suffering and maintenance of function.

The cure of disease and the relief of suffering, each representing a threat to human wholeness, have long been accepted as appropriate goals of medicine. Disease destroys the wholeness and integrity of the body, and pain and suffering can destroy the wholeness of the person. While medicine is well honed to combat pain, suffering is a more complex category, which may but does not necessarily involve the presence of pain. It is a particularly important problem in caring for the aged. Aging portends the dissolution of more than the body. "Suffering," Eric Cassell has written, "occurs when an impending destruction of the person is perceived; it continues until the threat of disintegration has passed or until the integrity of the person can be restored in some other manner." In the case of the aging, the threat will not pass. How can it be softened? Fear of the future, an acute source of suffering, will be an element in aging, particularly toward the end. There is no future, and that may be the hardest thing to accept. How is that to be tolerated? Cassell offers some helpful insights: "Meaning and transcendence offer two . . . ways by which the suffering associated with destruction of a part of personhood is ameliorated. Assigning a meaning to the injurious condition often reduces or even resolves the suffering associated with it. . . . Transcendence is probably the most powerful way in which one is restored to wholeness after an injury to personhood. When experienced, transcendence locates the person in a far larger landscape. The sufferer is not isolated

by pain but is brought closer to a transpersonal source of meaning and to the human community that shares those meanings." Cassell does not define "transcendence," but I would urge that a sense that one has lived out one's final years helping those who will remain is one important source of it.

A medicine oriented toward the relief of suffering will, in the case of the elderly, be a medicine that is concerned with the sick person, not the sickness of the person. The disease or combination of diseases that will be the actual cause of death and the source of pain can only be ameliorated, not cured; or, if it should be cured, it is understood that its place will soon be taken by another. The relief of pain may pose a special dilemma. For some at least, mental clarity in the presence of pain may be preferable to the drowsiness or stupefaction induced by pain relievers. For others, the terror of pain induced by some conditions may lead them in a different direction, such as heavy doses of morphine. In caring for a person who is trying to find meaning in a life coming to an end, different kinds of preference should be respected; it is the person as a whole who is the subject of treatment. But so far as possible, the goal of the physician should be to reduce the physical obstacles that impede the search for the meaning and transcendence which can make the suffering bearable. The further extension of life would then become a secondary goal, if a goal at all. The point is that life has now come to an end, and there is only one question of importance: what does a person need to secure at its closing the greatest possible integrity? Since more life as such is rarely the answer to that problem, then a high goal of a medicine for the aged will be the management of suffering. That this kind of medical care requires skills and understanding which go well beyond technical knowledge need not be stressed. That physicians and other health-care workers must here be prepared to spend time in talking with the elderly, and giving of themselves to them, is a prime duty.

What would a medicine be like that was oriented toward the relief of suffering rather than the deliberate extension of life? We do not yet have a clear answer to that question readily at hand, so long-standing, central, and persistent has been the struggle against death as a part of the self-conception of medicine. But the hospice movement is providing us with much helpful evidence. It knows how to distinguish between the relief of suffering and the extension of life. "The relief of suffering" means at least the control of pain and an active effort to promote physical functioning, mental alertness, and emotional stability. Medicine cannot by itself supply meaning and significance to the late years. That can be achieved only by the elderly person and by the larger society. But a life marked by pain, depression, and radical loss of physical function cannot be a life well positioned to seek a larger good. Those inflictions have a devastating way of turning one in upon oneself, of blotting out all other possibilities, and of inducing despair. A medicine that can relieve a heavy weight of that kind will be a splendid medicine. But can medical practice, as a general rule, play that role?

[. . .]

We are not required to continue chasing an indefinite life extension. We can settle for the achievement of a limited, natural life span. That would be sufficient, and would allow the possibility of concentrating on improving the quality of life prior to the end of that life span.

Unlike the goal of extending life, that of seeking to improve the quality of life of the elderly points to an important set of additional considerations which should be part of medicine's self-reflection. How should the good that is health, a primary good certainly, be understood in the constellation of other human goods? These include education, culture, economic prosperity, national defense, scientific research outside the health arena, and so on. Health itself, we sometimes need reminding, is a means and not an end. We can do nothing with good health itself; it makes other human goods possible. But we need to know what those goods are and how they are to be balanced against the value of health. A goal of the extension of life combined with an insatiable desire for improvement in health – a longer and simultaneously better life for the elderly – is a recipe for monomania and bottomless spending. It fails to put health in its proper place, fails to accept aging and death as part of the human condition, and fails to present to younger generations a model of wise stewardship. A goal of aging that stresses the needs of the future generations, not only those of the old, and a goal of medicine that stresses the avoidance of premature death and the relief of suffering would together provide an alternative to our present situation.

64

Going Blind

RAINER MARIA RILKE

She sat at tea just like the others. First
I merely had a notion that this guest
Held up her cup not quite like all the rest.
And once she gave a smile. It almost hurt.

When they arose at last, with talk and
    laughter,
And ambled slowly and as chance dictated
Through many rooms, their voices animated,
I saw her seek the noise and follow after,

Held in like one who in a little bit
Would have to sing where many people
    listened;
Her lighted eyes, which spoke of gladness,
    glistened
With outward luster, as a pond is lit.

She followed slowly, and it took much
    trying,
As though some obstacle still barred her
    stride;
And yet as if she on the farther side
Might not be walking any more, but flying.

65

The Decision to Have Reconstructive Surgery

MARGARET ALLOTT

In December 1989 a biopsy confirmed the presence of a malignant tumor in my left breast. Ironically, I had been prompted to visit my GP and was referred on to the hospital for a mammogram because I had located a pea-sized lump in my right breast – which turned out to be a harmless cyst.

At the time of the operation the possibility of reconstructive surgery had not crossed my mind. The trauma revolved around my chances of survival, which couldn't even be guessed at until the results of tests on the removed breast and lymph tissue were available, a week or so after the operation. The results indicated that there was a good chance the cancerous cells had not spread elsewhere and that neither chemotherapy nor radiotherapy were necessary. Great news. Chances were I would survive and even be enhanced – I believed (and still do) – by the experience of having to think deeply about my own mortality.

I hadn't consciously thought much about how my body would look minus a breast, but the day after the operation when the nurse removed the dressing she asked if I knew what to expect. I didn't and admitted to her that I now realized that I was afraid to look. She persuaded me that I should look at the wound and said in her experience many women had found it less upsetting than they had feared. She was right. The horizontal line of stitches running across my now flat left chest didn't seem too bad, indeed a small price to pay in exchange for life itself. I was discharged from hospital having been given a prosthesis with verbal instructions on how to place it and wear it inside my bra and a leaflet on a brand of underwear specializing in bras which would hold the prosthesis in place inside special pockets.

Months passed and I progressed well. At one of my many hospital check-ups the consultant mentioned breast reconstruction: providing I remained "clear" for a couple of years, he would offer me the possibility of reconstructive surgery. The seed was planted and this is when I began to consider the issues.

The first consideration was "Why would I (or anyone) want to go through reconstructive surgery?" After all, I was alive and healthy, the physical effects of the operation made no difference to those who knew me, they liked me or not, just as before. I had never had large breasts anyway and, in truth, I had always been more concerned about my more than ample-sized bottom than my flat-chestedness. By this time

I had been using the prosthesis for a year or so and was becoming more aware of its shortcomings. It "moved around" inside its pocket, thus not matching the shape or size of my other breast, and the bras available were always white, plain, old-fashioned, expensive "for what they were," and had to be ordered specially. Friends reassured me that they couldn't tell – and in any case, what difference did it make?

The first conclusion I came to is that a decision to have any sort of optional surgery must be made for oneself, not for how it looks or seems to others, but how it feels to you. Following this, I was forced to reappraise my own sense of body image. I'm a confident person with belief in my own intelligence and abilities – surely I didn't need a "perfect" body again to reassure me of this. But the body is the home of the mind and personal identity is rooted in the experience of body self-image.

On the practical side I knew life would be simpler if I didn't have to buy specially adapted items, and psychologically I knew I would regain some lost confidence if I could wear "normal" clothing. I realized that the reason for this was that each day when I used the prosthesis it *reminded* me of what had happened – that I'd had breast cancer and maybe it would come back. Each day began with that reminder and I began to believe that reconstructive surgery was a means of "putting me back" as far as possible to how I was, physically at least, before I had cancer. I knew of the possible risks involved and over a long period of time I read articles and books on the arguments around breast implant surgery and talked at length to the surgeon about his views and experiences, then decided to go ahead.

My family and close friends were, on the whole, against any form of reconstructive surgery involving implants because of the perceived risks. Almost daily, the newspapers carried reports of women suffering because of leakage, rejection, etc. Did I have a right to take a risk of this kind, however small I believed it to be, when if anything did go wrong it would be my husband and children who would suffer most?

Then there was the guilt about the cost to the NHS and taking up scarce resources for what could be seen as "cosmetic" surgery. Would someone go without a life-saving operation because of this? On the other hand, I told myself that I had worked and contributed all my life and was now *entitled* to any available treatment. The consultant was quite clear: reconstruction was not only a cosmetic exercise; he regarded it as a natural progression of the treatment for those who wanted it and viewed the psychological aspect of treatment for breast cancer as important as any other.

It took three years finally to put my name on the waiting list, and another year before I had the first operation. I thought about all these issues for a long time and came to the conclusion that whatever the dilemma I still wanted to go ahead, I had to do it for myself. For me, it was the right decision.

66

Survivor or Expert? Some Thoughts on Being Both

GILL DE LA COUR

I am a professional counsellor working with clients who have experienced sexual abuse as children. I am also a 'survivor' myself. When I was very young, I was sexually abused by a man who was, apparently, a close family friend. The abuse was extreme and traumatic. The way my family operated ensured that the experience was covered up and denied. The resulting feelings and terrors I suffered were consequently never acknowledged or dealt with during my childhood. It is only now I am an adult that I have been able to work through some of my feelings within the safety of my own personal therapy. I am an expert and a survivor; I have a foot in both camps. However, in this [chapter] I would like to question the validity of the very notion of these two camps and to examine what may be the significance of such polarised thinking, where this area is commonly perceived as consisting of two mutually exclusive groups.

The tendency to divide this area into work done by experts and work done by survivors themselves could be understood as the result of 'splitting'. In psychoanalytic theory, the process of splitting is seen as a primitive form of defence against overwhelming and unbearable fears and impulses. Melanie Klein has argued that the infant perceives the world in split terms of 'good breast' and 'bad breast', attributing to the bad breast all its own sadistic impulses and images of persecution and attack. This process serves the purpose of allowing the infant to disown such feelings, as they are seen to belong to something outside, to something 'other'. Unfortunately, once this has happened, the outside embodiment of these projected feelings becomes an extreme persecutor as it has been filled with all that is too unbearable to be contained within. Although this mechanism of defence originates from such an early stage of development, it is available to us and operative throughout our lives on both an individual and group basis. In short, we all do it!

Groups of any size will often use splitting to attribute fearful and destructive impulses to an outside enemy, thereby sparing themselves the painful task of owning, exploring and making reparation for destructive feelings which exist within. Such a mechanism is most likely to be used in situations which arouse a threatening level of anxiety. Childhood sexual abuse is obviously one such extreme and has consistently been responded to with the defences of splitting and denial.

This process can operate on a huge and sometimes obvious scale. While writing this,

I am struck by the ironic image of the crowds which gathered around the police van transporting the two boys found guilty of murdering and stoning James Bulger: the irony being that the crowd showed its anger and revulsion by hurling stones at the escorting police van. Splitting can also operate in a far more insidious and subtle form which colours and influences our relationships, our work and our ways of thinking. While the very reasoning behind the concept of this anthology results from the history of the way in which sexual abuse has previously been viewed, reacted to and written about, it also reflects an apprehension of reality which results from conscious and unconscious splitting.

By this process, 'experts' working with survivors will often deny their own survivor within. In such a divided world of us and them, we the experts are the ones who analyse, research and suggest treatment for our clients: it is only they outside who have such problems, it certainly is not us. Thus the outside group of clients/patients/survivors can be abused again unwittingly and apparently for their own good while the experts disown the fact that they may share difficult feelings and experiences. At one extreme a survivor attempting to communicate pain and distress through symptoms of life-threatening anorexia may be force-fed and rendered powerless. More commonly and pervasively, the survivor may be abused again in a far more subtle way by being generally doubted, feared, blamed and treated with disrespect. In the world of us and them, there is a powerful unconscious assumption at work that the two groups are mutually exclusive. So it is possible for a fellow professional to refer a client to me with an offensive remark like: 'Well, you know what it's like with these survivors, they often repeat the patterns of abuse with their own children. We're very worried about her baby...'

Such a remark could only be made to me by someone assuming that as I am a professional, therefore I cannot possibly be a survivor myself. The assumption that the problem belongs to 'that lot out there' is so pervasive and strong and the shame and stigma of abuse so great that the survivor within (and here I am clearly refer-

ring to myself) is gagged into silence. So far, under these circumstances, I have not been able to declare myself as not only one of us but also one of them too.

However, the survivor group can also fall into this same trap of split thinking. It is easy to see how this can happen around an issue which produces such high levels of fear and anxiety. While the Kleinian bad breast becomes an arch-persecutor embodying our disowned destructive impulses, the Kleinian good breast embodies our hopes and aspirations. Unfortunately this also represents a distorted reality, as over-idealisation can at best lead to disappointment and at worst provoke profound envy and confirm a sense of our own impoverishment and worthlessness. Clients often come into counselling with the conscious or unconscious assumption that they are coming to see someone who is psychologically perfect and flawless. Since a counsellor should not disclose their own material for many reasons, not least because the session is sacredly reserved for the client's needs and material, such an assumption would be largely unchallenged. Clients entering into counselling and psychotherapy are in a highly vulnerable position and so may need to believe that the person in whom they are placing their trust has greater expertise and is more perfect in every way than they are themselves. On the other hand, such vulnerability may provoke the opposite reaction and a client may need to rubbish their counsellor with the 'what would she know about it anyway' type of response. Clients may also have the need to believe that they have an untarnished-by-abuse professional to help them. A survivor who is going through the painful struggle of overcoming feelings of guilt and shame may need to avoid even the thought that their counsellor may be 'tarred with the same brush'. The admonition, 'Physician heal thyself!' has deep roots and reverberations.

In order to be a non-damaging and effective counsellor, all professionals owe it to themselves and their clients to be in a continual process of developing self-awareness and actively working on their own areas of personal difficulty through training and therapy. However, if we had our difficulties so well and easily resolved as to be psychologically perfect, then we would have very few feelings of genuine empathy with our clients. On the other hand, if we are so damaged by unresolved feelings that we take these out on our clients, then we will lack the objectivity to be able to offer the lack of fear and the impartiality which can be so helpful. As professionals we need to offer the genuine emotional response which comes from having experienced painful struggles of our own while at the same time being able to offer a dispassionate analysis which can provide our clients with safety and clarity. Furthermore, while I am working with a survivor I am always aware that their material and reactions may be utterly different from my own, even though I know that we share the experience of having been abused.

While there is a strong external reality which has given an historical need for the survivor to speak out in their own voice, to be their own expert, and to claim their own feelings, this may nevertheless be complicated by the distortions of an internal reality where unhelpful defences are at work. Personal change and development can be a disorientating and threatening experience. We often cling to what we know best. If we know how it feels to be held by the anguish of isolation, rage and despair and to relate to others with profound mistrust, then we may view the world in such a way that these feelings are perpetuated. Such patterns are not our fault and result from something that happened to us in the past but that may not be happening to us in the present. It may be possible to relinquish old and limiting ways of perceiving and relating in favour of new ways which, although more confusing, are more open and enriching. The world could indeed be more grey than we (survivors and experts alike) assume and far less black and white.

I therefore suggest that survivors may also be guilty of an 'us and them' split in the same way as experts. I once had the salutary experience of being emotionally attacked at a meeting by a representative from a women's survivors' group. As I was seen at the time to be in the expert camp, she made the assumption that I could not possibly know anything meaningful about sexual abuse. She saw me only as a professional

counsellor and to her this meant that I couldn't have the benefit of any first-hand experience. The setting would have been utterly inappropriate for any personal disclosure on my part and so I was unable to challenge the assumptions behind the exchange between us.

Until recently, I have unconsciously believed that these two groups are mutually exclusive and that I am guilty of some form of transgression by secretly belonging to both. Perhaps I am guilty of some dreadful act of duplicity by having a foot in each camp? I am still beset by fears that most survivors will recognise. Who should I tell? Who can I trust with this shameful secret and this double act? I must admit that it is far more comfortable for me to be seen as solely aligned with the professionals: that persona carries status, not stigma. Anyone I tell of my secret may imagine that I'm bound to abuse or collude with the abuse of my children. Similarly they may have fears that I'll abuse my clients. On a very deep level, I have these fears myself. As a counsellor, I may damage my clients; as a client I may manipulate my therapist into abusing me. The psychoanalytical precept that we all tend to repeat patterns of behaviour is loaded when it comes to abuse because of all the stigmatisation and fear of contamination which are involved.

Sometimes it is possible to learn a great deal by reminding ourselves of the obvious, so I'll state the obvious here. Being a person involves being more than any one thing. I am both a mother and a daughter. I am both a survivor working on my own pain in therapy and a counsellor undertaking therapeutic work with survivors. The assumptions of my colleagues and clients; the collective myths and fears of our society and my own feelings and fears of shame fuse together to make this a most uncomfortable and uneasy combination. But there is hope. As a trained and experienced professional, I have a wider view than that which could be gained purely from subjective experience. As a survivor I have real experience of how all this feels with an immediacy which could not possibly be learned from theoretical understanding alone. In both groups I feel different. In some ways, and especially on bad days, this can feel like being the odd one out and is upsetting. In other ways though, I know we are all different from each other anyway and working with difference can be the source of great creativity and growth.

I will conclude with the most crucial and painful dilemma that has emerged while writing this [chapter]. Can I own who I am? Can I let clients and colleagues identify this struggling double agent? What I am wrestling with, of course, is whether or not to sign my name. Perhaps this feels like 'coming out'. I am unsure whether I am more afraid of my own feelings or of other people's stereotypes and assumptions that may get dumped on me. I am afraid of the stigma which I know still surrounds survivors of sexual abuse. Why should I continue to feel ashamed of being a survivor? I would have no dilemma to work through if this [chapter] only showed me as an expert and I'm sure I would readily sign my name to it then! If I don't sign this, then fear will be compelling me to disown my survivor within. If I do sign, I'll be saying that this struggle has been mine and I'm proud of how far I've come with it. I will be acting on my rational belief that the two groups are not mutually exclusive and that it is possible to be both. I can own all of who I am. I can be proud of being me.

A Story About the Body

ROBERT HASS

The young composer, working that summer at an artist's colony, had watched her for a week. She was Japanese, a painter, almost sixty, and he thought he was in love with her. He loved her work, and her work was like the way she moved her body, used her hands, looked at him directly when she made amused and considered answers to his questions. One night, walking back from a concert, they came to her door and she turned to him and said, "I think you would like to have me. I would like that too, but I must tell you that I have had a double mastectomy," and when he didn't understand, "I've lost both my breasts." The radiance that he had carried around in his belly and his chest cavity – like music – withered, very quickly, and he made himself look at her when he said, "I'm sorry. I don't think I could." He walked back to his own cabin through the pines, and in the morning he found a small blue bowl on the porch outside his door. It looked to be full of rose petals, but he found when he picked it up that the rose petals were on top; the rest of the bowl – she must have swept them from the corners of her studio – was full of dead bees.

Part VIII

Continuing Contact: Chronic Illness, Disability, Deformity, Remission, and Relapse

Introduction

Long-term illness and disability present particular challenges equally for patients, carers, and professionals. Some of these challenges are evident enough. For the individual concerned, for example, and for his or her immediate family and friends, there is the plain problem of finding the courage to face the fact that there is no way back to full health. Jenny Lewis, in the opening chapter in this section, finds this courage, as many others have done, among her peers, "fellow women yet brave and practical / about their own survival." On a wider canvas, a problem of ever-growing prominence in day-to-day care is lack of resources. As Stuart Youngner graphically puts it in chapter 74, in relation to dementia, with a rapidly ageing population in Europe and America, "the avalanche is coming."

There are also more hidden challenges, though, many of which, in part just because they are less self-evident, may be even harder to meet. Rejection and stigmatization, in particular, are themes that run through the chapters in Part VIII. There is a paradox here. Chronic disease and disability are in many ways harder to bear than acute and time-limited illnesses, however devastating these may be at the time. Yet whereas acute illnesses elicit positive emotions – of care, concern, and so forth – chronic conditions tend to elicit negative emotions.

There is nothing new in this, of course. In chapter 69, writing of the skin as an organ of communication, Terence Ryan and Vineet Kaur remind us of the ill-treatment those with disfiguring disease have received all down the ages. We return to this chapter later. But a key point brought out in it, a point that goes to the heart of the paradoxical response to those with chronic conditions, is the extent to which, in many cultures and at many periods, disfigurement and disability have been equated with degeneracy. Leprosy, as Ryan and Kaur describe, is a "model for stigmatization and the inter-reaction between themes of cleanliness and the religious views of the Judaeo-Christian and Moslem literature of an earlier age;" and even today, on "skin wards, there is ritual bathing in which washing away the skin may still be perceived as equivalent to washing away the sin."

In our own time, AIDS is the paradigm of rejection and stigmatization of those with chronic disorders. This is in part because of the association between AIDS and what are still regarded as deviant, rather than merely different, modes of expression of human sexuality, notably homosexuality and promiscuity. Sex, never more freely available, is still morally suspect. Yet, as Virginia van der Vliet shows in chapter 70, "The Politics of AIDS," our prejudices are not sufficient to explain the moral opprobrium attaching to AIDS. For this extends to innocent and "guilty" alike. There is, in this, a complex interplay of values, individual and social, religious, financial, and political. This interplay, as van der Vliet describes, is coming to a new focus in a "politically charged debate . . . about the rights of HIV positive women to produce children." On the one hand in this debate there are women who may well be HIV positive and yet, in many cultures, are under extreme pressures to produce children; on the other, there is a growing concern about the number of babies who, at best, will be left orphaned, at worst, will die of the disease themselves. There are deep dilemmas here, both personal and social; indeed, as van der Vliet puts it, AIDS "has the unhappy knack of pitting 'individual rights' against 'public good'." The danger, though, she believes, as the number of AIDS cases continues to grow, is of a new eugenics pursued with reformist zeal, through which "policies could become . . . repressive."

The dangers of a repressive regime, zealously enforced, in situations of diverse and conflicting values, were highlighted in the Introduction to this volume (in our conclusion, "The Abuses of Absolutism"). As we noted there, these dangers have been nowhere more evident than in the abuses to which that most value-diverse area of healthcare, psychiatry, has been subject. There is no easy way to resolve conflicts of values, we argued, once absolutism is given up in favor of tolerance of diversity. But a key step to less abusive practices is to recognize that our powers of "second guessing" the values of others, particularly as between professionals and their clients and patients, are extremely limited. Hence it is fundamental, in such situations, to bring users (patients and carers) directly and substantively "into the loop."

The Avon Mental Health Measure, key parts of which are reproduced in chapter 71, is an example of a recent attempt to bring users into the loop in the area of needs assessment for the long-term mentally ill. In an early article in *Philosophy, Psychiatry, and Psychology*, the Oxford psychiatrist Max Marshall showed that existing instruments for measuring needs in this group consistently failed to reflect the values of those most directly concerned, i.e. users and carers (Marshall, 1994). The Avon Mental Health Measure allows users to represent their own views directly. More significantly, though, it was designed and developed by a team which included users on an equal basis with professionals. As can be seen, it is very clear and easy to use; it covers concerns that might not have occurred to the professionals on their own (e.g., that in expressing an "unmet need," a user might end up being discriminated against); it emphasizes strengths as well as problems; and it does not make false promises (it makes clear that some needs may not be met, and that professionals will not necessarily agree with a user's views of what they need). The Measure, therefore, reflects a philosophy of user–professional partnership, rather than either a professional-dominated or user-dominated model of service provision.

User–professional partnership is integral to the model of healthcare ethics outlined in the Introduction to this volume. In mental health in particular, but also in primary care in general, it is a central feature of healthcare ethics' response to the challenge of dealing with diversity of values in healthcare (Fulford, 1989: ch. 11). Besides diversity of values as such, however, chronic disease and disabling conditions show the importance in healthcare of conflicts between values of *qualitatively* different kinds. Thus, disease, imprudence, wickedness, ugliness, and so forth, are all negatively evaluated conditions. But the kinds of negative values they express are qualitatively different one from another.

Qualitative differences of values, as one of us has described in detail elsewhere (Fulford, 1989, especially Part 3), lie behind a wide range of ethically contentious questions in medicine. These are well illustrated by many of the problems discussed by Ryan and Kaur in chapter 69. Thus patients with unsightly skin conditions, for example, may be refused treatment on the grounds that the problem is merely "cosmetic." The (usually implicit) justification for such refusals is that although the condition is indeed a problem, it is not a problem with which doctors should be concerned because it is not, really, a disease (medical value) but a disfigurement (aesthetic value). In the case of AIDS, and other diseases associated with socially disapproved lifestyles (e.g. smoking, alcohol abuse), refusal of treatment may be justified either on the grounds that the person concerned does not "deserve" scarce resources (moral value), or that they are not capable of changing their ways and hence will squander resources (prudential value).

As with many other aspects of the value structure of medicine, the tensions between medical and other kinds of value are writ large particularly in mental health. "Mad or bad?" (medical or moral/legal value) is a familiar question in forensic psychiatry, e.g., with psychopathic personality disorder; "mad or sad?" (medical or personal value) is the corresponding question in civil proceedings involving involuntary treatment, e.g. for depression; "mad or foolish?" (medical or prudential value) is the counterpart question for self-defeating behavior, e.g. with alcohol or drugs.

Organic mental conditions, those due to gross pathology affecting the brain, have traditionally been regarded as an unambiguously proper focus of medical concern. Dementia is, in this sense, closer to bodily medical conditions than, say, hysteria. Yet as Elizabeth Forsythe describes in her account of her husband, John's, slide into Alzheimer's disease (chapter 72), the impact of such conditions on the moral faculties – emotion, desire, volition, motivation, and so forth – may be so profound as to strike to the very core of the person's identity, to their very soul one might say. Forsythe calls her piece "My Husband the Stranger;" and this is taken from a book with the title *Alzheimer's Disease: The Long Bereavement*. To some extent the changes in John were exaggerations of his previous personality: his "inner solitariness," for example, evolving into total isolation. Such changes are characteristic of slowly progressive organic mental disorders. All the same, their impact is so profound that for the patient's family and friends, it often seems that the person they knew is no longer there (Hope, 1994).

Dementia, in part because of its effect on personal identity, is a condition for which the support of carers who are not among the patient's family or friends, and hence have no memories of the person before the onset of their disease, may be particularly helpful. As Mary Howell puts it in chapter 73, writing on the role of caretakers in the care of the demented elderly, "Relatives of patients, reflecting on changes they see in personality, cognitive abilities, and relationships, grieve for their own sense of loss. ... But for anyone who gives direct care, each patient is at the same time *fully* a person" (emphasis in original). Howell lists the values of those who "do this work well with a sense of joy and accomplishment." At the top of the list is "A belief in the value of every living person." As Howell goes on to describe, whatever the codes and policies in place, it is the values of the care-givers directly concerned with individual patients, performing such daily routines as bathing and feeding, that crucially determine the quality of day-to-day care. These values are not fully explicit; they are perhaps incapable even of being fully articulated; but they are nonetheless crucial to the "craft skills" that distinguish good from bad clinical care.

We have several times emphasized the importance of hidden or implicit values in health-care ethics. In chapter 74, Stuart Youngner illustrates this in two further respects. The first is the way in which hidden values may be revealed by what people do in practice. Thus, Youngner is concerned with a proposal by D. J. Murphy, a doctor working in a long-term care facility, that professionals, rather than patients or relatives, should make decisions about "do not resuscitate" orders. Murphy, Youngner tells us, argues that these decisions should be made without reference to either the patient or his or her family, when the doctor believes that further intervention will be futile. But Murphy, Youngner notes, despite his theory, actually goes to great lengths in practice to involve all those concerned fully in such decisions. His practice, then, not his theory, reveals his true values. A deeper concern, though, coming to the second respect in which values are hidden in Murphy's proposal, is his (Murphy's) failure to recognize that "futile" in this context is not a purely technical but a deeply value-laden concept. Here, then, as in the case history of Simon described in chapter 20, we find crucial value judgments disguised as technical issues. "Under the guise of medical expertise," Youngner concludes, Murphy's proposal "encourages physicians to substitute their own value judgments for those of their patients."

Values, though, important as they are, are only one among a range of factors involved in understanding, as opposed merely to explaining, medical conditions. Meaning, significance, empathy, and insight, for example, are also important in this respect. Such factors are important in all areas of medicine. But they are vitally important in the context of chronic and disabling conditions. Consider empathy, for example. In mental disorder, difficulties of understanding may arise from gaps between the experiences of those concerned and everyday experiences. Dementia is, in a sense, understandable as an extension of everyday experiences of confusion and lapses of memory. To this (limited) extent, then, we are all capable of empathic insight into pathological forms of these experiences. And similar considerations apply to many other mental disorders, such as anxiety and depression.

Other mental disorders, though, may involve experiences which, at least at first glance, appear to be qualitatively different from everyday experiences. Such experiences, then, may not be (immediately) accessible to empathic understanding. This is the case, for example, with the seemingly bizarre symptoms of conditions such as schizophrenia and autism. How, for example, can we understand empathically the experience of schizophrenic thought insertion – thoughts that you are thinking (in this sense they are your own) and yet which you experience as the thoughts of someone else (Fulford, 1995). Karl Jaspers, indeed, to whom we owe a model of psychopathology expressly encompassing meanings as well as causes (Jaspers, 1913), defined such conditions in part by the fact that they are not readily understandable. Yet even with conditions such as these, as

Donna Williams's autobiographical account of her childhood autism shows (chapter 75), understanding is not only possible but essential to good clinical care. The seemingly pointless games she played as a young girl at school with her friend Sandra were attempts to make contact with others. They would "push [their] eyes in, in order to see colours, and we would scream and scream until our throats were red raw." But this was because "In the company of others my senses would cut off, and I would become so numb that, in order to experience something, I had to push myself to extreme limits."

Narrative accounts, as we noted in the volume Introduction, are among the most powerful ways of extending understanding and hence of providing content for a healthcare ethics which is based on respect for diversity of values. Narratives, though, as we also noted, are importantly complemented by a range of more formal methods. Among these, the contribution of phenomenology is illustrated in chapter 76 by Kay Toombs's account of the effects on her body of her progressive multiple sclerosis. Toombs is a philosopher who has specialized in phenomenology (see, e.g., her book, *The Meaning of Illness*, 1993). In our volume, she brings the skills of phenomenology to bear in showing the profound disturbance of agency, and hence both of self-identity and of one's relationship with the world, which result when "the body suddenly appears to have an opposing will of its own." She draws out in dramatic detail the impact on "one's whole way of being," not just of motor disorders, but of sensory disturbance, of loss of bladder and bowel control, and, most significant of all, of the disease itself. The varied and progressive lesions of multiple sclerosis produce a "paradoxical relation between body and self," which is "intrinsic to the experience of chronic illness and disability." The paradox is that "*My* body appears as other-than-me in that it continually opposes and frustrates my intentions; yet I *am* my body for I cannot escape my impaired embodiment" (emphases in original).

The importance of understanding each particular patient's experience, in bodily medicine as well as in psychiatry, is dramatically illustrated by the report from the *Guardian* newspaper, reproduced in chapter 77, of the "miracle" recovery of a young man, Geoff, diagnosed as suffering from persistent vegetative state (PVS). Geoff's story draws together many of the themes about chronic illness introduced in Part VIII: the importance of individual values (even when apparently unaware of his environment, Geoff was kept going by his love of music); the tension between the value of Geoff's life to himself and wider public-interest issues of resource allocation; the difficulty of defining "futility," even at a technical level (the statistics suggest that, conventional medical opinion notwithstanding, recovery from PVS is far from unusual); the crucial importance of including users in the decision-making process – it was Geoff's mother who was the first to realize that he was sometimes aware of what was going on.

Geoff's story, though, adds two important further dimensions to our understanding of chronic illness and disability. The first is the value of technology. Too often, technology is portrayed as the villain of the piece. In a healthcare model, though, as we showed in the Introduction to this volume, science and ethics are partners. The value of this partnership is illustrated in a very down-to-earth way by Geoff's story. Communication was the key to his (partial) recovery. But it was computer technology that was the key to establishing and developing a means of communication with him.

If the first dimension of understanding added by Geoff's story is the value of technology, the second is the value of disability itself. Thus Geoff, as reported in chapter 77, despite his extreme disablement, is described as "carrying on lively conversations" and communicating "regularly with his mother and friends." The point, and it is a point that is being made increasingly loudly by disabled people themselves (see Reading Guide), is that with chronic illness and disability, tragic as they may sometimes be, everything is far from being all doom and gloom. This positive message is well captured by the title of Sally French and John Swain's chapter, "Across the Disability Divide: Whose Tragedy?" French and Swain draw together both first-hand accounts and recent research, showing the extent to which the "tragedy view of disability is itself disabling." The "tragedy

view" reflects the values of non-disabled people, not those of the disabled. It assumes that "disabled people cannot be happy, or enjoy an adequate quality of life." Yet, as French and Swain describe, there are many examples of disablement, which, far from being a tragedy, carry with them positive advantages. Their examples range from the acquisition of particular skills (e.g. as physiotherapists, French, 1991) to a "more interesting sex life" (Shakespeare et al., 1996: 106). We should move, then, French and Swain conclude, away from the tragedy view "to better values including the celebration of differences."

With many progressive diseases, of course, there is little to celebrate. It is with such conditions, as we noted at the start of this Introduction, that the greatest challenges arise. And yet, even here, in facing these challenges, the best of human nature is often revealed. This is evident in every chapter in this section: Jenny Lewis's new found courage; the models "of good communication, of good behaviour, and of good practice in human relationships" provided by those concerned with skin diseases (chapter 69); the resourcefulness of those tackling the problem of AIDS education in non-western cultures described by van der Vliet; the positive strengths emphasized in the Avon Mental Health Measure; the lawyer whose practical help was so essential to Elizabeth Forsythe; and Dr Murphy's practice, despite his theory, in Stuart Youngner's chapter.

There is a final paradox here, then, a paradox to counter that of the stigmatization and rejection of chronic disorders with which we opened this Introduction. The final paradox is that it is with just such chronic conditions, the hardest to face, and the most stigmatized, that we find also the greatest goods in healthcare. As May Sarton, in our concluding poem (chapter 79) puts it, such conditions take us "into a new discipline . . . and a new grace."

REFERENCES

French, S. (1991) The advantages of visual impairment: Some physiotherapists' views. *New Beacon* 75/872: 1–6.

Fulford, K. W. M. (1989; repr. 1995 and 1999; 2nd edn forthcoming) *Moral Theory and Medical Practice* (Cambridge: Cambridge University Press).

Fulford, K. W. M. (1995) Thought insertion, insight and Descartes' cogito: Linguistic analysis and the descriptive psychopathology of schizophrenic thought disorder. In A. Sims (ed.), *Speech and Language Disorders* (London: Gaskell Press for the Royal College of Psychiatrists), ch. 12.

Hope, T. (1994) Personal identity and psychiatric illness. In A. Phillips Griffiths (ed.), *Philosophy, Psychology and Psychiatry* (Cambridge: Cambridge University Press), for the Royal Institute of Philosophy Supplement 37: 131–43.

Jaspers, K. (1913) *Causal and Meaningful Connexions Between Life History and Psychosis.* Repr. in S. R. Hirsch and M. Shepherd (eds.), *Themes and Variations in European Psychiatry* (Bristol: John Wright and Sons Ltd, 1974), ch. 5.

Marshall, M. (1994) How should we measure need? Concept and practice in the development of a standardised assessment schedule. *Philosophy, Psychiatry, and Psychology* 1: 27–36. (Commentaries by R. Crisp and J. Morgan, pp. 37–40.)

Shakespeare, T., Gillespie-Sells, K., and Davies, D. (1996) *The Sexual Politics of Disability* (London: Cassell).

Toombs, S. Kay (1993) *The Meaning of Illness: A Phenomenological Account of the Different Perspectives of Physician and Patient* (Dordrecht, The Netherlands: Kluwer Academic Publishers).

READING GUIDE

Ethical issues in long-term illness and disability are discussed in George Agich's *Autonomy and Long Term Care* (Oxford: Oxford University Press, 1993). Norman Daniels's *Just Healthcare* (Cambridge: Cambridge University Press, 1985) gives an authoritative discussion of a number of relevant issues, including equal access to care, prevention, treatment of the elderly, and the working relationship between practitioners and managers. Case examples of new patient-centered approaches to the development and delivery of healthcare (including disability) are given in K. W. M. Fulford, Steven Ersser, and T. Hope (eds.), *Essential Practice in Patient-Centred Care* (Oxford: Blackwell Science, 1995). For a thoughtful discussion of ethical issues in old-age psychiatry, see Tony Hope and Catherine Oppenheimer's "Ethics and the Psychiatry of Old Age," in R. Jacoby and C. Oppen-heimer, *Psychiatry in the Elderly*, 2nd edn (Oxford: Oxford University Press, 1997).

Balanced introductions to the themes of normalization and valorization in disability are given by W. Wolfensberger, in *The Principle of Normalization in Human Services* (Toronto: NIMR, 1972) and in "Social role valorization: A proposed new term for the principle of normalization," *Mental Retardation* 21 (1983): 234–9. Narrative accounts from the user literature include Peter Campbell's descriptions of his experiences of neuroleptic medication in "What we want from mental health services," in J. Read and J. Reynolds, *Speaking our Minds: An Anthology* (London: Macmillan Press, 1996), pp. 180–3. Recent work showing the importance of meaning and intention, particularly in "organic" brain disease, includes Steven Sabat and Rom Harre, "The Alzheimer's disease sufferer as semiotic subject," *Philosophy, Psychiatry and Psychology* 1 (1994): 145–63, and S. R. Sabat's *The Experience of Alzheimer's Disease: Life Through a Tangled Veil* (Oxford: Blackwell Publishers, 2001); also Pat Bracken's *Outside the Magic Circle: Meaning and Mental Illness in the Postmodern Age* (London: Whurr Publishers, forthcoming); and K. W. M. Fulford's "Disordered minds, diseased brains and real people," in *Philosophy, Psychiatry and Psychopathy: Personal Identity in Mental Disorder* (Avebury Series in Philosophy, in association with The Society for Applied Philosophy. Aldershot, England: Ashgate Publishing Ltd, 2000).

Philosophical work on the concepts of disorder relevant to understanding chronic disease and disability includes K. W. M. Fulford's analysis of incapacity as loss of agency in his *Moral Theory and Medical Practice* (Cambridge: Cambridge University Press, 1989; repr. 1995 and 1999; 2nd edn forthcoming) and Lennart Nordenfelt's *On the Nature of Health: An Action-theoretic Approach* (2nd edn forthcoming; Dordrecht; Holland: D. Reidel Publishing Company); this gives an in-depth analysis of the concept of health linking it directly to basic needs. Len Doyal and Ian Gough, *The Theory of Human Need* (London: Macmillan Press, 1991) is a careful analysis of the concept of need which combines ethical and economic theory. It covers disability, the interactions of social, political, and physical factors, and cultural diversity. A case example and discussion drawing together the ethical and conceptual issues raised by disability is Case 3.2, "Tom Benbow – Diagnosis and distributive justice", in D. Dickenson and K. W. M. Fulford's *In Two Minds: A Casebook of Psychiatric Ethics* (Oxford: Oxford University Press, 2000), pp. 67–76.

The *Philosophy and Medicine* book series, edited by H. Tristram Engelhardt and Stuart F. Spicker (Kluwer Academic Publishers), includes a number of relevant volumes. Besides Kay Toombs's *The Meaning of Illness* (noted above), see D. Leder (ed.), *The Body in Medical Thought and Practice* (1992); and R. M. Zaner (ed.), *Death: Beyond Whole-Brain Criteria* (1988).

The Way to Freedom
6th April, 1985

JENNY LEWIS

The arrows point to EXIT — the way to freedom —
beyond the ward and the car park. A new life.
And He tells me — the One in the white coat
that is — to find a new path to follow.

"Avoid stress," he says. "Or find better ways
to deal with it." And "Do things you want to do —
things that make you happy." But his meter is
 running.
Another patient waiting. I close his door behind me

and notice spears of sunlight piercing the dark
hospital corridor. Birds swoop outside the window.
A swordthrust of hunger reminds me the troops
need feeding if I'm going to win any battles.

So I forget the weekly shop and head
for a pub lunch — past a battleaxe of an orderly
and battalions of sad people shuffling towards
appointments. And I think of the one-breasted

Amazons; fellow women yet brave and practical
about their own survival who harnessed their
 energies
into living and dying with courage. And, suddenly,
I know that's what I want to do too.

So I follow the arrows.

Privacy and Display: Issues of Good Practice for Dermatologists

TERENCE J. RYAN AND VINEET KAUR

[. . .]

"Failure to communicate" is often given as a principal reason for breakdown in human relations within families or between nations. A communication failure is usually interpreted as verbal, but skin failure is a common cause of a similar breakdown in communication. Love at first sight, revulsion at disfigurement, and color prejudice are examples of communication that are necessary for human relationships in the classroom, in the practice of medicine, in prison, and between nations.

[. . .]

The Skin in its Social Context

Much of the following section is derived from the writings of Ray Jobling[1] and the quotes that he has given in describing the skin's social role. Jobling is Director of the Psoriasis Association (UK) and has psoriasis particularly in mind, but he also refers to the social, psychological, economic, and political implications of skin color and the negative social implications of dark pigmentation. In some countries, a tan is mis-takenly believed to be a sign of health. It is also a sign of being wealthy and socially privileged, being able to enjoy winter skiing or Mediterranean holidays, being socially attractive, and being respectable. Jobling also discusses in some detail the overlap between the cosmetic nature of many complaints.

One-third of all out-patient [dermatology] referrals from general practitioners may be deemed as unnecessary and half are sent for "social" rather than "clinical" reasons. Jobling quotes the British social anthropologist Vieda Skultans on blushing.[2] An inability to blush, according to one Victorian view, was said to provide an outward sign of inner failings including, most especially, moral weakness and lack of conscience. Excessive blushing, on the other hand, suggested clear "evidence of inner moral derangement and very often betrayed the chronic masturbator."

The role of the skin in signifying shame, he states, is well recognized in many cultures. The anthropologist Andrew Strathern[3] quotes the example of the Melpa of the Mount Hagen district of New Guinea's Western Highlands. They use the expression "shame is on the skin." When the Melpa feel shame they say that their skin has become too hot or too cold, or breaks out in a sweat. [. . .]

One may quote the Bible or the Koran, an example being Job's illness "my skin is broken and become loathsome" (Job VII: 5). On stage or in a film, clean skin is considered as evidence of a spotless character, whereas a blemish on the skin is often treated as evil and something to be blamed for. Such terms as face-saving, thick-skinned, thin-skinned, touchy, getting under the skin, or being stung to the quick, show that blows to one's self-esteem may be projected to the body's surface and consequently be symbolically expressed and experienced as injuries to the skin – disfiguring diseases – resulting in a lowering of self-esteem. [. . .]

Rees[4] describes cutaneous disease used as a representation of evil in the cinema, and while this is fiction, patients themselves may express similar views to the following one given in a letter to the Psoriasis Association: "it is not easy to live with psoriasis because it is in some ways a reflection of ourselves and we feel that we must be eternally on show as being miserable, wicked creatures with visible signs of inner wickedness." Jobling,[5] in a study of patients' subjective experiences of what is the worst thing about having psoriasis, gives many quotes of the word unclean, but shame is also frequently mentioned, as is an excessive attempt at cleansing. "Washing cleanses physically but also morally. The act of washing is a ritual purification."

The Stigma of Leprosy

Only the profession of leprology, which is now virtually unknown, knows better than dermatologists why leprosy is a model for stigmatization and the inter-reaction between themes of cleanliness and the religious views of the Judaeo-Christian and Moslem literature of an earlier age. It is well known that the biblical ambiguity between leprosy and psoriasis existed not merely in dermatological literature but also in the minds of many patients and their families. Probably the best description of the association and its management is in Leviticus, in which the prevention of uncleanliness gave rise to a whole host of regulations of the lives of communities, and there has been much discussion about the cultural or anthropological background to these concepts, i.e. the role of the priest in cleansing rather than curing or treating and the specifically male view of menstruation and bathing with a perception of competence. On any skin wards there is ritual bathing in which washing away the skin may still be perceived as equivalent to washing away the sin.

Awareness of the Skin as an Organ of Communication

A dermatologist is concerned with the feelings of rejection in all age groups. He or she manages the new born with a birth mark with understanding of its effect on the family and the influence of peers, school teachers, and employers.

Much can be learned about display by looking at the literature on hair, whether too much or too little, and considering concepts of disordered self-image and its management. For most, baldness is unacceptable, but the hair may be shaved to be "cool" or to debase people, as in the collaborators at the end of the last great war, or because it is sexually provocative, as in the case of shaving the new wives of an Orthodox Jew. The distinction between total alopecia and a shaved head can only be realized by those who have experienced it. The patient with alopecia may experience all kinds of interpretation: "I shave my head because I am small and with long hair I am perceived as soft and 'girly', with no hair I get more respect;" "It's a political statement having very close cropped hair, it is to do with identifying myself as a gay person;" "The style I have chosen to adopt is a very macho one with army overtones – almost identical to that adopted by skinheads, whose right-wing views are very different from my own;" "I go regularly to a Buddhist retreat and shave my head to cut off the self or ego."

Even more common, especially in schools, is the problem of acne: e.g. the adolescent who suffers from a degree of anxiety and depression, who cannot get through an interview, and who locks himself in a bathroom and hides from social situations. Helping such people to be confident is a very complex issue requiring empathy with those who have impairment of the skin. Even the most severe disfigurement can be bolstered by the effects of empathy; thus the "elephant man" became very confident, even vain, when Heads of State gave gifts which were of a cosmetic kind, and made him "quite a dandy." His caretaker, Stewart Treeves, provided cosmetic hair-brushes, combs, and scent, and with these the "elephant man" was clearly very delighted.

Not all problems are due to disease. The removal of tattoos or the treatment of wrinkles are other examples of problems which are often regarded as purely cosmetic. A young person's life can be totally ruined by tattoos applied 10 years earlier. One manages the so-called triviality of the cosmetic only because one knows that people's lives and their potential to achieve economically and socially may depend upon them. The professional model whose life is one of display must worry about shape, color, beauty, and a healthy image. The concept of the Greek ideal of beauty, the "confident nude," has a status which all would like to achieve as opposed to the Gothic shameful nude of Eve after the discovery.

The extreme of disfigurement is perhaps illustrated by burns. No amount of plastic surgery can restore those affected to looking good and such people have to learn to communicate when facing others. Solutions include workshops training people to communicate.[6] Sometimes we can use clothing or other systems of camouflage to restore people's confidence and there is a literature for cancer sufferers which is well developed.

In medicine we must help people without making their lives more difficult, and bring out the capacity to achieve by means other than appearance. Helping a child to achieve his or her potential is the job of the parent and the teacher. Handing yourself over to others is one aspect of that management. It is seen in the bonding of a parent and a child, the control of a class by an experienced school teacher, or the directing of soldiers by a platoon sergeant. One also sees it in the management of patients by doctors. In so doing we are developing the professional role of doctor–patient relationships, one person playing the sick role and the other

the provider of care, and one accepting a degree of institutionalization.

[. . .]

Bad Practice

The International Convention on Civil and Political Rights is a code of behavior about cruel, inhuman or degrading management of people, respect for autonomy, and protection of persons. Several of the quotes above indicate that persons may be degraded because of their appearance, "the little black sambo" of children's literature is believed to show color prejudice, as is the "gollywog." [. . .]

The author, on his first visit to Africa, viewed a demonstration of leprosy at two different leprosaria. One in which a nun introduced a young boy, fully clothed, by the name of Joseph and, before demonstrating his skin condition, described his gardening aptitude and successes. At another leprosarium one was issued with a passport at a guarded gate, the patient stood unclothed on a pedestal, was introduced as a number, and no communication took place as he was undressed to view. [. . .]

Case demonstrations have been central to the educational dermatologist for more than 100 years. Anything from 20 to 100 patients may be displayed to 20 to 500 dermatologists. The display may be without screens and patients may be placed on pedestals, photographed, prodded, and not spoken to. The question that is raised is "who should be in control of display?" Keenan,[7] writing of his experience as a prisoner in Lebanon for 4 years, has, on the front of his book, a crouched nude man. What he describes is survival and he emphasizes very strongly that clothing and nudity were always under his control. It was mostly he, and not his warders, who controlled how he looked. It was a very important part of his survival.

[. . .]

A Curriculum for Dermatologists

[. . .] Skin failure is a common cause of breakdown in communication and one end-point of health is to be able to display one's skin with confidence; indeed it should be a human right. Dermatologists should have great awareness of such an issue and be concerned not so much with disease as with health. They should not be ambivalent about the importance of the cosmetic. To be unwelcome in society is the worst disability, and it is one which the profession of dermatology can do much to relieve.

Spiro[8] suggests that medical schools squeeze empathy out of the students. It is the job of dermatologists to keep the skin in the foreground. It is so extraordinarily neglected that even the excellent article, based on the subject of empathy and making statements about the aesthetic, by Spiro in a journal as prestigious as the *Annals of Internal Medicine*, gives no mention of the skin. Skin simply has no profile in medical teaching. [...] Van Moeffaert[9] writes that many of the patients' perceptions are regarded, even by dermatologists, as minor compared with life threatening illnesses. Hence dermatologists may judge their patients' complaints to be exaggerated and may become irritated with an alopecia patient who cannot cope with baldness. Dawber[10] has described the primacy of "concern" when dealing with such problems.
[...]
The dermatologist must recognize ownership and know when the invasion of space becomes therapeutic. Stephen Ersser,[11] in searching for the therapeutic dimensions of the nurse–patient interaction, writes of the importance of the nurse's presence, the act of being with the patient. In dermatology practice being with the patient includes complete invasion of their space and how this should be used therapeutically is worthy of examination. [...] Dermatological nursing has to consider more complex issues. The patient who is isolated and feels the need to be touched may not benefit from being separated by a glove or a spatula. Professionalism and issues such as cross-infection control may require an explanation of why distancing is necessary. This has to be carried out without making the patient feel even more unclean. Ersser goes on to discuss attachment behavior and the tension that a patient may have between the need for privacy and the need to be with the

nurse. This leads on to the whole question of ritual and the way that, in the use of ritual to provide procedural action, a greater degree of confidence can be imbued. The examples of bad practice given above are mostly related to an absence of screening and a loss of privacy. To some extent they also relate to the aggression or arrogance of the doctor in power. [...]

Conclusions

To hide or display is a human right and that one end-point of health is to display with confidence. Dermatologists have much to contribute in providing a model of good communication, of good behavior, or of good practice in human relationships. [...] Tackling the issue of privacy versus display is a good beginning.

NOTES

1   Jobling, R., "Psoriasis and its treatment in psycho-social perspective," *Rev. Contemp. Pharmacother.* 3 (1992): 339–45.

2   Skultans, V., "Bodily madness and the spread of the blush," in J. Blacking (ed.), *The Anthropology of the Body* (London: Academic Press, 1977), pp. 145–60.

3   Strathern, A., "Why is shame on the skin?" in J. Blacking (ed.), *The Anthropology of the Body* (London: Academic Press, 1977), pp. 99–110.

4   Rees, V., "Dermatology in the cinema," *J. Am. Acad. Dermatol.* 33 (1995): 1030–5.

5   Jobling, "Psoriasis and its treatment."

6   Partridge, J., *Changing Faces: The Challenge of Facial Disfigurement* (London: Penguin Publishers, 1991).

7   Keenan, B., *An Evil Cradling* (Vintage) (London: Arrow, 1992), p. 296.

8   Spiro, H., "What is empathy. Can it be taught?" *Ann. Int. Med.* 116 (1992): 845.

9   Van Moeffaert, M. V., "Training future dermatologists in psycho-dermatology," *General Hospital Psychiatry* 8 (1986): 115–18.

10 Dawber, R. P. R. D. and Van Neste, D., *Hair and Scalp Disorders* (London: Martin Dunitz, 1995), p. 262.

11 Ersser, S., "A search for the therapeutic dimensions of nurse–patient interaction," in R. McMohan and A. Pearson (eds.), *Nursing as Therapy* (London: Chapman and Hall, 1991).

70

The Politics of AIDS

VIRGINIA VAN DER VLIET

[...]

A potentially [...] politically charged debate is beginning to surface about the rights of HIV-positive women to produce children at all. It centres on the issues of whether women have the right to give birth to 'doomed' babies, or to give birth when they themselves are 'doomed', and the baby will either die young or live to be a 'burden' on society once the mother, and usually the father, too, is dead. Even evidence which suggests that AZT, given to pregnant women, could reduce the number of paediatric transmissions, may be countered with the argument that this is simply producing healthy orphans.

With the exception of a small number of women in contemporary developed countries, the majority of the world's women appear to want to produce children. Since the future of any community depends on its physical need to reproduce itself, it is not surprising that the great majority of societies include strong pronatalist themes in both secular and religious teachings; Genesis' injunction to 'be fruitful, and multiply, and replenish the earth', is widely incorporated in reproductive norms. Similarly the pity, the scorn or the ostracism which 'barren' women experience make them eager to

fulfill the expectations of motherhood which marriage entails, not once, but usually repeatedly, and often at least until they produce a son. Many women in developed countries bear less than the 2.1 children necessary to replace population each generation, but in developing countries women continue to produce large numbers of children. In 1988, the women of China, notwithstanding its one-child population policy, produced on average 2.4 children, India 4.3 and Brazil 3.4. In much of sub-Saharan Africa, women had more than six with Nigeria averaging 7, Tanzania 7.1 and Kenya 8.1 (O'Connor, 1991: 47). The passage of bridewealth from husband's to wife's family often entails a contractual obligation for the woman – or a substitute provided by her family if she fails to fall pregnant – to produce a child. Childbirth often serves as a *rite de passage* into adulthood; a woman who does not produce may be in the same unenviable position as a man who never went through his society's mandatory male initiation process – a social failure. She risks being supplanted by a more fertile rival, particularly where polygyny is permitted. She will have no children to look after her in old age. When her husband dies he will have no legal heir; his land may revert to his family and she may have to leave the plot she cultivated. (The pro-natalist theme may also mean that a woman, barren or fertile, is inherited by her dead husband's brother. In areas where HIV is prevalent, such leviratic marriages may expose both of them to new risks of infection.)

There is a growing tendency to counsel couples who are at risk of producing an HIV-positive child to practise contraception or abortion. Dr Marvellous Mhloyi of the University of Zimbabwe's sociology department says that parents should be strongly advised to follow this advice. The risk of leaving orphaned children and of exposing older children to the additional trauma of losing a sibling to AIDS must be discussed. However, as he points out: 'These options are difficult within a cultural context where women derive status from maternity' (1991: 48).

An aspect of the problem often overlooked is that men, especially men from poor and marginalized communities, may also derive status from paternity. To prove one's manhood by fathering a child is often a purely biological statement; where the father is himself hardly more than a child, there is little capacity to assume social and financial responsibility for the action. Nevertheless, it may give him personal affirmation of his virility and enhance his status with his peers.

Where fertility has so many complex social corollaries, the counsel against having children offered to HIV-infected people may be little short of a personal disaster. Positive HIV status is often discovered during pregnancy, or when a child fails to thrive. Where fertility is important, where the woman is economically dependent on her husband, or where she fears violence or desertion should her husband know her HIV status, she may keep the information to herself. She may go ahead with a pregnancy, hoping that her baby will be spared. Dr Janet Mitchell, an obstetrician at New York's Harlem Hospital, says the medical profession's surprise at such seemingly irrational responses stems from their failure to see such decisions from the women's point of view. Even a 50% risk may seem acceptable. For women, childbearing may be seen as life-affirming, a window into the future, a reason to live.

While the woman in the remote village may not know she is HIV positive, in the developed world there is a good chance she may find out before she falls pregnant or early enough in her pregnancy to have a safe abortion. Increasingly, such women are being encouraged not to produce children. Ronald Bayer questions the whole ethic of such preventive intervention: 'the reformist zeal that so frequently has attended efforts to save children from their parents' misdeeds may merge with the eugenic tradition of challenging the absolute right of parents to bear children at high risk of congenital disorders'. He adds: 'That the women who are most at risk for bearing infected children are poor, black, and Hispanic, and most often intravenous drug users or their sexual partners, heightens the sense of disquiet about the prospect of a repressive turn in public policy'. Bayer argues that women are particularly vulnerable to the loss of their reproductive rights if it is believed to be in the public interest. He quotes, for instance, the 100,000 retarded women sterilized in the USA between 1920 and 1973 to prevent them transmitting their condition to their children. The gay demands for privacy, non-discrimination and non-repressive measures early on in the epidemic set a tolerant and voluntarist tone, but as the number of AIDS cases grows, policies could become more repressive.

Bayer writes that current counselling for couples with hereditary, genetic disorders essentially leaves the ultimate choice on childbearing in their own hands. The feminist movement has added an explicitly political dimension, insisting on the woman's right to control her own body. 'The notion of choice has served as an ideological cornerstone of the political program of the movement for reproductive rights and women's health'. Despite these developments, the poor or marginalized HIV-positive American woman is still likely to be advised against having a baby; some of the more strident critics of this approach have condemned it as 'a strategy for racial depopulation, as genocidal'.

Unlike other inherited diseases which may lead to the birth of a small number of disabled children each year, who will be dependent on parents or the State for care, AIDS is an epidemic, and a very costly one in every way. A child born to infected parents at worst will die in the first few months or years of life, at best will probably have to face life as an orphan. As in so many other areas, these hard facts are forcing even liberal thinkers to evaluate very carefully what constitutes appropriate HIV/ AIDS counselling. AIDS has the unhappy knack of pitting 'individual rights' against 'public good'. In spotlighting the paediatric epidemic, policy guidelines carry a whiff of eugenics disquieting to those who are concerned with issues of individual reproductive choice.

Such choices tend to be the prerogative of a minority of the world's women. Most neither know what options there are, nor have the resources to select from them if they do. How do you reach a poor, isolated, illiterate rural or urban woman, who is not at school, at work or at church or a clinic attender? The AIDS epidemic has, if nothing else, produced some innovative solutions. In Port au Prince, for instance, the hundreds of brightly painted beauty parlours dotted throughout poor neighbourhoods provide information to Haitian women; the proprietors act as effective educators and condom distributors, reaching three-quarters of the city's women. Elsewhere in the world, outreach programmes take the message to prostitutes, hawkers, commuters on buses and trains, people having lunch in the park. Musicians, drama groups, puppet-shows, videos, travel into dusty corners of the countryside with the AIDS message.

The message is only the first step. Armed with the facts, do women have the power, individually or as political pressure groups, to ensure they are allowed to practise safer sex?

71

The Avon Mental Health Measure

Editors' Introduction

Many attempts have been made to develop ways of assessing the needs of people with mental distress and disorder. In the past, these have generally been professional-centered but it is now widely recognized that it is essential to involve users of services and carers in the development of assessment measures. The Avon Mental Health Measure was designed for service users themselves to complete. It was developed by a team of 20 people in which users and professionals were equally represented. It is distinctive in being very clear and easy to use; it emphasizes strengths as well as difficulties, and it aims throughout to empower users and to indicate ways in which they can increase their control over their own care.

In this chapter we reproduce the "Guidance for Service Users" and the section of the form concerned with physical difficulties. Similar sections cover social problems, behavior, access, and mental health.

Guidance for Service Users

What is it?

The Avon Mental Health Measure is a document in which you can record your achievements and difficulties and describe what help you feel you want.

It allows you to build up a picture of yourself which should help you to gain more control of your life.

For example, if you have been ill, upset or distressed it should help you to say what services you need but are not getting at present.

What will it do for me?

- It gives you the opportunity to compile a profile of yourself and to explore your needs in many aspects of your life. This will be particularly useful if you want to have a Care Plan or Programme or if you want to ask for a review of the Care Plan you already have.

- It enables you to express your strengths, abilities, needs and concerns to mental health workers.
- Using the Measure at regular intervals will enable you to compare how you are coping at different times: People change and their needs change.
- It gives you a better understanding of yourself.

How will it be used?

You may want to fill in the Measure if you are to have a Care Plan (also called a Care Programme) or if your life has changed a lot. If you are in contact with a mental health worker, the Measure will help you to plan your future services as part of your Care Plan.

This means that you can have a real influence over what happens as part of your plan. You may find it useful to show to doctors who have difficulty in understanding your needs.

When you discuss your Care Plan, you should find it easier to explain your opinions and needs if you have filled in the Measure and written down some statements. At your Care Planning meeting, you can find out what can be done about your needs for support and advice. Any help which you need which cannot be provided for can be written down as 'unmet need'. This information is passed on and is used to plan for better services.

You need to fill in the information on each of the double pages. These are arranged under: Physical and Social Aspects, Behaviour, Access to services, and Mental Health.

Just choose the letter, A–E, for the column which best fits your life at present. There is also space for you to comment and to say if you want help to change your situation.

Your view of many of the topics is important since mental health workers do not always know about your social and physical situation. Your mental health worker will want to know about your opinions and comments. They can then try to meet your needs.

In some cases, you may not want to choose a letter, because you may be worried that your worker will recommend increasing medication or treatment. Your worker will want to know how best to help you, but should you prefer, you can leave a section blank.

Your workers will have had guidance about supporting you and not using the forms to either step up or take away services without a full discussion with you first. Preferably they will get your agreement to any changes. There is a section on page 14 which is for you to write down what help you are receiving at present and to comment on why it is important for you.

You might also want to use the Measure privately to think about yourself.

The Measure will NOT be used to assess benefits without your consent.

Should I ask for help to fill in the forms?

Filling in the topics on Behaviour and Mental Health may trigger memories of bad events and you may want to have someone with you who can give you support. You can ask for an advocate to help you.

An advocate is someone who can help you to think through your ideas and get them down onto paper. You could ask a friend, relative, or Carer to help you. You could also ask a member of a Patients Council or voluntary group who knows you well or a housing worker to act as an advocate to help you.

It is important that whoever you choose does not put you off from writing down what you want to say. Your needs may not be clear to the people who care for you.

Confidentiality – what happens with the information?

The information which you put down in the Avon Mental Health Measure will be used to write your Care Plan. One of the people in contact with you will write down what you have to say in a Summary Sheet. This will only be seen by the mental health workers who are in contact with you and by anyone else who you agree should see it.

You can keep your copy of the Measure. This may be useful if your situation changes and you want to ask for a review or to change the help you get.

Any information which is passed on to the people who plan services will not have your name attached to it. The sort of information which could be passed on is the percentage of people with mental health problems who have difficulty getting about or managing money.

Information about unmet need can also be used to plan new services.

What happens if my worker disagrees with my views?

You should be at the centre of your Care Plan or Care Programme. Your views are most important and you should be able to discuss any differences openly with your worker either before or during the Care Planning meeting.

The worker(s) may want to write down the letters for the columns which *they* think best describe your situation on the Summary Sheet. The Summary Sheet has a space for you to give your consent for it to be shown to mental health workers and to anyone else who you may choose, such as a Carer, who you may invite to your Care Planning meeting. The Summary Sheet also has a space for you to comment. This means that you can disagree with what has been written down or add any information or comments which you think have been left out. You should also be given a copy of the completed sheet.

What happens if I am still not happy?

You should make sure that you are happy with your Care Plan/Care Programme and not sign it unless you are. If you find you are not getting the services which your plan specifies, then you should contact your Care Co-ordinator who should be named on your plan.

Similarly if you are unhappy with the Summary Sheet, ask to have a copy of the sheet and ask if you can change it or add in extra information.

If you are still not satisfied you should ask for a leaflet which explains how to make a complaint.

Alternatively contact the Community Health Council or any Service User representative, Patients Council or Advocacy Worker to find out how to complain.

How do I go about filling in the Avon Measure?

You may be given the Measure while you are in hospital when your workers are beginning to think about setting up a Care Planning meeting for you.

If you have a copy in hospital, try to keep it safe, as much of the information you fill in will be very personal. You could ask for it to be put into a marked envelope with your notes when you are not using it.

You may find it easier to fill in part or all of the Measure on a day when you are feeling up to it. This is why there is a date space at the end of each section.

If when you look through the Measure, you feel you need help or support to fill it in, then ask a friend, relative or advocate to help you. (See 'Should I ask for help?' section.)

Read through each column for each topic and decide which best fits your situation. Write this down in the 'Letter chosen' column. You may want to write more than one letter down and some topics allow you to write down how you feel on a good day and a bad day.

The next space asks for further explanation if needed. This is your chance to explain your problems a bit more. If you run out of space, continue on blank page 18. The last space asks 'Do you need help to change things and if so what sort of help?'

Again your comments can make a real difference to the help you receive.

NOTE

Avon is an administrative area of South-West Britain. Copies of the Measure can be obtained from Publications Department, MIND, 15–19 Broadway, Stratford, London E15 4BQ, UK.

A	B	C	D	E	Letter chosen	Comments – further explanation if needed	Do you feel you need help to change things, if so what sort of help?
FOOD	**FOOD**	**FOOD**	**FOOD**	**FOOD**			
Frequently have little or no food for extended period (most of day) OR Frequently abuse food	Almost never eat regularly	Often skip meals or make do with snacks	Almost always eat regularly	Always eat regularly			

Abuse of food in A includes any problem with Anorexia or Bulimia. Not eating for long periods because you cannot afford to or you are not able to prepare and / or get food should be counted as A or B

A	B	C	D	E			
SHELTER / ACCOMMODATION	**SHELTER / ACCOMMODATION**	**SHELTER / ACCOMMODATION**	**SHELTER / ACCOMMODATION**	**SHELTER / ACCOMMODATION**			
Roofless or night shelter	Short term accommodation. e.g. friend's floor, or bed-sit	Accommodation unsuitable or poor quality	Accommodation could be better	Good accommodation. No worries about rent or security			

Quality refers to safety, warmth, lighting, sanitation etc

PHYSICAL HEALTH	**PHYSICAL HEALTH**	**PHYSICAL HEALTH**	**PHYSICAL HEALTH**	**PHYSICAL HEALTH**			
Physical health is very poor. e.g. Severe breathing / circulation problems	Often have physical health problems which cause regular difficulty	Some difficulties present most of the time	Occasional health problems	Physically fit and well			

Problems may include sight, hearing, moving about, breathlessness, epilepsy, skin problems, circulation problems etc. or generally feeling under the weather and having frequent colds or other infections

SELF-CARE	**SELF-CARE**	**SELF-CARE**	**SELF-CARE**	**SELF-CARE**			
Unable to fully care for myself	I hardly look after myself at all	I sometimes neglect to look after myself	I look after myself most of the time	I always take care of myself and my appearance			

e.g. unable to get out of bed. Self-care refers to hygiene: being able to wash, dress, presentation etc.

ILL EFFECTS OF TREATMENT	**ILL EFFECTS OF TREATMENT**	**ILL EFFECTS OF TREATMENT**	**ILL EFFECTS OF TREATMENT**	**ILL EFFECTS OF TREATMENT**			
Severe effects which are very upsetting. May include feeling 'foggy', slowed down, or having bad physical effects such as very dry mouth, constipation	Side effects are definite or marked and are sometimes upsetting	Mild side effects e.g. dry mouth, but not upsetting	Very occasional side effects	Do not notice any unwanted side-effects			

Only include side effects of treatment for mental health problems. Treatment includes medication, ECT and any talking treatment, e.g. talking about your problems may be upsetting

72

My Husband the Stranger: Part 1

ELIZABETH FORSYTHE

Large parts of John's life were always secret; I believe they remained hidden even from himself. Since his death, in 1986, I have come to see his illness and its conclusion as a development of the sort of person he was. [...]

I think that he was by nature a solitary person, although at times, on the surface, he seemed to enjoy being with people. During the war his talent for languages was of use in the intelligence service, and his attachment to various embassies helped him develop a role of easy sociability and charm which became useful later when he returned to business life. His inner solitariness seemed to need the protection of a superficial gregariousness. By the end of his life his solitariness was uppermost and in his dementia he became totally isolated and unreachable.

When we married, he was 45 and I was 28. To me he remained extraordinarily remote, in many ways essentially a stranger. He was a successful businessman and esteemed by his colleagues; yet there was always the sense that he was acting a role. He had expensive and immaculate business suits but would then wear a shabby tweed coat over the top and a rather battered felt hat. [...]

He had the expatriate Scot's longing to return to his homeland. In 1969 we bought some land and ruins in the far north-east of Scotland, and in due course built a beautiful house overlooking a harbour and the Moray Firth. I moved up there with our three children in 1973 and John should have retired and come to live there the following year; but sadly many things happened, including changes in his firm. He did not retire until five years later, though this was apparently not his decision.

It is difficult, looking back on the life of somebody who develops Alzheimer's disease, to be able to say, 'Yes, it started at such and such a time.' This was so in John's life. Hindsight makes it easy to say that John was not at all the same person outwardly when he retired in 1978 as he was when we made the decision to move to the far north of Scotland in 1969. Looking back now, I am sure that by 1978 his 'normal' solitariness had tipped into an abnormal sort of isolation which progressed into dementia.

Early that year, while John was still working in London and living in our earlier home near Cambridge, he suddenly developed a severe pain in his back. He stayed on his own in bed for a number of days before deciding to make the long journey north. He arrived on the night sleeper in Inverness and was exhausted, in a lot of pain and very depressed. He was admitted to an orthopaedic ward for diagnosis and treatment. After a week he was discharged in more or less the same state and came home to Caithness for a period of rest. Certainly he was in pain and in great distress; but he was also, quite uncharacteristically, depressed and tearful. He did not want me out of his sight and kept saying that he had spent all his life worrying about possessions and ignoring people. He seemed very sad that he had had so little time for his family during his working life. [...]

I shall never know whether these months prior to his return to London were the onset of Alzheimer's disease or a depressive illness; perhaps the distinction is unimportant. Certainly something profound and disturbing was occurring in John's mind. Although he was depressed while he was at home with his painful back, he had hopes and aspirations for his retirement which were different from his previous way of living. For many weeks we were extraordinarily close. It really did seem to be a turning point in his life and in our relationship.

I did not see John for several weeks after his return to London; when we did meet, he was once again a distant stranger and there was no more talk of spending time together.

In retrospect, some indication of his worsening condition might have been given by his attitude to money. John had had a substantial 'golden handshake' from his firm on his retirement. Early in 1978, during his week of 'depression', he had told me about the money and said that he intended to make two trusts: one to pay for the university education of our children and the other for an annuity for me because his work pension did not make provision for his widow, and with our age difference it was likely that I should outlive him.

After his return to London he spoke no more about these provisions. When two of the children started at university in the autumn of 1978, he said that he did not have enough money to help them and did not mention his capital sum or his earlier plans. He had always been secretive about money, and I had never known what his financial position was or how much he earned. From the time of the move to

Caithness I had always been short of money and did some part-time work to help with household bills. His sudden announcement that he was not able to make any contribution to our son and daughter's upkeep at university came as an amazing blow and I could think of no way of supporting them. [...]

The stranger with some sense of familiarity had gone and a stranger with a chilling feel of remoteness seemed to have arrived in his place. I found myself alone, very far from relatives and friends of long standing, with somebody who apparently wished to be entirely isolated both physically and emotionally. I became full of fear, for him, for the children, for myself and for the future. John now believed that I was responsible for any problems that he had in his retirement and this was because I was English.

Had he really changed, or was I different, and was there any way out of this nightmare? I could not find out, and at the end of 1980 I had a severe breakdown and went into hospital. John said that he wanted a divorce and did not want me to come home. I returned to the south on my own without job, money, home, husband, family, possessions or any understanding of what had been happening.

It was a time of great confusion and it did not then occur to me that John might be mentally disturbed, because I had been so obviously mentally ill myself.

From then on John made no contact with me. The following year he sold the house and moved to a London suburb to be near a cousin; but he did not send me money from the sale of the house, as he had previously agreed to do. I managed to get part-time work, rented a cottage, and the children continued at university without any financial support from John. He would not let me know his new address or his telephone number. I had no understanding of what had happened and in the end I tried not to think too much about him. I had to struggle with my own depression and work.

Two years later our son graduated from Edinburgh University and wanted both his parents to be at the ceremony. Peter had seen John at various times and found him a bit difficult and demanding. I had a shock when I met John that day. He looked a lot older: he was very preoccupied with his poor eyesight, and seemed convinced that he was going blind (he had always had very healthy eyes). John and I spent the afternoon together. Walking back to the hotel where I was staying, I realized that he was totally preoccupied with himself. These hours together had the sense of being in a dream and I seemed able to enter into his world and see it as he saw it.

It was a very frightening world. John believed that he was being pestered with people demanding money from him and sending him bills for things which he had never had. I do not know if I thought that this was the truth but I took everything he said as such because it was clearly what he believed to be true at that time. I had felt threatened by his strange view of reality but now I was no longer dependent upon him, and the physical and emotional distance made my understanding greater. [. . .]

A year after the meeting in Edinburgh, Peter was trying to equip a flat and asked John if he had any surplus household equipment. John said that he could take a van and meet him outside his flat. When Peter arrived, John said that he could only give him very little because all his possessions had been stolen. We thought that he was not being very generous and possibly even a little devious; now I realize that these delusions were an essential part of his dementia.

The 'crisis', the point at which some sort of intervention was unavoidable, came in the summer of 1985. He was still driving his car, and caused an accident. The police went to his flat to interview him but probably realized that he was not able to give evidence and finally dropped any charges against him. His driving licence was confiscated. His cousin kept in touch with me and finally wanted me to go and see him. I had not previously been to John's flat but it was immediately identifiable by all the locks, spy-holes on the door and strange signs and messages about where to put things. I could hear John walking about inside but it was about ten minutes before he came to the door. I could see him looking through one of the spy-holes and then he finally opened the door a crack while it was still chained. He did not appear to

recognize me and was very suspicious. I just kept talking and eventually he let me in.

It was the middle of a rather hot afternoon, but all the curtains were drawn, some of the windows were shuttered and the heating was on. He was partly dressed and took me all the way through the flat to the furthest room, which was his bedroom. It was blacked out, the electric lights were on and it was overpoweringly hot. The room was in a chaotic state, the bed unmade and the sheets filthy. He told me to sit down and indicated one of the two large director-type chairs in the room. Then he told me not to sit down but to put a towel on the seat first. He sat down and kept talking in a distracted way and looking at me with a puzzled expression but without recognition. I could not believe that this sad and mad old man was really my husband.

Eventually he went to a shelf, picked up a photograph of me, brought it over and thrust it at me, rather as a small child would, and told me that it was Elizabeth. I tried to explain that certainly it was a photograph of Elizabeth and that was me, his wife. He did not seem able to put these two ideas together. [. . .]

We walked the short distance to his cousin's together, but what two years previously had been a slow walk was now a shuffle. It was devastating.

John was obviously in need of help. His cousin was alone, following a series of bereavements, and wanted him to stay near her in his own flat, although his condition was deteriorating; but she did not want to have full responsibility for him. No one knew if he had any money, so that we were not able to employ help or begin to investigate the possibility of moving him to a home. I felt overwhelmed by the horror of the situation.

John had continued to go for private annual medical check-ups and always told his cousin that he was 100 per cent fit. He refused, however, to see his general practitioner. When I got home I telephoned the GP to see if he could suggest any solution. At first it was impossible to speak to him. I wrote and received no answer.

73

Caretakers' Views on Responsibilities for the Care of the Demented Elderly

MARY HOWELL

This [chapter] focuses on the perspective of day-to-day care of demented elderly persons. From this perspective, questions of ethical ambiguity take on immediacy and irrevocable consequences – for to act, in a situation of caretaking, is to decide.

The views expressed here reflect the experience of consulting on a nurse-run ward of mostly demented, mostly elderly patients. The majority of our patients have medically diagnosed chronic disorders that require skilled nursing care. In addition, most need assistance in every sort of physical function, from the spooning of pablum over trembling chins to the changing of diapers. None can take part in a connected discourse, and most can and do become assaultive intermittently and unpredictably. They eat notices posted on the walls, remove each other's condom catheters or cry out endlessly of what appears to be inconsolable disorientation. Most, in their earlier years, were successful, even distinguished, members of society; it is difficult to place them now into any explanatory scheme that tells us how to understand what has become of the person, the spirit.

In "The Network of the Imaginary Mother," the poet, Robin Morgan (1962), telling of her care of her aged and infirm mother, says, "The life comes first. There is no spirit without the form." In this expression, she rephrases a perspective of caretaking that we touch on daily: the essence of life is held in more than just personality, more than just spirit; it is held before all else in the form of the body. In our work, taking care of the body often stands as a metaphor for taking care of mind, spirit, the whole person. Taking care of the body is the vehicle through which we express medical and nursing competence, respect for the person in our charge, affection and tenderness, and our own self-esteem. "The life comes first. There is no spirit without the form."

We have heard of our demented elderly patients "the person is absent" or "gone." A recent documentary about Alzheimer's syndrome is entitled, "Someone I Once Knew." Relatives of patients, reflecting on changes they see in personality, cognitive abilities, and relationships, grieve for their own sense of loss, their awareness of what is no longer.

But for anyone who gives direct care, each patient is at the same time *fully* a person, of spirit and body both. In day-to-day caretaking, the emphasis is necessarily not on the emptiness of the half-full cup but on its relative fullness. Although Mr. X is different from the person he once was, and to those who knew him in past years may seem to be "less" of a person, to those who care for him day by day, he is a fullsome and substantial person, indeed. He requires care that is thoughtfully planned and executed; his social relationships are complex, difficult and often unpredictable – just as might be said of any of us – and his immediate needs range from those related to bare survival to remnants of mature and sophisticated development represented, for instance, by the enjoyment of music.

Caring for these demented, elderly patients is work of the most demanding sort. Let me remind you of what it is *not*.

It is *not* like caring for totally dependent small infants, although babies, like the demented elderly, need direct body care for all basic physical functions, from feeding to every form of waste elimination. We know that the baby will grow and develop, that our caretaking is time-limited, and that we will find pride and satisfaction in releasing the child from the intimacy of our care into autonomy. There is no such promise for the demented elderly patient. Barring miracles, we know that there will be only a greater and greater failure of independent function, a steadily increasing dependency.

It is *not* like taking care of developmentally delayed or mentally retarded persons, although the retarded, like the demented elderly, are slower to learn than most of us, and also are limited in their comprehension of the consequences of their behavior. We understand with most forms of retardation that the initial insult did its damage to the central nervous system on one catastrophic occasion; by learning to assess the competencies and capabilities of the individual retardate, we can tap into growth potentials that offer the patient – and ourselves as caretakers – vistas of new skills and new comprehensions. There is no such perspective for the demented elderly patient, whose central nervous system is progressively degraded and incapacitated.

It is *not* like taking care of patients with profound bodily injuries and handicaps, al-though the physically incapacitated, like the demented elderly, suffer deeply from the loss of formerly enjoyed abilities. With vigorous and imaginative rehabilitative efforts, the physically injured can substitute function, learn alternative ways of doing, and appreciate the expansion of previously undeveloped interests and talents. There are but few and scant rehabilitative avenues for lost functions – even though we *believe* that we can slow the loss of function with painstakingly attentive efforts.

It is *not* like taking care of the dying, even though the demented elderly are clearly moving toward the end of life. With patients who are actively aware of their engagement in the process of dying there is the possibility of offering support and relationship in the conduct of a thoughtful and deeply felt death experience. Just as we can work to orchestrate a "good" birth – one in which the helping persons, medical and otherwise, endeavor to sustain the authenticity and integrity of she who is giving birth and also of the borning baby – so too, we can engage ourselves in the orchestration of an authentic and integral death. To do so in the fullest sense, however, requires that the *patient* be planfull, present to contemporary relationships, and commemorative of past unfinished business. Once again, the elderly demented patient, himself apparently bereft of this social and spiritual presence, seems also to rob his caretakers of a role as a helping participant in the celebration of his death.

Having said what it is *not* like to care for the demented elderly, on a day-to-day basis, it is necessary, also, to position this work in the context of medical professionalism. After all, the highest standards of professional care are demanded in this work: balanced and substantiated judgment, attention to minute and myriad details in assessing the patient's well-being, co-ordination of complex and varied staffing patterns into a harmonious and effective whole, and the assumption of a profound and highly skilled responsibility for patients who usually are not able to speak for themselves and may also have no kin or friends to advocate on their behalf. But the competence of those who take care of the demented elderly is rarely, in my experience, acknowledged in any arena.

Whether they work in a teaching hospital, a general hospital, a long-term care facility or the patient's home, those who care for these lingering and derelict souls in their slowly disintegrating bodies are, themselves, demeaned and ignored. It is as if the disrespect of society – which is to say, the disrespect of each of us as individuals for the demented elderly – is extended, by association, to those who care for them.

Such neglect – and, sometimes, abuse – from individuals and institutions that look upon and, in some respects, have administrative and/or clinical control over one's caretaking efforts presents a stringent challenge to the individual caretaker's self-esteem. Interior questions: "How do I feel about aging?"; "How do I feel about my own parents, their aging and their deaths?"; "How do I feel about persons who must live in institutions, such as chronic-care wards and nursing homes?"; "Could this happen to me?" – questions like these interact with the most compelling query, "What am I doing, taking care of these crazy old folks?"

Among those who do this work well and with a sense of joy and accomplishment, I see these resources:

1. A belief in the value of every living person.
2. A willingness to become engaged and attached, not holding patients at a "clinical" or "objective" distance.
3. A deep pleasure and satisfaction in the skillful performance of complex *and* simple caretaking responsibilities – from making judgments about the promotion of well-being to the performance of the most elemental acts of intimate physical care.
4. An awareness and enjoyment of staff interactions – not only when they proceed smoothly and with comfortable communion, but also when they become scratchy and need to be worked on.
5. A tendency to unify individual and group energies in mobilization against a perceived "common enemy": all those who do not do this work, do not know how wearying it is, do not experience its urgencies and needs, and who treat staff and patients with either neglect or abuse.
6. A conviction – contrary to the conventional wisdom of medical professionalism – that this job is worth doing.
7. An enduring and compassionate sense of humor.

Before I say something about the responsibilities of those who are *not* direct care-providers in the support, sustenance and appreciation of those who *are*, I want to consider the ethical implications of these observations. Specifically, I want to examine some of the ethical dilemmas of decision-making at the level of the direct-care staff. I have chosen three such dilemmas as illustrations, not only of their problematic nature, but also of the particular and specific relationships between staff members, the nature of their work, and patients as persons.

Our first example is probably the most common and most overt instance of problematic decision-making. An elderly demented patient, virtually abandoned by his kinship family, but long and painstakingly cared for by his surrogate family of ward staff, is found apneic (not breathing) in his bed, 5 minutes after his vital signs had been checked. In some VA hospitals, it is not possible to order that there be no emergency resuscitation for such a patient no matter what may be the expressed wishes of the patient and his family. How quickly, then, with what reflective pause of seconds or minutes, does one move to notify other staff members and ultimately the emergency resuscitation team? Into the covert decision that determines the speed and efficiency of response will be poured all of the staff member's beliefs and ambivalences about this patient, the patient's family, the dementing disease, the aging process, and death itself. However we debate and codify the underpinnings and principles of ethical decision-making, this one life will hang in the balance for a few moments of hesitation by that solitary staff member, a hesitation that is determined essentially by private, intrapsychic perspectives.

As a second example, consider the understanding by direct-care staff that their information and their complaints are hugely instrumental in effecting medical-care decisions. An elderly demented patient whose feedings become more and more time-consuming, and who sometimes coughs during or after feedings, might be a candidate for placement of a gastrostomy tube. Depending on the philosophy and practice of the institution's consulting surgeons, these observations, made to the right person at the right time, may be enough to set into motion the gastrostomy procedure. But barring substantial weight loss, frank pulmonary infection, or the staff member's inability to complete other assigned tasks, the defining of this situation as a "problem" is subject – in real life practice – to quite individual judgement. Once again, the staff member's personal feelings and beliefs – about the risks and discomforts of surgical intervention, the desirability of "g-tube" feeding as opposed to more "normal" feeding, and the preferability of compounded chemical formulas as opposed to "real food," among other considerations – will influence the decision about whether this patient is reported to have a problem that needs attention and resolution.

As a third example, we might look at the delicate balance between the necessary acts of caretaking and the physical restraint of an aggressively uncooperative patient. As a general principle of patient's rights' surveillance, restraining a patient's arms or hands is permissible only in situations where there is a perceived danger of physical assault and injury to staff, to other patients, or to the assaultive patient himself. Suppose, on a given morning, an elderly demented patient who has been assaultive in the past refuses, by shouting and waving his arms, to cooperate with the staff member who is bathing and dressing him. There are other patients to be cared for; the patient needs to be dried and somehow covered; the commotion is setting up reactions of anxiety and anger among other patients on the ward. The amount of holding, its duration and firmness, and the words and tone of voice used by the staff member to complete the task of bathing touches the degree of restraint necessary to forestall assault. How this situation is "read" and acted upon will depend, once again, on the staff member's personal and idiosyncratic experience, beliefs and predilections.

I am not suggesting that the kind of discussion presented [here] – a discussion that all of us who are interested and engaged in this sort of work carry on at frequent intervals at our own places of work – has but limited relevance to the immediacy of care decisions. As we have noted, many, if not most, care decisions evolve out of a context of rational deliberation, the seeking of opinions other than one's own, even a search for consensus, if that is desired. I do want to point out that *some* decisions, fraught at their core with ethical perplexities, will always be made at the bedside, as it were, on no more than a moment's notice, and with no opportunity for consultation with anyone.

What we can do to bring these discussions and the day-to-day responsibilities of caretakers into close harmony is to ask caretakers to share with us the experience of such perplexing decisions, and ourselves to share perspectives brought from scholarly analysis. I want to emphasize the sense that both parties to this sharing – caretakers and consultants – have important words on these matters; this is by no means a one-sided offering by the consultant. With mutual respect we can sustain a forum that will be of help to all. It may be that the *process* by which direct caretakers make decisions of this sort cannot be greatly altered. But individual staff members may come to a greater understanding of their personal and common beliefs and feelings, especially in after-the-fact discussions of actions that impinged on a patient's rights or even affected the quality or duration of the patient's life span.

Staff interactions and relationships are of particular importance when patients are receiving chronic and total care. Time and space must be allotted so that adequate attention can be paid to tensions, misunderstandings and suggestions for improved team work. These meetings can be assisted, if staff wishes and so requests, by physicians who attend on the ward, or by consultants from nursing, social work, psychology, or psychiatry. No amount of consultation, however, can substitute for the provision of enough released time for staff to meet and talk together, free of the pressures of work undone.

I, for one, believe that a significant measure of our humanity as a society is found in the kind of care given to patients such as the demented elderly. Those who care for "the least of these" are carrying a burden for all of us, a burden that we might share in more fully. These caretakers deserve our expressed appreciation, at the very least.

When one's patients are marching toward a slow death, disintegrating and becoming daily more helpless and demented, it is sometimes difficult to appreciate the effects of one's care. We in medicine are, after all, trained to believe that curing is our business. The demented elderly will not be cured, nor can their status as healthy, functioning adults be more than marginally and temporarily improved. Medically we can only slow the progression of their dementia, disability and dysfunction. What then *is* accomplished by the direct-care staff in the responsible fulfillment of their daily tasks?

I know of no more satisfactory goal than to try to make each single moment of each day as gentle, as content, and as kindly as it can be. I suspect that those who work with the very old and infirm become especially good at this, for the anticipation and comprehension of inevitable death must make each of us want to savor every moment of now. Stephen Levine, in his book *Who Dies?*, quotes Zen master Suzuki Roshi: "'One should live their life like a very hot fire, so there is no trace left behind. Everything is burned to white ash.' Each act is done so fully and so completely there is *being* shared in each moment. There is nothing left to do but be" [emphasis added].

The core of caretaking and its support lies, I believe, in a perspective of life that values what is here, what we have, what exists. "The life comes first. There is no spirit without the form." Caretaking begins with physical care of the body, then expands, in the intensity of the caring and its focus, to become an attentive regard for *this* whole person existing in *this* time. Then time – time allotted, extended, strained, filled – becomes the raw symbol of ongoing life.

Galway Kinnell (1982) reminds us,

> Nobody likes to die
> But an old man
> Can know
> A kind of gratefulness
> Toward time that kills him,
> Everything he loved was made of it.

When death appears to be an almost infinitely slow march through time, as is often the case with the demented elderly, then the quality of caretaking significantly contributes to the quality of life.

REFERENCES

Kinnell, G. (1982) Spindrift. In *Selected Poems* (Boston: Houghton Mifflin), p. 61.

Levine, S. (1982) *Who Dies?* (New York: Anchor Press/Doubleday), p. 77.

Morgan, R. (1962) The network of the imaginary mother. In *Lady of the Beasts* (New York: Random House), pp. 63–88.

74

Who Defines Futility?

STUART J. YOUNGNER

For the past two decades, our society has struggled to identify the proper circumstances under which life-sustaining medical treatment should be limited. In fact, we seem to have reached a consensus on some aspects of the problem. It is generally agreed that a competent patient has the right to refuse life-sustaining treatment; when the patient is not competent, family members may limit treatment to serve the patient's best interests. [...] Under what circumstances can life-sustaining interventions be limited *without* the informed consent of the patient or family?

Murphy[1] notes correctly that cardiopulmonary resuscitation (CPR) is "rarely effective and in many cases futile" in the setting of a long-term-care facility, where many elderly patients are chronically ill or severely demented. He proposes a policy that "enables health care providers to make ethically sound, *unilateral* [emphasis mine] decisions regarding CPR." Physicians should only discuss the resuscitation decision with patients and families if resuscitation offers "some level of benefit" or the patient's prognosis is "at all equivocal."

Murphy argues that such a policy would avoid "futile" therapy that "can be harmful" because it prevents "a timely death." By acting unilaterally, physicians would avoid causing unnecessary suffering for the patient as well as an unfair "burden of guilt" for the family. Moreover, he argues, families' treatment decisions may be based on factors (e.g., guilt over not visiting the patient or fear of death) that have little to do with what the patient desired. (He believes, I assume, that health professionals are less likely than family members to have interests or values that potentially conflict with those of the patient.) Finally, he raises the question of whether society should provide the "substantial resources" that aggressive treatment of long-term-care patients would require.

Murphy justifies these claims with two ethical arguments. First, physicians' scientific knowledge and clinical experience enable them to recognize when a life-sustaining treatment is "futile." At this point, they should "reconsider the emphasis on autonomy" and exercise a strong paternalism that promotes patient (and family) well-being by limiting such treatment unilaterally and without even informing the patient and/or family. The second argument involves the broader social issue of the proper allocation of our nation's resources. In other words, does society have an interest in limiting "futile" interventions to divert limited resources to more productive use within, or even outside, the health care system? While these justifications have initial appeal, closer scrutiny reveals an alarming vagueness and confounding of issues.

The word "futile" has a categorical ring that masks a more subtle complexity. To delineate its meaning in specific situations, we must first examine the potential goals of the medical intervention in question.[2] For example, we can understand futility in purely *physiological* terms. Will a given vasopressor actually raise or maintain the patient's blood pressure? Will careful attention to fluid management be successful in maintaining electrolyte balance? Or, in the case of resuscitation, will CPR reestablish spontaneous heartbeat? We can also understand futility in terms of *postponing death*. We might, with diligent attention, be able to keep the serum sodium level within normal limits in a patient whose condition is rapidly deteriorating, but still fail to postpone death by even a few minutes. According to one standard, our efforts were futile; according to another, they were quite effective. *Length of life* represents another standard for judging futility. If our attention to fluid and electrolyte balance manages to postpone the patient's death for 24 hours, were our efforts futile? Many of the studies to which Murphy refers measure futility of CPR by whether or not the resuscitated patients lived to leave the hospital. Using this standard, CPR was futile if the patient lived a week, but died before discharge. And what about the *quality of life*? An intervention that kept a patient alive for six months might well be judged futile because it did not achieve an important goal of the patient – e.g., being able to walk and take care of his or her own personal hygiene. Finally, we might think of futility in terms of *probability*. A given intervention could be judged futile if the chance of achieving one or more of the goals just examined is not entirely absent, but is highly unlikely. But how low must the probability of success be before an intervention is judged futile? One percent? Five percent? Should statisticians define futility? When is an outside chance a chance worth taking?

Physicians are in the best position to know the empirical facts about the many aspects of futility. I would argue, however, that all, except for physiological futility and an absolute inability to postpone death, also involve value judgments. Physicians may be best suited to frame the choices by describing prognosis and quality of life – as well as the odds for achieving them. Physicians should not offer treatments that are physiologically futile or certain not to prolong life, and they could ethically refuse patient and family requests for such treatments. Beyond that, they run the risk of "giving opinions disguised as data."[3]

Living for five more days might give some patients the opportunity to say good-byes, to wait for the arrival of a loved one from another city, or to live to see the birth of a grandchild. For one patient, a life with extreme disability and pain might be quite tolerable; for another, it might be totally unacceptable. Risk takers might see a 3% chance as worth taking, while others might give more weight to the 97% chance of failure.

Nonetheless, the aggressive intervention of CPR in the event of cardiac arrest seems intuitively contraindicated in the long-term-care population described by Murphy. Murphy became understandably concerned when he discovered that only 10% of multiply impaired, very elderly patients had do-not-resuscitate orders. His solution (as opposed to his proposed policy) was eminently reasonable and extremely effective. He stopped avoiding discussion or using misleading euphemisms, such as, "Would you want us to do everything possible to save your life if your heart stopped beating?" Patients and families predictably answered this question by saying, "Why of course, doctor." He started talking turkey. He provided patients and family members with accurate descriptions of their medical conditions, poor prognoses, and the grisly realities of dying in a critical care unit. He presented the options as objectively as he could. The results were gratifying: 23 of 24 patients opposed resuscitation. None refused to discuss the tough issues because they felt uncomfortable. When patients were incompetent, all but one relative indicated that the patient would not have opted for resuscitation.

Why then does Murphy propose excluding patients and families from the decision-making process, and the even more radical step of not informing them of the do-not-resuscitate decision made unilaterally by the physician? Such a policy seems unnecessary; by communicating frankly with patients and families, he achieved the desired outcome. Why take the next step? Murphy seems to lapse back into an outdated (but perhaps yearned for) notion of paternalism. After giving ample evidence to the contrary, he worries that families will feel too guilty or will fail to "fully understand the implications of resuscitation despite detailed explanations." He goes on to say that making do-not-resuscitate decisions unilaterally and not informing patients and families will enable us to save time "better spent discussing other therapies and plans... that may have potential benefit." Acceptance of this position would also provide a justification for having physicians make unilateral and secret decisions about other "useless" therapies.

This latter reasoning becomes even more alarming when Murphy shifts from a paternalistic concern about what is best for the patient and family to a worry about how society should use its resources. He is not the first to be concerned about the massive resources consumed by the elderly in their final months, weeks, and even days of life – a problem that has been likened to a medical "avalanche."[4] As more and more elderly patients with chronic illnesses and severe dementia fill beds in long-term-care facilities in the decades ahead, the problem may become monumental.

While everyone seems to agree that the avalanche is coming, there is little consensus in our society about a national policy to handle the situation. Responsible persons, such as philosophers Daniel Callahan and Norman Daniels, as well as former Colorado Governor Lamm, have suggested that care to the elderly be limited; their ideas have met with loud and often harsh criticism. Public opinion polls and surveys reveal the ambivalence of the American public about these issues.[5] On one hand, they want more access to high-technology interventions, believe that we spend too little on health care, and generally are unwilling to limit health care to the elderly. On the other hand, Americans are not enthusiastic about paying more taxes to achieve these goals.

These are issues that must be decided at the public policy level. Americans may well choose explicitly to ration medical resources by denying them to those persons with the least chance of deriving benefit; other countries have chosen this course implicitly, by tradition. While rationing is always a painful process, the potential success of treatment may be a more ethically acceptable criterion than others, such as social worth or ability to pay.[6]

Until we reach a public consensus about how to deal with these very difficult issues, individual clinicians and institutions should continue to separate concerns about patient welfare from broader social and economic policy issues.[7] As professionals, we are there to serve our patients. As citizens, we can vote or lobby for policies that limit individual choice in the interests of a broader social good.

Murphy's proposal is a regressive step. Under the guise of medical expertise and concern for proper resource allocation, it encourages physicians to substitute their own value judgments for those of their patients. He urges physicians to cut off communication with patients and families about the futility of resuscitation, an intervention imbued with complex and powerful symbolism.[8]

His actions were much more appealing. By engaging in honest communication, he was able to use his clinical knowledge and judgment to help families and patients make wise choices about painful but inescapable issues. Physicians would do well to follow Dr Murphy's example – not his proposal.

NOTES

1 Murphy, D. J., "Do-not-resuscitate orders: Time for reappraisal in long-term-care institutions," *JAMA* 260 (1988): 2098–101.

2 Tomlinson, T., Brody, H., "Ethics and communication in do-not-resuscitate orders," *N. Engl. J. Med.* 318 (1988): 43–6.

3 McQuillen, M. P., "Ethics of life support and resuscitation," *N. Engl. J. Med.* 318 (1988): 1756.

4 Callahan, D., *Setting Limits: Medical Goals in an Aging Society* (New York: Simon and Schuster Inc. Publishers, 1987).

5 Evans, R. W., "Health care technology and the inevitability of resource allocation and rationing

decisions, part I," *JAMA* 249 (1983): 2047–52; "Health care technology and the inevitability of resource allocation and rationing decisions, part II," *JAMA* 249 (1983): 2208–19; Callahan, D., "Allocating health resources," *Hastings Cent. Rep.* 18 (1988): 14–20; Blendon, R. J. and Altman, D. E., "Public attitudes about health care costs: A lesson in national schizophrenia," *N. Engl. J. Med.* 311 (1984): 613–16.

6   Rescher, N., "The allocation of exotic medical lifesaving therapy," *Ethics* 79 (1969): 173–86; Childress, J., "Who shall live when not all can live?" *Soundings* 53 (1970): 339–55.

7   Angell, M., "Cost containment and the physician," *JAMA* 254 (1985): 1207.

8   Nolan, K., "In death's shadow: The meanings of withholding resuscitation," *Hastings Cent. Rep.* 17 (1987): 9–14.

75

Nobody Nowhere

DONNA WILLIAMS

At this primary school I learned to call myself mad. In my search for myself, when I was twenty-two I returned to the house I had grown up in. The woman there showed me something she had discovered written on the wall of my grandfather's shed. I remembered when I had written it. It was after my grandfather died. I was about six. It read: 'Donna is a nut.' Strangely, it took me four more years to realize that normal children refer to themselves as 'I'.

Whether other children were my friends was irrelevant. My first chosen school-friend was Sandra. I liked her smiling face, and she had dark shining hair. She was a big girl and she was jolly. Other children teased her. She became, in her words, 'my best buddy, old chum'.

Other children played school, mothers and fathers, doctors and nurses. Other children skipped ropes and played with balls or swap-cards. I had swap-cards. I gave them away in order to make friends, before learning that I was supposed to swap them, not give them away.

Sandra and I would play the same game every day. She'd laugh, I'd laugh, we'd laugh. We'd sit side by side and scream in each other's ear. It made me laugh because it tickled, and I really didn't care what it was that she was screaming; she was the first person to play my games.

Through playtime and lunchtime Sandra and I would drink as much water as we could, until we felt we would bust. We'd choke ourselves until we turned blue, coughing and struggling to breathe. We would try to push our eyes in, in order to see colours, and we would scream and scream until our throats were red raw.

I thought this was great fun. I had discovered that I could share physical sensation. In the company of others my senses would cut off, and I would become so numb that, in order to experience something, I had to push myself to extreme limits.

Sandra found another friend. I called her fat; she called me mad. Together, she and her new friend tried to include me. I did not know how to cope with having two friends at once. I solved the situation by rejecting them both.

I often played alone on the monkey bars, looking at my cards, climbing trees, pulling flowers apart, spinning around and around as I stared up into the sun. I would fall to the ground and watch the world spin. I was in love with life but I was terribly alone.

Other children were attracted to me. They would watch me in fascination, walking across the top of the monkey bars, swinging from a tree branch thirty feet up; in short, doing 'mad' things.

Though we went to the same school, my brother had nothing to do with me. Where he had once been protective towards me, I was now a nut, a spastic and an embarrassment. I really do not blame him. Just as I lived in my own world, he was doing fine in 'the real world'.

Classes seemed to be an extension of the playground, and the playground seemed to be an extension of the classes. The teacher soon learned not to let me go to the toilet by myself as I often wandered off and did not come back.

I'd be out in the playground enjoying myself. It seemed quite natural to me that if I did not like something I could find a way to avoid it. Looking back, I can imagine how strange it was for my teacher to be called out to the playground as one of her pupils was swinging and singing 'On Top of the World' as I hung by my knees from the top of one of the school's highest trees.

Everyone had gathered down below me. They shouted. I sang louder and louder and swung higher and higher. Finally I sensed their urgency and I got scared. Fearfully I climbed down. I still do not know if it was my actions which frightened me or the fear that someone might come up and get me. The teacher reassured me that I was not in trouble. Finally I came down. In dreams I replayed that day of defeat many times.

76

The Body in Multiple Sclerosis: A Patient's Perspective

S. KAY TOOMBS

The experience of illness means much more to the person who is ill than simply a collection of physical signs which define a particular disease state. Illness represents a distinct way of being in the world – a way of being which is characterized not simply by bodily dysfunction but by a concurrent disruption of self and the surrounding world (Toombs, 1988). This global sense of disorder is precipitated by a radical transformation in the relation between body and self. In health the body is, for the most part, taken for granted and ignored. Only occasionally do we pay explicit attention to our physical capacities, and then only in a fleeting manner. Normally we act in the world through the medium of our bodies in a largely unreflective fashion. We see, hear, speak, and move unthinkingly as we go about our business, simply accepting the cohesion of body and self. Illness disturbs this body/self unity. The malfunctioning body intrudes itself into our everyday existence, becoming the focal point and object of attention. In particular, the body presents itself as an oppositional force which curtails activities, thwarts plans and projects, and disrupts our involvements with the surrounding world. In various and varied ways the body is experienced as essentially alien, as that which is Other-than-me.

In this [chapter] I propose to examine the manner in which this experience of bodily alienation and disorder manifests itself in multiple sclerosis – an illness with which I have lived for sixteen years. In particular, I am concerned to show that, for the patient, the physical changes wrought by this disease represent much more than simply an objectively demonstrable neurological dysfunction. The breakdown in body is experienced as a fundamental transformation in one's whole way of being. This transformation includes not only a profound change in the relation with one's body, but also an alteration in one's sense of self and a disruption of the physical world.

I should perhaps, however, begin with a brief general description of M.S. in layman's terms for those who are not well acquainted with the illness. My purpose is simply to convey something of the way the disease manifests itself in the lives of those of us who have it, to note the wide variety and multiplicity of possible bodily disturbances, and to impart a little of the uncertainty, fear and distress which such a diagnosis necessarily evokes.

Multiple sclerosis is an incurable neurological disorder with its onset in early adult life (average age of onset is around age thirty, with more women affected than men). In the United States, after arthritis and trauma, it is the chief cause of major disability in adults of working age (Scheinberg, 1983a: 3). Since the disease involves multiple lesions scattered throughout the central nervous system, symptoms are varied and may include motor weakness (most often in one or both legs but sometimes in arms and face), spasticity, incoordination, tremor, paralysis of the lower extremities, loss of balance, speech disorder, sensory changes such as numbness or tingling, visual disturbances (blurred or double vision), loss of bowel and bladder control, sexual problems, and a generalized loss of energy which manifests itself as chronic and easy fatiguability (Scheinberg, 1983b). Clinically, multiple sclerosis may be categorized as being of the exacerbating-remitting type, in which discrete attacks of limited duration are followed by recovery – although recovery may well be incomplete leaving some residual disability – or the chronic progressive type, in which there is the steady accumulation of neurological deficit without remission. Chronic progressive multiple sclerosis usually evolves from exacerbating-remitting disease after a number of attacks, although approximately ten percent of patients have the chronic progressive form from the start (Weiner, 1987). The cause of M.S. is not known, the course of the disease is unpredictable, and at present there is no cure.

I was thirty years old when the disease was first diagnosed. In the beginning my illness was characterized by discrete attacks – the loss of vision in one or other eye, the loss of sensation in a leg, the sudden weakness of one or more limbs. Such attacks were sometimes followed by complete remissions. At other times they abated, leaving me with a new or increased disability. In recent years there have been fewer attacks (except for a recurrent optic neuritis which periodically robs me of sight). Rather there has been a slow, but relentless, gradual progression of disability in the course of which I

have (among other things) lost the full use of my legs, a good deal of upper body strength, my sense of balance, and normal voluntary control of my bowels and bladder. As is the case with many M.S. patients, the most visible manifestation of my illness is the result of motor dysfunction. Loss of coordination and weakness in both legs, together with the loss of equilibrium, have transformed my once normal-appearing manner of walking. I tend to stagger in a seemingly "inebriated" fashion, drag both of my feet, fall in embarrassingly public places, and bump into doorways and walls. Since I can now no longer walk further than thirty or forty yards, I use forearm crutches for short distances, and a wheelchair (or motorized scooter) for longer excursions.

This list of symptoms conveys, however, but a small part of my experience of multiple sclerosis. These varied and various bodily disturbances represent not only the loss of function but a profound change in my formerly comfortable relation with my body and in my sense of myself. In short, my once relatively orderly physical existence has been transformed into an uncertain and chaotic manner of being in the world. In reflecting upon this disordered manner of being which *is* my illness, I have come to recognize that the different bodily dysfunctions (motor, sensory, and so forth) have differing existential meanings. Each plays a distinct role in the creation and perpetuation of the disorder which now permeates my life. In addition, the nature of M.S. is such that the disease process itself carries a particular existential significance.

It is my purpose in this [chapter] to uncover such existential meanings and thereby convey something of the lived experience of multiple sclerosis. In what follows I shall analyze the specific disruptions caused by motor and sensory disturbances, and by such losses as the loss of bowel and bladder control (disorders which are typical of the disease and of my own experience). I shall then examine the impact of the disease process itself. In so doing I shall focus upon the manner in which the body is experienced as something which is essentially alien to the self, noting the specific implications of this change for those of us who are patients.

Motor Disorders

At the onset of any bodily malfunction the cohesive relation between body and self is profoundly disturbed. The body suddenly appears to have an opposing will of its own in that it refuses to yield to one's commands, frustrates one's intentions, and thwarts one's projects. Disturbances in motor function explicitly reveal the oppositional force of the body, rendering it primary. The simplest of actions such as changing location or picking up a coffee cup disclose the body's overt resistance. Instead of living my body unreflectively I may, for example, have to drag my leg forcefully across the room or explicitly compensate for the trembling of my arm as I reach for a cup. Rather than being that which enables me to carry out my projects in the world, the body presents itself as an obstacle to my intentions, as an impediment which must be overcome.

As H. T. Engelhardt, Jr. has pointed out, the neuromuscular system is the embodiment of action (Engelhardt, 1973: 136). Consequently, the disruption of this system through central nervous system damage represents an essential diminishment of one's capacity to function within the world. The possibilities for mundane action shrink. Habitual acts such as walking, running, lifting, sitting up, and so forth, can be performed only with effort or not at all. Indeed, the world itself takes on a different character. In health, the world presents itself as a field of practical significance. Objects are apprehended as manipulable or utilizable by the body (Merleau-Ponty, 1962: 81–2). With the breakdown of motor function, everyday objects present themselves as unaccustomed obstacles to the body. For the person with gait disturbance, for example, stairs which were formerly simply there "to be climbed" now represent obstructions "to be circumvented" or avoided. For the patient with a tremor, a glass of water presents itself as a concrete problem to be solved. Space constricts, not only in the sense that actions become severely circumscribed, but in the sense that the physical features of the surrounding world themselves assume a restrictive character. Slopes may be too steep to climb, sidewalks too uneven to walk on, doorways too narrow to navigate with a wheelchair.[1]

Furthermore, with motor dysfunction, the impaired body becomes the focus of attention. Since it is the principal means of one's interaction with the world, it must always be taken into account. It is a necessary precondition of one's plans and projects. For example, I must organize my daily activity in such a way as to compensate for the debilitating physical fatigue which accompanies motor weakness. To choose to do one project is, in effect, to ensure that I will not have enough energy to undertake another. For example, while I can walk the 30 yards from my office to the classroom, after lecturing for 50 minutes, I am quite unable to walk back. The most mundane of tasks – such as a trip to the grocery store or searching the library shelves for a particular reference – will produce a quite disproportionate exhaustion. Consequently, I must be constantly aware of my body's limitations if I am not to squander my very limited physical resources. While I do not brood about my illness, my disability remains always at the fringes of my consciousness. Indeed, I now view the world through the medium of my damaged body. My first impression of the Lincoln Memorial, for instance, was not one of awe at its architectural beauty but rather dismay at the number of steps to be climbed.

Moreover, the oppositional body poses an imminent threat to the integrity of the self. Life projects must be revised – and sometimes abandoned altogether – in light of physical disabilities. This revision necessarily incorporates a redefinition of one's self. Our sense of who we are is intimately related to the roles we occupy – professional and otherwise (wife, lover, provider) – and to those goals and aspirations we hold dear. Any permanent disruption of role causes one to feel diminished in person, as well as in body. Since the onset of multiple sclerosis occurs in early adulthood, it is usually the case that the illness strikes after important life choices and personal commitments have already been made (such as marriage, the establishment of a family, the building of a career). Consequently, the disruption of role and of self which accompanies neurological dysfunction is felt most profoundly. Even when disability is limited, the portent of the diagnosis (and the uncertainty which accompanies it) inevitably pose a threat to one's life plan. The future assumes an inherently problematic character. One can no longer make any definite assumptions with regard to one's future physical capabilities. Indeed, the diagnosis precipitates a fundamental change in the perception of self. One becomes a "person living with multiple sclerosis", "diseased" rather than "whole".

While the major impact of motor disturbances is to reveal the body as that which concretely opposes the self and disrupts one's involvements in the world, such disorders also effect a bodily alienation through the loss of corporeal identity. Each of us possesses a unique way of walking, talking, gesturing, which identifies the body as peculiarly "mine" (Merleau-Ponty, 1962). Motor disturbances destroy this familiar bodily way of being. For example, gait disorders not only cause mechanical difficulties in walking but also drastically alter appearance. In this disordered pattern of ambulation one no longer recognizes one's former bodily identity. The transformed manner of walking represents a fundamental change in body "style". The body is experienced as at once unfamiliar and uncomfortable. Furthermore, it is hard to accept this changed way of being not only because it incorporates an essentially alien corporeal style – after a couple of years I still have difficulty recognizing my increasingly peculiar gait as my own – but also because it represents an overwhelmingly negative body image. This is a culture which glorifies the body beautiful, placing great emphasis on physical fitness, sexuality and youth. Consequently, the type of changes in body style which accompany motor disorders represent not only an unfamiliar way of being but a diminishment of self-esteem.

Perhaps the most profound change in bodily identity occurs when one is forced to relinquish one's upright posture altogether and adopt an alternative mode of locomotion such as a wheelchair. While it is the case that any significant alteration in motor functioning represents a concurrent loss of autonomy (since one is no longer able to do certain things which were formerly unproblematic), the loss of upright posture symbolizes disability in a most profound way.[2] Verticality is directly related to autonomy (Sellers and Reiser, 1984: 27–8). Just as the infant's sense of independence is enhanced by his ability to maintain an upright posture and venture into the world unaided, so there is a corresponding loss of autonomy which accompanies the loss of uprightness. The loss of upright posture engenders feelings of helplessness and dependency. Moreover, it causes others to treat one as dependent. I have noticed, for example, that on those occasions when I use a wheelchair, strangers invariably address themselves to my husband and refer to me in the third person. "Would *she* like to sit at this table?", "What would *she* like to drink?", and so forth. Consequently, this particular change in one's bodily way of being incorporates a profound transformation in one's sense of self. In light of the loss of upright posture, one perceives oneself to be concretely disabled – a perception which is readily mirrored in the reactions of others.

Sensory Disorders

While motor disturbances effect a bodily alienation through the loss of corporeal identity and the establishment of the body as an oppositional force which is beyond the control of the self, the loss of tactual or kinesthetic sensation which may accompany neurological dysfunction is experienced as the radical disengagement of body from self. The immediately felt sense of position and movement is integral to the experience of the body as one's own. Kinesthetic sensations not only give the body an "interior", clearly identifying it as "mine", but combine with movements in such a way that I experience such movements as my own.[3] For example, when I reach for a cup I not only have an intuitive sense of the position of the arm, *my* arm, in space, but I concurrently experience this positioning of the limb as *my* bodily reaching. To lose this sense is to become disassociated from one's body and one's *actions*. It is "the" arm, rather than "my" arm, which moves.

In addition, the intuitive sense of the positioning of one's limbs allows one successfully to interpret the mundane demands of physical space. In stepping up onto the sidewalk, for instance, one unthinkingly positions one's leg to clear the height of the curb. Furthermore, one knows approximately where one's leg is in relation to the curb. The disturbance of this sense reveals the body's independence of *my* actions. The body deceives me. I step up knowingly as before, but now I trip and fall.

The loss of tactual sensation similarly effects a bodily detachment. A leg that is numb, that doesn't feel a prick when I jab it with a pin, just doesn't seem to belong to *me*. Engelhardt has noted that one can experience this otherness of body in the mundane experience of having one's leg go to sleep. The body is presented as *"something* to be *lived in*, to be enlivened". One massages the limb, desiring to feel in it and act with it (Engelhardt, 1973: 38). With the loss of sensation in M.S. the body is experienced as just that which *cannot* be enlivened.[4]

Bowel and Bladder Disorders

The disruption of voluntary bladder and/or bowel control is a most grievous effect of central nervous system damage. Such disorders have a distinct significance in the alienation of body from self. In particular, the body is experienced not merely as oppositional but as frankly malevolent, posing a constant threat to one's dignity and self-esteem. Bowel and bladder disturbances represent much more than simply a mechanical or neurological dysfunction. They signify the most elemental and profound loss of control over one's body. Incontinence reduces an adult to the status of a helpless infant. One is no longer master of even the most basic of bodily functions. This experience is deeply alienating. The body appears inherently untrustworthy. Not only does it fail me, but it is capable of causing me deep humiliation and shame.

Of course, one is not completely helpless. It is possible to develop strategies to minimize this particular bodily assault. Nevertheless, the very execution of such strategies provides a constant reminder of the tenuous control one exercises over one's body, and the ever-present threat it poses to one's dignity and self-respect. Indeed, so severe is this threat that many afflicted patients simply choose to withdraw from society rather than risk embarrassment and humiliation.

The Disease

In understanding the experience of M.S. it is important to recognize not only the differing impact of various bodily disorders (sensory, motor, visceral) but also the existential significance of the disease process itself. In the first place, since the disease is characterized by multiple lesions in the CNS, it produces a multiplicity of symptoms. This multiplicity of involvements represents a global loss of physical integrity. In it one senses the disorder and disintegration of one's whole body. Thus one experiences an all-encompassing loss of bodily control. Furthermore, since it is the central nervous system which is affected, one is unable to disassociate oneself from the diseased body part as one might with, say, an appendix which could be resected, or a heart valve which might be replaced. Consequently, one feels inescapably embodied, irrevocably attached to an essentially malfunctioning organism which promises to disrupt all one's involvements within the world. While the illness is not life-threatening, it is profoundly world-threatening. This sense of inescapable embodiment is further exacerbated by the long-term nature of the illness, the uncertainty of the prognosis, and the inability of biomedical science definitively to halt, or substantially alter, the course of the disease.

The relation with body in M.S. is, therefore, a paradoxical one. *My* body appears as Other-than-me in that it continually opposes and frustrates my intentions; yet I *am* my body for I cannot escape my impaired embodiment. This paradoxical relation between body and self is intrinsic to the experience of chronic illness and disability.[5] With permanent impairment the body undergoes a metamorphosis. It is transformed into a new entity, the "diseased body". The "diseased body", with its ongoing demands, necessarily stands in opposition to the self. Even when I have adapted to my bodily limitations I must – in one way or another – overtly take them into account as I go my way about the world. Thus, my body continually makes its presence felt. On a daily basis, whether I like it or not, I must compensate for its dis-abilities, hearken to its warnings, allow for its weaknesses, accede to its dictates. This constant taking-into-account, in turn, reveals the radical contingency and inescapability of my mode of embodiment. In essential ways this "diseased body", with which I am permanently identified, both shapes my existence and reflects my disordered manner of being in the world.

The experience of bodily alienation and disruption which characterizes M.S. is, thus, quite distinct from that mundane awareness of otherness of body which is sensed periodically in everyday life. From time to time we all must take into account our bodily resources and limitations. One knows, for example, that playing a long and vigorous game of tennis on a hot afternoon is likely to make one quite tired – too tired perhaps to carry out some other project. Yet when we take our bodies into account under such "normal" circumstances, we make the necessary adjustments largely unreflectively. Even if the body becomes the explicit focus of our attention, it does so only momentarily. Furthermore, the manner in which the body appears to such attention in "normal" circumstances is significantly different from the way it appears in illness. With the breakdown in organic function, the instrumentality of the body announces itself. For example, when I cannot see properly I perceive my eye as an instrument-for-seeing and, more particularly, as a *defective* instrument-for-seeing. My inability to walk provides a constant reminder of the inadequate performance of my limbs. Thus, with physical impairment, the damaged body appears primarily as a "faulty tool", or a malfunctioning mechanism – which is clearly not how it appears to us in health, even in those moments when we are aware of our bodily limitation.[6]

Moreover, in chronic illness, the metamorphosis to the "diseased body" incorporates a sort of Gestalt reversal, so that the expectation of bodily disruption becomes one's "normal" expectation and non-disruptive moments appear as somewhat fleeting anomalies. This is, perhaps, one of the important differences between chronic and acute illness. In acute illness there is an awareness that the experience of bodily disruption is *temporary* and one anticipates a return to some clearly defined level of "normal" functioning. Consequently, such a radical Gestalt reversal does not occur. Indeed, although acute illness may be "world-disrupting" it is, at some level, not "world-threatening" in the way that a chronic, progressive illness is. In the latter, not only is the bodily disruption ongoing and permanent (so that there can be no expectation of a return to "normal" functioning), but there are no clearly defined parameters of disability with which one can come to terms. It may, for example, ultimately be easier for one to adapt to *permanent* localized disruptions such as an amputated limb because one knows for certain the extent and nature of the disability. In a chronic, progressive illness such as M.S. the task of redefining the self in the face of bodily impairment is made more difficult by the uncertainty of the prognosis, the progressive nature of the illness, and the multiplicity of physical involvements. One is required to repeatedly redefine the self in the light of new or increased (and possibly increasing) disabilities. Thus, the experience of bodily alienation is particularly profound in illnesses such as M.S.

NOTES

I should like to thank Eric J. Cassell, M.D., and Steven Crowell, Ph.D., for their helpful comments on this essay.

1 As I have noted elsewhere, the lived body represents one's being-in-the-world. Thus, physical space is experienced primarily as functional space (that milieu within which one performs one's various activities). The breakdown in body results not only in the alienation of body from self but in the disruption of lived spatiality (Toombs, 1988: 210–12).

2 For an analysis of the significance of upright posture, see Erwin Straus's discussion on the constitution of lateral space. Straus shows that upright posture is "pregnant with a meaning not

exhausted by the physiological tasks of meeting the forces of gravity and maintaining equilibrium" (Straus, 1966: 137).

3 For an interesting discussion on Edmund Husserl's analysis of the role of kinesthetic sensation in the constitution of lived-body, see Engelhardt, 1977. Husserl argues that kinesthetic sensation not only gives the body an "interior", clearly distinguishing it from "merely" physical objects, but that there is an if-then relation between kinesthetic sensations and other tactual sensations such that every experience is necessarily a co-experience of sensations and the body as one's own.

4 Oliver Sacks (1984) has forcefully described this experience of being detached from one's body or one's limbs in his autobiographical account of his leg injury; see also this volume, ch. 59.

5 As phenomenologists such as Merleau-Ponty, 1962, Sartre, 1956, and Zaner, 1981 have noted, this paradoxical relation is fundamental to the structure of the lived body and is, therefore, not limited to the "diseased body". Nevertheless, the experience of illness (particularly chronic illness) explicitly reveals this relation.

6 Heidegger's analysis of the breakdown of the tool may provide a helpful analogy (1962: 102–7). The breakdown of the tool discloses certain fundamental intentional structures which are not normally made explicit. Furthermore, the broken tool becomes conspicuous and obstructive (as does the body in illness).

REFERENCES

Engelhardt, H. T. Jr. (1977) Husserl and the mind–brain relation. In D. Ihde and R. M. Zaner (eds.), *Interdisciplinary Phenomenology* (The Hague, Netherlands: Martinus Nijhoff), pp. 51–70.

Engelhardt, H. T. Jr. (1973) *Mind–Body: A Categorial Relation* (The Hague, Netherlands: Martinus Nijhoff).

Heidegger, M. (1962) *Being and Time*, trans. J. Macquarrie and E. Robinson (New York: Harper and Row).

Merleau-Ponty, M. (1962) *Phenomenology of Perception*, trans. C. Smith (London, UK: Routledge, Kegan Paul Ltd.).

Sacks, O. (1984) *A Leg to Stand On* (New York: Summit Books).

Sartre, J. P. (1956) *Being and Nothingness*, trans. H. E. Barnes (New York: Washington Square Press).

Scheinberg, L. (1983a) Introduction. In *Multiple Sclerosis: A Guide for Patients and Their Families* (New York: Raven Press), pp. 3–16.

Scheinberg, L. (1983b) Signs, symptoms, and course of the disease. In *Multiple Sclerosis: A Guide for Patients and Their Families* (New York: Raven Press), pp. 35–43.

Sellers, J. and Reiser, S. J. (1984) Stages of patienthood: Beyond autonomy and paternalism (unpublished presentation at the Rice University faculty symposium on metaphors and symbols of discourse on health, illness, and medicine, Houston, Texas).

Straus, E. (1966) *Phenomenological Psychology, Selected Papers*, trans. E. Eng (New York: Basic Books, Inc.).

Toombs, S. K. (1988) Illness and the paradigm of lived body. *Theoretical Medicine* 9: 201–26.

Weiner, H. L. (1987) COP 1 therapy for multiple sclerosis. *New England Journal of Medicine* 317/7: 442–4.

Zaner, R. M. (1981) *The Context of Self: A Phenomenological Inquiry Using Medicine as a Clue* (Ohio: Ohio University Press).

77

A Living Death

PETER LENNON

[In 1994] Geoff, a 19-year-old musician, was coming home by train from a party. No one knows what happened next. He had complained at the party of feeling ill and may have stuck his head out the window of the train to get some fresh air. The next time anyone saw him he was lying in the carriage with massive head and brain injuries.

The best that could be done was to repair the shattered skull; the injured brain was inoperable. His eyes open, but clinically unconscious, Geoff was pronounced to be in a Persistent Vegetative State.

Two years later, however, Geoff [was] carrying on lively conversations through a computer. As a result of this, and a number of other misdiagnosed cases revealed by Dr Keith Andrews, director of medical services at the Royal Hospital for Neurodisability, London, the case for reviewing the guidelines for the diagnosis of PVS has come under closer scrutiny.

Geoff's case highlights the difficulty of diagnosis. For six months he was believed to be mentally unaware. "But," says his mother Marie Applassany, "I was convinced he could hear me. None of the consultants would listen. They told me Geoffrey would never have any mental ability of any kind. You think they are

specialists and they know what they are saying. But I used to visit him two or three times a day; the consultant comes in once a month. I kept saying 'Geoffrey can hear me and sometimes he can see me.' But they said 'it's like a baby, he looks but there is no mental comprehension. It's just reflex action'."

Eighteen months later, when Geoff had been transferred to the Royal Hospital for Neurodisability, the senior clinical psychologist, Lesley Murphy, decided to experiment with a touch-sensitive buzzer. This recently developed device enables a paralysed patient to use the twitch of a muscle to buzz once for yes and twice for no. So, did Geoff understand? The buzzer sounded once. Characteristically a patient in a vegetative state is "awake but not aware." Geoff was fully aware.

Everything had to be re-thought. It was established that Geoff could communicate through a computer. This involves a laborious process whereby a nurse speaks out the letters of the alphabet and the patient makes his choice with single buzzes.

Geoff's first message was remarkable: "Geoff is cool!" the alleged vegetable wrote. For a year and a half, Geoff had been surrounded by people who believed he could neither see, hear, feel nor talk. "When I heard he could use the buzzer I could not believe it," says his mother: "I was told to ask him a question. I had been waiting nearly two years and now I didn't know what to ask my son. Then I asked a stupid question 'Geoff, do you know who I am?' Geoff buzzed 'Yes'."

He went on to describe his experience. So how did he feel? "Pretty awful, bored to tears." What kept you going? "Music." And later? "I was searching for my identity." He now communicates regularly with his mother and friends.

Four years ago, Dr Andrews became worried by the level of misdiagnosis in cases of PVS referred to him. "We did a retrospective study of our clinical records of the medical and occupational therapy departments between 1992 and 1995, and discovered that out of 40 patients referred as being in a vegetative state, 17 of them had been misdiagnosed. That is 43 per cent."

"Some," Dr Andrews said, "had been considered as vegetative for as long as four years. Since 60 per cent of brain damaged people are blind or visually badly impaired, this makes accurate diagnosis based on physical response very difficult."

Patients in these allegedly vegetative states can live as long as 20 or 30 years. "To be aware of your environment, but not to be able to communicate," Dr Andrews said, "must be an extremely distressing and horrifying sensation."

Dr Andrews says his study establishes that diagnosis cannot be made even by the most experienced clinician from a bedside assessment; neither can neurodiagnostic tests alone confirm the diagnosis of a vegetative state or predict the potential for recovery. Diagnosis, he says, requires the skills of a multidisciplinary team experienced in the management of people with complex disabilities. He wants this level of examination to become standard practice.

78

Across the Disability Divide: Whose Tragedy?

SALLY FRENCH AND JOHN SWAIN

Introduction

The divide we are discussing here is not in the categorization of people as disabled and non-disabled. Despite the evident personal, social, and political reality of this conception of a divide, we believe it is problematic in a number of ways, two of which are particularly pertinent to this chapter. First, a division cannot be made on the grounds of impairment. The divide between disabled and non-disabled people is not that one group has impairments while the other does not. Indeed, many non-disabled people have impairments, such as short and long sight, and impairment cannot be equated with disability. Secondly, the divide between two groups cannot be sustained on the basis that one is oppressed while the other is not. Non-disabled people are oppressed through poverty, racism, sexism, and sexual preference, as indeed are many disabled people. Whatever definition of oppression is taken, it will apply to some non-disabled as well as disabled people.

The divide we are addressing is in perceptions of disability, in terms of the meaning it has in people's lives. Perceptions, and the experiences on which they are founded, vary considerably, not least because many people become

disabled in later life having constructed understandings and lifestyles as non-disabled people. Nevertheless, there is a divide in perceptions that is most clearly related to a divide in experiences, being disabled or non-disabled.

Generally, non-disabled people do not want to be impaired or disabled, often equating the two. From this viewpoint, to be impaired (or, to be more specific, not to be able to walk, or see, or hear) would be a personal tragedy. There is a whole discourse of danger, risk, and even bravery and recklessness, which hinges on remaining non-disabled. The source of the divide is not, however, that this tragedy view of disability is applied by non-disabled people to themselves, but its extrapolation and application to disabled people.

There are a number of different possible explanations of this tragedy view of disability. It is sometimes thought to reflect a deep irrational fear of non-disabled people's own mortality (Shakespeare, 1994). A second form of explanation refers to dominant social values and ideologies, particularly through the association of disability with dependence (Oliver, 1993) and abnormality (Morris, 1991). There is a third type of explanation, however, which suggests that the tragedy perspective has a rational, cognitive basis constructed through experiences in disablist social contexts. Thus, so-called "irrational fears" can have a basis, in part, in a lack of knowledge about impairment and disability, engendered by lack of equal status contact between disabled and non-disabled people. They can also, particularly for parents of disabled children, be founded on beliefs about the benefits that non-disabled people have in education, work, and relationships. As we shall argue below, a non-tragic perspective, through experience and knowledge of disability, can be subjected to the same line of explanation – i.e. rational.

Notwithstanding explanations of the tragedy perspective, this divide in perceptions is far more than a matter of "agreeing to differ." The problem for disabled people is that the policies, practices, and interventions of non-disabled people are justified and rationalized by the non-disabled view of personal tragedy. The tragedy is to be avoided or eradicated, or non-disabled people are to be "normalized" by all possible means. Such are the negative presumptions held about impairment and disability that the abortion of impaired foetuses is barely challenged (Parens and Asch, 2000) and compulsory sterilization of people with learning difficulties was widely practiced in many parts of the world (Park and Radford, 1999). The erroneous idea that disabled people cannot be happy or enjoy an adequate quality of life lies at the heart of this response. The disabled person's problems are perceived to result from impairment rather than the failure of society to meet that person's needs in terms of appropriate human help and accessibility. There is an assumption that disabled people want to be "normal," although this is rarely voiced by disabled people themselves who know that disability is a major part of their identity (Mason, 2000). Disabled people are subjected to many disabling expectations, for example to be "independent," "normal," to "adjust" and "accept" their situation. It is these expectations that can cause unhappiness; it is rarely the impairment itself (French, 1994).

The aim of this chapter is to demonstrate, by reviewing the literature and drawing upon research, that being disabled need not be a tragedy, but may, on the contrary, enhance life or provide a lifestyle of equal satisfaction and worth. This perception of disability, which arises from the writings of disabled people themselves, challenges deeply held, negative presumptions about impairment and disability.

Who Needs Cure and Normality?

We turn, then, to examine what might be called a non-tragic view of disability. This has been developed, borne through experience of disability, along two lines: a social model of the problems faced; and appreciation of the quality of life that being disabled may bring. In the social model of disability, the difficulties and limitations that disabled people experience in their daily lives are explained in terms of the various barriers of institutionalized discrimination within society – structural, environmental, attitudinal – not in terms of personal tragedy.

The foundations of institutional discrimination are built at the *structural* level. Institutionalized discrimination is founded on the social divisions in society (Swain et al., 1998) and, in particular, hierarchical power relations between groups (disabled and non-disabled people). Inequalities in the distribution of resources, particularly economic, underpin hierarchical power relations, with many disabled people being marginalized from open employment and condemned to poverty (Burchardt, 2000). The concept of citizenship has also, in recent years, been drawn on in understanding structural barriers (Oliver, 1996). Disabled people, as a group, are denied political, social, and human rights that non-disabled people take for granted.

The *environmental* level of barriers is constructed, on these foundations, in the interaction between the individual and the collective, both socially and physically. These are the barriers confronted by disabled people in relation to rules, procedures, patterns of behavior, shared understandings, timetables, and so on (i.e. social organization), which are geared to the needs and norms of the non-disabled majority. The barriers are also created by aids that are geared to the needs and norms of non-disabled people (steps, taps, cars, buses, etc.), the needs and norms of disabled people being marginalized to "special" aids. Another focus for disabled people is in their relationship with service provision and professional practice, which can play such an important role in shaping their lives and enforcing dependency.

The third layer, *attitudinal*, which is built on the previous two, is constructed in the direct interactions between disabled and non-disabled people, as individuals or in groups. These barriers are manifest in the attitudes and personal prejudices of non-disabled people, their expectations and actions. They include the beliefs, feelings, and practices of individual professionals. These relate to, but can differ substantially from, collective professional practice at the environmental level.

In terms of quality of life, far from being tragic, being disabled can have benefits. If, for example, a person has sufficient resources, the ability to give up paid employment and pursue personal interests and hobbies, following an accident, may enhance that person's life. Similarly, disabled people sometimes find that they can escape class oppression, abuse, or neglect by virtue of being disabled. Martha, a visually disabled Malaysian woman we interviewed, was separated from a poor and neglectful family and sent to a residential special school at the age of 5. She states: "I got a better education than any of them [brothers and sisters] and much better healthcare too. We had regular inoculations and regular medicals and dental checks." She subsequently went to university and qualified as a teacher. Similarly, many visually disabled people became physiotherapists, by virtue of having their own "special" college, at a time when their working-class origins would have prevented them entering the profession. None of this is to deny, of course, that many disabled people who are educated in "special" institutions receive an inferior education and may, in addition, be neglected and abused (Corker, 1996; French and Swain, 2000).

A further way in which disability and impairment may be perceived as beneficial to some disabled people is that society's expectations and requirements are more difficult to satisfy and may, therefore, be avoided. A disabled man cited by Shakespeare et al. said: "I am never

going to conform to society's requirements and I am thrilled because I am blissfully released from all that crap. That's the liberation of disfigurement" (1996: 81).

Young people (especially women) are frequently under pressure to form heterosexual relationships, to marry, and to have children (Bartlett, 1994). These expectations are not applied so readily to disabled people, who may, indeed, be viewed as asexual. Although this has the potential to cause a great deal of anxiety and pain, some disabled people can see its advantages. Vasey states: "We are not usually snapped up in the flower of youth for our domestic and child rearing skills, or for our decorative value, so we do not have to spend years disentangling ourselves from wearisome relationships, as is the case with many non-disabled women" (1992: 74). Though it is more difficult for disabled people to form sexual relationships, because of disabling barriers, when they do, any limitations imposed by impairment may, paradoxically, lead to advantages. Shakespeare et al., who interviewed disabled people about their sexuality and sexual relationships, state: "Because disabled people were not able to make love in a straightforward manner, or in a conventional position, they were impelled to experiment, and enjoyed a more interesting sexual life as a result" (1996: 106).

For some people who become disabled their lives change completely, though not necessarily for the worse. One woman, quoted by Morris, states:

> As a result of becoming paralysed life has changed completely. Before my accident it seemed as if I was set to spend the rest of my life as a religious sister, but I was not solemnly professed so was not accepted back into the order. Instead I am now very happily married with a home of my own. (1989: 120)

The experience of disability may also lead to a heightened understanding of the oppressions endured by other people. French found that most of the 45 visually disabled physiotherapists she interviewed could find advantages in being visually disabled in their work. One important advantage was their perceived ability to understand and empathize with their patients and clients. As one said: "The frustrations of disability are much the same inasmuch as it is a physical limitation on your life and you think, 'if only'... Having to put up with that for so long, I know ever so well what patients mean when they mention those kinds of difficulties" (French, 1991: 1). Others believed that their visual disability gave rise to a more balanced and equal relationship with their patients, that patients were less embarrassed (for example about undressing) and that they enjoyed the extra physical contact the visually disabled physiotherapist was obliged to make. One therapist said: "Even as students when we had the Colles fracture class all round in a circle, they used to love us treating them because we had to go round and touch them. They preferred us to the sighted physios. I'm convinced that a lot of people think we are better" (ibid: 4).

As for non–disabled people, the quality of life of the disabled depends on whether they can achieve a lifestyle of their choice. This in turn depends on their personal resources, resources within society, and their own unique situation. Nevertheless, the writings of disabled people demonstrate that being born with an impairment or becoming disabled in later life can give a perspective on life which is both interesting and affirmative, and can be used positively.

From Tragedy to Identity

There is an ostensible contradiction in the non-tragic meanings of disability. Disability can, at one and the same time, be both oppressive and beneficial to people's daily lives. The resolution of this conflict lies for many disabled people in the affirmation of group and personal identity. This has been true for other oppressed groups, and is captured most dramatically by the phrase, "Black is Beautiful." Though it has not been a slogan of the Disabled People's Movement, the parallel, of course, is, "Disabled is Beautiful."

Group identity, through the development of the Disabled People's Movement, has addressed this contradiction in the following ways.

1. The development of a social model of disability has re-defined "disability" in terms of the barriers constructed in a disabling society rather than as a personal tragedy. Through group identity the discourse has shifted to the shared experience and understanding of barriers. "Personal tragedy" has been reconceptualized as frustration and anger in the face of marginalization and institutionalized discrimination.

2. Simply being a member of a campaigning group developing a collective identity is, for some disabled people, a benefit of being disabled in its own right.

3. Frustration and anger are being collectively expressed. They are expressed through the Disability Arts Movement and campaigns of the Disabled People's Movement, rather than being seen as personal problems to be resolved, say, through counseling.

4. Through group identity, it is recognized that just because there are benefits in being excluded from non-disabled society (which is capitalist, paternalistic, and alienating) it does not follow that disabled people should be excluded. From this way of thinking, disabled people enjoy the benefits of being "outsiders," but should not be pushed out – i.e. they should have the right to be "insiders" if they so wish.

5. Finally, group identity has been, for some, a vehicle for revolutionary rather than revisionist visions of change, often under the flags of "civil rights" and "equal opportunities" (Shakespeare, 1996). The inclusion of disabled people into the mainstream of society would involve the construction of a better society, with less sexism, better workplaces, better physical environments, and better values, including the celebration of differences. As Campbell and Oliver conclude in their history of the Disabled People's Movement: "In building our own unique movement, we may be not only making our own history but also making a contribution to the history of humankind" (1996: 180).

Nobody can predict the amount of tragedy or happiness a person will experience in life – there are thousands of interacting variables and, in addition, there are numerous ways of viewing any situation – and yet people feel confident to make such predictions about disabled people without asking them or conceiving of a society where disabled people are accepted. The inherent assumption is that disabled people want to be other than as they are, even though this would mean a rejection of identity and self. Disabled people, encouraged by the Disabled People's Movement, including the Disability Arts Movement, are creating positive images of themselves and are demanding the right to be the way they are – to be equal but different. Phillipe, Michlene, and Colin, all disabled, explain:

I just can't imagine becoming hearing, I'd need a psychiatrist, I'd need a speech therapist, I'd need some new friends, I'd lose all my old friends, I'd lose my job. I wouldn't be here lecturing. It really hits hearing people that a deaf person doesn't want to become hearing. I am what I am! (Phillipe, in Shakespeare et al., 1996: 184)

A few years later, at my special school, I remember one of the care staff loudly telling me that I should never give up hope because one day doctors would find a cure for my affliction, and I loudly told her that I did not want to be "cured." I remember this incident because of the utter disbelief this statement caused amongst all the non-disabled people present, and the delight this statement caused amongst my disabled friends. The school decided that I had "The Wrong Attitude" and that I should indeed go to Lourdes so that Jesus, the Virgin Mary and St Bernadette could sort me out. (Michlene, in Mason, 2000: 8)

We are who we are as people with impairments, and might actually feel comfortable with our lives if it wasn't for all those interfering busybodies who feel that it is their responsibility to feel sorry for us, or to find cures for us, or to manage our lives for us, or to harry us in order to make us something we are not, i.e. "normal." (Colin, in Tyneside Disability Arts, 1999: 35)

These perceptions of impairment are by no means confined to the disabled people of today. Talking of Helen Keller, who was born in 1880, Crow states: "It seemed that she could never fully satisfy people's curiosity for details nor could she reassure them entirely that she was content as herself. When the non-disabled world feted her courage, for Helen, her impairments were a natural, largely neutral condition" (2000: 854). Nor are they confined to people with physical and sensory impairments. Susan Wendell states: "I cannot wish that I had never contracted ME, because it has made me a different person, a person I am glad to be, would not want to have missed being, and could not relinquish even if I were 'cured'" (1996: 83). Similarly, Holliday Willey writes:

I do not wish for a cure to Asperger's Syndrome. What I wish for is a cure for the common ill that pervades too many lives, the ill that makes people compare themselves to a normal that is measured in terms of perfect and absolute standards, most of which are impossible for anyone to reach. (1999: 96)

Whose tragedy? For many disabled people the tragedy view of disability is in itself disabling. It denies their experiences of a disabling society, their enjoyment of life, and even their identity and self-awareness as disabled people.

REFERENCES

Bartlett, J. (1994) *Will You Be Mother? Women Who Choose To Say No* (London: Virago Press).

Burchardt, T. (2000) *Enduring Economic Exclusion: Disabled People, Income and Work* (York: Joseph Rowntree Foundation).

Campbell, J. and Oliver, M. (1996) *Disabling Politics: Understanding Our Past, Changing Our Future* (London: Routledge).

Corker, M. (1996) *Deaf Transitions: Images and Origins of Deaf Families, Deaf Communities and Deaf Identities* (London: Jessica Kingsley Publishers).

Crow, L. (2000) Helen Keller: Rethinking the problematic icon. *Disability and Society* 15/6: 845–59.

French, S. (1991) The advantages of visual impairment: Some physiotherapists' views. *New Beacon* 75/872: 1–6.

French, S. (1994) The disabled role. In S. French (ed.), *On Equal Terms: Working with Disabled People* (Oxford: Butterworth-Heinemann).

French, S. and Swain, J. (2000) Personal perspectives on the experience of exclusion. In M. Moore (ed.), *Insider Perspectives on Inclusion: Raising Voices, Raising Issues* (Sheffield: Philip Armstrong Publications).

Holliday Willey, L. (1999) *Pretending to be Normal: Living with Asperger's Syndrome* (London: Jessica Kingsley).

Mason, M. (2000) *Incurably Human* (London: Working Press).

Morris, J. (ed.) (1989) *Able Lives: Women's Experiences of Paralysis* (London: The Women's Press).

Morris, J. (1991) *Pride Against Prejudice: Transforming Attitudes to Disability* (London: The Women's Press).

Oliver, M. (1993) Disability and dependency: A creation of industrial societies? In J. Swain, V. Finkelstein, S. French, and M. Oliver (eds.), *Disabling Barriers – Enabling Environments* (London: Sage).

Oliver, M. (1996) *Understanding Disability: From Theory to Practice* (Basingstoke: Macmillan Press).

Parens, E. and Asch, A. (eds.) (2000) *Prenatal Testing and Disability Rights* (Washington: Georgetown University Press).

Park, D. C. and Radford, J. P. (1999) From the case files: Reconstructing a history of involuntary sterilisation. *Disability and Society* 13/3: 317–42.

Shakespeare, T. W. (1994) Cultural representation of disabled people: Dustbins for disavowal? *Disability and Society* 9/3: 283–99.

Shakespeare, T. W. (1996) *Disability, Identity, Difference*. In C. Barnes and G. Mercer (eds.), *Exploring the Divide: Illness and Disability* (Leeds: The Disability Press).

Shakespeare, T., Gillespie-Sells, K., and Davies, D. (1996) *The Sexual Politics of Disability* (London: Cassell).

Swain, J., Gillman, M., and French, S. (1998) *Confronting Disabling Barriers: Towards Making Organisations Accessible* (Birmingham: Venture Press).

Tyneside Disability Arts (1999) *Transgressions* (Wallsend).

Vasey, S. (1992) Disability culture: It's a way of life. In R. Rieser and M. Mason (eds.), *Disability Equality in the Classroom: A Human Rights Issue* (London: Disability Equality in Education).

Wendell, S. (1996) *The Rejected Body: Feminist Philosophical Perspectives on Disability* (London: Routledge).

79

AIDS

MAY SARTON

We are stretched to meet a new dimension
Of love, a more demanding range
Where despair and hope must intertwine.
How grow to meet it? Intention
Here can neither move nor change
The raw truth. Death is on the line.
It comes to separate and estrange
Lover from lover in some reckless design.
Where do we go from here?

Fear. Fear. Fear. Fear.

Our world has never been more stark
Or more in peril.
It is very lonely now in the dark.
Lonely and sterile.

And yet in the simple turn of a head
Mercy lives. I heard it when someone said
"I must go now to a dying friend.
Every night at nine I tuck him into bed,

And give him a shot of morphine,"
And added, "I go where I have never been."
I saw he meant into a new discipline
He had not imagined before, and a new grace.

Every day now we meet it face to face.
Every day now devotion is the test.
Through the long hours, the hard, caring
    nights
We are forging a new union. We are blest.

As closed hands open to each other
Closed lives open to strange tenderness.
We are learning the hard way how to mother.
Who says it is easy? But we have the power.
I watch the faces deepen all around me.
It is the time of change, the saving hour.
The word suddenly made new.
As we learn it again, as we bring it alive:

Love. Love. Love. Love.

Part IX

Continuing Contact: Dying

Introduction

Jenny Lewis's own narrative ended well, but the final poem in her volume, reproduced in chapter 80, is dedicated to those who "must go into the starless night alone." The sense of death not as the end but as "a moment between journeys," shared with the company of women past, is one of the most remarkable images in this wholly remarkable poem. Lewis has read her *Amazon* sequence at the San Francisco Art Rage Festival on breast cancer, as well as all cancer units of hospitals such as the Royal Marsden, raising money for Macmillan Cancer Relief. She writes that "the hugely positive response it receives from audiences gives it constant reaffirmation" for her.

By contrast, the sequence from Leo Tolstoy's *Death of Ivan Ilyich*, which comprises chapter 81, is filled with an abyss: the infinitely deep well of isolation and hopelessness into which Ivan Ilyich falls. Tolstoy describes Ilyich's suffering as not so much physical, or even mental: it is, rather, a moral agony. "What if my entire life, my entire conscious life, was *not the real thing*?" The inauthenticity of his life torments him with its utter conventionalism, but in acceding to his wife's wish that he should take the sacrament, he falls still deeper into convention, even if he has put his wife's wishes

first. Whereas Lewis's entire narrative is about connection, with heroic women predecessors and other, contemporary women, connection, for Ilyich, only brings more torment.

The philosopher Tom Buller has written an original article for this volume which tries to take what might be presented as Tolstoyan concerns about authenticity into account when considering advance directives. Suppose that an incompetent, demented woman of 63 – "Vera," a former historian who valued the intellectual life – develops pneumonia, which threatens the relatively happy life she appears to be living despite her dementia. She has an advance directive which stipulates that she would not want to be treated for the pneumonia in this case. Should we honor the directive, or respect the value of the contented but more limited life she now lives? As Buller puts it in chapter 82, "the first sacrifices the life of an incompetent, but contented woman on the basis of past interests that are no longer relevant; and the second commits Vera to the type of life that she had expressly sought to avoid when she was previously competent." The reason this has to do with authenticity is that we are forced to decide which set of desires represents the authentic wishes of the dying person. Summarizing the arguments of Rebecca Dresser, Buller notes that "autonomous decisions have authority only if they continue to be authentic, that is to say, that they continue to be reflective of the person's character and interests. And since the values and interests that applied when the person wrote an advance directive are no longer relevant (for example Vera's interest in her intellectual life in the case above), the directive no longer promotes the person's interests." Buller thinks that both alternatives suffer from temporal narrowness: they fail to take the whole narrative into account, ignoring in one case the future and in the other the past.

Chapter 83 is another poem, "Falls" by Edward Lowbury. Full of light paradoxes and literal reverses, it concerns "those on shaky limbs who fall in second childhood." We suggest the reader returns to it after reading the final chapter in this section, Pablo Neruda's "To the Foot from its Child," which shares many of its stylistic qualities, as well as its subject, but in an altogether more pessimistic manner.

There then follows a selection from the American Medical Association's Council on Ethical and Judicial Affairs. "Decisions Near the End of Life" is an abridged version of a report adopted by the delegates of the AMA at the 1991 annual meeting. It begins by charting the changing demography of death: where and when it occurs. Surveying the wide range of ethical questions that arise when life can be prolonged by modern technology, it then sets down some key "ground rules" for clinicians. Certain of these prescriptions can be and have been questioned, for example, the claim that there is no ethical distinction between withdrawing and withholding life-sustaining treatment. A survey of US and UK practitioners by one of the editors (Dickenson, 2000) found that only one in five respondents agreed or agreed strongly that withholding and stopping treatment are the same in ethical terms. More than three in five, 62 percent, disagreed or disagreed strongly with the statement. Overall, only US medical attending physicians are as likely to agree as disagree that there is no ethical difference. Every other group is more likely to disagree than agree with the "official" view

expressed in this AMA report, and also in similar guidelines laid down more recently by the British Medical Association (BMA, 1999). Of course practitioners' views could be dismissed as merely emotional or ignorant (Solomon et al., 1993), but conversely, one could also argue that the view that finds no distinction between withdrawing and withholding is too narrowly consequentialist.

We move on to a very poignant chapter: Kate Hill's "On the Suicide Threshold," from her book on the same subject, *The Long Sleep: Young People and Suicide*. Kate Hill wrote this book during her psychiatric training at the Warneford Hospital, Oxford; but the deeper motive for her concern was her brother's death by suicide. She herself died shortly thereafter of a cerebral haemorrhage. The excerpts that make up this chapter have been chosen by her father Don Hill, himself a medical ethicist.

Although Kate Hill's contribution is not actually a narrative, clearly it springs from narrative roots. Another actual first-person account, Elizabeth Forsythe's "My Husband the Stranger," is continued here from chapter 72 in Part VIII. The profoundly alienating nature of her estranged husband's illness, Alzheimer's disease, is somewhat transformed at his death here in a kind of reconciliation, but only after great suffering.

The concern with authenticity, first encountered in the Tolstoy chapter, recurs in chapter 87 in Martin Hollis's "A Death of One's Own." Hollis's starting point is a quotation from the poet Rilke: "The wish to have a death of one's own is growing ever rarer. Only a while yet and it will be just as rare to have a death of one's own as it is already to have a life of one's own." If this is so – and it could be seen as extreme individualism, rather than the sort of connectedness in which Lewis found hope – what is the rightful role of the doctor, "part mechanic and part priest"? Hollis comes round to a sceptical but not damning evaluation of the liberal notion that "A death of one's own is the ultimate in consumer choice."

The story of Ivan Ilyich continues in chapter 88, again dominated by the theme of inauthenticity, but this time not only the deception of Ivan Ilyich's own life: rather, that of his doctor, who enters "with a look on his face that seems to say: 'Now, now, you've had yourself a bad scare, but we're going to fix everything right away.' The doctor knows this expression is inappropriate here, but he has put it on once and for all, and can't take it off...Ivan Ilyich knows, for certain, beyond any doubt, that this is all nonsense, sheer deception, but when the doctor gets down on his knees, bends over him, placing his ear higher, then lower, and with the gravest expression on his face goes through all sorts of contortions, Ivan Ilyich is taken in by it." The attitude of Ivan Ilyich's wife seems no better to him: "Just as the doctor had adopted a certain attitude toward his patients, which he could not change, so she had adopted one toward him: that he was not doing what he should and was himself to blame, and she could only reproach him tenderly for this. And she could no longer change this attitude." As with his agreement to take the sacrament, for his wife's sake, so now Ivan Ilyich submits to examination by a second physician, although he knows his case is hopeless. His wife pre-empts his refusal by saying ironically, "So no arguments, please. I'm doing this for my sake." This is a double irony, and another deception, because it really is true, Ivan Ilyich feels: "Everything she did for him was done strictly for her sake; and she told him she was doing for her sake what she actually was, making this seem so incredible that he was bound to take it to mean just the reverse."

Ivan Ilyich might be said to be suffering from "total pain": "the conceptual linchpin in the philosophy of palliative care . . . the multidimensional experience of suffering that encompasses physical, social, psychological, and spiritual distress," as described by David Barnard in chapter 89, "The Coevolution of Bioethics and the Medical Humanities with Palliative Medicine." "The interpenetration of these dimensions of suffering results in the well-recognized phenomenon that prolonged, untreated physical pain can aggravate psychosocial or spiritual distress," and therefore palliative care, as pioneered by the hospice movement, is whole-person care. Barnard argues that medical humanities likewise takes the whole person as the focus of attention; we might argue that we are

attempting to do much the same in this volume, with its heavy concentration on narrative and literature.

Joanne Lynn's classic article, "Why I Don't Have a Living Will," reproduced here in chapter 90, prefigures Tom Buller's concerns, although she writes from the viewpoint of a physician rather than a philosopher. But whilst the doctor Joanne Lynn does use and support living wills for her patients, the person Joanne Lynn prefers not to have one for herself, "because I fear that the effects of having one would be worse, in my situation, than not having one." Is this just a form of medical paternalism, or, worse, hypocrisy? Lynn argues not: "A living will of the standard format attends to priorities that are not my own, addresses procedures rather than outcomes, and requires substantial interpretation without guaranteeing a reliable interpreter." More speculatively and profoundly, because they only pertain to the final stages of life, living wills reinforce the belief that there are the dying and there are the rest of us. That view needs to be challenged, not reinforced, Lynn asserts. Here the doctor and the person come together: "Working with persons with advanced years, advanced cancer, and advanced AIDS has illuminated the hubris of this cultural view.... We all are dying.... Pretending that there is a morally important demarcation between the merely mortal and the dying leads to harmful policies and practices generally." Lynn's critique extends to the hospice movement in so far as it serves "mostly relatively well-off cancer patients" in contrast with US society's failure to provide long-term care for those with chronic illness. One word of caution should be extended to UK readers: Lynn opts for living wills where no substitute decision-maker such as a family member can be found, but reliance on a substitute decision-maker is expressly prohibited in English law. Living wills, or information directives, might thus have a potentially larger role to play in the UK.

We return to literature toward the end of this section: first in chapter 91 with an extract on "the standing forth" from Gloria Naylor's extraordinary novel *Mama Day*. The extract is told in the words of Cocoa, an urbanized

African-American woman visiting a remote island off the Georgia coast where the supernatural traditions of the "conjure woman" – Cocoa's relative, Mama Day – still survive in the all-black community. The funeral of a 4-year-old child is an occasion to renew the community's commitment to a religion which, unlike Christianity, does not call for "a sermon, music, tears – the belief in an earthly finality for the child's life." Buoyed up by others' publicly spoken, yet mundanely phrased convictions of immortality, even the dead child's mother, Bernice, is able to stand up and forth: "When I first saw you, you were so very glad to be alive – new and declaring it to everyone. And when I see you again, you'll be forgiving of your old mama, who didn't remember for a moment that you were still here."

Guy de Maupassant's short story "The Devil" likewise concerns death in the old way, but it is a far more scathing account of traditional communities. Like the story of Ivan Ilyich, Maupassant's tale reminds us that although death in the old style was not medicalized, it was not necessarily something to be romanticized.

The final two chapters in this section, and the overall volume, are poems. John Stone's "Talking to the Family" is almost as clinical in its style and diction as the doctor's duty of breaking bad news, although there are odd, disturbing elements as well. Whilst the doctor is protected by his white coat, as a father what he is performing is a kind of surgery that can never be put right: "the cut ends of their nerves will curl."

By contrast, Pablo Neruda's "To the Foot from its Child" prefigures that later Latin American development, the world of magical realism, in which "the child's foot is not yet aware it's a foot, / and would like to be a butterfly or an apple." When it learns its fate, "this blind thing walks / without respite... / until the whole man chooses to stop."

And then it descended
underground, unaware,
for there, everything, everything was dark.
It never knew it had ceased to be a foot
or if they were burying it so that it could fly

or so that it could become
an apple.

REFERENCES

BMA (1999) *Guidelines on Withholding/Withdrawing Treatment* (London: BMA).

Dickenson, D. L. (2000) Are medical ethicists out of touch? Practitioner attitudes in the US and UK towards decisions at the end of life. *Journal of Medical Ethics* 26: 254–60.

Lewis, J. (2000) Personal communication to D. Dickenson.

Solomon, M. Z., O'Donnell, L., Jennings, B., Guilfoy, V., Wolf, S. M., and Nolan, K. (1993) Decisions near the end of life: Professional views on life-sustaining treatments. *American Journal of Public Health* 83: 14–23.

READING GUIDE

A more intensive treatment of the themes in this section, but with the same emphasis on first-person narratives and literary sources, can be found in Donna Dickenson, Malcolm Johnson, and Jeanne Samson Katz (eds.), *Death, Dying and Bereavement* (London: Sage, 2000, 2nd edn). The illustrated anthology edited by the philosopher Robin Downie, *The Healing Arts* (Oxford: Oxford University Press, 1994), also contains many classic literary texts on death and dying. The broader question of use of literature in medical students' courses is covered by the journal, *Medical Humanities*, co-published by the *British Medical Journal* group with its long-established sister journal, *Journal of Medical Ethics*.

The themes of authenticity and of individual values in a "death of one's own" are particularly acute in psychiatry. In dementia, for example, as Tony Hope has argued in "Personal identity and psychiatric illness," in A. Phillips Griffiths (ed.), *Philosophy, Psychology and Psychiatry* (Cambridge: Cambridge University Press, 1994), the loss of personal identity may be such that from the perspective of the carer, the person is already in effect dead to them, though they have not had the opportunity to grieve. Suicide and "psychiatric euthanasia" also raise key issues of authenticity, of the "true wishes" of the person concerned, and of rationality (see, in particular, Eric Matthew's introduction to a thematic issue of *Philosophy, Psychiatry, and Psychology*, on "Psychiatric Euthanasia": "Choosing death: Philosophical observations on suicide and euthanasia,"

Philosophy, Psychiatry, and Psychology 5/2 (1998): 107–12). The importance of the time dimension in advance directives is explored in Savulescu, J. and Dickenson, D., "The time frame of preferences, dis-positions, and the validity of advance directives for the mentally ill," *Philosophy, Psychiatry, and Psychology* 5/3 (1998): 225–46.

Epilogue: If You Must Go Into the Starless Night Alone

JENNY LEWIS

If you must go into the starless night alone,
have courage – we are with you; not angels,
saints or martyrs but ordinary women,
honouring kindness, mindful of the needs
of others. Our thoughts cradle the world,
comfort history against the shadow of chaos.

You'll throw off your coverlet of snowdrop
and primrose, run barefoot across the grass –
a child again, released into morning, into birdsong.

You'll hear the murmur of voices
like bees drowsing on the warm hillside –
follow the sound through the old garden,
past walls heavy with apricots; you'll inhale

scents of roses and lavender, just as we did.
Soon you'll find us, leaning on our spears,
facing the dawn – a brave tribe with our
wounds and battlescars; warriors, athletes,
poets, scholars – travellers in mind and body,
resting for a moment between journeys.

When you are refreshed, it'll be time to move on;
to venture out once more across the vast, cloudy
universe – solitary spirit, yet part of a thousand
indomitable armies whose voices you've heard
    calling,
telling you when it's time to leave, or to come,
    home.

Selection from *The Death of Ivan Ilyich*

LEO TOLSTOY

Another two weeks passed. Ivan Ilyich no longer got off the sofa. He did not want to lie in bed and so he lay on the sofa. And as he lay there, facing the wall most of the time, he suffered, all alone, the same inexplicable suffering and, all alone, brooded on the same inexplicable question: "What is this? Is it true that this is death?" And an inner voice answered: "Yes, it is true." "Then why these torments?" And the voice answered: "For no reason – they just are." Above and beyond this there was nothing.

From the start of his illness, from the time he first went to a doctor, Ivan Ilyich's life had been divided into two contradictory and fluctuating moods: one a mood of despair and expectation of an incomprehensible and terrible death; the other a mood of hope filled with intent observation of the course of his bodily functions. At times he was confronted with nothing but a kidney or an intestine that was temporarily evading its duty; at others nothing but an unfathomable, horrifying death from which there was no escape.

These two moods had fluctuated since the onset of his illness, but the farther that illness progressed, the more unlikely and preposterous considerations about his kidney became and the more real his sense of impending death.

He had merely to recall what he had been like three months earlier and what he was now, to remember how steadily he had gone downhill, for all possibility of hope to be shattered.

During the last days of the isolation in which he lived, lying on the sofa with his face to the wall, isolation in the midst of a populous city among numerous friends and relatives, an isolation that could not have been greater anywhere, either in the depths of the sea or the bowels of the earth – during the last days of that terrible isolation, Ivan Ilyich lived only with memories of the past. One after another images of his past came to mind. His recollections always began with what was closest in time and shifted back to what was most remote, to his childhood, and lingered there. If he thought of the stewed prunes he had been served that day, he remembered the raw, shrivelled French prunes he had eaten as a child, the special taste they had, the way his mouth watered when he got down to the pit; and along with the memory of that taste came a whole series of memories of those days: of his nurse, his brother, his toys. "I mustn't think about them – it's too painful," he would tell himself and shift back to the present. He would look at the button on the back of the sofa and the crease in the morocco. "Morocco is expensive, doesn't wear well; we had a quarrel over it. But there had been another morocco and another quarrel – the time we tore papa's briefcase and got punished, but mama brought us some tarts." And again his memories centered on his childhood, and again he found them painful and tried to drive them away by thinking about something else.

And together with this train of recollections, another flashed through his mind – recollections of how his illness had progressed and become more acute. Here, too, the farther back in time he went, the more life he found. There had been more goodness in his life earlier and more of life itself. And the one fused with the other. "Just as my torments are getting worse and worse, so my whole life got worse and worse," he thought. There was only one bright spot back at the beginning of life; after that things grew blacker and blacker, moved faster and faster. "In inverse ratio to the square of the distance from death," thought Ivan Ilyich. And the image of a stone hurtling downward with increasing velocity became fixed in his mind. Life, a series of increasing sufferings, falls faster and faster toward its end – the most frightful suffering. "I am falling..." He shuddered, shifted back and forth, wanted to resist, but by then knew there was no resisting. And again, weary of contemplating but unable to tear his eyes away from what was right there before him, he stared at the back of the sofa and waited – waited for that dreadful fall, shock, destruction. "Resistance is impossible," he said to himself. "But if only I could understand the reason for this agony. Yet even that is impossible. It would make sense if one could say I had not lived as I should have. But such an admission is impossible," he uttered inwardly, remembering how his life had conformed to all the laws, rules, and proprieties. "That is a point I cannot grant," he told himself, smiling ironically, as though someone could see that smile of his and be taken in by it. "There is no explanation. Agony. Death. Why?"

[...]

The doctor came at his usual time. Ivan Ilyich merely answered Yes or No to his questions, glowered at him throughout the visit, and toward the end said:

"You know perfectly well you can do nothing to help me, so leave me alone."

"We can ease your suffering," said the doctor.

"You can't even do that; leave me alone."

The doctor went into the drawing room and told Praskovya Fyodorovna that his condition was very bad and that only one remedy, opium, could relieve his pain, which must be excruciating.

The doctor said his physical agony was dreadful, and that was true; but even more dreadful was his moral agony, and it was this that tormented him most.

What had induced his moral agony was that during the night, as he gazed at Gerasim's broad-boned, sleepy, good-natured face, he suddenly asked himself: "What if my entire life, my entire conscious life, simply was *not the real thing*?"

It occurred to him that what had seemed utterly inconceivable before – that he had not lived the kind of life he should have – might in fact be true. It occurred to him that those scarcely perceptible impulses of his to protest what people of high rank considered good, vague impulses which he had always suppressed, might have been precisely what mattered, and all the rest not been the real thing. His official duties, his manner of life, his family, the values adhered to by people in society and in his profession – all these might not have been the real thing. He tried to come up with a defense of these things and suddenly became aware of the insubstantiality of them all. And there was nothing left to defend.

"But if that is the case," he asked himself, "and I am taking leave of life with the awareness that I squandered all I was given and have no possibility of rectifying matters – what then?" He lay on his back and began to review his whole life in an entirely different light.

When, in the morning, he saw first the footman, then his wife, then his daughter, and then the doctor, their every gesture, their every word, confirmed the horrible truth revealed to him during the night. In them he saw himself, all he had lived by, saw clearly that all this was not the real thing but a dreadful, enormous deception that shut out both life and death. This awareness intensified his physical sufferings, magnified them tenfold. He moaned and tossed and clutched at his bedclothes. He felt they were choking and suffocating him, and he hated them on that account.

He was given a large dose of opium and lost consciousness, but at dinnertime it all started again. He drove everyone away and tossed from side to side.

His wife came to him and said:

"*Jean*, dear, do this for me." (For me?)

"It can't do you any harm, and it often helps. Really, it's such a small thing. And even healthy people often . . ."

He opened his eyes wide.

"What? Take the sacrament? Why? I don't want to! And yet . . ."

She began to cry.

"Then you will, dear? I'll send for our priest, he's such a nice man."

"Fine, very good," he said.

When the priest came and heard his confession, he relented, seemed to feel relieved of his doubts and therefore of his agony, and experienced a brief moment of hope. Again he began to think about his caecum and the possibility of curing it. As he took the sacrament, there were tears in his eyes.

When they laid him down afterward, he felt better for a second and again held out hope of living. He began to think of the operation the doctors had proposed doing. "I want to live, to live!" he said to himself. His wife came in to congratulate him on taking the sacrament; she said the things people usually do, and then added:

"You really do feel better, don't you?"

"Yes," he said without looking at her.

Her clothes, her figure, the expression of her face, the sound of her voice – all these said to him: "*Not the real thing*. Everything you lived by and still live by is a lie, a deception that blinds you from the reality of life and death." And no sooner had he thought this than hatred welled up in him, and with the hatred, excruciating physical pain, and with the pain, an awareness of inevitable, imminent destruction. The pain took a new turn: it began to grind and shoot and constrict his breathing.

The expression on his face when he uttered that "Yes" was dreadful. Having uttered it, he looked his wife straight in the eye, and with a rapidity extraordinary for one so weak, flung himself face downward and shouted:

"Go away! Go away! Leave me alone!"

82

Subjective Values, Objective Good, and Incompetent Patients

THOMAS BULLER

Decisions concerning the ending of life-sustaining treatment for incompetent patients who were formerly competent present us with the following challenge: to what degree, if at all, should we take into account the interests and values that the patient had when she was competent? All of us care about how our lives go, and would view the prospect of becoming incompetent with fear and sadness; for incompetence means the loss of so much in our present lives that gives them value and makes them *our* lives – opinions, interests, value, memories, relationships with others. It is for this reason that many decide to write advance directives directing that life-sustaining treatment be withheld if they were to become incompetent, for there seems to be little value to a future life without these elements in it. However, the difficulty with this approach is that once we have become incompetent we might have a very different set of interests and values, as the following case attempts to show.

Vera Stuart is a 63-year-old nursing home patient who suffers from Alzheimer's dementia. Although incompetent, Vera seems quite content and could be described as "pleasantly senile." In particular, she appears to enjoy being read to (although she does not understand what is being read), sitting in the sunshine, and having her hair combed. Prior to the onset of dementia, Vera was an historian. An extremely knowledgeable person with a formidable memory, Vera loved the intellectual life that she led. The thought of becoming demented horrified her, and several years ago Vera wrote an advance directive requesting that she not receive life-sustaining treatment should she become incompetent. Vera has recently been diagnosed with pneumonia which is life-threatening if not treated immediately with antibiotics.[1]

We are thus faced with a choice between two options: we could decide to respect Vera's advance directive and withhold the antibiotics, or we could decide to override the directive and treat Vera with antibiotics. However, both of these options are problematic: the first sacrifices the life of an incompetent but contented woman on the basis of past interests that are no longer relevant; and the second commits Vera to the type of life that she had expressly sought to avoid when she was previously competent.

Unattractive though both these options might be, it seems difficult to imagine an alternative one, since we must either respect or reject the directive. Nevertheless, an important task remains, namely, to attempt to formulate an account that can provide a coherent explanation of which set of interests should take precedence, and thereby a means to resolve cases like Vera's.

Autonomy, Authenticity, and Identity

Recent discussions of the authority of advance directives have responded to the above challenge by wholeheartedly embracing one or other of the options. Examination of these accounts reveals the central point of contention to be whether a competent person's right to self-determination extends to the right to make future-binding treatment decisions should that person become incompetent; in other words, whether autonomy includes *precedent autonomy*. In their work, Ronald Dworkin, Norman Cantor, and Nancy Rhoden have presented various arguments to the conclusion that autonomy is both present and future directed, and hence a competent person can make future treatment decisions that apply to later incompetence.[2] In opposition to this view, Rebecca Dresser has consistently rejected the notion of precedent autonomy, arguing that the incompetent patient's prior interests when competent are now irrelevant, and, therefore, that treatment decisions must be based on the incompetent patient's current and future best interests.[3]

The disagreement between these two views can be understood as a disagreement over the scope and authority of autonomy, and the relationship between autonomy, authenticity, and identity. For example, according to Dworkin the value of autonomy is at least to some degree that it promotes *integrity* – it grants the freedom and responsibility to shape our lives according to our characters and our chosen interests and values. This value of autonomy is independent of the promotion of individual well-being, for the authority of an autonomous decision is derived not from whether the decision is in the

person's best interest, but whether the decision is the product of a "recognized and coherent scheme of value." In other words, the authority of a decision is derived in considerable part from its authenticity – whether it is consistent with the person's character and her chosen interests and values. On Dworkin's account, this integrity view of autonomy will apply to both contemporaneous and future decisions, for "it seems essential to someone's control of his whole life that he be able to dictate what will happen to him when he becomes incompetent."[4] Thus a person who writes a living will is making a decision that is both reflective of his interests and values, and a "judgment about the overall shape or character of the kind of life he wants to lead."[5] A decision of this type, therefore, has greater authority, and thus takes precedence over the contemporaneous interests of the later incompetent patient, which reflect neither authenticity nor integrity.

For her part, Rhoden defends an "active" sense of persons where persons are understood as (almost literally) self-creators, rather than "passively" as merely the experiences of sensations.[6] A central element in Rhoden's account is the notion of agency: persons are moral agents and agency is necessarily future-orientated; for a decision to choose a certain course of action such as writing an advance directive necessarily depends on being able to conceive of the effect this decision will have upon us in the future. The person who writes the directive imagines herself in an unwanted future state (from her present perspective) as an incompetent patient, and on the basis of this image decides to direct future treatment. Moreover, according to Rhoden, prior directives have authority over the later interests of the incompetent patient because of a hierarchical difference in value between a person's moral and spiritual values, and the later purely physical interests of the incompetent patient.

Thus for both Rhoden and Dworkin, the notion of precedent autonomy logically follows from a view of personal identity that sees the competent and incompetent person as the same person, despite the loss of those psychological characteristics that are defining of who we are and the basis of our interests. This is not to suggest in any sense that personal identity is constituted by continuity of the physical, rather than the psychological; rather, it is to claim that when we look at a person's psychological life in terms of the progression from competence to incompetence, the critical interests that define and identify what is of importance to us do not have to be presently held to retain their authority.[7]

Dresser's rejection of precedent autonomy is based on a rather different understanding of autonomy. For her, autonomy implies the capacity to be autonomous: we can correctly regard a person to be autonomous if, and only if, that person retains the capacity to make autonomous decisions; and since the incompetent person clearly lacks this capacity, it is inappropriate to allow the incompetent person to make treatment decisions. "Precedent autonomy" is, therefore, a fiction. A second element in Dresser's rejection of precedent autonomy is her view that autonomous decisions have authority only if they continue to be authentic, that is to say, that they continue to be reflective of the person's character and interests. And since the values and interests that applied when the person wrote an advance directive are no longer relevant (for example, Vera's interest in her intellectual life in the case above), the directive no longer promotes the person's interests. As Dresser says:

> They [incompetent patients] cannot now exercise autonomy, and their former remarks on death and dying (if any exist) constitute only a piece of the puzzle, for their situations and experiences are now vastly altered. As a result, choices on their treatment are not like the choices competent persons make about life-sustaining treatment. What makes them different is the altered consciousness of the incompetent person who experiences the consequences of the treatment decision.[8]

A third reason for rejecting precedent autonomy is that the conditions of personal identity in cases like Vera's are no longer met. The neurological damage that has rendered Vera incompetent has destroyed her psychological characteristics, and thus her advance directive lacks authority not only because it is based on now irrelevant interests that counter her present best interests, but also because the former competent Vera can be thought of as a different self. Dresser supports the view that a person's life can be thought to be composed of a series of "successive selves," and thus she would refer to the incompetent patient as a separate, "later self" rather than a different person. Thus, for Dresser, by respecting the prior wishes of the patient when competent, we abandon the now incompetent patient and our moral obligation to care for the best interests of those unable to look after themselves.

Despite the differences between the two accounts, I think that, ironically, they suffer from similar problems of temporal narrowness: the autonomy model ignores the future; the best interests model ignores the past. The autonomy model of Cantor, Dworkin, and Rhoden treats all incompetent patients as severely incompetent individuals with profoundly diminished lives and ignores the fact that some incompetent patients, such as Vera, have relatively coherent likes and dislikes that contradict earlier interests and values, and a sense of self. Consider if, instead of the level of incompetence that Vera presently has, she were to be in a persistent vegetative state. As far as the autonomy model is concerned, there is no difference between a profoundly incompetent or a moderately incompetent Vera. It might appear that this would not be the case if Vera's dementia were minimal, for Dworkin is prepared to admit that a mildly demented patient may retain to some degree at least the capacity for integrity and authenticity.[9] But notice that this analysis depends on viewing the incompetent Vera in terms of her putative autonomy, rather than on her current best interests; in other words, Dworkin is prepared to grant that the interests of the incompetent patient have value, and may even take precedence over the former competent person's interests, only if the incompetent patient can present a legitimate claim for autonomy.

There are other reasons for thinking that the current best interests of the incompetent patient matter more than the autonomy model allows. Imagine the not-too-distant possibility that we have discovered a drug, *cognazol*, that can reverse to some extent the ravages of Alzheimer's, and this discovery has occurred after Vera became incompetent. The effect of *cognazol* would be to improve Vera's condition so that she would be only mildly demented, although she will never regain the interests, values, and character that she had before the onset of the disease. Regardless of whether Vera knew of, or anticipated, such a possibility when she was competent, should we give Vera the drug? Since the effect of the drug would be to strengthen the interests of the incompetent Vera over her former competent self, it seems plausible to contend that the autonomy model would argue against improving Vera's cognitive status. However, if the integrity value of autonomy presents a claim against actions that seek to interfere with a person's autonomy, such as overriding an advance directive, then on a principle of moral symmetry it would also present a claim against actions that seek to prevent the possibility of autonomy, such as respecting the directive.[10]

The best interests model ignores the future by seeing no distinction between those incompetent patients who were previously competent and those who were never competent, for the prior competent life of the now incompetent patient is thought to be irrelevant. To see this we might consider the following two cases.

Mike Jones is a 67-year-old lifelong Jehovah's Witness who is incompetent as a result of suffering a moderate cerebral stroke two days ago. Mike has an advance directive stating that he does not wish treatment to be performed should it require the use of blood or blood products. A week prior to suffering the stroke, Mike met with his physician to confirm his wishes. Mike's condition is irreversible, but he has retained sufficient ability to be able to recognize his family and caregivers. The decision at hand is whether to perform surgery in an attempt to relieve the pressure on his brain in order to attempt to prevent further strokes.

In the second case, Larry Smith is a 67-year-old man with an IQ of approximately 10 who has lived in state institutions for most of his life. He has recently been diagnosed as having acute myeloblastic monocytic leukemia. Recommended treatment is chemotherapy, which can bring remission for between two months and a year, but it has serious side effects, such as anemia and infection. In addition, the probability of remission is less for patients over the age of 60.

As far as the best interests model is concerned, the cases of Vera, Mike, and Larry are alike, for any treatment decision made should be on the basis of the patient's current best interests. It is ultimately unimportant that Mike's incompetence has only lasted a week and that he had such clear and well-known prior religious views, for if his current interests would be furthered by further treatment, then this is what we should do. Part of Dresser's objection to the autonomy model is epistemic – that we frequently have only a confused idea of what the patient would have wanted – and for this reason we may, like the US Supreme Court, feel that we are lacking in "clear and convincing" evidence of what the patient wants in the absence of an advance directive.[11] But even when such evidence is presented, this information would not be sufficient for Dresser to trump the interests of the incompetent patient.

Additionally, recall that part of Dresser's objection to the autonomy model is that she claims that the neurological event that has rendered Vera incompetent has also disrupted the psychological characteristics necessary for personal identity. Imagine that an improved *cognazol* can reverse the ravages of dementia and restore Vera to her former competent state. Would Dresser argue that it would be wrong to sacrifice the interests of the incompetent Vera for those of her former, and now future, competent self? It would seem that Dresser would have to draw this conclusion, for there is no greater psychological connection between the incompetent Vera and her former competent self than between the incompetent Vera and her future competent self. I suspect that Dresser would provide Vera with the drug that reverses the dementia, and the justification would be that dementia is not simply a different psychological state from our normal cognitive one, but a *worse* one – dementia involves the loss of much of what gives life meaning.

A Reductionist, Psychological Account

In order to overcome the narrowness of the autonomy and best interest models, Buchanan and Brock have attempted to formulate an account that accommodates the differences in the three cases outlined in the previous section, and recognize that not all cases involving incompetent patients are the same.[12] They have argued that the advance directive has authority to make future non-treatment decisions on the basis of autonomy, but that the directive can be overridden in those cases where the competent and incompetent persons are psychologically discontinuous and have radically different interests in the continuation of life-sustaining treatment. As a basis for their view, Buchanan and Brock support a particular theory of personal identity and the authority of autonomous decisions:

1. A person's identity is constituted by a set of psychological characteristics (memories, intentions, beliefs, dispositions, etc.) and the identity of a person over time consists in an overlapping chain of these psychological characteristics; furthermore, these characteristics hold to different degrees: as a person ages, the psychological characteristics that constituted his early character will diminish.
2. The authority of a person to make decisions that affect her at a later time "tracks" the degree of psychological continuity between the person at these times; in other words, the more closely psychologically connected Vera at $t1$ is with Vera at $t2$, the more weight we should ascribe to her prior decisions.

This theory is a reductionist, psychological one, because it claims that there is nothing to a personal identity over and above the psychological connections. Since these connections can be held to different degrees, we can plausibly describe the later Vera as "less or more" the same person as the earlier Vera. We can refer to this theory as RP.[13]

Buchanan and Brock are clear in their support for RP and specifically address the notions that personal identity consists only of psychological continuity, and that the strength of our obligation to respect the advance directive corresponds in considerable part to the degree of psychological continuity:

First, all else being equal, the greater the degree of psychological continuity between A, the competent person who issued the directive, and B the (incompetent) individual whose body (and brain) are spatio-temporally continuous with A's, the greater the moral authority of the advance directive, i.e., the more *weight* A's wishes, as expressed in the advance directive, should be accorded in determining what is to be done for B.[14]

The obligation to respect the directive corresponds only *in part* to the degree of psychological continuity, for Buchanan and Brock argue that there is a threshold level of psychological continuity at which personal identity becomes an "all-or-nothing" matter and does not admit of degrees. Once this threshold level has been reached, the advance directive has full moral force. However, as the level of psychological continuity falls below this threshold,

the moral authority or force of the advance directive diminishes correspondingly. In other words, for cases that fall *below* the threshold level...the more readily the advance directive may be overridden by competing moral considerations, including our concern for the well-being of the incompetent individual.[15]

Buchanan and Brock's position remains a reductionist one, despite the inclusion of a threshold concept of psychological continuity, for by establishing a threshold level they are not claiming that there is anything to personal identity other than psychological continuity; rather, they are merely placing an upper boundary on the degree of psychological continuity necessary for the directive to have full authority.

There is some similarity between Buchanan and Brock's position and that of Dresser, for both support a reductionist psychological view of personal identity that ties the authority of prior decisions to the degree of psychological continuity. However, these two accounts differ in an important aspect: whereas Buchanan and Brock set the level of psychological continuity necessary for personal identity low, Dresser would set the level high. The upshot of this is that if we consider a case where there has been a substantial change in psychological characteristics, interests, and values, whereas Dresser would maintain that the later incompetent patient is a different self or person, Buchanan and Brock would regard the incompetent patient as the same self or person, other things being equal. In other words, a greater degree of alteration or destruction of psychological characteristics is necessary on Buchanan and Brock's account for loss of personal identity than on Dresser's.

In *Deciding for Others*, Buchanan and Brock discuss what they term the "slavery argument," which is, essentially, the objection to advance directives raised by Dresser:

(i)   One person's advance directive has no moral authority to determine what is to happen to *another person*.

(ii)   In some cases of severe and permanent neurological damage, for example, that due to advanced Alzheimer's dementia, psychological continuity is so disrupted that the person who issued the advance directive no longer exists.

(ii′)   The individual who remains after neurological damage has destroyed the person who issued the directive is a (different) *person*.

(Therefore)

(iii)   In such cases the advance directive has no moral authority to determine what is to happen to the individual who remains after neurological damage has destroyed the person who issued the advance directive.[16]

Buchanan and Brock's response to the slavery argument is to maintain that the neurological damage that has destroyed personal identity had also destroyed *personhood* – the incompetent patient is no longer a person – and if the patient is no longer a person, then clearly he cannot be a different person; hence the authority of the advance directive is intact. This response depends on establishing that the level of psychological continuity necessary for personal identity should be set low, such that the interference in a person's psychology that would be sufficient to destroy personal identity would also be sufficient to destroy personhood. Buchanan and Brock seek to establish this by arguing that if we set the required level high, then we would be faced with the "severe disruption of basic social practices and institutions," for there would be many cases where personal identity but not personhood has been lost. Furthermore, they contend that despite the loss of personhood and personal identity, the competent person's interests in not receiving life-sustaining treatment survive. The basis for this claim is that since interests can survive death (a grandparent may have an interest in her grandchildren getting married, even though this might occur after her death), so interests can survive the loss of competence.

If we return to the historian Vera, neither Buchanan and Brock nor Dresser would maintain that she needs to have the *same* beliefs, desires, and memories as the demented Vera in order for us to say that she is one and the same person; however, they would disagree as to when the incompetent Vera ceases to be the same person or self as the competent Vera. The conditions of authenticity and identity are stricter for Dresser than for Buchanan and Brock, since in order for a decision to have authority there must be a greater degree of psychological continuity.

Psychological Continuity and the Authority of Prior Decisions

Does RP, in conjunction with surviving interests, provide a defense of the authority of advance directives, as Buchanan and Brock intend: namely, to distinguish those cases where the directive should be respected from those in which it should be overridden on the basis of the lack of psychological continuity?

As a preliminary to answering this question, it is worthwhile to briefly consider the relationship between personal identity and personhood as understood by Buchanan and Brock. When we talk about something or someone at one time as being the same as something or someone at a later time, it is imperative to specify the same *what*.[17] It is clear from their response to the "slavery argument" that Buchanan and Brock understand the *what* to be "person." If we consider the necessary and sufficient conditions of "being the same person as," it is clear that one of the necessary conditions must be being a person; for if Vera is no longer a person once she has become profoundly demented, then she certainly cannot be the same person as the person who wrote the directive. It is this consideration that presumably underlies Buchanan and Brock's motivation to set the level of psychological continuity necessary for personal identity low, and allows them to defend the authority of advance directives in cases of profound dementia. However, this leaves untouched those cases like Vera's where the dementia is less severe. Here, Buchanan and Brock have ruled out the option of classifying Vera as a "non-person" by setting the level of psychological continuity so low. Thus, if they are to defend the view that Vera's advance directive can be overridden on the basis of minimal authority due to lack of psychological continuity, this cannot be on the grounds that Vera is not the same person. The locus of discussion, therefore, is over what is meant by the degree of psychological continuity between the competent person who issued the directive and the incompetent individual.

To return to the matter of the success of RP, let us imagine the gradual progression of Vera's dementia from its onset, $t2$, until its final stage, $t4$. Furthermore, for the sake of argument, let us suppose that when Vera is at the stage described in the original case above she is at some mid-point in her progressive dementia, $t3$. According to Buchanan and Brock, once Vera's psychological characteristics have been disrupted to the extent that they no longer meet the threshold level necessary for personal identity, the authority of her advance directive will be proportional to the degree of psychological

continuity between her former competent self and her present incompetent self. We can assume that once Vera has reached the midpoint stage, $t3$, she is below the threshold level.

The first important point to notice on Buchanan and Brock's account is that since Vera's dementia will progressively rob her of the psychological characteristics that constitute her identity, and the authority of the directive is proportional to the level of psychological continuity, the authority of Vera's directive will *decrease* as Vera's dementia *increases*. This decrease will continue until just before the endstage, when Vera ceases to be a person and her surviving interests come into effect. As this chapter has intended to show, the most troubling cases for supporters of advance directives are those such as Vera, where we appear to have rival sets of psychological characteristics and interests; less troubling are those cases where the level of incompetence is far greater, for in these cases the person's psychology and interests will be much reduced, and there is greater agreement as to the incompetent patient's best interests. Yet on Buchanan and Brock's account it seems that as Vera's condition worsens, and with it the loss of both rival and non-rival psychological states, so the directive loses its authority. Whether one supports advance directives or not, their intention is to prevent having to spend one's last months or years as a profoundly demented individual; it is this type of existence that alarms us, I would contend, rather than an existence like Vera's. But on Buchanan and Brock's account, apart from the very last stages of incompetence, the directive will have least force when perhaps it is most important and most needed.[18]

In fact, it seems as though Buchanan and Brock have two answers to the question of when the directive is at its weakest. Consider Vera's psychological status at $t3$ (the case described above) and her status at $t4$ (the endstage). On the one hand, the authority of the directive is greater at $t3$ than at $t4$, for whereas Vera has at least some of the relevant psychological connections with her former competent self at the mid-point in her dementia, she has no such connections once she has reached the endstage of her dementia; however, on the other hand, the authority of the directive is greater at *t4* than at *t3*, for at *t4*, despite the loss of both personal identity and personhood, and thus any rival psychological characteristics, Vera's prior interests in non-treatment survive. If the preferred answer is that the directive is stronger at *t4* than at *t3*, then this provides the following strategy for caregivers who are supporters of directives: wait until the patient's dementia has reached its end-stage. It appears as if Vera's ability to control future non-treatment will depend greatly on the time in her dementia at which she requires life-sustaining treatment. If she requires such treatment at the onset of the dementia, then on one reading of Buchanan and Brock, she would have a better chance of having the directive respected than at the end-stage. This raises the further objection that the authority of the directive appears to be overly dependent on chance.

Can Buchanan and Brock justify overriding Vera's directive at *t3*? If the contention is that the moral authority of the directive is at its weakest at this time due to minimal psychological continuity, then it would appear that the directive could be overridden to defend the incompetent Vera's best interests. The difficulty with this approach is that there is a very fine line between the case where Vera's psychological continuity with her former competent self is so low that the directive has minimal authority, and the case where Vera ceases to be a person at all. If Buchanan and Brock support RP and permit the directive to be overridden at *t3* because of minimal psychological continuity, then this is very close to the situation where the conditions for personal identity are not met. And since the loss of personal identity is linked to the loss of personhood, this would mean that Vera would no longer be a person. However, if Vera is no longer a person, then there is no justification for overriding the directive, for on the above analysis the wishes of past competent persons take precedence over the interests of current non-persons.

This is not to say that Buchanan and Brock are forced to give up linking the loss of personal identity with the loss of personhood if they permit the directive to be overridden at *t3* on the grounds of lack of psychological continuity.

But it is easy to imagine that Vera might lose more connections with her former self whilst at the same time enjoying the sunshine and contentedly living her life; and there will come a point when we might feel obliged, like Dresser, to claim that Vera is no longer the same person. But this option is only open to Buchanan and Brock if they are then prepared to claim that Vera is no longer any person.

The challenge comes from the fact that although being a person is necessary for being the same person, it is obviously not sufficient, and as Vera's case shows (and also perhaps cases involving patients suffering from multiple personality disorders), we can conceive of a loss of identity without a loss of personhood.[19]

A Non-Reductionist Argument for Advance Directives

I hope the above discussion has shown that there are considerable problems in attempting to tie the authority of advance directives with a reductionist psychological theory of personal identity. Part of the problem of this approach is that it appears to pay too little attention to the fact that the future dementia is going to happen to *me*. When a person writes an advance directive, she is contemplating a future in which *her* mind has been seriously impaired and *she* has become incompetent; she is not contemplating a future with some other, incompetent person in it. Thus, in writing the directive, Vera is attempting to control her future by preventing herself from living the life of an incompetent, albeit pleasantly senile, woman.

As Bernard Williams asks, "Why should I hinder my future projects from the perspective of my present values rather than inhibit my present projects from the perspective of my future values?"[20] Williams's answer is that these projects are in some sense constitutive of who I am, in that they provide me with reasons for living. Furthermore, it is only because a person sees herself as someone whose values and interests will change over time that the person identifies her present values as primary and grants them the authority over later ones. In other words, Vera is fully aware that once she has become incompetent she may well have a different set of interests and values; and it is because she is aware of this that she is able to recognize the importance of her present value of not wanting to receive life-sustaining treatment and to seek to prevent receiving such treatment should she become incompetent.

The conclusion to be drawn is that we have to understand Vera's decision to write the directive when she was competent as the decision of someone who deliberately and expressly attempts to make her present values control her future ones, because she believes that it will be *she* who will be demented. If Vera did not believe this, it is difficult to explain her decision.

It might be objected that in order for a desire to retain its authority it must continue to be authentic, that is to say, it must continue to be the case that the person has that desire. Another way of saying this is to claim that Vera's desire for future non-treatment is contingent on its own existence: Vera's desire for non-treatment at some future time only makes sense if she continues to desire non-treatment at this future time. In response to this objection, one might contend that Vera's desire for non-treatment is a *categorical desire*, and as such is not contingent on its own persistence. Since Vera's desire for non-treatment determines whether she lives or dies, this desire, therefore, determines whether she is going to have any desires at all. In other words, her desire cannot be contingent on her continuing to have this desire, since the desire settles the very question of whether she has any desires at all. If this is correct, then it is appropriate to regard Vera's advance directive as a categorical desire, for an advance directive determines whether Vera is going to live or die, and whether she has future desires. Thus the directive is not contingent on whether Vera continues to have the desire for non-treatment. Hence it is no objection to say that the directive lacks authority because she no longer has the desire for non-treatment, for the authority of the directive is not contingent on the persistence of the desire.

Does this mean that advance directives should be respected no matter what? I don't think that this is an appropriate conclusion to draw, for in doing so we would be granting future non-treatment decisions greater force than contemporaneous ones. I think that it is helpful to consider the conditions under which we think that it would be justified to override the contemporaneous non-treatment decision of an autonomous person. In broad terms, we could justify such paternalistic intervention on two grounds: either we believe that the person will later consent to our intervention, or we believe that the harm caused by our intervention is less than the harm that would result if we did not intervene. I suggest that these should be our justifications when we seek to override a valid advance directive. We should do so only if we believe in good faith that either the competent person would have agreed to such an intervention, or we believe that the harm that will befall the incompetent patient should the directive be respected is greater than the harm involved in overriding an autonomous decision.

The success of this view depends on whether one can avoid quantifying the amount of harm on the basis of the degree of psychological continuity: it is less harmful to override Vera's directive at *t3* than at *t2* since there is less continuity with the former competent person. If this view is successful, then I think we would have some way of deciding what to do in cases such as Vera's without abandoning the fact that she has expressly desired not to receive life-sustaining treatment. This strategy has the advantage of simplicity, since we do not have to determine whether the competent and incompetent Vera are, or to what degree they are, the same person or self in order to determine the authority of the directive, and it has the advantage of charity since it recognizes that we care how our lives go and that we might rationally choose not to want to be kept alive should we become incompetent.

NOTES

1   This case is based on a description in Allen E. Buchanan and Dan W. Brock, *Deciding for Others: The Ethics of Surrogate Decision-Making* (New York: Cambridge University Press, 1989), p. 108.

2 Ronald Dworkin, *Life's Dominion: An Argument About Abortion, Euthanasia, and Individual Freedom* (New York: Alfred A. Knopf, 1993); Norman Cantor, *Advance Directives and the Pursuit of Death with Dignity* (Bloomington: Indiana University Press, 1993); Nancy K. Rhoden, "The limits of legal objectivity," *North Carolina Law Review* 68/5 (1990): 845–65.

3 Rebecca Dresser, "Dworkin in dementia: Elegant theory, questionable policy," *Hastings Center Report* 25/6 (1995): 32–8; "Missing persons: Legal perceptions of incompetent patients," *Rutgers Law Review* 46/2 (1994): 609–719; Rebecca Dresser and Peter J. Whitehouse, "The incompetent patient and the slippery slope," *Hastings Center Report* 24/4 (1994): 6–12; Rebecca Dresser, "Autonomy revisited: The limits of anticipatory choices," in Robert H. Binstock, Stephen G. Post, and Peter J. Whitehouse (eds.), *Dementia and Aging: Ethics, Values, and Policy Choices* (Baltimore, MD: Johns Hopkins University Press, 1992), pp. 71, 85.

4 Ronald Dworkin, "Autonomy and the demented self," *The Millbank Quarterly* 64/2 (1986): 7.

5 Ibid: 11.

6 Rhoden, "The limits of legal objectivity;" see also Christine Koorsgaard, "Personal identity and the unity of agency: A Kantian response to Parfit," *Philosophy and Public Affairs* 18/2: 101–32.

7 Presumably, supporters of the autonomy model would hold that the competent person and incompetent patient *are* the same person on the basis of overlapping psychological connections.

8 Dresser, "Missing persons," pp. 610–11.

9 Dworkin, "Autonomy and the demented self," p. 9.

10 For further discussion of the moral symmetry principle, see Michael Tooley, *Abortion and Infanticide* (Oxford: Clarendon Press, 1993), pp. 184–241.

11 Dresser, "Missing persons," p. 622; *Cruzan* vs. *Missouri Department of Health*, 497 US 261 (1990).

12 Allen E. Buchanan and Dan W. Brock, *Deciding for Others* (New York: Cambridge University Press, 1989).

13 RP is an example of the type of the account proposed by Derek Parfit in *Reasons and Persons* (Oxford: Oxford University Press, 1986).

14 Buchanan and Brock, *Deciding for Others*, p. 179.

15 Ibid.

16 Ibid: 182.

17 David Wiggins, *Identity and Spatio-Temporal Continuity* (Oxford: Basil Blackwell, 1967).

18 One could contend that the directive is most needed here on the grounds that at this stage we would have little evidence of the incompetent patient's current interests.

19 A recent, thorough discussion of this topic can be found in Jennifer Radden, *Divided Minds and Successive Selves* (Cambridge: MIT Press, 1996).

20 Bernard Williams, "Persons, character and morality," in Amelie Oksenberg Rorty (ed.), *The Identities of Persons* (Berkeley: University of California Press, 1976), p. 206.

83

Falls

EDWARD LOWBURY

Pulled by the sky's gravitation
Smoke falls upwards;
The money-spider floats, in perfect balance;
And a child on shaky limbs
Drops into its mother's arms,
Or falls light – no need to fear the fall
When earth is near and motherly.

But no maternal arms
Reach out to save those on shaky limbs
Who fall in second childhood.
The earth is hard and far away beneath
    them,
The bones are brittle
And every fall brings pain or injury –
Until, at last, light
As smoke, they feel once more
The gravity of the sky
And learn to fall upwards.

84

Decisions Near the End of Life

COUNCIL ON ETHICAL AND JUDICIAL AFFAIRS, AMERICAN MEDICAL ASSOCIATION

Over the last 50 years, people have become increasingly concerned that the dying process is too often needlessly protracted by medical technology and is consequently marked by incapacitation, intolerable pain, and indignity. In one public opinion poll, 68% of respondents believed that "people dying of an incurable painful disease should be allowed to end their lives before the disease runs its course."[1] A number of comparable surveys indicate similar public sentiment.[2]

Since the [early twentieth] century, there has been a dramatic shift in the places where people die. Sixty years ago, the vast majority of deaths occurred at home. Now most people die in hospitals or long-term care facilities. Approximately 75% of all deaths in 1987 occurred in hospitals and long-term care institutions,[3] up from 50% in 1949, 61% in 1958, and 70% in 1977.[4] This transition from the privacy of the home to medical institutions has increased public awareness and concern about medical decisions near the end of life. "Since deaths which occur in institutions are more subject to scrutiny and official review, decisions for death made there are more likely to enter public consciousness."[5]

The development of sophisticated life support technologies now enables medicine to intervene and forestall death for most patients. Do-not-resuscitate orders are now commonplace.[6] [...] This growing capability to forestall death has contributed to the increased attention to medical decisions near the end of life.[7] [...] The report will focus on competent patients in nonemergency situations.

Definitions

The decisions near the end of life examined in this report are those decisions regarding actions or intentional omissions by physicians that will foreseeably result in the deaths of patients. In particular, these decisions concern the withholding or withdrawing of life-sustaining treatment, the provision of a palliative treatment that may have fatal side effects, euthanasia, and assisted suicide.

Life-sustaining treatment is any medical treatment that serves to prolong life without reversing the underlying medical condition. Life-sustaining treatment may include, but is not limited to, mechanical ventilation, renal dialysis, chemotherapy, antibiotics, and artificial nutrition and hydration. At one time, the term *passive euthanasia* was commonly used to describe withholding or withdrawing life-sustaining treatment. However, many experts now refrain from using the term passive euthanasia.

The provision of a palliative treatment that may have fatal side effects is also described as *double-effect euthanasia*. The intent of the treatment is to relieve pain and suffering, not to end the patient's life, but the patient's death is a foreseeable potential effect of the treatment. An example is gradually increasing the morphine dosage for a patient to relieve severe cancer pain, realizing that large enough doses of morphine may depress respiration and cause death.

Euthanasia is commonly defined as the act of bringing about the death of a hopelessly ill and suffering person in a relatively quick and painless way for reasons of mercy. In this report, the term euthanasia will signify the medical administration of a lethal agent to a patient for the purpose of relieving the patient's intolerable and incurable suffering.

Voluntary euthanasia is euthanasia that is provided to a competent person on his or her informed request. *Non-voluntary euthanasia* is the provision of euthanasia to an incompetent person according to a surrogate's decision. *Involuntary euthanasia* is euthanasia performed without a competent person's consent. This report will not examine involuntary euthanasia further, since it clearly would never be ethically acceptable.

Euthanasia and assisted suicide differ in the degree of physician participation. Euthanasia entails a physician performing the immediate life-ending action (e.g., administering a lethal injection). *Assisted suicide* occurs when a physician facilitates a patient's death by providing the necessary means and/or information to enable the patient to perform the life-ending act (e.g., the physician provides sleeping pills and information about the lethal dose, while aware that the patient may commit suicide).

Discussions about life-ending acts by physicians often refer to the patient's "competence" or "decision-making capacity." The two terms are often used interchangeably. However, *competence* can also refer to a legal standard regarding a person's soundness of mind. *Decision-making capacity* signifies the ability to make a particular decision and is not considered a legal standard. "Competence" for the Council's purposes will mean "decision-making capacity."

The evaluation of a person's decision-making capacity is an assessment of the person's capabilities for understanding, communicating, and reasoning. Patients should not be judged as lacking decision-making capacity based on the view that what they decide is unreasonable.[8] People are entitled to make decisions that others think are foolish as long as their choices are arrived at through a competently reasoned process and are consistent with their personal values.

Ethical Framework

Determining the ethical responsibilities of physicians when patients wish to die requires a close examination of the physician's role in society. Physicians are healers of disease and injury, preservers of life, and relievers of suffering. Ethical judgments become complicated, however, when these duties conflict. The four instances in which physicians might act to hasten death or refrain from prolonging life involve conflicts between the duty to relieve suffering and the duty to preserve life.

The considerations that must be weighed in each case are: (1) the principle of patient autonomy and the corresponding obligation of physicians to respect patients' choices; (2) whether what is offered by the physician is sound medical treatment; and (3) the potential consequences of a policy that permits physicians to act in a way that will foreseeably result in patients' deaths.

Patient autonomy

The principle of patient autonomy requires that competent patients have the opportunity to choose among medically indicated treatments and to refuse any unwanted treatment. Absent countervailing obligations, physicians must respect patients' decisions. Treatment decisions often involve personal value judgments and preferences in addition to objective medical considerations. We demonstrate respect for human dignity when we acknowledge "the freedom [of individuals] to make choices in accordance with their own values."[9]

Sound medical treatment

The physician's obligation to respect a patient's decision does not require a physician to provide a treatment that is not medically sound. Indeed, physicians are ethically prohibited from offering or providing unsound treatments. Sound medical treatment is defined as the use of medical knowledge or means to cure or prevent a medical disorder, preserve life, or relieve distressing symptoms.

This criterion of soundness arises from the medical ethical principles of beneficence and nonmaleficence. The principle of *nonmaleficence* prohibits physicians from using their medical knowledge or skills to do harm, on balance, to their patients, while the principle of *beneficence* requires that medical knowledge and skills be used to benefit patients.

Generally, a treatment that is likely to cause the death of a patient violates the principle of nonmaleficence, and a failure to save a patient's life is contrary to beneficence. However, for these decisions near the end of life the patient does not consider his or her death to be an absolutely undesirable outcome.

Practical considerations

Policies governing decisions near the end of life must also be evaluated in terms of their practical consequences. The ethical acceptability of a policy depends on the benefits and costs that result from the policy. In addition to the impact on individual cases (e.g., patients will die according to their decision to have life supports withdrawn), there are likely to be serious societal consequences of policies regarding physicians' responsibilities to dying patients.

Withholding and Withdrawing Life-sustaining Treatment

The principle of patient autonomy requires that physicians respect a competent patient's decision to forgo any medical treatment. This principle is not altered when the likely result of withholding or withdrawing a treatment is the patient's death. [...]

Decisions that so profoundly affect a patient's well-being cannot be made independent of a patient's subjective preferences and values.[10] Many types of life-sustaining treatments are burdensome and invasive, so that the choice for the patient is not simply a choice between life and death. When a patient is dying of cancer, for example, a decision may have to be made whether to use a regimen of chemotherapy that might prolong life for several additional months but also would likely be painful, nauseating, and debilitating. Similarly, when a patient is dying, there may be a choice between returning home to a natural death, or remaining in the hospital, attached to machinery, where the patient's life might be prolonged a few more days or weeks. In both cases, individuals might weigh differently the value of additional life vs the burden of additional treatment.

The withdrawing or withholding of life-sustaining treatment is not inherently contrary to the principles of beneficence and nonmaleficence. The physician is obligated only to offer sound medical treatment and to refrain from providing treatments that are detrimental, on balance, to the patient's well-being. When a physician withholds or withdraws a treatment on the request of a patient, he or she has fulfilled the obligation to offer sound treatment to the patient. The obligation to offer treatment does not include an obligation to impose treatment on an unwilling patient. In addition, the physician is not providing a harmful treatment. Withdrawing or withholding is not a treatment, but the forgoing of a treatment.

[...]

Withdrawing or withholding some life-sustaining treatments may seem less acceptable than others. The distinction between "ordinary" vs "extraordinary" treatments has been used to differentiate ethically obligatory vs ethically optional treatments.[11] In other words, ordinary treatments must be provided, while extraordinary treatment may be withheld or withdrawn. Varying criteria have been proposed to distinguish ordinary from extraordinary treatment. Such criteria include customariness, naturalness, complexity, expense, invasiveness, and balance of likely benefits vs burdens of the particular treatment.[12] The ethical significance of all these criteria essentially is subsumed by the last criterion – the balance of likely benefits vs the burdens of the treatment.[13]

When a patient is competent, this balancing must ultimately be made by the patient. As stated earlier, the evaluation of whether life-sustaining treatment should be initiated, maintained, or forgone depends on the values and preferences of the patient. Therefore, treatments are not objectively ordinary or extraordinary. For example, artificial nutrition and hydration have frequently been cited as an objectively ordinary treatment which, therefore, must never be forgone. However, artificial nutrition and hydration can be very burdensome to patients. Artificial nutrition and hydration immobilize the patient to a large degree, can be extremely uncomfortable (restraints are sometimes used to prevent patients from removing nasogastric tubes), and can entail serious risks (for example, surgical risks from insertion of a gastrostomy tube and the risk of aspiration pneumonia with a nasogastric tube).

Aside from the ordinary vs extraordinary argument, the right to refuse artificial nutrition and hydration has also been contested by some because the provision of food and water has a symbolic significance as an expression of care and compassion.[14] These commentators argue that withdrawing or withholding food and water is a form of abandonment and will cause the patient to die of starvation and/or thirst. However, it is far from evident that providing nutrients through a nasogastric tube to a patient for whom it is unwanted is comparable to the typical human ways of feeding those who are hungry.[15] In addition, discomforting symptoms can be palliated so that a death that occurs after forgoing artificial nutrition and/or hydration is not marked by substantial suffering.[16] Such care requires constant attention to the patient's needs. Therefore, when comfort care is maintained, respecting a patient's decision to forgo artificial nutrition and hydration will not constitute an abandonment of the patient, symbolic or otherwise.

There is also no ethical distinction between withdrawing and withholding life-sustaining treatment.[17] Withdrawing life support may be emotionally more difficult than withholding life support because the physician performs an action that hastens death. When life-sustaining treatment is withheld, on the other hand, death occurs because of an omission rather than an action. However, as most bioethicists now recognize, such a distinction lacks ethical significance.[18] First, the distinction is often meaningless. For example, if a physician fails to provide a tube feeding at the scheduled time, would it be a withholding or a withdrawing of treatment? Second, ethical relevance does not lie with the distinction between acts and omissions, but with other factors such as the motivation and professional obligations of the physician. For example, refusing to initiate ventilator support despite the patient's need and request because the physician has been promised a share of the patient's inheritance is clearly ethically more objectionable than stopping a ventilator for a patient who has competently decided to forgo it. Third, prohibiting the withdrawal of life support would inappropriately affect a patient's decision to initiate such treatment. If treatment cannot be stopped once it is initiated, patients and physicians may be more reluctant to begin treatment when there is a possibility that the patient may later want the treatment withdrawn.[19]

While the principle of autonomy requires that physicians respect competent patients' requests to forgo life-sustaining treatments, there are potential negative consequences of such a policy. First, deaths may occur as a result of uninformed decisions or from pain and suffering that could be relieved with measures that will not cause the patient's death. Further, subtle or overt pressures from family, physicians, or society to forgo life-sustaining treatment may render the patient's choice less than free. These pressures could revolve around beliefs that such patients' lives no longer possess social worth and are an unjustifiable drain of limited health resources.

The physician must ensure that the patient has the capacity to make medical decisions before carrying out the patient's decision to forgo (or receive) life-sustaining treatment. In particular, physicians must be aware that the patient's decision-making capacity can be diminished by a misunderstanding of the medical prognosis and options or by a treatable state of depression. It is also essential that all efforts be made to maximize the comfort and dignity of patients who are dependent on life-sustaining treatment and that patients be assured of these efforts. With such assurances, patients will be less likely to forgo life support because of suffering or anticipated suffering that could be palliated.

The potential pressures on patients to forgo life-sustaining treatments are an important concern. The Council believes that the medical profession must be vigilant against such tendencies, but that the greater policy risk is of undermining patient autonomy.

Providing Palliative Treatments that may have Fatal Side Effects

Health care professionals have an ethical duty to provide optimal palliative care to dying patients. At present, many physicians are not informed about the appropriate doses, frequency of doses, and alternative modalities of pain control for patients with severe chronic pain.[20] In particular, inappropriate concerns about addiction too often inhibit physicians from providing adequate analgesia to dying patients. Physicians should inform the patient and the family that concentrated efforts to relieve pain will be a priority in the care of the patient, since fear of pain is "one of the most pervasive causes of anxiety among patients, families and the public."[21]

The level of analgesia necessary to relieve the patient's pain, however, may also have the effect of shortening the patient's life. [...] A competent patient must be the one who decides whether the relief of pain and suffering is worth the danger of hastening death. The principle of respect for patient autonomy and self-determination requires that patients decide about such treatment.

The ethical distinction between providing palliative care that may have fatal side effects and providing euthanasia is subtle because in both cases the action that causes death is performed with the purpose of relieving suffering. The intent of the former is to relieve suffering despite the fatal side effects, while the intent of the latter is to cause death as a means by which relief of suffering is achieved. Most medical treatments entail some undesirable side effects. In general, the patient has a right to decide either to risk the side effects or to forgo the treatment. It does not follow from this reasoning that a patient also has a right to choose euthanasia as a medical treatment for their suffering.

An important concern is that patients who are not fully informed about their prognosis and options may make decisions that unnecessarily shorten their lives. In addition, severe pain might diminish the patient's capacity to decide whether to choose a treatment that risks death. Caution when determining decision-making capacity in this situation, therefore, must be exercised, and patients should be fully informed.

Euthanasia

Euthanasia is the medical administration of a lethal agent in order to relieve a patient's intolerable and untreatable suffering. Whether or not a physician may use the skills or knowledge of medicine to cause an "easy" death for a patient who requests such assistance has been debated as early as the time of Hippocrates. Recently, euthanasia has been gaining support from the public and some in the medical profession. In the Netherlands, while physician-performed euthanasia remains illegal, physicians have not been prosecuted since 1984 when they follow certain criteria.[22] These criteria include that (1) euthanasia is explicitly and repeatedly requested by the patient and there is no doubt that the patient wants to die; (2) the mental and physical suffering is severe with no prospect for relief; (3) the patient's decision is well-informed, free, and enduring; (4) all options for alternative care have been exhausted or refused by the patient; and (5) the physician consults another physician.[23] The frequency of euthanasia in the Netherlands has been estimated to range from 2000 to 20000 persons per year.[24] [...]

Though the principle of patient autonomy requires that competent patients be given the opportunity to choose among offered medical treatments and to forgo any treatment, it does not give patients the right to have a physician perform a treatment to which the physician has objections. Though patients have a right to refuse life-sustaining treatment, they do not have a right to receive euthanasia. There is an autonomy interest in directing one's death, but this interest is more limited in the case of euthanasia than in the case of refusing life support.

The question remains whether it is ethical for a physician to agree to perform euthanasia. To approach this question one must look to the principles of beneficence and nonmaleficence and to the larger policy implications of condoning physician-performed euthanasia.

Can euthanasia ever constitute sound medical treatment? Any treatment designed to cause death is generally considered detrimental to the patient's well-being, and therefore unsound. However, proponents of euthanasia argue that euthanasia is a sound treatment of last resort for the relief of intolerable pain and suffering. From the perspective of competent patients who request euthanasia in the face of such suffering, death may be preferable, on balance, to continued life.

On the other hand, most pain and suffering can be alleviated. The technology of pain management has advanced to the point where most pain is now controllable. The success of the hospice movement illustrates the extent to which aggressive pain control and close attention to patient comfort and dignity can ease the transition to death.[25]

There may be cases, however, where a patient's pain and suffering is not reduced to a tolerable level and the patient requests a physician to help him or her die.[26] If a patient's pain and suffering are unrelievable and intolerable, using medical expertise to aid an easy death on the request of the patient might seem to be the humane and beneficent treatment for the patient.

However, there are serious risks associated with a policy allowing physician-performed euthanasia. There is a long-standing prohibition against physicians killing their patients, based on a commitment that medicine is a profession dedicated to healing, and that its tools should not be used to cause patients' deaths. Weakening this prohibition against euthanasia, even in the most compelling situations, has troubling implications.[27] Though the magnitude of such risks is impossible to predict accurately, the medical profession and society as a whole must not consider these risks lightly. Two noted ethicists have expressed the role of this prohibition:

> The prohibition of killing is an attempt to promote a solid basis for trust in the role of caring for patients and protecting them from harm. This prohibition is both instrumentally and symbolically important, and its removal would weaken a set of practices and restraints that we cannot easily replace.[28]

If euthanasia by physicians were to be condoned, the fact that physicians could offer death as a medical treatment might undermine public trust in medicine's dedication to preserving the life and health of patients.[29] Some patients may fear the prospect of involuntary or nonvoluntary euthanasia if their lives are no longer deemed valuable as judged by physicians, their family, or society.[30] Other patients who trust their physicians' judgments may not feel free to resist the suggestion that euthanasia may be appropriate for them.[31]

Another risk is that physicians and other health care providers may be more reluctant to invest their energy and time serving patients whom they believe would benefit more from a quick and easy death. Caring for dying patients is taxing on physicians who must face issues of their own mortality in the process, and who often perceive such care as a reminder of their failure to cure these patients.[32] In addition, the increasing pressure to reduce health care costs may serve as another motivation to favor euthanasia over longer-term comfort care.

Allowing physicians to perform euthanasia for a limited group of patients who may truly benefit from it will present difficult line-drawing problems for medicine and society. In specific cases it may be hard to distinguish which cases fit the criteria established for euthanasia. For example, if the existence of unbearable pain and suffering was a criterion for euthanasia, the definition of unbearable pain and suffering could be subject to different interpretations.

Furthermore, determining whether a patient will benefit from euthanasia requires an intimate understanding of the patient's concerns, values, and pressures that may be prompting the euthanasia request. In the Netherlands, physicians who provide euthanasia generally have a lifelong relationship with the patient and the patient's family, which enables the physician to have access to this vital information.[33] In the United States, however, physicians rarely have the depth of knowledge about their patients that would be necessary for an appropriate evaluation of the patient's request for euthanasia.

More broadly, the line-drawing necessary for the establishment of criteria for euthanasia is also problematic. If competent patients can receive euthanasia, can family members request euthanasia for an incompetent patient? Would it be acceptable for physicians to perform euthanasia on any competent individuals who request it? Furthermore, since it will be physicians and the state who ultimately answer these questions, value judgments about patients' lives will be made by a person or entity other than the patients.

Since it is unclear at this time where these lines should be drawn, the proposition of allowing euthanasia is particularly troublesome. A potential exists for a gradual distortion of the role of medicine into something that starkly contrasts with the current vision of a profession dedicated to healing and comforting.

[...] Before euthanasia can ever be considered a legitimate medical treatment in this country, the needs behind the demand for physician-provided euthanasia must be examined more thoroughly and addressed more effectively. A thorough examination would require a more open discussion of euthanasia and the needs of patients who are making requests. The existence of patients who find their situations so unbearable that they request help from their physicians to die must be acknowledged, and the concerns of these patients must be a primary focus of medicine. Rather than condoning physician-provided euthanasia, medicine must first respond by striving to identify and address the concerns and needs of dying patients.

Physician-Assisted Suicide

[...]

There is an ethically relevant distinction between euthanasia and assisted suicide that makes assisted suicide an ethically more attractive option. Physician-assisted suicide affords a patient a more autonomous way of ending his or her life than does euthanasia. Since patients must perform the life-ending act themselves, they would have the added protection of being able to change their minds and stop their suicides up until the last moment.

However, the ethical objections to physician-assisted suicide are similar to those of euthanasia since both are essentially interventions intended to cause death. Physician-assisted suicide, like euthanasia, is contrary to the prohibition against using the tools of medicine to cause a patient's death. Physician-assisted suicide also has many of the same societal risks as euthanasia, including the potential for coercive financial and societal pressures on patients to choose suicide. Further, determining the criteria for assisting a patient's suicide and determining whether a particular patient meets the criteria are as problematic as deciding who may receive euthanasia.

While in highly sympathetic cases physician-assisted suicide may seem to constitute beneficent care, due to the potential for grave harm the medical profession cannot condone physician-assisted suicide at this time. The medical profession instead must strive to identify the concerns behind patients' requests for assisted suicide, and make concerted efforts at finding ways to address these concerns short of assisting suicide, including providing more aggressive comfort care.

Conclusions

- The principle of patient autonomy requires that physicians must respect the decision to forgo life-sustaining treatment of a patient who possesses decision-making capacity. Life-sustaining treatment is any medical treatment that serves to prolong life without reversing the underlying medical condition. Life-sustaining treatment may include, but is not limited to, mechanical ventilation, renal dialysis, chemotherapy, antibiotics, and artificial nutrition and hydration.

- There is no ethical distinction between withdrawing and withholding life-sustaining treatment.

- Physicians have an obligation to relieve pain and suffering and to promote the dignity and autonomy of dying patients in their care. This includes providing effective palliative treatment even though it may foreseeably hasten death. More research must be pursued examining the degree to which palliative care reduces the requests for euthanasia or assisted suicide.

- Physicians must not perform euthanasia or participate in assisted suicide. A more careful examination of the issue is necessary. Support, comfort, respect for patient autonomy, good communication, and adequate pain control may decrease dramatically the demand for euthanasia and assisted suicide. In certain carefully defined circumstances, it would be humane to recognize that death is certain and suffering is great. However, the societal risks of involving physicians in medical interventions to cause patients' deaths is too great in this culture to condone euthanasia or physician-assisted suicide at this time.

NOTES

1 Associated Press/Media General. *Poll No. 4* (Richmond, VA: Media General, February 1985).

2 Wanzer, S. H., Federman, D. D., Adelstein, S. J., et al., "The physician's responsibility toward hopelessly ill patients," *N. Engl. J. Med.* 320 (1989): 844–9.

3 National Center for Health Statistics. *Vital Statistics of the United States, 1987, II: Mortality, Part A* (Washington, DC: US Public Health Service, 1990).

4 *Deciding to Forego Life-Sustaining Treatment: A Report on the Ethical, Medical, and Legal Issues in Treatment Decisions* (Washington, DC: President's Commission for the Study of Ethical Problems in Medicine and Biomedical and Behavioral Research, 1987).

5 Capron, A. M., "Legal and ethical problems in decisions for death," *Law Med. Health Care* 14 (1986): 141–4.

6 Lipton, H. L., "Do-not-resuscitate decisions in a community hospital," *JAMA* 256 (1986): 1164–9.

7 Capron, "Legal and ethical problems in decisions for death."

8 Buchanan, A. E. and Brock, D. W., *Deciding for Others: The Ethics of Surrogate Decisionmaking* (New York: Cambridge University Press, 1989).

9 *Guidelines on the Termination of Life-Sustaining Treatment and the Care of the Dying: A Report by the Hastings Center* (Briarcliff Manor, NY: Hastings Center, 1987).

10 Brock, D. W., "Death and dying," in R. M. Veatch (ed.), *Medical Ethics* (Boston, MA: Jones and Bartlett Publishing Inc, 1989).

11 Beauchamp, T. L., Childress, J. F., *Principles of Biomedical Ethics*, 3rd edn (New York: Oxford University Press, 1989).

12 Ibid; Lynn, J. and Childress, J. F., "Must patients always be given food and water?" *Hastings Cent. Rep.* (October 1983): 17–21.

13 Beauchamp and Childress, *Principles of Biomedical Ethics*.

14 Ramsey, P., *The Patient as Person* (New Haven, CN: Yale University Press, 1970), pp. 113–29.

15 Lynn and Childress, "Must patients always be given food and water?"

16 Schmitz, P. and O'Brien, M., "Observations on nutrition and hydration in dying patients," in J. Lynn (ed.), *By No Extraordinary Means: The Choice to Forego Life-Sustaining Food and Water* (Bloomington, IN: Indiana University Press, 1986); Billings, J. A., "Comfort measures for the terminally ill: Is dehydration painful?" *J. Am. Geriatr. Soc.* 33 (1985): 808–10.

17 *Deciding to Forego Life-Sustaining Treatment; Guidelines on the Termination of Life-Sustaining Treatment and the Care of the Dying*; Beauchamp and Childress, *Principles of Biomedical Ethics*.

18 Ibid.

19 *Deciding to Forego Life-Sustaining Treatment.*

20 Rhymes, J., "Hospice care in America," *JAMA* 264 (1990): 369–72.

21 Wanzer et al., "The physician's responsibility toward hopelessly ill patients."

22　De Wachter, M. A. M., "Active euthanasia in the Netherlands," *JAMA* 262 (1989): 3316–19.

23　Rigter, H., "Euthanasia in the Netherlands: Distinguishing facts from fiction," *Hastings Cent. Rep.* 19 (suppl) (1989): 31–2.

24　De Wachter, "Active euthanasia in the Netherlands."

25　Rhymes, "Hospice care in America."

26　Wanzer et al., "The physician's responsibility toward hopelessly ill patients"; Rhymes, "Hospice care in America."

27　Sprung, C. L., "Changing attitudes and practices in forgoing life-sustaining treatment," *JAMA* 263 (1990): 2211–15; Lifton, R. J., *The Nazi Doctors: Medical Killing and the Psychology of Genocide* (New York: Basic Books Inc, 1986).

28　Beauchamp and Childress, *Principles of Biomedical Ethics.*

29　Kass, L. R., "Neither for love nor money: why doctors must not kill," *Public Interest* 94 (1989): 25–46.

30　Ibid.

31　Ibid; Orentlicher, D., "Physician participation in assisted suicide," *JAMA* 262 (1989): 1844–5; Kamisar, Y., "Some non-religious views against proposed 'mercy-killing' legislation," *Minn. Law Rev.* 42 (1958): 969–1042.

32　*Deciding to Forego Life-Sustaining Treatment; Guidelines on the Termination of Life-Sustaining Treatment and the Care of the Dying.*

33　Battin, M. P., "Remarks at University of Florida Colleges of Medicine and Nursing conference: Controversies in the care of the dying patient," Orlando, FL, February 14, 1991.

85

On the Suicide Threshold

KATE HILL

The Suicide Spectrum

Somewhere in the region of 44,000 young people under the age of 25 turn up each year in the casualty departments of general hospitals throughout the UK, having injured or poisoned themselves. [...]

News of a suicide poses ominous questions. A common reflex is the need to know whether a young person really *meant* to do it. This element of choice gives suicide its peculiar potency and draws us, moth-like, to the dead person's state of mind. [...]

Was this a *real* suicide attempt, onlookers may ask, or was it just a cry for help? Unfortunately the logical assumptions behind this question – firstly that young people who 'attempt suicide' *know* what they want, and secondly that what they want is *either* life *or* death – are often inappropriate to the confusion of young people who behave self-destructively. Those who overdose or injure themselves are often afraid and desperate, states which do not encourage clear thinking. [...] Those who *have*, at times, longed for death or contemplated suicide, may be uncertain that they really wanted to die as a result of a 'suicide attempt'. [...] The desire to die is a mercurial element. Varying between individuals, fluctuating over time and intensifying during a crisis, it frequently conflicts with a desire to go on living.

The tenuous link between self-destructiveness and death may make it difficult for some young people to fathom their own behaviour.

> I tried to commit suicide four times. I slashed my hands, wrists and arms. I just felt so much mental pain inside. [...] I think maybe I just really, really wanted to hurt myself. (MAXINE)

Maxine associated self-mutilation with suicidal behaviour, and since suicidal behaviour invokes death, felt that she had tried to 'commit suicide'. [...]

As Maxine's experience suggests, self-harm is often preceded, not by thoughts about dying, but by a build-up of intolerable tension.[1] As one survivor of sexual abuse observed: 'Self-harm is not about suicide, it is about surviving and getting through each moment.'[2] When powerful feelings of anger, frustration or despair threaten to overwhelm, this survival strategy provides a way of maintaining control. [...] In a similar way, young people may overdose as a desperate survival strategy, swallowing pills as some people down alcohol – to temporarily escape or blot out intolerable feelings of misery and anxiety.[3]

[...] Functioning also as an SOS flare, when other forms of communication fail, such behaviour signals the inability to cope.[4] [...]

Somewhere between one-fifth and one-third of young people who take overdoses – which accounts for the vast majority of young people's suicide attempts – say their goal was death.[5] In all other cases young people say that they overdosed meaning to survive or they did not care whether they lived or died.[6] [...] The gamble between death, and a life which is a little improved, a little changed, a little closer to happiness perhaps, may seem a risk worth taking if the present feels intolerable.

[...However,] the suicide attempts of some young people are motivated by a clear wish to be dead. Lorraine had wanted to die for some months before she finally took an overdose, aged 20. After a childhood marred by her father's alcoholism and violent behaviour, she had had to cope with her older sister's death in a traffic accident. [...]

It's a terrible thing when you wake up in the morning and you *don't want to be alive*. I genuinely wanted to die. [...]

The motives of young people who overdose or injure themselves are often wide-ranging. The *suicide spectrum* comprises the range of actions which carry connotations of suicide. At the near end of this spectrum is self-harm, often regarded as suicidal gesturing. At the far end is that unambiguously suicidal behaviour motivated by a desire for death. [...]

Young People's Ideas about Death and Dying

[...] I thought Hell must be like a grave; like lying awake all day in a grave. Heaven was a big green field with pink cherry blossoms, with lots of people singing. (SUSIE)

Gleaning an understanding of death and dying is one of life's more pensive necessities. All children and adolescents think and fantasise about death as part of their natural development. Young children regard it as a temporary state, like sleep, and have difficulty comprehending its causes and finality.[7] [...] Children invariably visualise death as similar to life.[8] The dead mimic the living – eating, drinking and playing with toys, perhaps – but they do so in a new location. The question, 'where do people go when they die?' reflects a need to clear up the logistics. The somewhere else of death may be associated with Heaven, Hell, the sky or underground places.[9] Cheryl recalled trying to make a telephone call, as a child, to her dead grandmother: 'She had died and the phone was disconnected, but I thought I could get through.'

Between the ages of about five and ten children begin to recognise the possibility of their own death, and the death of people around them, but they have yet to grasp its finality.[10] [...]

The permanence of death is not usually fully understood until early adolescence. Half of children aged 6–11 in one study believed death was reversible.[11] [...] The average adolescent comes to understand the finality and biological causes of death by the age of 13.[12]

Conceptions of death are naturally subject to cultural influences and religious dictates. In the absence of spiritual consensus or prescriptive teachings, today's children and adolescents must develop a personal understanding of death with relatively little guidance. The raw material from which they must derive this understanding is often perplexing. [...] The abundant screen deaths of modern entertainment appear as rewindable as the video machine: 'Television and the movies regularly depict reversible, clean deaths as characters are killed in one show and reappear on another.'[13] Despite these decoys, the scientific consensus of Western culture proposes that death brings physical and psychological cessation.

Yet for many adolescents more contentious death lore offers the prospect of immortality.[14] [...] One in three British adolescents (aged 12–18) believes in life after death and one in three believes in Heaven and Hell.[15] [...] Where Heaven is a big, green field with cherry blossoms there may be every reason to go there.

Death may appear desirable because of what it is *not*.

> Death was a state where there was no tension, where everything was fine. It was just the end of trauma, the end of being upset and of crying and having to live with these horrible people. It would stop this racing round in my head and it would have just been sleep and I'd be going to Heaven. (CHERYL)

[...]

As one might expect, suicidal children are more preoccupied with death than others. Thoughts and dreams linger on their own imagined death, the deaths of family members and how people die in general.[16] Not only is death a greater concern to such young people but it is perceived to be more benign: 'Many suicidal children believe that death is a temporary, pleasant state that will relieve all tensions.'[17] A study of 13–16-year-olds in the USA found that those with frequent thoughts of suicide were more likely than other children to believe in the reversibility of death and/or to believe that they would remain cognizant after they had died.[18] By contrast, non-suicidal children are more likely to understand that death is final.[19]

[...]

[Yet] under pressure, young people's perceptions of death may fluctuate, to the extent that their basic understanding becomes distorted. A child who has understood in happier times that death lasts for ever may lose sight of its irrevocability when distressed: 'Suicidal children may understand that death is final, but when stressed they begin to believe that death is temporary.'[20] The emotional meanings associated with death – punishment, reunion, separation – change with a young person's experience and emotional needs.[21] Lorraine became deeply suicidal two years after her sister's death. She suspected death was 'nothingness', but the possibility that it might reunite her with her dead sister fed her suicidal resolve: 'I think death is just like nothing. But I was thinking I might catch up with my sister somewhere. [...]' Infused with new emotional meanings, death becomes more attractive.

[...] The real thing may be more frightening, and fear can protect.[22] Half an hour after taking an overdose Debbie was overwhelmed by panic: 'I was almost hysterical with the actual physical fear – what is going to happen between now and death?' Her instinct was entirely appropriate. 'Humans,' noted one writer, 'are hard to kill.' [...] Permanent brain damage, a broken back, respiratory failure, coma and organ damage are some of the more appalling outcomes of non-fatal suicide attempts. [...] Susie betrayed little sense of the physical havoc that must be wrought on a young and healthy body to rid it of life: 'I'd heard of people dying of alcohol poisoning. I thought drinking would be a nice way because it makes your head all floaty.' A relative ignorance of biology may aid the young in their evasiveness.

Running Out of Answers: The Suicide Solution

A young person's attraction to death is nurtured by how he or she feels about life. Debbie was a deeply depressed 12-year-old when she took a large overdose. Like many young people who attempt suicide, she had been struggling to cope with her feelings and problems for some time prior to her overdose. Yet none of the strategies by which Debbie tried to improve her lot proved to have a lasting effect. Her suicide attempt represented an end-point in an unsuccessful search for other, less desperate solutions:

> The bullying started off as being spat at and then it got to being beaten up occasionally. I didn't want to go to school ever. I remember my parents just saying, 'It's not that bad – you'll have to go.' And my brothers used to beat me up. They got bullied at school, so they bullied me in turn. [...]
>
> I was pretty big. One day I was sitting there eating this big bag of crisps. I was shovelling them into my mouth. And suddenly I realised I eat like that. I don't know why – for comfort probably. At the age of 11, I put on three stone, very suddenly. [...]

I thought one of the things I had to do before I killed myself was to try and get help. I really tried, but I couldn't find it. I remember endlessly going to see [a teacher]. I cried a lot. I would tell her how awful I felt and she would tell me there were all these things to live for. I got the feeling she didn't believe me.

But they sent me to a psychiatrist before I tried to kill myself. I told him everything. [...] I had two sessions with him and then he said: 'Everything's fine. She's a normal, healthy little girl.'

They don't take you seriously. [...] The only reason they wanted me to live was because they were so scared of death. [...]

I was trying to see if there was any reason at all that I should live and I couldn't find one. [...] I remember writing lists with the pros and cons of each [way of dying] – slit your wrists, jump off a bridge...

By the time of her overdose Debbie had exhausted her ability to cope and felt powerless to defend herself against the anxieties and hurts of living. She attempted suicide when she had 'tried everything' and run out of alternatives. [...]

The sense of powerlessness described by Debbie is common among young people who are suicidal. Struggling to cope with problems and feelings that will not go away, often in isolation, a young person will feel increasingly helpless. Those who attempt suicide, in general, appear to experience the events and feelings in their life as less under their control than others.[23] [...]

Usually adolescents develop coping skills – or ways of handling stress – between the ages of about 11 and 15 and these often stay with them long into adult life.[24] [...] [They] may come to *include* self-harm, suicidal fantasies, talking of suicide and, finally, acting. Suicidal behaviour may represent a desperate 'solution' to all problems, but a solution nevertheless. [...] As young people grow more despairing, and as their self-esteem slips with their sense of control, suicidal 'solutions' become more comforting and attractive.[25]

Suicidal Thinking: Fantasies and Motives

I see myself lying in the casket. I am in my blue dress and my hands are folded over my chest. I can see my parents and friends around me. They are crying.[26]

The punitive childish fantasy – 'You'll be sorry when I'm dead' – reflects a child's growing awareness that death has an impact on others. It exerts extraordinary influence and commands full attention.[27] [...]

Barry felt his regular fantasising about suicide, during early adolescence, provided both an exemption clause for failure and retribution against those who had left him feeling neglected and isolated:

I just saw it as a way out; a cop–out from everything. If I couldn't do my schoolwork I'd think, 'Well it doesn't matter, because I'm going to commit suicide next week.' And I felt angry as well, because no one could see. [...] It seemed like they didn't want to see it. [...]

[...] Around 60 per cent of adolescents are reported to have given suicide serious consideration at least once, suggesting that thoughts of suicide are common enough at times of stress.[28] In a survey of American schoolchildren 8.9 per cent reported suicidal ideation, compared to 2 per cent who had either threatened suicide or made attempts.[29]

[...] Yet suicidal fantasies may grow less potent with use and, if a young person's circumstances do not improve, the temptation to enact fantasy will grow.

Suicidal Talk, Suicidal Plans and Impulsive Suicidal Acts

Once he said he was going to kill himself. And one time he said he was going to blow his head off. He didn't really mean it at the time. But in the back of my mind I thought – why is he saying that? [...]

This time I could tell in his eyes. He had a frightened look. A very frightening look. It was frightening me and he was also very frightened. That was why I knew he was going to do it because of his fear of what he was going to do. He was petrified I think. He was petrified that he was going to do it. He kept on repeating himself, saying: 'I'm going to commit suicide, I'm going to commit suicide.' (JANICE, MARK'S SISTER)

[...] As the suicidal process intensifies, those with explicit plans may threaten suicide. Six months before he shot himself Mark talked about doing so to his sister. At this point, the suicide threat lacked urgency and seemed improbable. [...] In the months following her brother's death Janice felt, with the torturous benefit of hindsight, that Mark's earlier talk of suicide had been a plea for help.

Clues, warnings, threats are commonly given by those who are suicidal to people close to them. Talk of suicide may be indirectly expressed, since shame, guilt and fear of rejection forge strong prohibitions on such communications. [...] Warnings may be similarly obscure, only recognised as such after a death. On the day of his death 20-year-old Steven turned down an invitation from his sister to come to dinner saying, 'I shan't be coming Viv. I shan't be here.' [...] Yet many young people make quite explicit references to their self-destructive feelings and intentions. Feelings – 'I want to die' – and plans – 'I am going to kill myself' – can be expressed very directly.

[...] And for some, silence may reflect determination to go through with it. The wish to die may be so strong that they simply will not risk the intervention of others. The majority of young people who take their lives however *do* express their suicidal feelings and intentions beforehand.

He was talking about suicide, kind of jokingly. Me and a friend were in his car and he was saying: 'The best way to kill yourself is gassing.' I said: 'No it ain't. The best way to kill yourself is pills.' I thought he was just talking. It's unbelievable – only 19 – a good friend of mine. Then he actually said he

was going to kill himself. He said he was going to jump off a tall building. (CLIF-FORD, EARL'S FRIEND)

[...] A suicide attempt can be a carefully planned action, or one that occurs with a suddenness that takes even the attempter by surprise.

[...]

Something came to a head very quickly that day. It was a very spontaneous thing she did. I think she did it in a fit of anger. (PATRI-CIA, ELAINE'S MOTHER)

A suicidal urge may culminate in death with terrible rapidity. [...] Particularly among the youngest victims, suicides may appear to have been rapidly conceived, often carried out in anger shortly after a 'last straw' event.[30] These events themselves are rarely very different from those experienced by adolescents in general.[31]

[...] In one study of young people who had taken an overdose, fewer than half of those recovering in hospital said they considered the overdose for more than 15 minutes beforehand.[32] Only 8 per cent thought about it for over 24 hours.[33] In another study, few children's overdoses (5–7 per cent) showed evidence of premeditation, and these tended to be amongst the most depressed and suicidal.[34]

[... Yet] young people who try suicide are likely to have gone over the idea in the past, a thought process that has been called a 'cognitive rehearsal' for suicidal behaviour.[35] They may have fantasised about suicide, imagined its effects on others, wondered which method they would choose and the circumstances in which they might use it. A suicide threat or warning suggests that such a 'rehearsal' is going on. [...]

Suicidal Danger Signs

That last Saturday he said to me, 'I want to be free. I want to be free.' He had tears in his eyes. When he said he wanted to be free I thought he meant free of college, of work. I put my arms round him and gave him a hug. And he suddenly said to me: 'I'm just having a last go on my computer. I don't want it any more. And d'you think you can get rid of my leather jacket?' I said, 'Why me? You can sell it. It'll give you a bit of money.' He said to me, 'I've written it all down.' And he did leave a letter. But when he said these things I never thought he was going to take his own life. (ANGELA, TERRY'S MUM)

Suicidal young people do *not* fit an identikit list of warning signs, since their depression and despair have many guises. One adolescent's vulnerability may be masked by angry and defiant behaviour, another's may resonate with the subdued hopelessness more commonly associated with despair. The contrast between impulsive and premeditated youth suicides suggests the difficulties of generalising about suicidal crises. Nevertheless a number of warning signs may help identify young people who are moving towards a life-threatening crisis. Talk of suicide is a common one. More rarely a young person may give away possessions. [...] This putting in order of personal affairs suggests a very imminent danger. So too may a sudden lift in mood, following a long depression. [...] Sadly, after prolonged emotional pain and struggle, deciding to kill oneself may bring a sense of relief. [...]

[...] Signs of depression double as danger signals for suicide. Social withdrawal, changing sleep patterns, lethargy, loss of interest and concentration problems, changes in appetite or weight, neglected appearance are common signs of depression. [...] Certain signs of depression and suicidal depression may unfortunately be regarded by others as symptomatic of adolescent rebellion or bad conduct rather than deep unhappiness. Excessive drinking or drug-taking may reflect an adolescent's need to escape overwhelming feelings and relieve depression, yet this may not be recognised. When a young person gets conspicuously drunk, plays truant from school, fights and bullies, steals, gambles or generally 'acts up', his or her vulnerability may be masked whilst others become increasingly disapproving and alienated. The vulnerable 'troublemaker' may receive short shrift.

[...] Research suggests that mental health professionals may often overlook the despair of suicidal adolescents whose behaviour is aggressive and defiant, whilst recognising internalised, resigned depression.[36] [...]

Finally, suicide may occur just as a young person appears to have been 'getting better' following a severe mental health crisis. [...] Restored insight may bring with it fear and a cruel sense of hopelessness about the future. The months after discharge from psychiatric hospital are known to be a high-risk time for suicide.[37] A young person emerging from a mental health crisis will remain extremely vulnerable for some time to come. [...]

Suicide Attempts: Meaning to Die and Knowing How

[...] I remember being in my room crying and trying to suffocate myself with my pillow. I was eight or nine. [...] (BARRY)

I have often thought of a variety of ways of killing myself such as the guillotine. I would go to France and have it done. (A 12-year-old, quoted by Cynthia Pfeffer in *The Suicidal Child*)

Meaning to die and knowing how are distinct, and the need to draw this distinction is nowhere more vital than in responding to suicidal behaviour among the young. [...] There may be a wide gulf in young minds between deadly intentions and lethal know-how. [...] If the wish to die remains intact, a lethal suicide attempt becomes more probable as know-how increases. [...]

Some young suicide attempters mean to die but survive. Others mean to survive but end up dead. [...] In her study of young people who took an overdose Sally O'Brien observed: 'Whether people actually died or survived did not depend on how determined they were to die.'[38] [...] Children and adolescents are unlikely to choose drugs with any knowledge of their pharmacological properties. Most younger children who overdose use tablets found at home. The chosen drug is the one within arm's reach, as in Barry's case: 'There were always pills in the house, left over from when my mother died. No one had ever got round to throwing them out.'[...] In hospital receiving treatment for liver damage, the survivors of para-cetamol overdoses, many of them adolescents, were asked by researchers what they knew about the drug. Few had known that it was dangerous to the liver and most said they would not have taken the drug if they had realised what its conse-quences would be.[39][...] *Any* act of self-harm or attempted suicide in the young must be regarded as extremely serious.

NOTES

1 Simpson, M. A., "The phenomenology of self-multilation in a general hospital setting," *Can-adian Psychiatric Association Journal* 20 (1975): 429–34.

2 Harrison, D., *Self Harm: The Visible Hurt* (South West MIND Newsletter, No 18, 1993).

3 Hawton, K., Cole, D., O'Grady, J., et al., "Mo-tivational aspects of deliberate self-poisoning in adolescents," *British Journal of Psychiatry* 141 (1982): 286–91.

4 Eldrid, J., *Caring for the Suicidal* (London: Con-stable, 1988).

5 Hawton, Cole, O'Grady, et al., "Motivational aspects of deliberate self-poisoning in adoles-cents."

6 White, H., "Self-poisoning in adolescents," *British Journal of Psychiatry* 124 (1974): 24–35; Hawton, Cole, O'Grady, et al., "Motivational aspects of deliberate self-poisoning in adoles-cents."

7 Nagy, M., "The child's view of death," *Journal of Genetic Psychology* 73 (1948): 3–27.

8 Stillion, J. and Wass, H., "Children and death," in H. Wass (ed.), *Dying: Facing the Facts* (Wash-ington DC: Hemisphere Publishing Corpor-ation, 1979).

9 Orbach, I., *Children Who Don't Want to Live* (San Francisco: Jossey-Bass, 1988).

10 Piaget, J., *The Child's Concept of the World* (Pat-terson, NJ: Littlefield Adams, 1960).

11 McIntyre, M. S., Angle., C. R., and Struppler, L. J., "The concept of death in mid-western children and youths," *American Journal of Dis-eases of Children* 123 (1972): 527–32.

12 Anthony, S., *The Discovery of Death in Childhood and After* (London: Penguin, 1971); Pfeffer,

C. R., *The Suicidal Child* (New York: Guildford Press, 1986).

13 Curran, D. K., *Adolescent Suicidal Behavior* (New York: Hemisphere Publishing Corpor-ation, 1987).

14 Pfeffer, *The Suicidal Child*.

15 McIntyre, Angle, and Struppler, "The concept of death in mid-western children and youths"; Furnham, A. and Gunter, B., *The Anatomy of Adolescence: Young People's Social Attitudes in Britain* (London: Routledge, 1989).

16 Pfeffer, *The Suicidal Child*.

17 Ibid.

18 McIntyre, Angle, and Struppler, "The concept of death in mid-western children and youths."

19 Orbach, I. and Glaubman, H., "Suicidal, aggres-sive and normal children's perceptions of per-sonal and impersonal death," *Journal of Clinical Psychology* 34 (1978): 850–7; Orbach, I., "As-sessment of suicidal behaviour in young chil-dren: Case demonstrations," in R. F. W. Diekstra and K. Hawton (eds.), *Suicide in Ado-lescence* (Dordrecht: Martinus Nijhoff, 1987).

20 Pfeffer, *The Suicidal Child*.

21 Ibid.

22 Orbach, "Assessment of suicidal behaviour in young children."

23 Paykel, E. S., Prusoff, B. A., and Myers, J. K., "Suicide attempts and recent life events: A con-trolled comparison," *Archives of General Psych-iatry* 32 (1975): 327–33.

24 Hanser, S. T. and Bowlds, N. K., "Stress, coping and adaptation," in S. S. Feldman and G. R. Elliott (eds.), *At the Threshold: The De-veloping Adolescent* (Cambridge, MA: Harvard University Press, 1990).

25 Quinnet, P., *Suicide: The Forever Decision* (New York: Continuum Publishing Company, 1992).

26 Ibid.

27 Hawton, K., *Suicide and Attempted Suicide in Children and Adolescents* (Newbury Park, Califor-nia: Sage, 1986); Orbach, *Children Who Don't Want to Live*.

28 Ross, C., "School and suicide: Education for life and death," in R. F. W. Diekstra and K. Hawton (eds.), *Suicide in Adolescence* (Dordrecht: Marti-nus Nijhoff, 1986).

29 Pfeffer, *The Suicidal Child*.

30 Hoberman, H. and Garfunkel, B. D., "Com-pleted suicide in youth," in C. R. Pfeffer (ed.), *Suicide Among Youth* (Washington DC: Ameri-can Psychiatric Press, 1989).

31 Ibid.

32 Hawton, Cole, O'Grady, et al., "Motivational aspects of deliberate self-poisoning in adolescents."

33 Ibid.

34 Kerfoot, M., Personal communication (1993).

35 Hawton, *Suicide and Attempted Suicide in Children and Adolescents.*

36 Harrington, R. C., *Depressive Disorders in Childhood and Adolescence* (Chichester: John Wiley, 1993).

37 Goldacre, M., Seagroatt, V., and Hawton, K., "Suicides after discharge from psychiatric inpatient care," *Lancet* 342 (1993): 283–6.

38 O'Brien, S., *The Negative Scream: A Story of Young People Who Took an Overdose* (London: Routledge and Kegan Paul, 1985).

39 Gazzard, B. G., Davis, M., Spooner, J., et al., "Why do people use paracetamol for suicide?" *British Medical Journal* 1 (1976): 212–13.

86

My Husband the Stranger: Part 2

ELIZABETH FORSYTHE

In September 1985 I spent a few days with one of my wisest friends, whose mother had had dementia. It was three days before I could bring myself to speak about John because I felt so distressed and guilty about the whole problem. She helped enormously by telling me, among other things, about power of attorney and the Court of Protection.

I had still not managed to speak to John's doctor. Apart from my own judgement that his mind was disturbed, I had no medical or any other professional support.

Eventually I managed to make an appointment to see John's GP. I discovered that at each medical check-up there had been comments about John's deteriorating mental state, but his doctor said that as there was nothing he could do to help he had not contacted him. He was not enthusiastic about getting a psychogeriatrician to him. Nothing was settled.

John began wandering at night. The police brought him back to his cousin, who telephoned me. I suggested that it might be better if, instead of having him back in his flat, he might be persuaded to go into a nursing home. She refused to say to anybody apart from myself that she could not cope.

Finally I consulted a very compassionate solicitor, the first professional person I had met who actually knew what he was doing and could bring all the relevant problems together and begin to resolve them. John's doctor had to sign a form to say that John was not capable of managing his own affairs. This he would not do and the delay ran into months. I telephoned and wrote to him but he continued to procrastinate.

The legal profession cannot act until the medical profession commits itself to a diagnosis and signs forms to that effect. Eventually I did persuade John's general practitioner to arrange a home visit from a psychogeriatrician. It was confirmed that John had some sort of dementia. The question of whether he should be temporarily admitted to a mental hospital was discussed with the consultant, but no decision was taken.

It became clear that John could no longer live on his own. After a visit from a social worker, it was arranged that he should be taken to a mental hospital. The GP had finally been persuaded to sign the papers for the Court of Protection. While John was in hospital I managed to get down to his flat and, with the help of a social worker, go through some of his things and begin to get his financial affairs into some semblance of order. We realized that he could afford to go into a comfortable nursing home. I decided that as John's cousin wanted him to be near her, we should look for a nursing home in that area. We found one which appeared to be good and comfortable. He could have a large, ground-floor room with his own furniture, bathroom and a door into a walled garden.

Three weeks after John had been admitted, the agreed fee which I was paying rose sharply without any prior information. I felt an unease which later showed itself to be justified. I contacted the nursing home and discovered it had changed hands. A medical friend told me about a recently opened mental nursing home in Norfolk which had an excellent reputation. I went and saw it and was most impressed with the staff and the general atmosphere.

Suddenly I knew what had to be done in John's best interests and I had a great sense of urgency. It is a pity that I had not had the confidence to make John's interests of paramount importance long before this. I arranged for a medical agency to move him from one nursing home to the other – a considerable distance. The director thought that an ambulance might frighten John and sent his own car with two nurses, one of whom was a trained mental nurse; the other acted as driver. I went down with them. When I went into the nursing home I did not recognize John. He was totally rigid, could barely shuffle, was unable to swallow, so that his saliva was running down his face, and he was a strange sallow colour. He looked like a living corpse. [. . .]

The journey took about four hours but it seemed never-ending. He was so rigid that we had to bend him quite hard to get him into the car. I sat beside him on the back seat and kept looking at him to see if he was still breathing. It was very difficult to see if he was or not. His face was expressionless and the only signs of life was the slightest flicker of his eyelids from time to time.

In previous years we had spent a lot of time in Norfolk on holiday. As we started driving through Thetford Forest, I was aware of some sort of increased life in John. He did not move his head but his eyes seemed to be looking through the windows and I told him where we

were and reminded him of all the previous times when we had driven along that road. We arrived at the nursing home and he was welcomed and made comfortable. The matron was horrified by the state he was in and thought that he had probably had too many drugs. This was later confirmed by their doctor. He had drug-induced Parkinsonism.

John lived for another six months. I think that for much of that time he was reasonably happy and at times I caught glimpses of a smile of recognition. Three years later I wish that I had abandoned every other activity and just spent as much time as possible with him during those months, I think that it is important to spend time with somebody who is dementing – for your own sake, if not for theirs. It is easy to say that John did not know who I was. I understand now that every small thing I did for him during those last months helped me sort out my own confused feelings about him. In the simple acts of feeding him or helping him dress or just sitting and holding his hand, I could rekindle some of the love and tenderness I had once felt for him.

One problem was that he became very spiteful as he became more active. Sometimes he would do nothing but hit, punch and pinch. Obviously I found this very distressing. He did talk a little, but it was almost impossible to understand anything of what he was saying, although at times a few words were clear.

His physical deterioration accelerated, and in October 1986 he died. Although he had not known who I was for more than a year, during his dying I know that he knew who I was, and could understand something that I wanted to say to him before we parted. His dying brought us back together again after many years of difficulty and much distress.

Three years later, I am better able to understand the damage that was done to John, to me, to our family and friends through ignorance about dementia – my own ignorance, and also that of John's GP. That ignorance perpetuated my own confusion, guilt and inability to believe that I was capable of doing anything positive. John's disintegration was a threat to my own integrity: accepting that this was so has brought the opportunity to understand a great deal about myself, and in so doing to improve my relationships with those around me. Watching the disintegration of somebody close and experiencing it within yourself is painful, but in the end all the anguish need not be a waste.

87

A Death of One's Own

MARTIN HOLLIS

The wish to have a death of one's own is growing ever rarer. Only a while yet and it will be just as rare to have a death of one's own as it is already to have a life of one's own. (Rainer Maria Rilke)

Rilke's remark conjures up an officious array of well-meaning persons bent on completing our orderly passage from cradle to grave. They tidy our files cosily about us, inject us with extreme unction and slide us into the warm embrace of the undertaker. At the forefront of the array stands the doctor, part mechanic and part priest. His main task is to repair the living with resources whose effective and impartial allocation is a chief topic of medical ethics. But his role is not that of an impartial allocator: his patients want his partisan support. This builds a moral tension into a role played out where system meets patient, and one made instructively plain in the care of the dying. The system no doubt prefers death to be cheap and orderly but this thought may not move someone like Rilke wanting a death of his own. The doctor is then caught between his general duty to patients at large and his particular duty to the patient in front of him, a tension tautened for a Hippocratic promoter of health and life by a patient in search of an exit.

To put flesh on the theme, let us start with an awkward case for the doctor. George is an old man, a widower, in hospital after a stroke. Although fairly well recovered, he is still fragile and has poor balance. But he is clear-headed, especially about his wish to go home. He says firmly that he could manage on his own; and so he probably could, if he had enough support. Otherwise there is a real danger of his falling, fracturing a leg and being unable to summon help. There is a risk of hypothermia. He may easily become dirty, unkempt, emaciated and dehydrated, since it is not plain that he can dress, toilet and feed himself for long. He may not manage to comply with his medication. He might perhaps even become a risk to others by leaving his fire unattended or causing a gas explosion. None of this would be worrying, if there was a supporting cast. But his house is not suited to his condition. His only relative is his daughter, living elsewhere, with her own job and family and not willing to take George on. His neighbours are unfriendly. Social Services can offer something – perhaps a home help, meals on wheels, a laundry service, day care, an alarm service. But this does not truly cover nights and weekends and, anyway, George is liable not to eat the meals and not to accept the day care. Meanwhile the advice from social services is that he should stay in hospital. It is good advice for the further reason that there will be no second chance. Often one can allow a patient a try at looking after himself, knowing that he can be scooped up and returned to hospital, if necessary. But George is too fragile and too alone for this to be a promising option. Yet he is in no doubt that he wants to go home and denies that he needs any of the missing support.

[...] How much self-determination should George be allowed, given that his insight is poor? How much responsibility does the doctor shoulder, if he colludes with George's wishes? Both questions sound easy, if one begins by disputing their assumption that they can be posed primarily from the doctor's point of view. Or so I supposed, until I tried the familiar philosophical tactic of challenging the assumptions and found that the still waters run awkwardly deep. In what follows, I shall open with George's point of view and try to extract a line which gives the doctor clear guidance. Having duly failed, I shall then address the tension between system and patient as claimants on the doctor's integrity, before finally reverting to George's own wishes for his life or death.

The first question was how much self-determination George should be allowed, given that his insight is poor. As a preliminary, the story, as told, does not guarantee that George's insight is poor at all. It could be that he has a pretty shrewd idea that he will not last long on his own but simply wants to go home to die. Being also shrewd enough to know that he cannot expect the doctor's co-operation on those terms, he takes on the conventional patient's role in a well-tried dramatic dialogue between confident patient and concerned doctor. It is both polite and politic to offer the doctor clean hands by persuading him that the patient has the determination to cope. It is both polite and politic for the doctor to collude in what is, after all, not exactly the doctor's business, once he has been offered enough to satisfy any later enquiry into negligence. Under the surface of the conventional dialogue another has been conducted. George's questions about his true condition, asked and unasked, have been answered and advice given. George has rejected the advice, absolving the doctor of private and public responsibility. Honour has been satisfied on both sides.

I raise this possibility as a way of ushering in what one might call a decent liberalism. Traditionally the doctor's role is attended with more paternalism than a liberal doctor may relish. The liberal reminds us that today's doctor is no longer God and should not play God. He is the patient's servant, not his master. If George really did want to live out a full, self-sufficient life and was suffering from illusions, brought on perhaps by resentment at the humiliations of hospital routine, then the doctor might have a duty to be obstructive. But a good servant accepts his master's wishes and, in so far as George is weary of the world, the doctor is not his judge. Doubts about George's autonomy, a liberal would say, should be resolved in George's favour and a discreet way found of avoiding scandal. George's insight is not *outrageously* poor and there is a chance that it is not poor at all.

[...] What makes this traditionally liberal is less its general view that, as J. S. Mill put it, there is a circle round each individual human being, which it is not the job of government or anyone else to invade, and more its particular presumption (also to be found in Mill) that a person is a mind, who owns a physical machine whose disposal is up to the owner. The liberal line becomes trickier, if, as has become fashionable of late, one reverts to the ancient view that patients are not bodies but *persons*, and adds that a person is not a mind lodged in a body like a pilot in a vessel or motorist in a car. This subverts the idea that the doctor is just a mechanic and hence subverts one neat way of denying that the doctor is God. The other liberal route to granting the patient's autonomy thus starts from an idea of respect for *persons*. For all its greater current plausibility, it is stonier, however, and I am not sure that it gets there. Here are some of the complications.

George's chances of coping on his own seemed at first to depend merely on the support available for his rickety physical machine. But, if George is thought of as a *person*, we shall have to notice that psychological and social factors matter too. To discuss the social factors would take me too far afield. So let me just say that George's chances of recovering manageably from a stroke may vary with his class, gender, income and previous occupation, and that strokes may belong in a mysterious category, along with, for example, cot deaths and schizophrenia, where it looks as if social factors may even be causal. Meanwhile there is the obvious social point that he would get on better if he had friendly neighbours. In brief, the likely health of *persons* cannot be assessed in social isolation.

More directly relevant are the psychological factors. George's chances depend on his state of mind – his desires, beliefs and strength of will – which the doctor who treats George as a person must take into account. An instant complication is that the doctor's diagnosis or prognosis can affect George's chances. For an extreme case reflect on the common tale that in cultures which believe in witchcraft the knowledge that he has been cursed is enough to make a man curl up and die. In George's case there is an obvious risk that, in establishing his chances of survival, the doctor will upset his precarious balance and thus improve his insight at the expense of his health. [...] George may need his self-confidence and a doctor, who believes in improving people's insight, may be something of a health risk.

The point becomes less quirky in relation to desires, as opposed to beliefs. Having it borne in on him just how lonely, friendless and helpless he is can seriously damage George's will to live. The doctor cannot assess the situation by, so to speak, hidden camera and one-way mirror alone. He must interact with George, must probe his determination or apathy and, in short, must prod the roots of the plant to see how well they withstand prodding. This is also a comment on the earlier thought that George may be wholly clear about consequences but too diplomatic to say so: the doctor cannot act on the mere possibility that it is so. If George started with an unresolved mixture of hope for an independent life and weariness of a lonely one, he may well finish with a newly defined wish to go home to die. To put it too starkly, no doubt, respect for persons threatens sometimes to mean killing them off.

It is rapidly becoming unclear whether we are concerned with George's wants or George's interests. Which of the two is indicated by the maxim that patients should be treated as persons? The easier answer is the economist's: let there be consumer sovereignty for George's *wants*. If he still wants to go home after becoming clear about the risks, then the doctor has no business to obstruct him further. A merit of the answer is that it avoids having to tangle with the awkward concept of interests. Who can say that it is in George's interest to drift on into an institutionalized decline rather than to shorten his loneliness by returning home? The doctor is to probe the difference between considered and unconsidered wants. Having established what George truly wants, he need not worry about whether the preferred outcome is in George's interests. [...]

The suggestion, generalized, is that the doctor's role should be patient-centred, with patients sovereign and doctors their servants. A death of one's own is the ultimate in consumer choice. When generalized thus, however, this version of liberalism runs into difficulty. [...]

The classic liberal spokesman on the sovereignty of the individual words the case in terms of interests. The argument of Mill's *On Liberty* is that it is in our *interests* to be left to pursue our own good in our own way (so long as we do not interfere with the liberty of others). In *The Principles of Political Economy* he maintains that individuals are the best judges of their own *interests*. This at once raises a question about whether individuals' *wants* are sovereign, when they conflict with their interests. Mill gives a clear answer – No. In *On Liberty* he insists that the only liberty worth the name is that of pursuing our own good in our own way and argues that neither legal nor physical force may be used to compel or obstruct this pursuit. But he has no scruples about applying social pressure to ensure that we use the liberty to achieve the individuality and autonomy, which he holds to be in our interests, whatever our foolish wishes to the contrary. In the *Principles* (Book V, Chapter 11) he considers seven exceptions to the general maxim that individuals are the best judges of their own interests and bids government take action in each of them to make sure that what is done is truly in individuals' interests. Among them are cases where the individuals concerned are not mature and sane adults in full possession of their faculties, and where an individual attempts 'to decide irrevocably now what will be in his interest at some future time'. [. . .]

Death is, in general, an awkward case for a liberal debate about what is in someone's interests. If death is the end of a person, then it closes his profit and loss account, making it hard to maintain that he will be better off, if he no longer exists. Even the thought that his life would be in the red, were he around to live it, becomes awkward with senile dementia. On the other hand, if death is not the end, then who knows how to adjust the profit and loss account for another world? Yet a fully patient-centred approach would need a view on these enigmas. [. . .]

At any rate, my point is that a patient-centred approach cannot avoid tangling with questions of *interests* as soon as patients start wanting what is bad for their health. This is not to say that good health is always an overriding interest – doctors are sometimes asked to support people doing dangerous or exhausting tasks which shorten their lives. But no doctor is required to help masochists suffer more pain in the name of consumer sovereignty. The most libertarian version of a liberal-inspired patient-centredness on offer is one which gives the patient the benefit of the doubt when it is not clear that his wants are in his interests.

Patient-centredness is thus not the enemy of paternalism that one might suppose. It invites us to decide in the patient's interests but leaves the doctor often the better judge of them. All the same, I imagine that sympathies still lie with George, old, lonely, uncared for and wanting release. The first question was how much self-determination he should be allowed, given that his insight is poor. Treating George as a person will, I imagine, be held to imply only that the doctor should make sure that his insight is not so poor as to frustrate his clear interests. So far, presumably, George goes home.

But I have almost commanded this answer by asking about a single patient and exploiting the obvious attractions of patient-centredness as a guide to medicine. The other question was how

much responsibility the doctor shoulders, if he colludes with George's wishes. A natural thought is that, if the answer to the first question is to give George the decision, then the doctor must be morally in the clear for the purposes of the second. But, on reflection, it is not so simple. Even a patient-centred approach saddles the doctor with moral responsibilities which are not exhausted by serving George's interests. I open my case by asking which patient is to be at the centre of a patient-centred approach.

It is time that the doctor had a name too. Resisting a revealing temptation to call him Dr Smith, I shall christen him Henry. (In what follows Henry is a hospital doctor overseeing George's treatment and discharge. But, since the moral relationship which I want to discuss is a professional yet personal one better typified by a GP, he can be thought of as George's GP also. This elasticity, I trust, will not spoil the argument.) It is a trick of the example to suggest that Henry is involved only as George's medical adviser and that only Henry is involved in the decision. Henry has other patients beside George and belongs to a medical profession most of whose patients are not Henry's. [. . .]

George is occupying a hospital bed. There are other people waiting for beds and George does not really need one. At first sight this is not Henry's problem, partly because it is not his fault that there is a lack of outside support to keep George going and more generally because ordinary hospital doctors and GPs are not responsible for the overall allocation of resources. But this is too formal a way of looking at a doctor's responsibilities. If Henry is an experienced and respected GP, he has a *de facto* power to call up social service support or to secure hospital beds, while his credit remains good. His credit is staked on every case and depends on his not staking it too casually. He can mortgage it for any one patient but, if his fellow professionals do not agree that the case merited the resources by comparison with other cases, it will be that much harder for Henry to secure help for his next patient. Hence Henry's considered pronouncement on George may have costs and benefits to Henry's other patients.

To serve *all* his patients he needs a good reputation among those who allocate resources which cannot meet all claims by all doctors. George, let us assume, simply wants the best result for himself. Henry aims more widely at the best for all his patients. These aims can conflict.

Moreover Henry is not solely the champion of his own patients. He has a doctor's concern for all the sick, shared with fellow doctors and with others in the work of promoting health. That opens up an interesting ambiguity in the notion of patient-centred care. Should each doctor care for his own patients (and, more broadly, each professional for his own parish)? Or should each behave as a member of a group whose aim is the good of all patients? These alternatives do not yield the same result. Just as Henry's 100 per cent effort on George's behalf may do what is best for George at the expense of Henry's other patients, so Henry's 100 per cent commitment to his own patients may be at the expense of other patients. Similarly, a powerful consultant, administrator or health team can get more than proportional resources for their own parish if their own parish is what counts. Patient-centredness is ambiguous on the point. [. . .]

If Henry is an experienced, effective doctor who knows how to work the system better than most, then equality of patients' need seems to mean that he should *not* do his best for his patients. To block this odd conclusion, we might try envisaging the care network as a system of checks and balances. Henry is to do his best for his own patients but other professionals, with their rather different concerns, do their best to stop him getting away with unfair allocations. [. . .]The best efforts of each in his own parish can then sum to the best which the system can deliver as a whole. But this is to take a very idealized view of the social world about us. [. . .]

The general puzzle is one of professional duty in a world of imperfect compliance. It is not one of legal obligation, since Henry can see to it that his back is covered whatever he does. He can steer George either back home or back into his hospital bed and cover himself by the wording of his professional judgment. Ethically, however, we still want to know how much responsibility is his if he steers George home, knowing that the social work support really available is not really enough. It is not his responsibility to provide enough support to free George's hospital bed with a clear conscience. But he has a moral decision to make and he is answerable for it in a way which George is not and which is not trumped by George's wish to go home. He might consider, for instance, encouraging George to go home partly because this is one way of putting pressure on those who allocate the budget to social services. This would be for the future benefit of others in need but hardly for the present benefit of George. This sort of consideration is endemic in the ethics of professional roles when played out among roles which mesh imperfectly, and it is one on which patient-centredness gives no guidance.

A final ambiguity about 'patient-centred' is found by asking whether it means 'answerable to the patient'. The initial reaction is probably that it does. The doctor–patient relationship is usually deemed one-to-one, in that it is a confidential relation of trust between a doctor and a patient with a right to his undivided commitment. [. . .] The broader question is whether even a patient-centred practice is not answerable to a wider tribunal. [. . .] The doctor is answerable to the community at large. [. . .] How much responsibility does Henry shoulder if he colludes with George's wishes? The question is incomplete: how much responsibility *to whom*?

It has emerged by now, I hope, that if we try for something patient-centred, to the effect that the doctor's duty is to his patient, the idea is thoroughly ambiguous. Even concentrating on the particular patient of the immediate case we find that the duty is to serve the patient's interests as a person rather than his declared wants for his physical machine. Liberal notions of autonomy leave the patient's wishes the benefit of the doubt as a guide to his interests but override them when his insight is clearly lacking. Meanwhile patient-centredness cannot be construed thus one-to-one. Henry is answerable for more people than George and to more people than George. He is responsible at least for his other patients; perhaps, as a member of the caring professions, for the overall welfare of those in need of care. Equally he is responsible not only to George and other patients but also to fellow professionals and ultimately the community at large. As soon as resources are short or roles mesh imperfectly, Henry's best efforts for George have a price paid elsewhere. 'Patient-centred' starts with George but cannot mean simply 'George-centred' and gives no guidance on where to stop. George is still inescapably Henry's patient. So far I have turned a simple plea by an old and lonely widower for a death of his own into an intricate set of questions about Henry's duties. That is rough on George but, all the same, I propose to say a bit more about professional integrity as a factor in medical ethics before returning to death as a proper exercise of consumer sovereignty.

This difficult notion comes with some philosophical baggage which needs to be unloaded. Integrity, as a general moral concept, is commonly invoked as an objection to consequentialist ethics: even if it would save the Health Service a pile of money to let George die off quietly, Henry should refuse to be party to such base calculation. This admonition may be made from either of two points of view. One belongs to the kind of deontological or duty-based ethics which opposes principle to consequence and bids us do right and damn the consequences. From this point of view the Hippocratic oath is a sort of categorical medical imperative which forbids doctors all compromise with lack of resources or any other obstacle to the patient's good health. Integrity demands acting on pure principle with the moral consistency of a rhinoceros. My short comment is that principle and consequence cannot be so starkly opposed. On the one hand utilitarians are applying a principle when they adopt whatever solution makes for the greater welfare of the greater number. On the other there are always questions of whether a principle is appropriate to a situation and of how it is to be applied – questions which demand care for results. Hence integrity does not provide independent leverage on what is right or best to do. It demands only that, having identified the right or best thing to do, the agent goes ahead and does it.

The other common use of integrity is to appeal against all systematic ethics, whether of principle or of consequence. The *locus classicus* is the existentialist idea of authenticity which forbids the agent to accept *any* general guidance in advance of a situation, on pain of 'bad faith'. [. . .] My short comment is that we can agree in refusing to let the doctor hide behind an unexamined conscience but cannot possibly construe professional integrity as *carte blanche* for a professional to do whatever he finds most 'authentic' at the moment of choice.

That leaves two unmistakable tensions involved in the notion of professional integrity, both concerned with the relation of self to role. One has to do with conflicts between a doctor's personal beliefs and the demands of his office. The other has to do with the degree for which he is personally responsible, when the duties of his role are overridden by other pressures.

[. . .]

The dilemmas of professional integrity are distinct both from personal dilemmas (shall I betray my country or my friend?) and from professional dilemmas (shall Henry improve George's insight at the expense of his health?) They cross the line between personal and professional. Presumably no one thinks that the doctor should hang up his conscience along with his hat and obey all possible orders by the authority which hands out his stethoscope. In that case he might as well take the job of medical assistant to a team of torturers. But integrity can seem so much a personal notion that the opposite view is tempting. Should he ever compromise his private conscience and, if so, when and why?

The easy part of the answer is that private conscience is not infallible and where it is just another term for personal convictions, not safe from bigotry. A doctor may not eject patients from his surgery as he might visitors from his living room. He cannot refuse them on grounds of their race, sex, religion or politics. But, on the other hand, total moral neutrality is not what we ask of doctors. We expect them to uphold a professional code, whose rationale is their special situation in relation to a broader ethic of concern for others. The broader ethic cannot be wholly bland and its special application to medicine is bound to conflict from time to time with what a doctor personally thinks right. Mismatch can occur in both directions. For example official guidance for doctors on abortion, on severely handicapped infants, on patients long comatose and on the incurably senile can strike some as too strict and others as too lax. Then there will be tension because we need the doctor's personal moral commitment but not too much of it.

The same goes for the other kind of tension, when scarcity of resources interferes with the doctor's duty. The National Health Service had hoped originally to avoid this difficulty by giving doctors a free hand in prescribing what they thought best. But it is clear by now that the medical task is expanding, not shrinking, and cannot possibly be fully resourced. Two typical ways of applying the cork are to limit the doctors' efforts (for instance by restricting the list of prescribable drugs or by letting queues form) and to put decisions about allocation in non-medical hands (as with the rationing of kidney machines by committees of citizens). However it is done, doctors are then asked to acquiesce in what they may think a betrayal of their calling. They may wonder whether they are absolved from guilt, when their patients die of treatable renal failure, by the undoubted fact that they did not decide the allocation between health and roadbuilding.

[...]

So let us draw the threads together, answer the question about Henry's responsibility, if he colludes with George, and lets the poor fellow go home at last. I have been offering an oblique comment on a natural approach to medical ethics, which goes, so to speak, top down. One starts with a broad aim for the system, like maximizing welfare subject to constraints of justice, and tries to translate it into policies for allocating resources and applying them to individual patients. I do not think this is a false approach and I have not tried to belittle the problems it identifies, which are typically to do with scarcity of resources and the need to weigh the claims of medicine against other priorities. My comment is that, however well one works things out top down, there is an ineliminable moral friction where top down meets bottom up. Where policy meets patient, the doctor has moral choices to make which no code of medical ethics can reduce to routine. Since a system of care is to be judged finally at its point of delivery, it is crucial to think about it from bottom up as well as from top down.

[...] I imagine that most doctors will think it best to let George go and will find this responsibility easiest to shoulder. Indeed, I think that they must, as more people live longer into a fragile and confused old age. But responsibility is not here lessened on the ground that letting die is not killing. Having learnt to postpone death, we have set ourselves problems of when to cut short the losses of an extended life. We have a collective responsibility for what Henry decides but Henry is responsible for his decision. Although he can cover his back by recording a clinical judgment that George's insight and prospects were adequate, he knows that there is more to the moral question than clinical judgment.

At any rate, George goes home. He remains on his doctor's conscience as he is carried out a month later to a forgotten grave. But so he would have done also, languishing on in a hospital bed. Without hoping to make it easier to see in the twilight, let me end with a patient-centred prayer, also from Rilke:

O Herr, gib jedem seinen eignen Tod,
Das Sterben, das aus jedem Leben geht,
Darin er Liebe hatte, Sinn und Not.

Even when a death of one's own is a poor consumer choice, it is a proper exercise of human dignity.

88

Selection from *The Death of Ivan Ilyich*

LEO TOLSTOY

It was morning. He knew it was morning simply because Gerasim had gone and Pyotr, the footman, had come, snuffed out the candles, drawn back one of the curtains, and quietly begun to tidy up the room. Morning or night, Friday or Sunday, made no difference, everything was the same: that gnawing, excruciating, incessant pain; that awareness of life irrevocably passing but not yet gone; that dreadful, loathsome death, the only reality, relentlessly closing in on him; and that same endless lie. What did days, weeks, or hours matter?

"Will you have tea, sir?"

"He wants order, so the masters should drink tea in the morning," thought Ivan Ilyich. But he merely replied: "No."

"Would you care to move to the sofa, sir?"

"He wants to tidy up the room and I'm in the way. I represent filth and disorder," thought Ivan Ilyich. But he merely replied: "No, leave me alone."

The footman busied himself a while longer. Ivan Ilyich stretched out his hand. Pyotr went up to him obligingly.

"What would you like, sir?"

"My watch."

Pyotr picked up the watch, which was lying within Ivan Ilyich's reach, and gave it to him.

"Half-past eight. Are they up?"

"No, sir. Vasily Ivanovich (the son) went to school and Praskovya Fyodorovna left orders to awaken her if you asked. Shall I, sir?"

"No, don't bother," he said. "Perhaps I should have some tea," he thought, and said: "Yes, tea . . . bring me some."

Pyotr headed for the door. Ivan Ilyich was terrified at the thought of being left alone. "What can I do to keep him here?" he thought. "Oh, of course, the medicine."

"Pyotr, give me my medicine," he said. "Why not?" he thought. "Maybe the medicine will still do some good." He took a spoonful and swallowed it. "No, it won't help. It's just nonsense, a hoax," he decided as soon as he felt that familiar, sickly, hopeless taste in his mouth. "No, I can't believe in it anymore. But why this pain, this pain? If only it would let up for a minute!" He began to moan. Pyotr came back. "No, go. Bring me some tea."

Pyotr went out. Left alone Ivan Ilyich moaned less from the pain, agonizing as it was, than from anguish. "The same thing, on and on, the same endless days and nights. If only it would come quicker! If only *what* would come quicker? Death, darkness. No! No! Anything is better than death!"

When Pyotr returned with the tea, Ivan Ilyich looked at him in bewilderment for some time, unable to grasp who and what he was. Pyotr was disconcerted by that look. Seeing his confusion, Ivan Ilyich came to his senses.

"Yes," he said. "Tea...good. Put it down. Only help me wash up and put on a clean shirt."

And Ivan Ilyich began to wash himself. Pausing now and then to rest, he washed his hands and face, brushed his teeth, combed his hair, and looked in the mirror. He was horrified, particularly horrified to see the limp way his hair clung to his pale brow. He knew he would be even more horrified by the sight of his body, and so while his shirt was being changed he avoided looking at it. Finally it was all over. He put on a dressing gown, wrapped himself in a plaid, and sat down in an armchair to have his tea. For a brief moment he felt refreshed, but as soon as he began to drink his tea he sensed that same taste again, that same pain. He forced himself to finish the tea and then lay down, stretched out his legs, and sent Pyotr away.

The same thing again and again. One moment a spark of hope gleams, the next a sea of despair rages; and always the pain, the pain, always the anguish, the same thing on and on. Left alone he feels horribly depressed, wants to call someone, but knows beforehand that with others present it will be even worse. "Oh, for some morphine again – to sink into oblivion. I'll tell the doctor he must think of something to give me."

One hour then another pass this way. Then there is a ring in the entranceway. The doctor perhaps? The doctor indeed – fresh, hearty, stocky, cheerful, and with a look on his face that seems to say: "Now, now, you've had yourself a bad scare, but we're going to fix everything right away." The doctor knows this expression is inappropriate here, but he has put it on once and for all and can't take it off – like a man who has donned a frock coat in the morning to make a round of social calls.

The doctor rubs his hands briskly, reassuringly. "I'm chilled. Freezing cold outside. Just give me a minute to warm up," he says in a tone implying that one need only wait a moment until he warmed up and he would set everything right.

"Well, now, how are you?"

Ivan Ilyich feels the doctor wants to say: "How goes it?" but that even he knows this won't do, and so he says: "What sort of night did you have?"

Ivan Ilyich looks at the doctor inquisitively as if to say: "Won't you ever be ashamed of your lying?" But the doctor does not wish to understand such a question.

"Terrible. Just like all the others," Ivan Ilyich said. "The pain never leaves, never subsides. If only you'd give me something!"

"Yes, you sick people are always carrying on like this. Well, now, I seem to have warmed up. Even Praskovya Fyodorovna, who's so exacting, couldn't find fault with my temperature. Well, now I can say good morning." And the doctor shakes his hand.

Then, dispensing with all the banter, the doctor assumes a serious air and begins to examine the patient, taking his pulse, his temperature, sounding his chest, listening to his heart and lungs.

Ivan Ilyich knows for certain, beyond any doubt, that this is all nonsense, sheer deception, but when the doctor gets down on his knees, bends over him, placing his ear higher, then lower, and with the gravest expression on his face goes through all sorts of contortions, Ivan Ilyich is taken in by it, just as he used to be taken in by the speeches of lawyers, even though he knew perfectly well they were lying and why they were lying.

The doctor is still kneeling on the sofa, tapping away at him, when there is a rustle of silk at the doorway and Praskovya Fyodorovna can be heard reproaching Pyotr for not informing her of the doctor's arrival.

She comes in, kisses her husband, and at once tries to demonstrate that she has been up for some time, and owing simply to a misunderstanding failed to be in the room when the doctor arrived.

Ivan Ilyich looks her over from head to toe and resents her for the whiteness, plumpness, and cleanliness of her arms and neck, the luster of her hair, and the spark of vitality that gleams in her eyes. He hates her with every inch of his being. And her touch causes an agonizing well of hatred to surge up in him.

Her attitude toward him and his illness is the same as ever. Just as the doctor had adopted a certain attitude toward his patients, which he could not change, so she had adopted one toward him: that he was not doing what he should and was himself to blame, and she could only reproach him tenderly for this. And she could no longer change this attitude.

"He just doesn't listen, you know. He doesn't take his medicine on time. And worst of all, he lies in a position that is surely bad for him – with his legs up."

And she told him how he made Gerasim hold his legs up.

The doctor smiled disdainfully, indulgently, as if to say: "What can you do? Patients sometimes get absurd ideas into their heads, but we have to forgive them."

When he had finished his examination the doctor glanced at his watch, and then Praskovya Fyodorovna announced to Ivan Ilyich that whether he liked it or not, she had called in a celebrated physician, and that he and Mikhail Danilovich (the regular doctor) would examine him together that day and discuss his case.

"So no arguments, please. I'm doing this for my sake," she said ironically, letting him know that she was doing it all for his sake and had said this merely to deny him the right to protest. He scowled and said nothing. He felt that he was trapped in such a mesh of lies that it was difficult to make sense out of anything.

Everything she did for him was done strictly for her sake; and she told him she was doing for her sake what she actually was, making this seem so incredible that he was bound to take it to mean just the reverse.

At half-past eleven the celebrated doctor did indeed arrive. Again there were soundings and impressive talk in his presence and in the next room about the kidney and the caecum, and questions and answers exchanged with such an air of importance that once again, instead of the real question of life and death, the only one confronting Ivan Ilyich, the question that had arisen concerned a kidney or a caecum that was not behaving properly, and that would soon get a good trouncing from Mikhail Danilovich and the celebrity and be forced to mend its ways.

The celebrated doctor took leave of him with a grave but not hopeless air. And when Ivan Ilyich looked up at him, his eyes glistening with hope and fear, and timidly asked whether there was any chance of recovery, he replied that he could not vouch for it but there was a chance. The look of hope Ivan Ilyich gave the doctor as he watched him leave was so pathetic that, seeing it, Praskovya Fyodorovna actually burst into tears as she left the study to give the celebrated doctor his fee.

The improvement in his morale prompted by the doctor's encouraging remarks did not last long. Once again the same room, the same pictures, draperies, wallpaper, medicine bottles, and the same aching, suffering body. Ivan Ilyich began to moan. They gave him an injection and he lost consciousness.

When he came to, it was twilight; his dinner was brought in. He struggled to get down some broth. Then everything was the same again, and again night was coming on.

89

The Coevolution of Bioethics and the Medical Humanities with Palliative Medicine, 1967–97

DAVID BARNARD

Attending and accompanying with the patient in his dying is, in fact, the oldest medical ethics there is.

Paul Ramsey, *The Patient as Person* (1970)

The Common Matrix of Concern

It would be an oversimplification to point to any single factor as *the* stimulus for the modern development of bioethics or the medical humanities. David Rothman has described many social, institutional, and scientific strands of this story: e.g., the increasing social distance between doctor and patient, the rise of the modern hospital, the explosion of biomedical research (and research funding) after World War II, and the rapid proliferation and expense of medical technology.[1] Life-prolonging technologies such as mechanical ventilators and dialysis machines were particularly significant in this story, and it is no exaggeration to say that problems arising near the end of life were crucial to the birth of bioethics and the other disciplines of the medical humanities.

Arguably the first significant texts in the nascent field of bioethics were *Morals and Medicine* by Joseph Fletcher, first published in 1954, and *The*

Patient as Person by Paul Ramsey, published in 1970.[2] (Both Fletcher and Ramsey were theologians. Philosophers were latecomers to the debates about humanistic and ethical issues in medicine, generally following in the footsteps of ministers and historians.) The care of the dying figures prominently in both books. Fletcher devotes separate chapters to the question of truthfulness in medicine (the problem of breaking bad news) and to euthanasia. Ramsey's long chapter on the care of the dying anticipates every significant theme in today's debates about withholding and withdrawing treatment, pain management, physician-assisted suicide, and euthanasia. To both Fletcher and Ramsey, the way modern scientific medicine had technologized and professionalized healing in the mid-twentieth century threatened to eclipse medicine's moral and humanistic core. Near the beginning of his book Fletcher cites with approval Francis Peabody's 1927 essay on "The Care of the Patient." Fletcher then continues,

The moralist's interest in the ethics of medicine has to do with *the care of the patient*, not with the treatment of a disease. We are concerned with medical care rather than with medical treatment. Dr. Peabody's phrase captures the heart of the matter; the care of a patient "must be completely personal."...What is this, but to say that a patient's moral and ethical rights and interests must weigh as heavily as his physical needs and condition?[3]

Ramsey begins the preface to his book with the following words:

This volume undertakes to examine some of the problems of medical ethics that are especially urgent in the present day. These are by no means technical problems on which only the expert (in this case, the physician) can have an opinion. They are rather the problems of human beings in situations in which medical care is needed. Birth and death, illness and injury are not simply events the doctor attends. They are moments in every human life. The doctor makes decisions as an expert but also as a man among men; and his patient is a human being coming to his birth or to his death, or being rescued from illness or injury in between....Resonating through [the doctor's] professional actions, and crucial in some of them, will be a view of man, an understanding of the meaning of the life at whose first or second exodus he is present, a care for the life he attends in its afflictions.[4]

The factors that spurred the development of the modern hospice movement are strikingly similar. Four aspects of medical care in the industrialized West are particularly significant in this regard:

1. Medical technology has blurred the line between life and death, leaving many people attached to invasive mechanical life support and enduring pain, helplessness, and expense throughout their last weeks and days of life.
2. The devaluation of symptom control in medical education and practice has caused

caregivers to concentrate narrowly on the pathophysiology and cure of disease, rather than on the patient's experience of illness, resulting in a great burden of preventable but unnoticed suffering.
3. A loss of extended family ties and community has caused the physical and emotional burdens of caring for a dying person to fall more heavily on the members of isolated nuclear families (and disproportionately on women).
4. Strained and evasive relationships frequently increase the loneliness, and therefore the suffering, of the dying and bereaved.

These factors have created a strong public demand for improved care near the end of life, frequently expressed in the slogan "dying with dignity." This phrase has come to mean very different things to different people, including (especially in the United States) the increasingly popular preference for legalizing physician-assisted suicide. David Roy, Director of the Center for Bioethics at the Clinical Research Institute of Montreal, has provided the following definition of dying with dignity. His definition not only captures the essential goals and characteristics of hospice care and palliative medicine, it also demonstrates the essentially humanistic emphasis of those disciplines:

*   dying without a frantic technical fuss and bother to squeeze out a few more moments or hours of biological life, when the important thing is to live out one's last moments as fully, consciously, and courageously as possible;
*   dying without that twisting, racking pain that totally ties up one's consciousness and leaves one free for nothing and for no one else;
*   dying in surroundings that are worthy of a human being who is about to live what should be one's "finest hour." The environment of a dying patient should clearly say: the technical drama of medicine has receded to the background to give way to the central human drama of a unique human being "wrestling with his God";
*   dying in the presence of people who know how to drop the professional role mask and

relate to others simply and richly as a human being.[5]

Course work in death and dying, the nature of suffering, and other humanistic perspectives on issues near the end of life figured very prominently in the earliest bioethics and humanities curricula in medical schools.[6] By the early 1980s, most U.S. medical schools had at least some elective course offerings in both death and dying and bioethics. Some schools created full-fledged humanities programs that brought literary, historical, religious, philosophical, and cultural perspectives to bear on medical concerns.

These educational trends paralleled the development of professional organizations for hospice and palliative care and the growing scientific and professional literature for these fields. The table of contents of the *Oxford Textbook of Palliative Medicine* (first published in 1993) reinforces the point that the humanities and bioethics are what might be termed "tributary disciplines" to the larger field of palliative medicine, in much the same way as fields such as pharmacology, psychiatry, and radiotherapy can be so described.[7]

It would be a mistake, however, to assume that the relationship between the humanities and palliative care is unidirectional, i.e., that humanistic concepts and methods have influenced palliative care with no reciprocal influence of palliative care on the humanities. Indeed, it is their very engagement with the realities of clinical practice that has kept the academic disciplines of the humanities from spinning off into ever more esoteric and irrelevant mind games. Stephen Toulmin's 1982 article, "How Medicine Saved the Life of Ethics,"[8] makes this point, although he, too, was anticipated by Joseph Fletcher in 1954. Fletcher commented that "moralists who spend little or no time in the terminal wards of a modern city hospital cannot contribute much in the way of realistic opinion or relevance to the subject of euthanasia. They need to examine the facts, or to reexamine them, not only statistically but clinically."[9]

Some philosophers and theologians subtly devalue the physical, fleshly aspects of medical and nursing care by viewing them in the ultim-

ate contexts of human finitude and spirituality. From this point of view, the care of the body and alleviation of its pain are *only* or *merely* the care of the body, whereas attention to the spirit – to the realms of community, destiny, and meaning – is somehow closer to the true nature of care. Yet there are times when the gentle and skillful touch of a doctor or nurse is the only medium we have to express community and love, and it often sets an example for friends and family who may be too frightened to caress the dying person's cheek or hand.

Ramsey understood and articulated the inherent linkage between humanistic concern and the technical acts of palliative care. As Ramsey points out, these dimensions are inextricably connected, which is why ethics, the humanities, and palliative medicine sprang so easily and naturally from their common matrix of concern.

It is true that death is now accepted [Ramsey wrote in *The Patient as Person*]; and it is no longer opposed. This makes room for appropriate caring actions which are means to no future consequence. These actions are fulfillments of the *categorical* imperative: Never abandon care! Perhaps they should not be called means at all, since they effectuate or hasten the coming of no end at all. Upon ceasing to try to rescue the perishing, one is then free to care for the dying. Acts of caring for the dying are deeds done bodily for them which serve solely to manifest that they are not lost from human attention, that they are not alone, that mankind generally and their loved ones take note of their dying, and mean to company with them in accepting this unique instance of the acceptable death of all flesh.[10]

The Elaboration of the Concept and Practice of "Whole Person Care"

In 1963 Cicely Saunders asked one of her patients to "tell me about your pain." The woman responded, "Well doctor, it began in my back but now it seems that all of me is wrong....I could have cried for the pills and the injections but I knew that I mustn't. It seemed as if all the world was against me and no one understood how I felt. My husband and son were marvelous but they were having to stay off work and lose their money. But it's so wonderful to begin to feel safe again."[11]

Saunders commented that this patient had just described "total pain." Total pain is the conceptual linchpin in the philosophy of palliative care. It refers to the multidimensional experience of suffering that encompasses physical, social, psychological, and spiritual distress. The interpenetration of these dimensions of suffering results in the well-recognized phenomenon that prolonged, untreated physical pain can aggravate psychosocial or spiritual distress, just as depressed or existentially anguished patients frequently report increased pain intensity and require increased doses of analgesics, even in the absence of disease progression.

From the beginning, every definition of palliative care has made reference to the physical, psychological, and spiritual aspects of suffering, and the importance of attending not only to the patient but also to the patient's family. In other words, the aim of palliative care is care for the whole person, who is understood to consist of body, mind, and spirit, and to live (and die) in a particular family, social, and cultural context. Illness and death are biographical as well as biological processes.

Accordingly, palliative care and palliative care education have embraced three broad areas: (1) the science and techniques of pain management and symptom control; (2) the psychological, social, and spiritual aspects of dying and grieving; (3) self-knowledge on the part of caregivers, especially regarding personal attitudes toward death and emotional reactions to loss. Palliative care is whole person care not only in the sense that the whole person of the patient is the object of attention. Palliative care also demands that the whole person of the caregiver be involved. Palliative care is, par excellence, care that is given through the medium of a human relationship. Education for palliative care is education for building and sustaining relationships, and for the use of the self as a primary diagnostic and therapeutic modality.[12]

In an identical fashion, the medical humanities have taken the whole person as the focus of their attention. The disciplines of the humanities, particularly the fields of literature, history, religious studies, and cultural studies, have addressed the personal experience of illness (as opposed to the strictly biophysiologic aspects of disease), the social and cultural contexts of sickness and help-seeking behavior, and the moral and existential concerns that people face when they are critically ill – and that caregivers face when they form close relationships with the sick and the dying. The history of the medical humanities since the 1960s is the history of progressively richer, subtler, and more clinically relevant portrayals and analyses of these dimensions of health care.

Summaries of the current state of the art in the humanities' contributions to medical education were the focus of a special issue of *Academic Medicine* published in September 1995. In their introduction to this issue, guest editors Rita Charon and Peter Williams wrote:

> Medicine and the humanities have always been interwoven. Great literature has been written by and about physicians. Medical practice has always operated with the guidance of ethics, law, and religion. The work and science of healing have ever been a focus of philosophers and historians; care of the sick and dying has reciprocally called the attention of sensitive physicians to the meaning and chronicles of human life. To integrate the study of the humanities in medical school is not to provide doctors with a civilized veneer but to allow them to reach to the heart of human learning about meaning, life, and death.[13]

The Era of Public Policy and Corporate Medicine

With a few notable exceptions (e.g., participation on the Harvard Ad Hoc Committee to Examine the Definition of Brain Death in

1968, and the National Commission for the Protection of Human Subjects of Biomedical and Behavioral Research, from 1974), the first generation of scholars in bioethics and the medical humanities worked in relative isolation from the halls of policy making or government. The majority of their contributions were in the form of scholarly publications or teaching in academic medical centers. By the early 1980s, however, this began to change.

In 1982 the President's Commission for the Study of Ethical Problems in Medicine and Biomedical and Behavioral Research began to issue a series of comprehensive reports on topics that included access to health care, informed consent, and decisions to forego life-sustaining medical treatment. Both the Commission and its professional staff included representatives from the bioethics community. More recently, the National Bioethics Advisory Committee has assumed a similar, congressionally mandated role in analyzing the ethical issues arising from biomedical research and practice and recommending regulatory and/or legislative actions. During the 1990s, bioethicists and other medical humanities scholars also have participated on many task forces and commissions at the state level. Two examples with direct relevance to end-of-life care are the New York State Task Force on Life and the Law[14] and the Michigan Commission on Death and Dying.[15]

The increasingly public dimension of work in bioethics and the medical humanities reflects the increasing complexity and pluralism of U.S. society – demographically, culturally, and morally. It is not sufficient to articulate finely wrought conceptual arguments or to inspire empathy for patients' experiences through fiction, poetry, or personal narrative. More and more, concern for the social and ethical dimensions of health care requires entry into the political arena. Policies on organ procurement and distribution, assisted reproduction, and abortion are salient examples. Issues that are especially relevant to palliative care include the regulation of the prescription of narcotics, the use of advance directives, and physician-assisted suicide. In all of these instances, clinicians and their bioethics and humanities colleagues are called to political action and

negotiation in order to develop policies that are consistent – to the greatest extent possible – with the values and preferences of patients and the consciences of health professionals.

Notwithstanding the importance of the issues mentioned above, at present the most significant public policy challenges for bioethics and humanities derive from the changes in the financing and organization of health care that are taking place today. In the words of Dan Brock,

New graduates of medical school or residency training face a system dramatically different from that faced by their counterparts one or two decades ago. . . . Serving patient needs is being replaced by strategic planning to capture profitable market segments and shed unprofitable operations. With the dramatic rush to consolidation and merger in the health care industry over the last couple of years, a trend to greater concentration of economic power is likely to continue, and the professional autonomy of physicians employed by these large complex organizations will continue to erode.[16]

Caregivers in hospice and palliative care are also in the thick of the debates over the future of health-care financing, professional autonomy, and patient welfare. Just as eloquent and insightful scholarship in the humanities has had to be supplemented by participation in policy making, so have the palliative care physician's skill and compassion had to be augmented by political action. The future of palliative care in the United States will be determined as much by economic and political decisions as by practitioners' competence.[17] Already there has been successful lobbying for an experimental ICD-code for palliative care, intended to facilitate access to palliative care for hospitalized patients.[18] Continued pressure will be needed to move from the research phase of this experiment to its implementation by the Health Care Financing Administration. Managed care companies' increasing share of the health-care market likewise has major implications for hospice and palliative care.[19]

Bioethics, the medical humanities, and palliative medicine have thus arrived at very similar stages in their coevolution. Conceptual, analytical, and scholarly achievement has brought these fields to a mature state. To reap the benefits of their combined, synergistic focus on whole person care near the end of life, however, practitioners in these fields must press beyond the familiar parameters of their professional and intellectual traditions, and learn to participate in the political arena. In doing this, palliative care physicians can draw on the ancient traditions of humanism and advocacy for patient welfare that have helped shape the modern medical profession. And scholars in bioethics and humanities can contribute their own long traditions of values exploration and rhetorical power. An example of both is provided by the Jewish philosopher of religion, Rabbi Abraham Joshua Heschel. Heschel addressed the Annual Convention of the American Medical Association in June 1964. His address was entitled "The Patient as a Person." Not only did his title anticipate that of Paul Ramsey's seminal book on medical ethics; Heschel also gave us further proof that the concerns of today (in this case the economic threats to patients' welfare) have been dealt with profoundly for decades. His address included these words:

> The doctor is not simply a dispenser of drugs, a computer that speaks. In treating a patient he is morally involved. What transpires between doctor and patient is more than a commercial transaction, more than a professional relationship between a specimen of the human species and a member of the American Medical Association. Medicine is not simply merchandise, and the relationship between doctor and patient is blasphemously distorted when conceived primarily in terms of economics: the doctor a merchant, the patient a customer. What comes to pass in the doctor's office is a profoundly human association, involving concern, trust, responsibility.[20]

NOTES

1   Rothman, D. J., *Strangers at the Bedside: A History of How Law and Bioethics Transformed Medical Decision Making* (New York: Basic Books, 1991).

2   Fletcher, J., *Morals and Medicine* (Boston: Beacon Press, 1960); Ramsey, P., *The Patient as Person: Explorations in Medical Ethics* (New Haven: Yale University Press, 1970).

3   Fletcher, *Morals and Medicine*.

4   Ramsey, *The Patient as Person*.

5   Roy, D., "Ethics and aging: trends and problems in the clinical setting," in J. E. Thornton and E. R. Winkler (eds.), *Ethics and Aging: The Right to Live, the Right to Die* (Vancouver: University of British Columbia Press, 1988).

6   McElhinney, T. K. (ed.), *Human Values Teaching Programs for Health Professionals* (Ardmore, PA: Whitmore, 1981).

7   Doyle, D., Hanks, G. W. C., and MacDonald, N. (eds.), *Oxford Textbook of Palliative Medicine*, 2nd edn (Oxford: Oxford University Press, 1998).

8   Toulmin, S., "How medicine saved the life of ethics," *Perspect Biol. Med.* 25 (1982): 736–50.

9   Fletcher, *Morals and Medicine*.

10   Ramsey, *The Patient as Person*.

11   Saunders, C., "Introduction," in C. Saunders and N. Sykes (eds.), *The Management of Terminal Malignant Disease*, 3rd edn (London: Edward Arnold, 1993).

12   Kearney, M., "Palliative medicine: Just another specialty?" *Palliative Med* 6 (1992): 39–46; Novack, D. H., Suchman, A. L., Clark, W., et al., "Calibrating the physician: Personal awareness and effective patient care," *JAMA* 278 (1997): 502–9.

13   Charon, R., Williams, P., "Introduction: The humanities and medical education," *Acad. Med.* 70 (1995): 758–60.

14   The New York State Task Force on Life and the Law, *When Death is Sought: Assisted Suicide and Euthanasia in the Medical Context* (Albany, NY: Health Research, 1994).

15   Final Report of the Michigan Commission on Death and Dying. Legislative Service Bureau, State of Michigan (Lansing, MI: Michigan Commission on Death and Dying, 1994).

16   Brock, D. W., "Ethical responsibilities of academic health centers in the new health care market," in M. Osterweis, C. J. McLaughlin, H. R. Manasse, et al. (eds.), *The U.S. Health Workforce: Power, Politics, and Policy* (Washington, DC: Association of Academic Health Centers, 1996).

17   Field, M. J., Cassel, C. K. (eds.), *Approaching Death: Improving Care at the End of Life*. Report

of the Committee on Care at the End of Life, Institute of Medicine (Washington, DC: National Academy Press, 1997).

18 Cassel, C. K., Vladeck, B. C., "ICD-9 code for palliative or terminal care," *N. Engl. J Med.* 335 (1996): 1232–4.

19 Miles, S. H., Weber, E. P., and Koepp, R., "End-of-life treatment in managed care: The potential and peril," *West J Med.* 163 (1995): 302–5; Morrison, R. S., Meier, D. E., "Managed care at the end of life," *Trends Health Care Law Ethics* 10 (1995): 91–6.

20 Heschel, A. J., "The patient as a person," in A. J. Heschel, *The Insecurity of Freedom* (Philadelphia: Jewish Publication Society of America, 1966), pp. 24–38.

90

Why I Don't Have a Living Will

JOANNE LYNN

For a dozen years, my clinical practice has been largely with dying patients, my academic pursuits have focused on medical ethics, and my public service has been mostly at the interface of medicine and law. One would think that I would have "done the right thing" long ago and signed a living will. I have not. This [chapter] is meant to illuminate my reasons. Some of my reasons may apply to others, and I will also mention some concerns that affect others but not me. However, I do not oppose the growth and development of advance directives. Rather, I hope to open the public and professional discussion of how to make decisions for incompetent adults in order to include more varieties of formal and informal advance directives and to force policy-makers to consider how to make decisions for incompetent adults who have no advance directives.

As a physician, I do use advance directives, both formal and informal, with many patients in all of my clinical settings. I have supported the Patient Self-Determination Act[1] and the distribution of living wills by Concern for Dying, and I have pushed for health care durable power of attorney legislation in my local jurisdictions. My endorsement of and enthusiasm for advance directives might well lead some to think that I am merely extraordinarily inefficient and imprudent in regard to my own affairs when they discover that I do not have a living will. While I may have these flaws of character, this particular behavior is not evidence for them.

I do not have a living will because I fear that the effects of having one would be worse, in my situation, than not having one. How could this be? A living will of the standard format attends to priorities that are not my own, addresses procedures rather than outcomes, and requires substantial interpretation without guaranteeing a reliable interpreter. Of course, a highly individualized formal advance directive might be able to escape these concerns, as is addressed below. First, however, I will consider the merits of a "standard" living will, such as is available in stationery stores and through the mail.

On its face, a "living will" purports to instruct caregivers to provide no life-sustaining treatment if the person signing it ever were on the verge of dying, with or without treatment, and were unable to make decisions for himself or herself. On the one hand, this is hardly a surprising instruction. Some combination of short life, interminable personal suffering, and adverse effects upon others is enough that virtually all persons would prefer to have had the opportunity to avoid this outcome, even at the cost of an earlier death. I have seen enough suffering that I can readily list all manner of existences that would induce me to accept death rather than have medical treatment to extend life. Not just in my case but in most cases, the text of a living will in standard format rarely tells the physician anything that was not nearly as likely to be true without it. The fact that a person took the time and trouble to sign one and get it to the physician does imply something about that person's character and the seriousness with which he or she approaches these issues, but not much about the individual's preferences and priorities.

As a physician, I use the fact that a person presents a standard-format living will as an opportunity to explore what he or she really means to avoid, what is really feared and hoped for, and who would be trusted to make decisions. This use is exceedingly valuable, but requires no legal standing for the document and does not require that it be treated as the definitive statement of what should be done.

However, many persons believe that they accomplish some very different ends by signing a living will. They believe they keep themselves from ever ending up like Nancy Cruzan or Karen Quinlan, or like a family member who had a particularly gruesome end of life in an intensive care unit. That belief is wrong. The public use of the standard living will is largely premised on an implicit promise that the document cannot ensure. Standard form living wills *should* have virtually no impact upon the care of persistent vegetative state patients, persons receiving vigorous therapy for potentially reversible physiologic imbalance, or persons with no clearly progressive and irreversible course toward imminent death, for none of these people clearly meet the requirement of dying soon irrespective of treatment. When people feel, as they commonly seem to, that having signed a living will serves to ensure that they will avoid medical torment of all sorts, they are misconstruing the document.

Nevertheless, sometimes living wills do have an impact upon the care plan of all sorts of patients because physicians and other providers inattentively overgeneralize. All too commonly,

someone who has a living will is assumed to have requested hospice-type care including a "Do not resuscitate" order, to prefer not to use intensive care, and to have refused curative treatments. This assumption can obviously shape the care plan without there being explicit confirmatory discussion with patient or surrogate. Thus, the living will can also lead to errors of undertreatment.

The standard form living will is thoroughly disappointing as a legal document. It does not reliably shape the care plan as intended and carries risks of affecting the care plan adversely. Unless it is used as a trigger for further communication, it has little justification. As a patient, I do not believe I will need to have that trigger.

The "standard-form" living will may be an unfair target for my critique, as there have been many efforts made to personalize and expand living wills,[2] especially by incorporating the designation of a proxy (which has conventionally been perceived as part of the durable power of attorney). While some of these are quite good, all entail some serious remaining difficulties that would preclude my using them and that should occasion some care in their use by others.

For example, a living will entails a construction of reality that identifies, at any one time, a group of persons who are "dying." The rest of us, in this conception, are not. Only if one is among the dying is the living will in effect. I cannot accept this construction of reality. Working with persons with advanced years, advanced cancer, and advanced AIDS has illuminated the hubris of this cultural view. Classifying some persons as "dying" does function to protect people, most of their lives, against recognizing that there is a death in store for each of us. The boundary between being merely mortal (like all humans) and being in the "dying" category is a boundary that people want desperately to find (and to find themselves in the "non-dying" group).

However, the schism simply does not exist. We all are dying. As the likely time of death comes closer, some issues tend to be more important, but there is no clear dividing line. Sometimes persons far from death are mainly concerned with comfort or spiritual concerns; sometimes persons facing death in the next few hours are still completing business deals. Pretending that there is a morally important demarcation between the merely mortal and the dying leads to harmful policies and practices generally. One stunning example is the societal support for hospices through Medicare which serves mostly relatively well-off cancer patients with homes, in contrast with the societal denial of adequate support for long-term care for those who are severely disabled and alone.

Also, the way that living wills have generally come to be constructed has focused attention on the patient's status (dying soon no matter what is done) and the procedures to be forgone (those that are artificial and "only" serve to prolong dying, sometimes expressed as a list of medical procedures). These two attributes of the standard living will subtly distort good decision-making. Good decision-making rests primarily in pursuing the best possible future, from among those plans of care that can be effectuated, and with the "best possible" being defined from the patient's perspective to the extent possible. Nothing in this model needs to turn on the proximity to death or the nature of the procedure involved, except as these considerations shape the desirability of various future courses to the patient. Sometimes ventilators are morally required, but sometimes even changing the sheets is contraindicated. For someone to be asked to decide in advance whether he or she would want dialysis, ventilator, or feeding tubes, without knowing what using these procedures would yield, is incomprehensible.

In addition, the issues that have become conventional to deal with in extended-version living wills are but a frail reflection of the concerns that very sick patients actually express. In fact, some of their real concerns have almost completely lost a place in the discussion of any kind of formal advance directives. Many patients are concerned about the emotional, physical, and financial burdens that their prolonged existence might entail for family. So often one hears, with real sincerity, "I don't want to be a burden," and so often we fail to have the ability, within this culture, to acknowledge and explore that

sentiment. Perhaps, if we all learned how to carry on the discussions, many persons would be found to be more concerned about the issues around imposing burdens on others than are concerned about the ignominy of persistent vegetative state or the torment of long-term ventilator use. Certainly, I would. However, this we do not talk about and we do not include in conventional advance directives.

Many people may also have a high preference for being able to choose a course of care that will never look foolish. Many persons seem to be more concerned to do the conventional thing, to be supported by friends and family as having "done his best," and never to have to feel that one bears much of the responsibility for the outcomes that one must endure. For example, I accepted a widely-used protocol for the treatment of a family member's illness, even though I knew that there was no data to support using some of the particularly onerous components of the protocol. The reason was largely because refusing those components would leave me bearing the responsibility for any adverse outcome. Even a maximally creative living will is likely to have difficulty expressing this particular sentiment; the formal prose itself tends to make the author look silly.

A number of factors that are known to affect decision-making are not regularly given voice through living wills. How is a person to write a living will that would ask for his family to seek divine guidance in prayer, or to ensure that her death is as dramatic and public as the rest of her life has been? Certainly, doing so would be difficult with any form that I have seen. In fact, much of what people ordinarily take to be important in their other choices is shunned in the conventional living will and the process of writing it. There is little passion or pathos, only the clean, sterile, black and white of choices made and enforced. Perhaps that is not how some, or most, of us would choose to die, if all choices were available. I, for example, would hope that my family would be emotional about the choices to be made, not simply concerned with the application of my advance directives to my situation.

Although my personal concerns do not include the first of these, two special classes of patient refuse to be involved in living will ne-gotiations because of a fundamental discord be-tween their model of how life is to be lived and the decision-analysis model that informs ad-vance directives discussions. A substantial number of patients simply find it incomprehen-sible or distasteful to imagine that their choices have an impact upon the length of life. Even if this counts as a denial of the facts of the situ-ation, it still is cause for concern that there are a lot of people who refuse to "play the game" for what amounts to religious reasons. Such per-sons commonly state, "It's up to God." Surely they do not therefore gain the obligation to be tormented by modern medicine; but, at least under some legal conditions, that is their only option if they lose competence without giving advance directives limiting life-sustaining treat-ment.[3]

The other group who refuse to be involved in advance directives includes those who simply want to be able to live in the moment and to have a community and family that is trust-worthy about making future choices. I person-ally have a great deal of sympathy with this claim. Why is it that the society wants individ-uals to get clear about their preferences and priorities and to express them in detail – only about life-sustaining medical treatment? Why can potential future patients not just trust that caregivers and family will make "about" the right choice? I prefer to believe that the "system" is caring and compassionate rather than that it is a cafeteria of services that can freely be chosen or forgone. One might well want to imagine that one's "circle of friends" would be affected by one's plight and motivated to ensure that the best possible choices were made. A survey of the competent residents of a nursing home that I served found that none of the residents' advance decisions (formal or in-formal) were known to all relevant caregivers and decision-makers, yet every resident was highly confident that the right choices would be made. Is this a less good state of affairs than if as many decisions as possible were made in advance and these choices were well-known and documented, but the system of care was feared by the clients? I think not. Of course, perhaps we can have trustworthy systems of care *and*

formal advance directives; but, very likely, re-quiring formal advance directives before reason-able plans of care can be implemented for a variety of situations will prove an obstacle to a sense of trustworthiness.

I, and surely some other patients, prefer family choice *over* the opportunity to make our own choices in advance. The patient himself or herself may well judge the family's efforts less harshly than he or she would judge his or her own decisions made in advance or by the pro-fessional caregivers. I have had a number of seriously ill patients say that their next of kin will attend to some choice if it comes up. When challenged with the possibility that the next of kin might decide in a way that was not what the patient would have chosen, the patient would kindly calm my concern with the observation that such an error would not be very important. High[4] found that patients prefer family deci-sion-making even if they have never discussed preferences with the family. Perhaps this is an important finding, one that should be enabled to find expression in advance directives if that is one mechanism that allows patients to express their views.

This is not the only way that the current focus on advance directives is troubling to a vigorous concept of family life. Families are those who grieve for the patient's suffering and death, who have a history of making deci-sions that account for the well-being of all con-cerned, and about whom the patient most likely would have had the most concern. Somehow to imagine that the society *could*, or *should* set up systems that remove the family from decision-making is almost outrageous. What if Nancy Cruzan had written a living will that stated that she wanted all treatment stopped if ever she were rendered unconscious for more than three days? Would the society really want care-givers to be obliged to stop treatment then, if her family vigorously objected?

Suppose that Justice Scalia, who wrote force-fully to encourage the requirement that life be sustained in the *Cruzan* case,[5] were afflicted with a terrible, lingering dying, relying upon all manner of medical torment to sustain life. Suppose also that his family claimed that they knew better what he would have wanted than do those who interpret his public writings and that they want treatment stopped. Should this society really establish systems of care that require that the family's voice be silenced? Surely not. While they might have to discuss their views at some length, surely the voice of a loving family should be prominent.

The idea of family decision-making is further constrained by the common requirement in durable powers of attorney and proxy statutes that there be one solo decision-maker designated. For many families, making a unitary designation is contrary to the family's history of making conjoint decisions and imposes the possibility of generating an unnecessary discord, as someone must be granted disproportionate authority.

The question at this point might well be "Why do I use advance directives at all?" rather than "Why do I not have one?" I have found four good uses for formal advance directives. First, for anyone for whom a legally-sanctioned surrogate either does not exist or might be controversial (e.g., should it be the mother or the long-term mate of an AIDS patient), a durable power of attorney is quite valuable. Provided that the person has at least one other person willing and capable of serving as surrogate, having that person properly designated can ease a great deal of administrative and legal concerns. In Virginia and the District of Columbia for persons whose next-of-kin are appropriate surrogates, they are automatically granted the authority.[6] However, in many jurisdictions, even patients with close family would be well-served by having a durable power of attorney.

For a much smaller number of people, I use durable powers of attorney to document unusually specific preferences or unusual preferences. Thus, a person who never wants to be in a particular hospital again, or to have a particular treatment again, or to be treated for pain, might well benefit by carefully documenting this preference.

For another group of patients and families, anxieties are best laid to rest by generating a formal advance directive. The formal document might be more weighty and enduring than any one surrogate or caregiver. Also, the discussion about priorities and preferences might most naturally and easily be organized around the task of writing a formal advance directive.

For patients and families that would use a next-of-kin surrogate (which is legally authorized without additional formalities in my jurisdiction), who have fairly conventional preferences about the goals and burdens of advanced illness, and who are most comfortable with informal agreements, I do not encourage formal advance directives. These criteria fit my situation.

What should I do? Clearly, I could not use a living will in any of its standard formats. What I should do is to write a durable power of attorney naming my husband as surrogate (if I were to become incompetent outside of Virginia and the District of Columbia) and asking that all concerned defer to his judgment, however he comes to it, unless they feel that his decision amounts to abuse. Specifically, I would not want any judge or other person to overrule my family's choice on the basis of anything I have written or said about medical treatment (including anything else that I have said in this [chapter]!). I believe I have a trustworthy family and a supportive circle of friends. I would prefer to endure the outcome if they "err" in predicting my preferences, or even if they choose to ignore my preferences other than the preference for family decision-making, rather than to remove from them the opportunity and the burden of making the choices. I do not want anyone else presuming to impose what are taken to be my desires as expressed elsewhere upon that family.

Once signed and witnessed, that last paragraph can serve as my advance directive.

NOTES

1 The Patient Self-Determination Act, Sections 4206, 4751, of the Omnibus Budget Reconciliation Act of 1990, P.L. 101–508 (Nov. 5, 1990).

2 President's Commission for the Study of Ethical Problems in Medicine and Biomedical and Behavioral Research, *Deciding to Forego Life-sustaining Treatment* (Washington, DC: US Government Printing Office, 1983); The Hastings Center, *Guidelines for the Termination of Treatment and the Care of the Dying* (Bloomington, IN: Indiana

University Press, 1987); Emanuel, L. L. and Emanuel, E. J., "The medical directive. A new comprehensive advance care document," *J. Am. Med. Asso.* 261 (1989): 3288–93; L. J. Schneiderman, J. D. Arras, "Counseling patients to counsel physicians on future care in the event of patient incompetence," *Ann Intern. Med.* 102 (1985): 693–8; Gibson, J. M., "National Values History Project," *Generations* XIV (1990): 51–64; *Your Health Care Choices: A Guide to Preparing Advance Directives for Health Care Decisions in Arizona* (The Dorothy Garske Center and Arizona Health Decisions, 4250 East Camelback Road, Suite 185K, Phoenix, AZ 85018, October 1990).

3 *In re* O'Connor 72, N.Y.2d 517, 531 N.E.2d 607, 534 N.Y.S.2d 886 (1988); *Cruzan v. Harmon*, 58 L.W. 4916, June 26, 1990; *In re* Christine Busalacchi, Missouri Court of Appeals No. 59582, March 5, 1991.

4 High, D. M., "All in the family: Extended autonomy and expectations in surrogate health care decision-making," *Gerontologist* 28 (1988) (suppl): 46–52.

5 *Cruzan v. Harmon*, 58 L.W. 4916, at 4924, 6-26-90 (Scalia, J, concurring).

6 Health Care Decisions Act of 1988, The District of Columbia, 35 DCR 8653, D.C.Code Ann. Chap. 21-2210; VA Code Sections 54.1-2981 to -2992 (1988 and Supp. 1990).

91

Mama Day

GLORIA NAYLOR

We were at it again only for about an hour when they stopped working, almost in mass. But no one had given a signal, that I understood at least. "It's time to go to the standing forth." I followed them through the fields in back of the stores at the bridge junction to a little wooden church — and what they meant was a funeral. No flowers. No music. People were coming from all directions, each dressed apparently in whatever they were wearing when they knew the time had come. The men who had been working on the bridge in dirty overalls with tar under their fingernails. Miss Reema in her blue smock from the beauty parlor. One woman with her hair shampooed and a towel around her head. One had on a house coat and fuzzy slippers. Even Bernice and Ambush weren't in special clothes, but black wasn't needed to set them apart.

We filed into the pews, facing the simple pine coffin set up in the front. The minister was there, but he had little to say. When the rustling and moving had quieted, he cleared his throat and said, Charles Kyle Duvall, 1981 to 1985. Who is ready to stand forth? He sat back down and for a while there was silence. And then Miss Reema got up and walked to the front of the church and stood looking down at the closed coffin: When I first saw you, she began, you

were wearing a green bunting, being carried in your mama's arms. You had a little fuzzy patch of hair on your head and your mouth was open to let out a squall. I guess you were hungry. And when I see you again, she said, you'll be sitting at my dining table, having been invited to dinner with the rest of my brood. It went on like that, person after person. Dry eyed and matter of fact. The minister calling out, Who is ready to stand forth? Someone had seen him in a stroller and would see him again in his own car. If they first saw him walking, they would see him running. Dr Buzzard got up and had first seen him sucking away on a pacifier, and when he saw him again he'd be more than ready for a handful of his special ginger candy. Always addressing the coffin, and sometimes acting as if they expected an answer back. You liked my toy whistles, didn't you? the owner of the general store asked him. Well, when I see you again, you'll be buying my silver earrings for a sweetheart of yours.

Why did I get the feeling that this meeting wasn't meant to take place inside of any building? The church, the presence of the minister, were concessions, and obviously the only ones they were going to make to a Christian ritual that should have called for a sermon, music, tears – the belief in an earthly finality for the child's life. His parents weren't even crying and I could have cut Ambush's grief with a knife. He was the next to rise: You were bunching up your fists, angry and small. And I thought I had a fighter on my hands. A golden glove champ, maybe. And when I see you again, you'll be fighting for the place you deserve among other great men. Surely, Bernice couldn't take part in this. The woman had gone out of her mind when that child died. But she also stood up, trembling. Her voice could barely be heard. And she turned to the coffin with an air – could it be? – of apology: When I first saw you, you were so very glad to be alive – new and declaring it to everyone. And when I see you again, you'll be forgiving of your old mama, who didn't remember for a moment that you were still here.

And that was it. It took only two men to carry the coffin because it was so small. It was laid into the open grave that was waiting behind the church and covered up. They began to disperse as calmly as they came. I stood there immobile by the fresh grave, trying to sort out the meaning of all this in my mind. Dr Buzzard's callused hand applied gentle pressure to my arm. Come on, he said, we got us a bridge to build.

92

The Devil

GUY DE MAUPASSANT

The peasant was standing opposite the doctor, by the bedside of the dying old woman, and she, calmly resigned and quite lucid, looked at them and listened to their talking. She was going to die, and she did not rebel at it, for her life was over – she was ninety-two.

The July sun streamed in at the window and through the open door and cast its hot flames onto the uneven brown clay floor, which had been stamped down by four generations of clodhoppers. The smell of the fields came in also, driven by the brisk wind, and parched by the noontide heat. The grasshoppers chirped themselves hoarse, filling the air with their shrill noise, like that of the wooden crickets which are sold to children at fair time.

The doctor raised his voice and said: "Honoré, you cannot leave your mother in this state; she may die at any moment." And the peasant, in great distress, replied: "But I must get in my wheat, for it has been lying on the ground a long time, and the weather is just right for it; what do you say about it, mother?" And the dying woman, still possessed by her Norman avariciousness, replied *yes* with her eyes and her forehead, and so urged her son to get in his wheat, and to leave her to die alone. But the doctor got angry, and stamping his foot he said:

"You are no better than a brute, do you hear, and I will not allow you to do it. Do you understand? And if you must get in your wheat today, go and fetch Rapet's wife and make her look after your mother. I *will* have it. And if you do not obey me, I will let you die like a dog, when you are ill in your turn; do you hear me?"

The peasant, a tall, thin fellow with slow movements, who was tormented by indecision, by his fear of the doctor and his keen love of saving, hesitated, calculated, and stammered out: "How much does La Rapet charge for attending sick people?"

"How should I know?" the doctor cried. "That depends upon how long she is wanted for. Settle it with her, by Jove! But I want her to be here within an hour, do you hear."

So the man made up his mind. "I will go for her," he replied; "don't get angry, doctor." And the latter left, calling out as he went: "Take care, you know, for I do not joke when I am angry!" And as soon as they were alone, the peasant turned to his mother, and said in a resigned voice: "I will go and fetch La Rapet, as the man will have it. Don't go off while I am away."

And he went out in his turn.

La Rapet, who was an old washerwoman, watched the dead and the dying of the neighborhood, and then, as soon as she had sewn her customers into that linen cloth from which they would emerge no more, she went and took up her irons to smooth the linen of the living. Wrinkled like a last year's apple, spiteful, envious, avaricious with a phenomenal avarice, bent double, as if she had been broken in half across the loins, by the constant movement of the iron over the linen, one might have said that she had a kind of monstrous and cynical affection for a death struggle. She never spoke of anything but of the people she had seen die, of the various kinds of deaths at which she had been present, and she related, with the greatest minuteness, details which were always the same, just like a sportsman talks of his shots.

When Honoré Bontemps entered her cottage, he found her preparing the starch for the collars of the village woman, and he said: "Good evening; I hope you are pretty well, Mother Rapet."

She turned her head round to look at him and said: "Fairly well, fairly well, and you?"

"Oh! as for me, I am as well as I could wish, but my mother is very sick."

"Your mother?"

"Yes, my mother!"

"What's the matter with her?"

"She is going to turn up her toes, that's what's the matter with her!"

The old woman took her hands out of the water and asked with sudden sympathy: "Is she as bad as all that?"

"The doctor says she will not last till morning."

"Then she certainly is very bad!" Honoré hesitated, for he wanted to make a few preliminary remarks before coming to his proposal, but as he could hit upon nothing, he made up his mind suddenly.

"How much are you going to ask to stop with her till the end? You know that I am not rich, and I cannot even afford to keep a servant-girl. It is just that which has brought my poor mother to this state, too much work and fatigue! She used to work for ten, in spite of her ninety-two years. You don't find any made of that stuff nowadays!"

La Rapet answered gravely: "There are two prices: Forty sous by day and three francs by night for the rich, and twenty sous by day, and forty by night for the others. You shall pay me the twenty and forty." But the peasant reflected, for he knew his mother well. He knew how tenacious of life, how vigorous and unyielding she was. He knew, too, that she might last another week, in spite of the doctor's opinion, and so he said resolutely: "No, I would rather you would fix a price until the end. I will take my chance, one way or the other. The doctor says she will die very soon. If that happens, so much the better for you, and so much the worse for me, but if she holds out till tomorrow or longer, so much the better for me and so much the worse for you!"

The nurse looked at the man in astonishment, for she had never treated a death as a speculative job, and she hesitated, tempted by the idea of the possible gain. But almost immediately she suspected that he wanted to juggle her. "I can say nothing until I have seen your mother," she replied.

"Then come with me and see her."

She washed her hands, and went with him immediately. They did not speak on the road; she walked with short, hasty steps, while he strode on with his long legs, as if he were crossing a brook at every step. The cows lying down in the fields, overcome by the heat, raised their heads heavily and lowed feebly at the two passers-by, as if to ask them for some green grass.

When they got near the house, Honoré Bontemps murmured: "Suppose it is all over?" And the unconscious wish that it might be so showed itself in the sound of his voice.

But the old woman was not dead. She was lying on her back, on her wretched bed, her hands covered with a pink cotton counterpane, horribly thin, knotty paws, like some strange animal's, or like crabs' claws, hands closed by rheumatism, fatigue, and the work of nearly a century which she had accomplished.

La Rapet went up to the bed and looked at the dying woman, felt her pulse, tapped her on the chest, listened to her breathing, and asked her questions, so as to hear her speak: then, having looked at her for some time longer, she went out of the room, followed by Honoré. His decided opinion was, that the old woman would not last out the night, and he asked: "Well?" And the sick-nurse replied: "Well, she may last two days, perhaps three. You will have to give me six francs, everything included."

"Six francs! six francs!" he shouted. "Are you out of your mind? I tell you that she cannot last more than five or six hours!" And they disputed angrily for some time, but as the nurse said she would go home, as the time was slipping away, and as his wheat would not come to the farmyard of its own accord, he agreed to her terms at last:

"Very well, then, that is settled; six francs including everything, until the corpse is taken out."

"That is settled, six francs."

And he went away, with long strides, to his wheat, which was lying on the ground under the hot sun which ripens the grain, while the sick-nurse returned to the house.

She had brought some work with her, for she worked without stopping by the side of the dead and dying, sometimes for herself, sometimes for the family, who employed her as seamstress also, paying her rather more in that capacity. Suddenly she asked:

"Have you received the last sacrament, Mother Bontemps?"

The old peasant woman said "No" with her head, and La Rapet, who was very devout, got up quickly: "Good heavens, is it possible? I will go and fetch the curé"; and she rushed off to the parsonage so quickly, that the urchins in the street thought some accident had happened, when they saw her trotting off like that.

The priest came immediately in his surplice, preceded by a choir-boy, who rang a bell to announce the passage of the Host through the parched and quiet country. Some men, working at a distance, took off their large hats and remained motionless until the white vestment had disappeared behind some farm buildings; the women who were making up the sheaves stood up to make the sign of the cross; the frightened black hens ran away along the ditch until they reached a well-known hole through which they suddenly disappeared, while a foal, which was tied up in a meadow, took fright at the sight of the surplice and began to gallop round at the length of its rope, kicking violently. The choir-boy, in his red cassock, walked quickly, and the priest, the square biretta on his bowed head, followed him, muttering some prayers. Last of all came La Rapet, bent almost double, as if she wished to prostrate herself; she walked with folded hands, as if she were in church.

Honoré saw them pass in the distance, and he asked: "Where is our priest going to?" And his man, who was more acute, replied: "He is taking the sacrament to your mother, of course!"

The peasant was not surprised and said: "That is quite possible," and went on with his work.

Mother Bontemps confessed, received absolution and extreme unction, and the priest took his departure, leaving the two women alone in the suffocating cottage. La Rapet began to look at the dying woman, and to ask herself whether it could last much longer.

The day was on the wane, and a cooler air came in stronger puffs, making a view of Epinal, which was fastened to the wall by two pins, flap up and down. The scanty window curtains, which had formerly been white, but were now yellow and covered with fly-specks, looked as if they were going to fly off, and seemed to struggle to get away, like the old woman's soul.

Lying motionless, with her eyes open, the old mother seemed to await the death which was so near, and which yet delayed its coming, with perfect indifference. Her short breath whistled in her throat. It would stop altogether soon, and there would be one woman less in the world, one whom nobody would regret.

At nightfall Honoré returned, and when he went up to the bed and saw that his mother was still alive he asked: "How is she?" just as he had done formerly, when she had been sick. Then he sent La Rapet away, saying to her: "Tomorrow morning at five o'clock, without fail." And she replied: "Tomorrow at five o'clock."

She came at daybreak, and found Honoré eating his soup, which he had made himself, before going to work.

"Well, is your mother dead?" asked the nurse.

"She is rather better, on the contrary," he replied, with a malignant look out of the corner of his eyes. Then he went out.

La Rapet was seized with anxiety, and went up to the dying woman, who was in the same state, lethargic and impassive, her eyes open and her hands clutching the counterpane. The nurse perceived that this might go on thus for two days, four days, eight days, even, and her avaricious mind was seized with fear. She was excited to fury against the cunning fellow who had tricked her, and against the woman who would not die.

Nevertheless, she began to sew and waited with her eyes fixed on the wrinkled face of Mother Bontemps. When Honoré returned to breakfast he seemed quite satisfied, and even in a bantering humor, for he was carrying in his wheat under very favorable circumstances.

La Rapet was getting exasperated; every passing minute now seemed to her so much time and money stolen from her. She felt a mad inclination to choke this old ass, this headstrong old fool, this obstinate old wretch – to stop that short, rapid breath, which was robbing her of her time and money, by squeezing her throat a little. But then she reflected on the danger of doing so, and other thoughts came into her head, so she went up to the bed and said to her: "Have you ever seen the Devil?"

Mother Bontemps whispered: "No."

Then the sick-nurse began to talk and to tell her tales likely to terrify her weak and dying mind. "Some minutes before one dies the Devil appears," she said, "to all. He has a broom in his hand, a saucepan on his head and he utters loud cries. When anybody had seen him, all was over, and that person had only a few moments longer to live"; and she enumerated all those to whom the Devil had appeared that year: Josephine Loisel, Eulalie Ratier, Sophie Padagnau, Séraphine Grospied.

Mother Bontemps, who was at last most disturbed in mind, moved about, wrung her hands, and tried to turn her head to look at the other end of the room. Suddenly La Rapet disappeared at the foot of the bed. She took a sheet out of the cupboard and wrapped herself up in it; then she put the iron pot on to her head, so that its three short bent feet rose up like horns, took a broom in her right hand and a tin pail in her left, which she threw up suddenly, so that it might fall to the ground noisily.

Certainly when it came down, it made a terrible noise. Then, climbing on to a chair, the nurse showed herself, gesticulating and uttering shrill cries into the pot which covered her face, while she menaced the old peasant woman, who was nearly dead, with her broom.

Terrified, with a mad look on her face, the dying woman made a superhuman effort to get up and escape; she even got her shoulders and chest out of bed; then she fell back with a deep sigh. All was over, and La Rapet calmly put everything back into its place; the broom into the corner by the cupboard, the sheet inside it, the pot onto the hearth, the pail onto the floor, and the chair against the wall. Then with a professional air, she closed the dead woman's enormous eyes, put a plate on the bed and poured some holy water into it, dipped the twig of boxwood into it, and kneeling down, she fervently repeated the prayers for the dead, which she knew by heart, as a matter of business.

When Honoré returned in the evening, he found her praying. He calculated immediately that she had made twenty sous out of him, for she had only spent three days and one night there, which made five francs altogether, instead of the six which he owed her.

93

Talking to the Family

JOHN STONE

My white coat waits in the corner
like a father.
I will wear it to meet the sister
in her white shoes and organza dress
in the live of winter,

the milkless husband
holding the baby.

I will tell them.

They will put it together
and take it apart.
Their voices will buzz.
The cut ends of their nerves
will curl.

I will take off the coat,
drive home,
and replace the light bulb in the hall.

94

To the Foot from Its Child

PABLO NERUDA

The child's foot is not yet aware it's a foot,
and would like to be a butterfly or an
    apple.

But in time, stones and bits of glass,
streets, ladders,
and the paths in the rough earth
go on teaching the foot that it cannot fly,
cannot be a fruit bulging on the branch.
Then, the child's foot
is defeated, falls
in the battle,
is a prisoner
condemned to live in a shoe.

Bit by bit, in that dark,
it grows to know the world in its own
    way,
out of touch with its fellow, enclosed,
feeling out life like a blind man.

These soft nails
of quartz, bunched together,
grow hard, and change themselves
into opaque substance, hard as horn,
and the tiny, petalled toes of the child
grow bunched and out of trim,
take on the form of eyeless reptiles

with triangular heads, like worms.
Later, they grow calloused
and are covered
with the faint volcanoes of death,
a coarsening hard to accept.

But this blind thing walks
without respite, never stopping
for hour after hour,
the one foot, the other,
now the man's
now the woman's,
up above,
down below,
through fields, mines,
markets and ministries,
backwards,
far afield, inward,
forward,
this foot toils in its shoe,
scarcely taking time
to bare itself in love or sleep;
it walks, they walk,
until the whole man chooses to
    stop.

And then it descended
underground, unaware,

for there, everything, everything was
   dark.
It never knew it had ceased to be a foot

or if they were burying it so that it could fly
or so that it could become
an apple.

Index

Compiled by Meg Davies (Registered Indexer, Society of Indexers)

Note: Tables and figures are indicated by page references in italics. Both American and British spelling are used in this volume; the index uses American spelling. Names of contributors to this volume are not indexed, except where their work is cited in other contributions.